THE PREGNANCY BOOK FOR TODAY'S WOMAN

Also by Howard I. Shapiro

THE BIRTH CONTROL BOOK
THE NEW BIRTH CONTROL BOOK

The PREGNANCY BOOK *for* TODAY'S WOMAN

SECOND EDITION

HOWARD I. SHAPIRO, M.D.

HarperPerennial

A Division of HarperCollins*Publishers*

Source of radiation chart which appears on page 333, source: National Council on Radiation Protection and Measurement, from *The New York Times*, Nov. 20, 1987. Reproduced by permission of *The New York Times*.

HarperCollins books may be purchased for educational, business, or sales promotional use. For information, please write: Special Markets Department, HarperCollins Publishers, Inc., 10 East 53rd Street, New York, NY 10022.

FIRST EDITION

Designed by Ruth Kolbert

Library of Congress Cataloging-in-Publication Data

Shapiro, Howard I., 1937–
    The pregnancy book for today's woman / Howard I. Shapiro. — 2nd ed.
       p.   cm.
    Includes bibliographical references and index.
    ISBN 0-06-273030-4
    1. Pregnancy—Popular works.   2. Childbirth.   3. Pregnant women—Health and hygiene.   I. Title.
RG121.S495   1993
618.2'4—dc20   92-53284

94 95 96 97 AC/RRD 10 9 8 7 6 5 4 3

TO
JEAN PIKE
for her extraordinary nursing skills,
friendship, humor, and loyalty.
Thank you for extending your one week visit to 23 years.

TO
SUZANNE AND MARJORIE SHAPIRO
for the happiness they have given me
and for the love and laughs we have shared.

TO
BETTE
the love of my life,
whose devotion and encouragement inspired me
to write this book.

▮▮▮ *Contents* ▮▮▮

⌷⌷⌷ *Tables* ⌷⌷⌷

ııı *Preface* ııı

Since 1983, when *The Pregnancy Book for Today's Woman* was originally published, the discovery, development, and refinement of technology has advanced faster in obstetrics than in any other medical specialty. Procedures considered routine for the pregnant woman today, such as the biophysical profile, vaginal ultrasound, and chorionic villus sampling (CVS), were not even mentioned in the first edition of this book. PUBS, amnioinfusion, MRI, and echocardiography are but a few terms from the new obstetrical vocabulary—one that may sound confusing but is actually quite easy to learn. As I hope I proved in the 1983 edition, there is no medical subject so complex that it can't be explained in language anyone can understand.

During the past decade we have come to the sad realization that no one is immune from the deadly AIDS virus. A virtually unknown entity when the first edition of this book was written, AIDS has become the ninth leading cause of death among children 1 to 4 years of age. Other sexually transmitted diseases such as herpes, chlamydia, HPV, hepatitis, and penicillin-resistant gonorrhea continue to wreak havoc on pregnant women and their babies. Effective prevention and the latest methods of diagnosing and treating these diseases are fully discussed in Chapter 6.

The profile of women of childbearing age has also changed significantly since 1983. It is estimated that more than 70% of American women of reproductive age currently work outside the home. Based on present fertility rates, more than 1 million pregnancies can be expected among these women each year. Medical concerns of pregnant workers run the gamut from the dangers of physical and emotional stress to the potential hazards of cigarette smoke and chemical pollutants in the workplace. Recent reports linking prolonged exposure to computer terminals with a higher incidence of miscarriage and fetal anomalies has caused great concern. In addition to medical problems, important social issues confronting today's working woman include legislation dealing with employee rights, maternity leave, and the illegality of job bias simply because she is pregnant or of child-bearing age.

Many of today's working women have responded to the demands of career advancement by delaying childbirth. Women over 30 now give birth to more than one-fourth of all babies born in the United States. Throughout the book I elaborate on these many issues confronting the pregnant woman over 30.

When today's pregnant woman is not working she is likely to be enjoying her leisure time in a variety of ways. In this edition, I report on the new and valuable knowledge which has been gained about the effects of different sports and aerobic exercises on the fetus. I also present updated information on vacation travel, Lyme disease, sexuality, dangerous new recreational drugs, radon, and a host of other important issues. The chapter on medication has been expanded to discuss the myriad of new drugs that have been introduced since 1983.

Obstetrical technology is growing by leaps and bounds, but science without humanity makes all this progress meaningless. The patient-doctor relationship remains the most important determinant of a rewarding birth experience, and today's woman has brought a new sense of equality, assertiveness, consumerism, and skepticism to this relationship. A recent survey of thousands of women found that the most significant factors in choosing and staying with a doctor are the doctor's communicative skills, short waiting periods for appointments, and convenient office hours.

Women and men will enjoy the childbirth experience to its fullest when accurate medical information is made available to them in language that can be easily understood. The first edition of *The Pregnancy Book for Today's Woman* was successful because it was written for patients, not doctors. Once again, my purpose is to share my knowledge of pregnancy and childbirth with the reader. I have maintained the question and answer format because I believe it helps to achieve this goal while also serving as a quick reference for specific concerns. The vast majority of these questions are those of the many women I have had the privilege to treat during the past 25 years. This project, therefore, belongs to them as well as me. My greatest hope is that those who read this book will consider it to be the best and most accurate source for information on pregnancy and childbirth.

Acknowledgments

The author is once again indebted to Dawn Perkins for the many hours spent and the care taken in typing and preparing the manuscript. We have worked harmoniously and steadily through four books over the past twelve years, despite the ever growing size of her family.

I am especially thankful to my agent and friend, Russell Galen, for his patience, knowledge, and sound advice.

I am fortunate to have had Carol Cohen as my editor once again. Her knowledge of the subject, her intelligence, and her enthusiasm have added immeasurably to the successful completion of the book. Thanks also to Sarge, who put all the pieces together and let me add those last few crucial paragraphs.

My friend Joe Podrat, Director of the Department of Pharmacy at Norwalk Hospital, played a vital role in updating and clarifying the information in the Medication chapter. Debra Rosner, R.D. provided invaluable help in preparing the Nutrition chapter, while Sheila Calle, Senior Physical Therapist, Outpatient Service, shared her vast knowledge of prenatal exercises with me.

I am pleased I had the opportunity to devote the necessary time, effort, and research to this book over the past four years. I am proud of the finished product.

Finally, the encouragement I received from my beautiful wife Bette and my delightful daughters Suzanne and Marjorie will always be cherished.

DISCLAIMER

The purpose of this book is to make you aware of the normal progress of pregnancy and the problems that may arise. You will need to consult your doctor to assess any problems or questions you may have; proper diagnosis and treatment of all symptoms connected with pregnancy call for careful attention to your concerns from your doctor.

1

CONTRACEPTION
and
CONCEPTION

*N*o method of birth control is 100% effective, and accidental pregnancies occur even with the most reliable techniques. (Often it is not the method of contraception which is at fault, but the failure of the individual who teaches or uses a particular technique.) Serious problems can arise when pregnancy follows contraceptive failure. All methods, including the Pill, intrauterine devices (IUDs), surgical sterilization, spermicides, and even rhythm, have been reported to entail significant fetal and maternal risks. This chapter analyzes the various problems associated with pregnancy following contraception and sterilization failure, and the correct methods of diagnosing and treating each complication.

 ## BIRTH CONTROL PILLS

If a pregnancy occurs when I am on the Pill, is it more likely to be in the tube rather than in its normal location in the uterus?

This depends on the type of birth control pill you take. A pregnancy located outside the uterus is called an ectopic pregnancy. By far the most common type of ectopic pregnancy is one in the fallopian tube, called a tubal pregnancy. Rupture of the wall of the tube by an ectopic pregnancy can result in severe intraabdominal hemorrhage and even death. Tubal pregnancies may also pass out of the open end of the tube, which does not attach

directly to the ovary. This condition is known as a tubal abortion. In extremely rare circumstances, the fetus will implant in the abdominal cavity and continue to grow after it has passed out of the tube. Rarer still, an abdominal pregnancy may go to term.

No reports suggest that users of combination-type oral contraceptives (those that contain a synthetic estrogen combined with chemicals called progestogens or progestins) are more likely than other women to suffer from an ectopic pregnancy if they accidentally conceive. However, data from at least 18 separate studies strongly suggest a higher incidence of ectopic pregnancy among women who conceived while using the progestin-only minipill. One group of researchers suggested that the progestin norgestrel, the type found in Ovrette, was more likely to be responsible; other studies have implicated norethindone, which is found in both NorQD and Micronor. In contrast, a progestin named lynestrenol, which is manufactured in Europe, has not been found to increase a woman's risk of ectopic pregnancy. The mechanism by which a minipill makes one more susceptible to an ectopic pregnancy is unknown, but it is theorized that the progestin slows down the transport of the fertilized egg through the fallopian tube. As a result, it attaches itself within the tube rather than in its normal location within the endometrium of the uterus.

Your doctor should always consider the possibility of an ectopic pregnancy if you develop abdominal pain or have a positive pregnancy test while on a progestin-only minipill.

If I continue to take birth control pills without realizing I am pregnant, is there a chance that the genitals of my female fetus may be masculinized?

Yes, though it is a remote possibility. The reason why this can happen is that the progestin in the Pill is a synthetic hormone more closely related to the male hormone testosterone than to the female hormone progesterone. The formation of a grossly enlarged clitoris, resembling a male penis, and a labia majora, or outer vaginal lips, resembling a male scrotum, is believed to be caused by the passage of progestins across the placenta at the time that these organs are being formed, between the seventh and twelfth weeks of pregnancy. If you stop the Pill before the seventh week, you can be assured that your female offspring will not be masculinized.

Since all birth control pills used today contain only a fraction of the progestin found in older formulations, the risk of masculinized genitals, even if the Pill is taken after the seventh week, is extremely small. Birth control pills currently mar-

keted in the United States contain one of seven progestins: levonorgestrel, norgestrel, ethynodiol diacetate, norethindrone acetate, norethindrone, norgestimate, and norethynodrel. By far the most potent and, theoretically, the one most likely to masculinize a female fetus is levonorgestrel, found in Levlen, Nordette, and Triphasil. Norgestrel, the progestin in Ovral, Lo/Ovral, and Ovrette, contains exactly one-half the masculinizing potential of levonorgesterol, but Lo/Ovral, for example, with 0.3 milligrams of norgestrel, is identical in its fetal effects to the 0.15 milligrams of levonorgestrel contained in Levlen and Nordette. The progestins ethynodiol diacetate, norethindrone, norethindrone acetate, norgestimate, and norethynodrel, found in a variety of birth control pills, have much lower fetal masculinizing potential than either levonorgestrel or norgestrel.

To avoid fetal anomalies, isn't it best to wait three months from the time I stop the Pill until the time I conceive?

This is one of the most prevalent misconceptions surrounding the use of birth control pills. It is based on one outdated 1970 report showing an increased incidence of chromosomal defects in spontaneously aborted fetuses of women who had conceived within three months after stopping the Pill. Several subsequent studies have failed to find such chromosomal defects, nor is there an increased likelihood of spontaneous abortion, ectopic pregnancy, or congenital anomalies when a woman conceives immediately after she stops the Pill. Unfortunately, many doctors continue to believe and to disseminate this misinformation.

Some studies have concluded that women who conceive soon after stopping the Pill have lower miscarriage and stillborn rates and a greater likelihood of giving birth to both identical and fraternal or nonidentical twins. In one report from Israel, doctors found that the number of infants born with heart defects was 1.7 per 1,000 for recent Pill users, compared with 3.7 per 1,000 for nonusers.

Another study, published in 1986, compared the outcome of 2,859 pregnancies in women who conceived within three months of using the Pill with a group of 7,000 nonusers. The overall incidence of congenital anomalies was 2.83% in Pill users compared to 2.95% in nonusers.

The only justification for waiting to conceive after you stop the Pill is that it will be easier for you and your doctor to determine your date of conception, since periods tend to be irregular for the first three months after stopping the Pill. However, this should present no great problem since ultrasound is readily available for accurately determining fetal age.

Are birth defects more common among women who inadvertently use birth control pills early in pregnancy?

There is a great deal of controversy about this subject, but the majority of today's authorities are far more optimistic than earlier researchers. Between 1973 and 1980 several reports concluded that inadvertent use of birth control pills early in pregnancy predisposed the fetus to a wide variety of congenital anomalies. Many of these studies were flawed because they lumped all hormones together instead of distinguishing between birth control pills and other estrogen and progestin preparations. Also, many studied too few patients to be statistically reliable.

The current prevailing opinion is that inadvertent use of the Pill early in pregnancy may increase your risk of giving birth to a baby with a congenital heart defect. Fortunately, this risk is probably no greater than 1 per 1,000 births above the usual incidence of 7 to 8 per 1,000 births. Your risk of giving birth to a baby with other defects is no higher than that of the general population. The most recent and optimistic article dealing with this question was published in the *Journal of the American Medical Association* in 1986. Doctors at the Centers for Disease Control in Atlanta, Georgia, studied first-trimester hormone exposure among

mothers of 1,091 infants with Down syndrome and 1i other malformations. They concluded that there is no statistically significant association between any malformation category and oral contraceptive exposure. Most experts would agree that the risk of a birth defect is so low for a woman who accidentally takes birth control pills early in pregnancy that it is not necessary for her to consider abortion.

The problem can be avoided in just about all cases if the absence of pregnancy is confirmed before oral contraceptives are started. This may sound like a simple suggestion, but it is violated repeatedly by women and their doctors. Second, hormones should not be used as a method of bringing on a late period unless a sensitive pregnancy test, performed in a laboratory or doctor's office, first proves to be negative. Finally, if you miss one or more birth control pills during a cycle and then skip a period after the last pill is taken, get a pregnancy test before starting a new box of pills.

If I take birth control pills in high doses as a "morning-after" pill, is my risk for birth defects higher if it isn't successful and I become pregnant?

A variety of estrogen compounds have been used as postcoital, or "morning-after," pills to prevent pregnancy following unprotected intercourse at midcycle (see page 13). The combination of 0.050 milligrams of ethinyl estradiol and 0.5 milligrams of norgestrel, the components of Ovral, have been demonstrated to be a highly effective postcoital contraceptive. In a recent study, 608 women received two Ovral tablets within 72 hours of unprotected intercourse, followed by two tablets 12 hours later. The pregnancy rate was a remarkably low 0.16%.

Unfortunately no studies have been conducted on the fetal effects of such a high dose of oral contraceptives taken so early in pregnancy. However, based on other studies one would surmise that the risk of an anomaly or defect should be no greater than that quoted for inadvertent Pill use early in pregnancy (see previous question). In fact, it may actually be lower since "morning-after" Ovral is taken for only a 12-hour time span at a point in pregnancy long before the fetal organs start to develop.

Can birth control pills cause vitamin or mineral deficiencies that may be harmful to a pregnancy which occurs soon after the Pill is stopped?

Probably not. Several studies have suggested that the estrogen in oral contraceptives may prevent the intestine from absorbing certain important vitamins and minerals such as vitamin B_{11} (folic acid), vitamin B_6 (pyridoxine), vitamin B_{12} (cobalamin, cyanocobalamin), vitamin B_2 (riboflavin), vitamin E (alphatocopherol), vitamin C (ascorbic acid), and zinc. However, there has never been a definitive scientific study demonstrating that the use of oral contraceptives causes any clinically apparent vitamin *deficiency* in a woman who is on an adequate diet. There is no real evidence to show that oral contraceptive users need to take vitamin supplements; vitamin and mineral supplements are indicated only when deficiency symptoms become apparent and can't be corrected through dietary adjustments.

Is it true that a woman is more likely to give birth to a girl if conception occurs soon after birth control pills are discontinued?

No. In 1974, the English medical journal *Lancet* reported a nearly 2-to-1 female-to-male birth ratio when conception occurred immediately following use of oral contraceptives, but the study involved fewer than 200 pregnancies. A large study in 1976 from the Harvard School of Public Health noted the female-to-male ratio to be 1-to-1 among 6,000 recorded births which followed oral contraceptive use. In a 1986 study of more than 10,000 women, males accounted for 52% of the infants born to both recent Pill users and nonusers. Another interesting finding was that the average birth weight of infants born to former Pill users was slightly, though not significantly, higher (3,224 grams versus 3,217 grams) than that of infants born to women who did not use the Pill.

Are there certain medical problems which, if they occur while I am on the Pill, are more likely to happen again during pregnancy?

Yes. Often a doctor can predict which of his patients will encounter difficulties during pregnancy based on their reactions to the Pill. The development of diabetes is a perfect example. Most investigators agree that oral contraceptives can have a detrimental effect on blood sugar and blood insulin in healthy as well as diabetic women. It has been proven that the progestin, even in the lower amounts found in the minipill, is the culprit in worsening glucose metabolism and plasma insulin levels. Several researchers over the past five years have discovered to their surprise that the oft-maligned estrogen component of the Pill can ameliorate and even totally reverse the harmful changes in plasma and insulin levels caused by the progestins. Preliminary research has demonstrated that the new triphasic birth control pills (three separate progestin levels) might not adversely affect glucose and insulin levels because they contain a lower total dose of progestin in each Pill cycle. It is also believed that the progestin norgestimate (Ortho-Cyclen), newly introduced in 1992, is less likely than other progestins to cause metabolic abnormalities.

Among women with normal glucose (sugar) tolerance tests before using the Pill, approximately 10% develop abnormal reactions to such tests while taking the Pill. This "chemical diabetes" produces no symptoms and reverts to normal when the Pill is no longer used. But this abnormality may reappear when predisposed individuals are subjected to the hormonal stimulation and stress of pregnancy. Pregnancy-induced or gestational diabetes requires strict dietary control and often insulin in order to prevent fetal complications (see page 309). It is important for your doctor to routinely test for this condition one or more times during pregnancy, especially if you showed an abnormally high blood-sugar level when using birth control pills.

High blood pressure, or hypertension, develops in approximately 3 to 5 percent of all women who use the Pill and usually drops to normal within three months after the Pill is stopped. The rise in blood pressure accompanying use of oral contraceptives is directly related to the strength of the estrogen they contain and the number of years a woman has been taking the Pill. Even the newest low-dose formulations containing 0.030 to 0.035 milligrams of estrogen have the capacity to raise the blood pressure. Only very recently have scientists come to learn that progestin strength and dosage may also affect a woman's blood pressure, but to a lesser degree than the estrogen component. During pregnancy, an elevation of blood pressure during the last three months, termed preeclampsia or toxemia, appears more likely among women susceptible to a significant rise in blood pressure while using oral contraceptives. If you have a history of hypertension while using the Pill, you should be carefully watched during your pregnancy.

Both the Pill and pregnancy are responsible for alterations in blood platelets and certain blood substances called clotting factors. This in turn may subject a very small percentage of susceptible women to inflammatory conditions of the veins of the legs and pelvis, a condition called thrombophlebitis. Thrombophlebitis of the deep veins of the legs and pelvis often presents a real threat to a woman's life because these clots can become dislodged and travel through the circulatory system to a vital organ such as the lung, causing instant death. If you have a history of previous deep-vein thrombophlebitis while on the Pill, your obstetrician may want to consider anticoagulation, or medical thinning of the blood, with a drug called heparin (see page 298).

Approximately 3 out of every 100,000 women using the Pill each year develop a benign though potentially fatal liver tumor called hepatocellular adenoma, or hepatoma. The growth of these tumors appears to be linked to the estrogen in the Pill, and those oral contraceptives with the highest doses of estrogen are the most dangerous. Some investigators believe it is the combined effect of the progestin and the estrogen which is to blame for this problem. Women who are most susceptible are those over 30 who have used the Pill for more than four years. Rupture of a hepatoma results in massive intraabdominal hemorrhage, and often the only symptoms preceding this catastrophe are the suggestion of a mass (enlargement) or fullness and slight pain under the right rib cage or on the right upper side of the abdomen. A hepatoma can usually be diagnosed before rupture through an x-ray scan of the liver. After the birth control pills are discontinued, the tumor generally diminishes in size and remains dormant.

However, reactivation of hepatocellular adenoma is possible days or even years later if the Pill is restarted or if pregnancy occurs. Several deaths from ruptured adenomas have been reported during the pregnancies of women with previous histories of Pill-induced hepatoma. If a woman with a history of hepatoma does conceive, it is vital that her doctor see her often and palpate her abdomen for enlargement or upper abdominal pain during each prenatal visit. Pregnancy must be terminated at the first indication that the tumor has recurred in order to avoid the risk of continued enlargement and a potentially fatal rupture. Some doctors recommend delivery by cesarean section for women with a history of Pill-induced hepatoma, even if there are no clinical signs or symptoms that the tumor has recurred. This recommendation arises from a fear that the bearing-down maneuvers during the final stage of labor may create excessive tension on a small, undiagnosed hepatoma. Since rupture of a hepatoma requires replacement with large volumes of blood, observation in a well-equipped hospital with a modern blood bank is essential. It is not known if cutting out a hepatoma prior to pregnancy will guarantee a problem-free gestation, since smaller tumors may grow under the influence of the pregnancy hormones. Furthermore, surgery of this type, even under the best circumstances, is extremely difficult and potentially very dangerous.

Are there certain skin diseases which can appear during Pill use as well as during pregnancy?

Intense generalized itching, occasionally associated with jaundice or yellowing of the skin, has been reported in a small number of women on the Pill. This condition, known as cholestatic pruritis and jaundice, is the result of the accumulation of bile in the circulatory system. While the progestin is probably the main culprit, estrogen has also been implicated in this problem. The only known method of treating cholestatic pruritis is to stop using the Pill. Unfortunately, affected women note its recurrence when they become pregnant because of the increased release of estrogen and progesterone.

Spider nevi, or liver spots (*telangiectasias*), are tiny red spots occasionally found on the upper chest, neck, and face of fair-skinned Pill users. They result from the estrogen-induced dilation of tiny, fragile skin capillaries and are totally harmless. Susceptible women develop many more spider nevi during pregnancy because of the extremely high levels of estrogen secretion.

Chloasma, or melasma, is the presence of dark-brown pigmented areas on the face, believed to be caused by sensitivity to the marked increase in estrogen hormone production during pregnancy as well as to the estrogen component of the Pill. Melasma involving the cheeks, upper lip, and forehead is commonly called "the mask of pregnancy" (see page 204). It is often accompanied by brown coloration of the nipples and linea nigra, a dark, thin line that runs from the navel to the pubic hairline. Freckles and brown moles or nevi (pigmented areas) on the skin also darken as a result of these hormonal changes. It has been theorized that the hyperpigmentation of chloasma occurs when

estrogen stimulates the pituitary gland to release large amounts of melanocyte-stimulating hormone (MSH). MSH in turn induces cells on the skin's surface, called melanocytes, to increase in number and secrete greater amounts of the skin pigment melanin. Exposure to sunlight while on the Pill or during pregnancy, especially in fair-skinned individuals, intensifies chloasma. Although many women with chloasma are often distressed by their appearance, the condition is harmless, and it improves following childbirth or discontinuation of the Pill.

Of far greater concern than chloasma is the question of whether the Pill and pregnancy increase a woman's risk of malignant melanoma. This potentially fatal form of cancer originates in the melanocytes within a pigmented mole on the skin and then reproduces at an abnormally rapid rate and spreads to other parts of the body. Its incidence in the general population is 9 to 13 per 100,000, and it is more common among fair-skinned individuals and those exposed to excessive amounts of sunlight over a period of years.

To date, a majority of studies links Pill use to malignant melanoma, but investigators have not adequately accounted for a host of variables such as a woman's personal and family history of cancer, her skin and hair coloring, the climate in which she lives, and the amount of time she spends in the sun. Pending further research, the relationship between use of birth control pills and a woman's predisposition to malignant melanoma remains inconclusive. To be safe, anyone with a history of this disease, even if it occurred years before, should use alternative methods of contraception. Similarly, if a woman develops melanoma while using birth control pills, she should discontinue the Pill immediately and forever.

Whether or not the hormonal changes of pregnancy cause an increase in the incidence and severity of malignant melanoma remains controversial. Though MSH does alter skin pigmentation in pregnancy, a direct association between this observation and the occurrence of melanoma has not been documented. There is, however, enough circumstantial evidence to suggest that hormonal factors have some bearing on the tumor's biological behavior and rapidity of spread. Some experts believe that a woman with a history of melanoma should avoid pregnancy. Other doctors recommend a waiting period of three to five years following treatment.

The best melanoma treatment is prevention.

Avoidance of excessive sun is critical. If you notice changes in the size, shape, or color of a skin mole, immediately call it to the attention of your doctor. Ulceration, pain, bleeding, or the presence of a new mole adjacent to one already present are all cause for concern. The location of a mole is also critical—those on the soles, palms, trunk, and external genitals require the closest observation.

NORPLANT

What are the effects of the new Norplant contraceptive on the developing fetus?

Norplant is a long-acting, reversible, hormonal contraceptive for women that was first approved by the Food and Drug Administration (FDA) in 1990. It consists of six capsules, each 34 millimeters long (the length of a matchstick) and each containing 35 milligrams of the progestin levonorgestrel. All six Norplant capsules are easily inserted under the skin of a woman's upper arm under local anesthesia and can be removed in the same fashion. The slow release of 30 micrograms of levonorgestrel daily provides excellent contraception for up to five years,

with pregnancy rates less than 1 percent annually.

The 30-microgram dosage of levonorgestrel released daily from the six Norplant capsules is only 20 percent of the 150-microgram dose found in a single low-dose combination birth control pill such as Nordette or Levlen. As a result, little if any of the drug enters the fetal circulation in the event of an accidental pregnancy. Therefore, it is unlikely to affect female fetal genital development in ways that have been associated with progestin use (see page 2) or to cause birth defects. Nevertheless, the capsules should be removed immediately if pregnancy occurs and a woman has opted not to undergo an abortion.

IUDS

What is an IUD?

An IUD, or intrauterine device, is inserted into the uterine cavity and left there for various periods of time for the purpose of contraception. There are more than 2 million women in the United States currently using the IUD for contraception. As a result of adverse publicity surrounding IUD use, it is estimated that it is used by only 3 percent of women versus 7 percent five years ago. Since 1909,

gynecologists seeking immortality have had IUDs of various sizes and shapes named after them. Names such as Grafenberg, Hall, Stone, Birnberg, Marguiles, Lippes, and Majzlin are remembered fondly by some women and vilified by a great number of others. There are currently two IUDs approved for use in the United States; the copper-containing ParaGard and the progesterone-containing Progestosert.

All IUDs have a nylon tail, or strings, which protrude from the cervix into the vagina. By touching the tail or viewing it with a speculum, you and your doctor can usually be assured that the IUD is in place. Since each IUD has a characteristic tail, a doctor can determine the type of IUD you have even if he or she did not insert it.

How does an IUD prevent pregnancy?

Several theories exist. For example, the presence of an IUD in the uterine cavity is known to stimulate an inflammatory reaction. As a result, large microscopic cells called macrophages are released. These are believed by some researchers to be capable of destroying sperm before they can get into the fallopian tube to fertilize the egg. Medicated IUDs containing copper and progesterone are believed to further enhance the hostility of the uterine lining, or endometrium. In addition, it is believed that progesterone thickens mucus within the cervix so that sperm are unable to penetrate it. However, some researchers and others with philosophical and religious objections to IUDs insist that macrophages destroy an already fertilized egg each month, thereby causing an early abortion.

Another theory of IUD action is that its presence in the uterus as a foreign object increases the motility of the fallopian tubes and thus stimulates the movement of the egg down the tube at a rate which is faster than would normally occur. (Copper in high concentrations is known to enhance this increase in tubal motility.) As a result, an egg too immature to implant into the uterine lining reaches the endometrium.

Is ectopic pregnancy more common in women wearing an IUD?

No. But, since the IUD prevents pregnancy in the uterus and not in the tube, any woman wearing an IUD who has a positive pregnancy test should strongly suspect an ectopic pregnancy. In fact, about 3 to 4 percent of all pregnancies conceived among IUD wearers are ectopic, meaning that they are outside the normal location in the endometrial cavity. While the fallopian tube is overwhelmingly the most common site for an ectopic pregnancy, for unknown reasons there is a significant increase among IUD users in the percentage of ectopics located in the ovary. Regardless of the location of an ectopic pregnancy, early diagnosis and treatment is vital in preventing severe abdominal hemorrhage and even death (see page 61).

In the past, researchers believed that present and former IUD users were at a significantly greater risk of an ectopic pregnancy, with progressively higher rates reported the longer the IUD was worn. This was believed to result from a greater likelihood of tubal infection and scarring, thereby hindering the fertilized egg from passing down the tube to its normal destination in the endometrium. However, more recent data clearly show that the IUD does not increase a woman's risk of an ectopic pregnancy, but only appears to do so since it is so effective in preventing a normal pregnancy from occurring. In other words, it is a relative rather than an absolute increase in the percentage of ectopic pregnancies that we see among IUD users who accidentally conceive. The most recent and convincing study exonerating prior use of a copper IUD as a cause of subsequent ectopic pregnancy was published in the *American Journal of Obstetrics and Gynecology* in 1989. In this report, 1,051 women were found to have no greater likelihood of ectopic pregnancy in gestations following removal of their copper-containing IUD.

Certainly, if you conceive while using an IUD, your doctor should strongly consider the diagnosis of ectopic pregnancy. Symptoms of pregnancy accompanied by lower abdominal discomfort and a slight amount of dark vaginal bleeding can indicate an ectopic pregnancy. With such a pregnancy, movement of the cervix, either through intercourse or pelvic examination, usually elicits extreme pain in the lower abdomen. Occasionally it is possible for your doctor to detect an enlargement in the tube containing the ectopic pregnancy. If only a minimal amount of tissue along with the IUD is removed during an abortion on an IUD user with a positive pregnancy test, ectopic pregnancy again should be strongly suspected.

Often women suffering from an ectopic pregnancy will not have the typical symptoms of pregnancy, and the possibility of this diagnosis may be overlooked by the examining doctor. In one study of 70 women eventually diagnosed as having an ectopic pregnancy associated with an IUD, the symptoms of bleeding and pelvic pain at first were often attributed to the mere presence of the IUD and not the undetected pregnancy. In more than 50 percent of these patients, the IUD was removed between one and eight weeks before the definitive diagnosis of ectopic pregnancy was made at surgery, presumably in the hope that the removal or changing of the IUD would alleviate the symptoms. If you continue to experience pain and bleeding after your IUD is removed, the diagnosis of ectopic pregnancy should be strongly considered and a pregnancy test obtained.

An alert physician should be able to diagnose practically all ectopic pregnancies prior to rupture. New vaginal ultrasound techniques make it possible to distinguish between an intrauterine and ectopic pregnancy within one to three weeks of a woman's missed period (see Chapters 2 and 11). In addition, a highly sensitive pregnancy test, combined with laparoscopy, has significantly increased the percentage of unruptured ectopic pregnancies that are diagnosed each year. The benefits of this new technology are reflected in a fourfold decline in the death rate from ectopic pregnancies over the last decade. In addition, it is much easier to repair and preserve the fallopian tube, rather than remove it, if surgery is performed prior to rupture.

What should I do if I become pregnant while using an IUD?

Regardless of the type of IUD you have, if you decide to continue with the pregnancy, the device should be removed immediately. By doing this, your risk of miscarriage is reduced to approx-

imately 30 percent, compared to 50 percent if the IUD is left in place. (The risk of miscarriage is normally 10 to 15 percent.) The likelihood of losing a pregnancy when removing an IUD is often determined by the IUD's position in relation to the pregnancy, or gestational, sac. IUDs located below the sac can usually be safely removed, while those above will often precipitate a miscarriage. The position of the IUD in relation to the gestational sac can be accurately determined by ultrasound examination.

If the IUD strings cannot be seen, you can assume that the device has either been expelled without your knowledge, has been taken up into the uterus with the pregnancy, or has perforated the uterus earlier and is now in the myometrium or muscle of the uterus or the abdominal cavity. Again, ultrasound can resolve this question. Since even a single x-ray taken early in pregnancy to locate an IUD causes undue radiation exposure to the fetus, x-ray is not recommended unless ultrasound is unavailable. In a 1988 report, doctors at the Albert Einstein College of Medicine in New York reported that they were able to successfully retrieve seven of eight missing IUDs early in pregnancy by using a uterine-viewing instrument called a hysteroscope placed through the cervix. The seven IUDs removed were all located below the gestational sac, and manipulation of the hysteroscope was accomplished under video guidance. This technique may have great potential for women facing the dilemma of carrying a pregnancy in the presence of an IUD.

If it is determined that the IUD is in the uterus but cannot be removed, it is the obligation of your obstetrician to warn you that you may develop a severe and even life-threatening infection during the pregnancy. The option of therapeutic abortion with removal of the IUD should be presented to all women in this predicament.

How can an IUD cause infection during pregnancy? What are the symptoms, and how is the infection treated?

A great variety of bacteria normally inhabit the vagina and are often found on the IUD strings as well. When these strings are taken up into the enlarging uterus during pregnancy, the bacteria they contain have the potential in a small percentage of women to cause a severe infection within the uterine cavity. Such an infection may then spread through the muscles of the uterus and into the lower pelvis. During the infectious process, the fallopian tubes and ovaries may become matted together in a ball of pus called a tubo-ovarian abscess. Rupture of such an abscess is associated with very high mortality rates. The toxins, or poisons, from the bacteria may also enter the bloodstream and attack distant organs, producing an overwhelming reaction and a drop in blood pressure called toxic, or septic, shock, which may also be fatal. IUD-associated infections during pregnancy are more apt to happen during the first six months. The risk of a second-trimester spontaneous abortion is increased twenty-six-fold among women carrying pregnancies in the presence of an IUD. Even more frightening is the fiftyfold increase in the maternal death rate.

Sadly, IUD infections during pregnancy are often extremely difficult to diagnose. In many of the reported cases, the women did not develop symptoms specific to the pelvis until late in the course of the disease. Instead, the initial symptoms often appeared only as a general feeling of tiredness, with possibly some respiratory symptoms accompanied by generalized muscle aching, fever, chills, headache, and other flu-like symptoms. These symptoms often rapidly progressed within a matter of hours to irreversible septic shock. When symptoms are present in the pelvis, more than half the women with infection experience tenderness over the uterus accompanied by a pus-filled vaginal discharge. Other common symptoms are bleeding and leakage of infected amniotic fluid from the vagina.

Some doctors have suggested that if suspicious symptoms develop but the diagnosis remains uncertain, an amniocentesis (see Chapter 11) should be performed immediately and the sample of amniotic fluid examined for evidence of infection. Regardless of the length of the pregnancy, the diagnosis of toxic or septic shock (infection associated with a sudden drop in blood pressure) resulting from an IUD requires immediate termination of the pregnancy and aggressive antibiotic therapy. Though this may appear to be harsh treatment in a pregnancy that has progressed to six months, if it is not done the infection will rapidly spread to a point where even a hysterectomy will not be able to contain it.

Can an IUD cause injury to the fetus?

No. Excluding fetuses lost as a result of miscarriages caused by the presence of an IUD in the uterus, it has been estimated that 20,000 infants survive and are successfully born each year to American women wearing IUDs. It is only natural that these women express fears that the IUD may harm or cause deformity of the fetus by entangling a limb or other parts of the body. Fortunately, this does not happen, since the IUD always lies outside the gestational or pregnancy sac of the baby. Of greater concern is our inability to predict the potential dangers of chemicals such as progesterone and copper lying in close proximity to the developing fetus.

To date, there have been no malformations reported among infants following exposure to the Progestasert IUD (which contains progesterone) in utero, though the number of infants born under such circumstances is still too small to draw definite conclusions. It is not totally accurate to compare the fetal effects of progesterone released from the Progestasert with the synthetic progestins contained in birth control pills. Most authorities agree that the latter have a far greater potential for causing anomalies than progesterone, a hormone which is present in abundance in all pregnancies. Experimental IUDs containing progestin rather than progesterone are now being evaluated. I am far more concerned about the close proximity of these devices to the developing fetus than I am about the progesterone which is found in the Progestasert device.

A 1975 report in the *British Medical Journal* described two women who conceived while using IUDs containing copper. Both gave birth to infants with similar limb defects in which some of the bones in the leg, arm, hand, and foot were missing. Contrary to this is a 1976 study from the Population Council of New York. This large project involved 157 women carrying pregnancies to completion in the presence of copper-containing IUDs. Only one minor congenital anomaly was noted among the offspring of these women, and this was a benign growth on the vocal cords of one of the babies. There were no limb deformities in any of the offspring. Other studies measuring copper levels of spontaneously

aborted fetuses exposed to a copper-containing IUD in utero revealed no increase in copper in the fetal brain, liver, or kidneys. A 1990 study measuring copper levels in electively aborted fetuses exposed to copper-containing IUDs in utero revealed no malformations and no traces of copper deposits in the fetal brain, liver, kidneys, or placenta. Finally, and most importantly, in a study conducted by scientists from the Centers for Disease Control, mothers of 96 infants born with shortened and deformed limbs over a six-year period were interviewed and compared with two control groups. The results, published in *Fertility and Sterility*, indicated that there was no significant increase in the occurrence of limb reduction deformities among babies exposed to the IUD at the time of conception.

 SPERMICIDES

Can contraceptive spermicides used by a woman harm her fetus?

Vaginal spermicides, or sperm-killing preparations, are readily available without prescription in most drug stores in the form of creams, gels, aerosol foam, tablets, suppositories, the TODAY Vaginal Contraceptive Sponge, and VCF, or Vaginal Contraceptive Film. Spermicides are also used in conjunction with the diaphragm and cervical cap. Some of the newer brands of condoms contain the same spermicide found in the majority of products used by women. All spermicide preparations consist of a spermicidal agent and an inert base which physically blocks the sperm and disperses the spermicide. Nonoxynol-9 and octoxynol-9 are the names of the spermicides found in practically all of these preparations. (Spermicides in the past contained mercury and chemicals called hydroquinones. There was con-

cern that these compounds might affect the genetic material in the sperm, leading to conception with birth defects, or be absorbed into the bloodstream, causing toxicity in women using them. As a result, these agents were taken off the market in the late 1960s.)

Until the early 1980s, it was believed that currently used spermicides were completely innocuous. However, at that time several investigators reported an increased incidence of spontaneous abortion, lethal chromosomal abnormalities, limb reduction deformities, and low birth weight complicating the pregnancies of women using a spermicide at the time of conception or in the months prior to conception. It was theorized that because spermicides damaged but didn't necessarily kill sperm cells, they allowed abnormal sperm to fertilize an egg. Other scientists speculated that absorption of spermicides into the bloodstream produced direct damage to the egg before conception. This theory was supported by scientific observation from Germany demonstrating that 1.5 percent of a measured amount of nonoxynol-9 was found in the urine samples of women 20 minutes after it was applied vaginally. Longer exposures produced a urine concentration of 10 percent.

Many knowledgeable scientists and epidemiologists have questioned the validity of these findings, and the preponderance of subsequent information has totally exonerated all currently used spermicides. One investigation, conducted by doctors at the Centers for Disease Control in 1983, compared two groups of mothers who gave birth to infants with birth defects; one group had used spermicides at the time of conception and the other had not. They found no specific anomaly patterns in the spermicide group and concluded that there was no evidence of a link between spermicides and chromosomal abnormalities or birth defects. Dr. James L. Mills and his associates at the National Institute of Child Health and Human Development (NICHD) studied the outcome of pregnancies in more than 8,000 women who had used spermicides either before or after their last menstrual period. Their research, published in *Fertility and Sterility* in 1985, evaluated the incidence of malformations, low birth weight, premature delivery, and spontaneous abortion among these women. They compared their results with those obtained from pregnancies among women who had been using other methods of contraception either immediately before or soon after they conceived. The malformation rates were found to be slightly higher in the women who had not been exposed to spermicides.

Two additional NICHD-supported studies, published in the *New England Journal of Medicine* in 1987, lend further support to the safety of spermicide use. Dr. Dorothy Warburton and her colleagues at Columbia University obtained information from 13,729 women undergoing am-

niocenteses regarding their specific use of spermicides at the time of conception as well as during the months and years preceding conception. They found that the incidence of Down syndrome and other chromosomal abnormalities was equal among spermicide users and nonusers. In the second study, doctors at Boston University School of Medicine and the University of Iowa evaluated the effects of spermicides on five separate groups of infants: 265 with Down syndrome, 396 with a defect of the male genitalia known as hypospadias, 146 with limb reduction defects, 116 with malignancies, and 215 with neural tube defects such as spina bifida and anencephaly. These infants were compared to a control group of more than 3,000 infants with a variety of other malformations. Although spermicide exposure was noted both before and during early pregnancy in many of the cases studied, the doctors found that the risks for specific defects were not related in any way to the timing or duration of spermicide use. Further confirmation of these findings was provided in 1988 by Barbara Strobino and her associates at New York Medical College, who concluded that spermicide use near the time of conception was not associated with any change in the sex ratio at birth, the weight of a newborn, or the presence of a major anomaly.

Based on a thorough review of all data, medical experts have concluded that there is no relationship between spermicide use and an abnormal pregnancy outcome. Furthermore, it is comforting to know that pregnancy termination is not warranted if pregnancy follows spermicide failure. As stated in a 1988 opinion of the American College of Obstetricians and Gynecologists, "There is now clear scientific consensus that vaginal spermicides are not associated with increased risks of malformation in offspring of women who become pregnant either while using these agents or after discontinuing usage just prior to pregnancy."

⇒ POSTCOITAL, OR "MORNING-AFTER," CONTRACEPTION ⇐

What is the "morning-after" pill?

"Morning-after," or postcoital, contraceptives are hormones which, when taken within 72 hours of unprotected coitus at ovulation, are highly effective in preventing survival of the fertilized egg. Though several hormonal preparations have been used effectively as postcoital contraceptives, most gynecologists associate the "morning-after" pill with the infamous drug diethylstilbesterol, or DES. Unlike other estrogens, DES is classified as a nonsteroidal synthetic estrogen. This is a fancy way of saying that it is made in the laboratory and not in the body, and is of a chemical structure totally different from the steroidal shape of natural estrogens and those contained in birth control pills.

In addition to DES, many other hormonal preparations have proven to be highly effective in preventing the survival of the fertilized egg when administered within 72 hours following unprotected intercourse at the time of ovulation. Currently the most popular of these products is Ovral, a commonly prescribed birth control pill. This pill contains the synthetic estrogen ethinyl estradiol and the progestin norgestrel. Ethinyl estradiol is the estrogen component of most other oral contraceptives manufactured today. It has been used alone, without the progestin, as a highly successful "morning-after" pill. Similarly, the progestin norgestrel has been used alone as a postcoital contraceptive. However, Ovral remains the most popular postcoital contraceptive because it is readily available in most pharmacies and is less likely to cause unpleasant side effects, such as nausea and vomiting, than other products. In addition, its rate of success is 99 percent.

"Morning-after" hormones act as interceptors, meaning that they prevent implantation of the egg after fertilization has taken place.

What is the "morning-after" IUD?

Insertion of an IUD after unprotected intercourse effectively prevents pregnancy almost 100 percent of the time. Since fertilization takes place in the tube and is followed by a three-day journey of the egg to the endometrium, the IUD usually sets up an inflammatory reaction in the endometrium that is capable of destroying the egg as it reaches its destination. Used in this way, the IUD probably causes early abortion.

In one study, 97 women had a copper-containing IUD inserted following unprotected intercourse. Seventeen women had them inserted within 27 hours, 30 within 48 hours, 17 within 72 hours, 17 within 96 hours, 14 within 120 hours, and 2 within 144 hours. There were no pregnancies. The advantage of an IUD over DES and other "morning-after" medications is that it causes no nausea or vomiting. In addition, it may be left in the uterus for contraception during future cycles.

What effects will "morning-after" hormones have on the developing fetus if they fail to intercept the pregnancy?

The effects of postcoital hormones on a fetus that is only a few hours old are unknown, but, since organ development does not take place for several weeks, it is highly unlikely that they would be responsible for causing anomalies. (In the case of postcoital Ovral, the incidence of deformities is believed to be far less than previously anticipated [see page 3].) However, when postcoital hormones are inadvertently taken after pregnancy is already a few weeks along, the risk of fetal anomalies increases significantly.

In the highly publicized experience with DES, both male and female fetuses have been reported to suffer a wide range of congenital abnormalities when the drug was taken after the seventh week from the last menstrual period. An advantage of using ethinyl estradiol, conjugated estrogens, and other steroidal estrogens is that they are not likely to initiate the changes characteristic of nonsteroidal estrogens such as DES.

How is DES given to a mother related to vaginal cancer in her daughter?

Practically all medication given to a mother crosses the placenta and reaches her fetus. Between 1940 and 1971, DES was widely used to prevent miscarriage, especially for women with a poor obstetrical history, diabetes, and others who experienced vaginal bleeding early in pregnancy. It has been estimated that approximately 2 million pregnant women took either DES or one of two other equally harmful nonsteroidal estrogens, dienestrol and hexestrol. In most instances, treatment with these substances began in the seventh week of pregnancy. Coincidentally, that is the time when vaginal and cervical development and demarcation become most active in the female fetus.

In 1972, three Boston physicians noted a sudden increase of young women in the number of previously rare cancers of the vagina and cervix called clear-cell adenocarcinomas. Upon further investigation they discovered that the majority of the mothers of these young women had taken nonsteroidal estrogens during their pregnancies. In addition, benign though highly abnormal changes were observed in the cervix and vagina of many of the daughters exposed to DES, dienestrol, and hexestrol. The Registry of Clear-Cell Adenocarcinoma of the Genital Tract of Young Females was formed in 1972 with the purpose of reporting all such tumors in women born in the United States and abroad after 1940. In 1977, the name of the Registry was changed to the National Cooperative Diethylstilbestrol Adenosis Project, or DESAD.

Adenosis is a term used to describe the presence of strawberry-red, mucus-secreting, glandular tissue on the outer part of the cervix and vagina. These glands are normally located inside the cervix and are usually not readily seen with a speculum. Using sophisticated diagnostic techniques, including colposcopy (microscopic viewing of the cervix), skilled gynecologists have noted adenosis in anywhere from 80 to 97 percent of daughters exposed in utero to DES.

Though adenosis is a benign condition, epidemiologists have concluded that in rare instances, adenosis cells can change into malignant vaginal and cervical adenocarcinomas. To date, approximately 500 vaginal and cervical adenocarcinomas have been reported among the estimated 2 million DES-exposed daughters. Use of nonsteroidal estrogens by the mothers has been confirmed in approximately 65 percent of the cases. More than 50 of these women have died of adenocarcinoma, while others have undergone radical and mutilating operations to prevent the spread of the disease. Fortunately, our worst fears of an epidemic of genital cancer have not been realized. The risk of developing clear-cell cancer is estimated to be no more than 1.4 per 1,000 and possibly as few as 1.4 per 10,000 exposed daughters. Though DES-exposed women with clear-cell adenocarcinoma have ranged in age from 7 to 34 years, the peak incidence appears to occur at the age of 19, with a precipitous decline noted after the age of 24. The occurrence of clear-cell adenocarcinoma after the age of 27 is extremely rare.

At the present time it is impossible to know what effect, if any, the use of DES will have on the granddaughters of women who first used it during their pregnancies. However, animal research at Michigan State University in 1987 is somewhat disconcerting. In preliminary studies, 13 of 40 "granddaughter," or third-generation, mice developed cancers of their reproductive tracts. No such cancers were found in the third generation of mice whose grandmothers were not exposed to DES.

What are the benign cervical and vaginal changes caused by DES?

In addition to adenosis, the cervix in approximately 40 to 50 percent of DES-exposed daughters often appears characteristically deformed, so that the diagnosis of maternal DES ingestion can be made simply by viewing its unusual shape during a routine examination. One of these distorted shapes, called a vaginal hood or collar, is seen as a circular fold in the upper vagina into which the cervix containing adenosis appears to merge. Another is the classic cock's comb, a small triangular protuberance seen at the upper pole of the cervix. In addition to abnormalities of the cervix and vagina, in 1977 doctors at Baylor College of Medicine described uterine abnormalities, including underdevelopment of the uterus combined with a peculiar T-shaped configuration of the uterine cavity and constricting bands in the cavity along the horizontal arm of the T. These abnormalities are easily found by hysterosalpingogram, a technique in which dye injected through the cervix outlines the uterine cavity and fallopian tubes. More recent investigation has determined that the presence of irregular or "shaggy" margins of the endometrial cavity outline that show up on x-ray is often associated with prenatal exposure to DES. About two-thirds of DES-exposed women have uterine anomalies that are detected by hysterosalpingogram, even though the external configuration of the uterus may appear normal when viewed through a laparoscope. In one study of DES-exposed women, 86 percent of those with characteristic cervical anomalies were noted on x-ray to have a uterine defect.

Do abnormalities of the cervix and uterus in DES daughters adversely affect their chances of a successful pregnancy?

While the question of infertility among DES-exposed women remains controversial, experts agree that the pregnancy of a DES-exposed woman must be classified as high-risk. In July 1978, Dr. Donald Goldstein of Harvard Medical School reported on the pregnancies of five women exposed to DES in utero. All had typical abnormalities of the cervix and all experienced symptoms characteristic of an incompetent cervix, one that is weakened and unable to carry the weight of a growing pregnancy (see previous discussion). An incompetent cervix usually results in a spontaneous and premature dilation, or opening, of the cervix, followed by miscarriage during the second or third trimester. Dr. Goldstein attributed this to underdevelopment (hypoplasia) of the cervixes of these women and suggested that the chances of successful pregnancy could be enhanced by suturing the cervix just after the twelfth week of pregnancy, before it begins to dilate. A suture placed around the cervix in this fashion is called a cerclage. In a 1987 study from the Hospital of the University of Pennsylvania, Dr. Jack Ludmir and his associates prophylactically sutured the cervix of 26 DES-exposed women between the twelfth and fourteenth week of pregnancy and managed an identical group of 36 women expectantly, suturing the cervix only if it appeared to be dilating prematurely during one of the many vaginal examinations conducted during pregnancy. The average length of pregnancy in the former group was more than three weeks longer and no babies were lost. In contrast, five infant deaths from premature birth occurred in the group that did not undergo prophylactic cerclage. In addition, 16 women, or 44 percent, in this group required an emergency cerclage of the cervix at some point in their pregnancies. Dr. Ludmir and his colleagues concluded that there is no reliable method for detecting those DES-exposed women at greatest risk for an incompetent cervix. For this reason, they suggested that routine placement of a suture early in pregnancy should be given strong consideration for all DES-exposed women.

Depending on which of the many studies you read, the incidence of cervical incompetence among DES daughters has been estimated at anywhere from 1.6 to 43 percent. It is obvious that routine suturing of the cervix of all DES daughters will subject many women to a surgical procedure which may be unnecessary. In an attempt to eliminate this problem, doctors are evaluating the role of frequent ultrasound surveillance in order to detect the earliest signs of cervical dilatation and shortening, or effacement. In a 1989 study, published in *Obstetrics and Gynecology*, doctors at Wayne State University followed their DES-exposed women with serial ultrasounds and found that only 5 of 21 required cerclage. In addition, there were no missed diagnoses of cervical incompetence. This led them to conclude that routine cerclage is not recommended when skillful ultrasound technology is available for making the early diagnosis of cervical change.

In a 1980 study, Dr. Goldstein and Dr. Merle J. Berger reported a dismal 31 percent spontaneous abortion rate among DES-exposed women, a 5 percent incidence of ectopic pregnancy during the first trimester, and an additional 18 percent miscarriage rate during the second trimester. Sadly, only 34 percent of all the DES-exposed women in two recent studies eventually achieved a successful full-term pregnancy.

In a 1984 project that combined the research of doctors from Baylor College of Medicine and the Mayo Clinic, 676 DES-exposed women underwent hysterosalpingogram. The pregnancy outcome for almost half of these women was related to the severity of their uterine defects noted on x-ray. The presence of a T-shaped uterus, uterine constrictions, or a "shaggy" appearance of the endometrium were all associated with a higher incidence of premature birth, ectopic pregnancy, and an overall unfavorable pregnancy outcome when compared to women with normal uterine x-rays. Even with a normal uterine configuration, a DES-exposed individual was slightly more likely than other women to have an unfavorable pregnancy outcome. In an excellent review of this subject, published in the January 1988 issue of *The Journal of Reproductive Medicine,* doctors at Harvard Medical School analyzed the records of 200 women exposed to DES and 12,240 unexposed women to evaluate the relation between maternal DES expo-

sure and pregnancy outcome. They found a statistically greater likelihood of ectopic pregnancy, bleeding during the first three months, low birth weights, premature labor, premature rupture of the membranes, placenta previa, toxemia, and breech position of the baby among DES-exposed women. Of interest was a reversal in the usual birth ratio of more males than females. In 1990, Dr. John M. Thorpe, Jr., and his associates at the University of North Carolina School of Medicine published their data on the deliveries of 45 women having a history of in utero DES exposure. When compared to a control group, DES-exposed women were more likely to undergo cesarean, require manual removal of the placenta, and experience hemorrhage in the postpartum period. One interesting and unexplained observation was that the labor patterns and cervical dilation rates were more normal in those DES-exposed women having their first babies than in those who had previously given birth.

On the brighter side, up to 80 percent of all the DES-exposed women in two recent studies eventually achieved a successful pregnancy. This encouraging fact should be conveyed to all women who were exposed to DES in utero: Even if you fail to carry one or two pregnancies successfully, the odds are still in your favor that your persistent attempts will be rewarded. Another cause for optimism is a study from Boston's Beth Israel Hospital, in which doctors found that some of the vaginal and cervical abnormalities attributed to DES may decrease spontaneously and even disappear in time.

Since the DES-exposed woman is at an increased risk for an unfavorable reproductive outcome, she must be carefully monitored throughout her pregnancy. This monitoring should include frequent office visits, periodic pelvic examinations to detect premature cervical dilation or effacement, and serial ultrasound studies, if available. If it is determined that the cervix is prematurely dilating or effacing, cerclage should be strongly considered.

If I inadvertently take DES without realizing that I am pregnant, what are the chances of my daughter developing adenosis?

This situation could theoretically occur if a woman with irregular periods uses DES as a "morning-after" pill without realizing she is pregnant. Table 1 demonstrates the likelihood of adenosis based on when in the pregnancy DES was first taken.

Surprisingly, the amount of DES ingested is of less importance than when in pregnancy it was begun. For example, adenosis has been known to develop after women used very small amounts of DES for only a few days during the critical seventh week of pregnancy.

If I take DES early in pregnancy and then give birth to a son, what problems may I anticipate?

Research conducted at the University of Chicago in 1981 on 308 DES-exposed men has revealed abnormalities of the genital tract in 31 percent. Of these, approximately half had cysts of the epididymis, the tube that carries sperm from the testes. Other genital defects noted were abnormally

TABLE 1

PERCENTAGE OF WOMEN WITH ADENOSIS BASED ON WEEK DES WAS STARTED

Week of Pregnancy DES Started	Percentage
1–6	Close to 0
7–8	100
9–10	89
11–12	70
13–14	20
15–16	Less than 15
16–19	Less than 5
After week 19	None

SOURCE: *Compiled by author.*

small testes, undersized penises, and thickening of the capsule of the testicle. Moreover, 18 percent showed severe pathologic changes in sperm shape, concentration, and motility, compared with only 8 percent in a control group. Similar findings have been noted in a smaller study by doctors at New York's Beth Israel Medical Center. It is still too early to determine whether lesions comparable to vaginal and cervical adenocarcinoma will develop in these males, though it appears unlikely. However, 65 percent of the DES-exposed men with abnormally small testes had a history of undescended testes, and it has long been known that such men may be at increased risk of developing cancer of the testes at a later date. In a report published in the *Journal of the American Medical Association* in 1983, doctors from Tufts-New England Medical Center in Boston described the case of a 28-year-old DES son who was found to have a malignant testicular tumor called a seminoma. Though this one case does not constitute epidemiological evidence of a relationship between DES and testicular cancer, the peak incidence of this tumor occurs when men are in their 30s. Since DES use was most prevalent in the late 1950s and 1960s, it is possible that the group at greatest risk would be expected to contract cancer in the early 1990s.

By far the most encouraging report concerning exposure of males to DES in utero was published by doctors from the Mayo Clinic in 1984. They compared 828 exposed men and 676 controls for genito-urinary anomalies, infertility, and testicular cancer and found no differences between the two groups. In trying to explain why their findings were in such contrast to those of other groups, the Mayo Clinic doctors theorized that the study designs of previous programs were faulty in several ways. In addition, the men in their study might have been exposed to lower doses of DES than men in other studies who were found to have low sperm counts and congenital anomalies.

The suggestion of doctors at the University of Chicago and Beth Israel Hospital is that all DES-exposed men undergo a complete urological examination. Although data are scarce, researchers have found no evidence of effects on a third generation of males following DES exposure.

A psychosexual study conducted at Stanford University on boys exposed to DES in utero concluded that they were significantly "less masculine" than a comparative group not exposed to this drug. Psychiatrists rated 6- and 20-year-olds according to masculinity factors, such as athletic coordination, behavioral movements, heterosexual experience, masculine interests, and aggression-assertion attitudes. While the potential inaccuracies and biases of such a study are readily apparent, it does suggest that hormones may be capable of influencing some aspects of postnatal psychosexual development in boys.

In 1983, the *British Journal of Obstetrics and Gynaecology* published the findings of doctors at Radcliffe Infirmary, who had studied 264 sons and 266 daughters of women who had taken DES during their pregnancies. They found that DES offspring had a higher incidence than unexposed individuals of a wide range of psychiatric illness, including depression, anxiety, and anorexia. Larger studies are needed to confirm or refute these findings.

 THE RHYTHM METHOD

What is the rhythm method?

The rhythm method is a birth control technique based on limiting intercourse only to those times of the month thought to be free from the possibility of pregnancy. It is the only contraceptive technique sanctioned by the Catholic Church. Many proponents of the rhythm method consider its name to be obsolete and believe that the terms "natural family planning" and "fertility awareness" best describe the various techniques encompassed by this form of contraception. Despite the large sums of money devoted to the promotion and development of natural family planning methods, no significant inroads have been made in gaining new advocates or in drastically reducing the relatively high failure rates associated with their use.

Most people who either practice or teach natural methods of family planning are morally and religiously opposed to the use of other means of birth prevention during the fertile days of the menstrual cycle. Strict adherents of "pure" natural family planning stress the importance of abstinence and self-control during these days in order to preserve the "naturalness" of the method and to strengthen the bond of shared responsibility, dedication, and faithfulness between couples. Many natural family planning supporters are adamant about the importance of intercourse only within the marriage and the acceptance of a child should a pregnancy occur. While I appreciate and respect this position, I am also aware of the realities and frailties of today's society. Since this book is intended for the majority of individuals seeking practical advice in such matters, I recommend alternative methods of contraception during the fertile days of the month, when pregnancy is most likely to occur.

Calculation of the safe and unsafe times of the month can be achieved by one of three techniques: the calendar technique, daily basal body temperatures, and the sympto-thermal method. The calendar method, rarely used today, is based on the length of previous menstrual cycles. More accurate is the daily basal body temperature method, which is based on the fact that a woman's temperature rises soon after ovulation and stays elevated until menstruation begins. This elevation of temperature results from the release of progesterone by the ovary following ovulation. Since it is presumed that an egg is incapable of being fertilized 24 hours or longer after ovulation, the elevation of temperature for three consecutive days practically always means that pregnancy will not take place if a woman has intercourse after that time.

The sympto-thermal method, the most accurate, combines the use of daily basal body temperatures with changing bodily symptoms indicative of ovulation. The most important of these symptoms is the evaluation of the mucus secreted by the glands of the cervix. As ovulation approaches, the glands of the cervix under the influence of estrogen secrete a progressively more abundant amount of thin, watery, lubricative, and stretchable mucus. Spinnbarkeit is the name given to the ability of the mucus to stretch, while "peak symptom" describes the raw-egg consistency and appearance of the mucus at ovulation. Typically, ovulation occurs within a day or two before or after the peak symptom and maximum Spinnbarkeit. When the mucus stretches to a length of approximately 4 inches, ovulation is imminent or has just occurred. Following ovulation, the mucus becomes thick, tacky, and opaque, and it lacks Spinnbarkeit. This results from the effect of progesterone produced by the corpus luteum in the ovary. To avoid conception, abstinence is necessary from the time the thin mucus is first noted until four days after the peak symptom. This method of rhythm, based on analyzing changes in the cervical mucus, is also known as the "ovulation method," "fertility awareness," and the "Billings method," for Evelyn L. Billings and John J. Billings, two ardent proponents who pioneered its use.

Aren't there newer tests which make the rhythm method almost 100 percent effective in preventing pregnancy?

No. Perfecting the rhythm method has challenged scientists for many years. To date, the goal of finding a rapid, inexpensive, accurate, self-administered method of precise ovulation predic-

tion has remained elusive. Over the past ten years a variety of inventors and charlatans have devised exotic instruments, computerized digital thermometers, electrical devices, complicated calendars, and "fertility kits" in attempts to measure more precisely body temperature, the exact day of ovulation, and changes in the consistency and stretchability of a woman's cervical mucus. Most of these devices have proven less than satisfactory. Despite the proliferation of such gadgets, no method has proven more accurate than the careful observation by a woman who has taken the time to familiarize herself with the cyclic hormonal and physical changes that take place in her body each month.

One accurate, although fairly expensive, new method of pinpointing ovulation is the determination of the luteinizing hormone (LH) surge, which occurs prior to ovulation. Several companies have manufactured test kits that can measure the sudden surge of LH, which always precedes ovulation by 24 to 38 hours. Manufacturers of kits that measure the LH surge are not permitted to advertise their product as a means of enhancing the rhythm method, but you may nonetheless find them helpful for this purpose.

There have been no scientific studies to show whether the use of ovulation test kits for the presence of LH can improve the success rate of the rhythm method. But if used in conjunction with the sympto-thermal method, one can only assume that the kits will add to the effectiveness of this method. Two notable disadvantages are the time required to run the tests daily, sometimes twice a day as ovulation approaches, and the cost of one or two new kits each month.

The CUE Ovulation Predictor is another promising new device that can predict and confirm ovulation with an accuracy of 93 to 100 percent, according to its manufacturer, Zetek, Incorporated, of Aurora, Colorado. Unlike other ovulation prediction kits, which detect changes in LH levels, the CUE device electrically measures subtle differences in the salivary and vaginal secretions of sodium, potassium, and chloride as ovulation approaches. Although the CUE device was originally approved by the FDA in 1985 for couples seeking pregnancy, it is likely to be helpful to women in improving the accuracy of the rhythm method.

If pregnancy occurs while using the rhythm method, are there any dangers to the fetus?

There is some evidence to suggest that a wide range of medical problems, such as spontaneous abortion and birth defects, may be related to the use of the rhythm method. It has been demonstrated that the best chance for normal pregnancy occurs when fertilization of the egg takes place just at the time of ovulation. Users of the rhythm method are more likely to abstain from intercourse at that time and for the few days prior to ovulation. Coitus 12 to 24 hours after ovulation is more likely to expose an overripe, unhealthy egg to fertilization. Whereas fertilization normally takes place in the portion of the fallopian tube closest to the ovary, late fertilization does not occur until the egg has traveled some distance along the tube or has entered the uterine cavity. This has been termed "postovulatory," "tubal," or "intrauterine" overripeness. In the second type of overripeness, termed "preovulatory" or "follicular," the egg is retained in the ovary beyond the normal time. As a result, structural defects take place in the egg which may produce an abnormal fetus when ovulation and fertilization finally occur. Both types of overripeness have been held responsible for pregnancy problems.

Down syndrome and several other chromosomal abnormalities most often occur when a pair of chromosomes fail to separate as they normally should when the egg is being formed just prior to fertilization. This phenomenon, called nondisjunction, results in an extra chromosome in the embryo. For unknown reasons, eggs that are not fertilized soon after ovulation and those in women over 30 are more likely to experience nondisjunction. In addition, a 1982 study from Europe has found that seasonal factors play a role, with nondisjunction more apt to occur in February through April conceptions. Aging sperm have also been implicated as a cause of problem pregnancies among couples using the rhythm method. Though sperm older than 48 hours are usually unable to fertilize an egg, there are notable exceptions to this rule. In fact, some hearty sperm have been known to live for seven days, leading investigators to speculate that pregnancies conceived with these old sperm are more apt to be abnormal.

Statistical data from three different studies conducted in New England have indicated a significantly higher rate of congenital central nervous system defects in the Catholic population than in the Protestant population. In the September 16, 1978, issue of the medical journal *Lancet*, two researchers noted an association between infrequent intercourse and an increased incidence of Down syndrome. The October 21, 1978, issue of *Lancet* published a letter from Marie T. Mulcahy, from the State Health Laboratory Services in Perth, Australia, suggesting that the findings could probably be attributed to the rhythm method of contraception. Ms. Mulcahy cited an epidemiological study of Down syndrome patients who were born in western Australia between 1966 and 1975 that showed the incidence among births to Catholic women to be more than double that found in all other religions. Ms. Mulcahy noted that this high incidence remained more or less constant throughout the ten-year period, that it was apparent in all maternal age groups, and that it was not related to birth rank or to ethnic origin of either parent.

Dr. Richard Juberg, in a 1983 study published in *Human Genetics*, reported the effects of delayed fertilization among 33 parents having children with chromosomal abnormalities such as Down syndrome. Dr. Juberg found 22 instances in which there was definite evidence of delayed fertilization. While other variables may certainly be responsible, it appears likely that the rhythm method may play a role in causing some of these chromosomal abnormalities.

MENSTRUAL EXTRACTION AND ABORTION

What is the difference between menstrual extraction and first-trimester abortion?

A first-trimester abortion, one which is performed during the first three months of pregnancy, is most effectively carried out with a small flexible plastic cannula (tube) or curette (loop or ring) attached to a suction machine. Menstrual extraction, also known as menstrual regulation and mini-abortion, is usually performed within three weeks beyond the missed period, on a woman with a slightly enlarged or normal-sized uterus. At this early stage, the cervix rarely has to be dilated, and a suction cannula with a very small diameter may be used to evacuate the uterine contents. A woman requesting menstrual extraction is usually one whose period is late and who is fearful of pregnancy but prefers not to know if she is pregnant. It must be emphasized that the criterion for calling a procedure a menstrual extraction rather than an abortion is not whether the pregnancy test is positive or negative.

Do menstrual extraction and first-trimester elective abortion always terminate a pregnancy?

A woman undergoing menstrual extraction or early elective abortion should understand that her pregnancy may not be terminated in a small percentage of cases. This may occur because the pregnancy sac is so small that it may be missed by the suction apparatus. In addition, the smaller cannulas used for menstrual extraction are less likely to create suction which adequately dislodges the fetal sac from the uterine wall. One study found that the pregnancy remained intact in 3 percent of all women undergoing menstrual extraction. When the small 4-millimeter cannula was used, the incidence of this complication rose to 5 percent. However, with the slightly more uncomfortable 6-millimeter cannula, the continuing pregnancy

rate was a very low 0.7 percent. Regardless of the cannula size used, all tissue should be studied for microscopic confirmation of an early pregnancy. If such confirmation is not obtained, a pregnancy test and re-examination should be performed immediately in order to be certain that the pregnancy has been terminated.

If I decide to continue with my pregnancy after a failed menstrual extraction or first-trimester abortion, will the pregnancy have complications?

Fetuses surviving a failed menstrual extraction or first-trimester abortion will practically always have an intact gestational or pregnancy sac, and you need not fear deformity or injury. Ultrasound confirmation of a good heartbeat and a healthy fetus is often reassuring. However, the insertion of instruments into the uterine cavity at the time of the attempted procedure can occasionally cause a severe infection of the pregnancy tissues. Symptoms of this complication usually appear within a week and include a temperature higher than 38°C (100.4°F), a foul-smelling vaginal discharge which may be blood-tinged, and lower abdominal cramps. If not treated rapidly, the infection may spread to the lower pelvis, the tubes, and the ovaries, causing permanent damage, adhesions, and impaired future fertility. Bacteria may also enter the bloodstream and attack other organs and even cause death. These potentially dangerous complications can be avoided with immediate hospitalization, high doses of antibiotics, and termination of the pregnancy with a dilatation and curettage (D and C). Attempts at salvaging a pregnancy in the presence of a uterine infection are foolhardy and doomed to failure.

All Rh-negative women should receive an intramuscular injection of immune globulin (RhoGAM, Gamulin Rh, or Rho-D Immune Globulin) within 72 hours after a menstrual extraction or abortion in order to prevent the formation of antibodies against Rh-positive babies during future planned pregnancies. The one exception to this is if the father is known to be Rh-negative, in which case the medication need not be given. If you are Rh-negative and the menstrual extraction or abortion did not terminate your pregnancy, be assured that the injection of Rh-immune globulin will not cause harm. In fact, it will probably help in preventing you from forming antibodies against your Rh-positive fetus.

Isn't a woman's risk of infertility and ectopic pregnancy greater following an elective abortion?

Theoretically, if an abortion is complicated by a severe postoperative pelvic infection involving the fallopian tubes, the result could be tubal occlusion, higher rates of infertility, and tubal pregnancies. You can prevent this complication by immediately reporting a postabortion fever, abdominal pain, or foul-smelling discharge and by seeking appropriate antibiotic treatment from your doctor.

Fortunately, these complications rarely occur. Seven separate studies have failed to demonstrate a relationship between abortion and subsequent infertility. In fact, doctors from Harvard Medical School, in a 1984 report published in *Obstetrics and Gynecology*, found that pregnancy rates were increased for women reporting three or more induced abortions. The authors of the study attributed this to the probability that these women frequently resorted to abortion as a result of their greater than average fertility. Similarly, a Columbia University College of Physicians and Surgeons report in 1986 noted no association between elective abortion and future ectopic pregnancy. Despite these facts, there appears to be a prevailing myth among doctors and patients that elective abortion poses great risks to future successful pregnancies. In fact, I know of several instances in which women have decided to continue with an unplanned and unwanted pregnancy because they feared that an abortion would lead to infertility or a hazardous outcome of a future planned pregnancy.

What complications might be encountered during a pregnancy that follows a first-trimester abortion?

To avoid most complications, the ideal time to perform a first-trimester abortion is probably between the seventh and ninth weeks of pregnancy, as measured from the last menstrual period. After the tenth week, complications such as hemorrhage, retained placental fragments, and infection increase significantly.

A great controversy currently exists among gynecologists over the important question of whether dilatation of the cervix at the time of an abortion is responsible for an incompetent, or weakened, cervix during subsequent pregnancies. A woman with an incompetent cervix will suffer from repeated second-trimester spontaneous abortions and premature births because her cervix will be unable to support the weight of her growing uterus (see discussion on DES, page 15). Though the cause of cervical incompetence is usually unknown, trauma in the form of forceful dilatation may be the problem in some women, and several researchers believe that women who undergo repeated abortions are more likely to have an incompetent cervix.

In an experimental study reported in the *British Journal of Obstetrics and Gynaecology*, dilators were passed through the cervixes of surgically removed uteri in an attempt to detect the stage of dilatation at which microscopic tissue rupture could first be detected. In almost 50 percent of the specimens tested, evidence of tissue damage was apparent at a dilatation of 9 to 11 millimeters. The investigators concluded that use of a dilator 8 millimeters or less caused a harmless dilatation of the cervix, while dilators larger than that critical size were more likely to cause damage.

Although it is possible to question the applicability of these experimental data, the lesson to be learned is obvious: The smallest possible dilators should be used for a suction curettage if the potential problem of an incompetent cervix is to be avoided. The effects of midtrimester (second-trimester) abortion on future cervical incompetence are of greater concern than those of first-trimester abortion, since greater dilatation of the cervix is required in the former.

Clinical studies investigating the relationship between first-trimester abortion and subsequent spontaneous abortion and premature labor are somewhat contradictory. In an impressive study from the University of Washington in 1977, researchers compared the obstetrical records of more than 500 women who had previously had an induced abortion and a similar control group who had not experienced the procedure. They concluded that there were no significant differences between the two groups. Furthermore, the incidence of spontaneous abortion and premature birth was not affected by the number of previous abortions or by the week of pregnancy in which the previous abortion was performed. A 1980 report from Hawaii, involving more than 2,000 women, reached similar conclusions but noted that the risk of miscarriage was far greater when pregnancy occurred within one year after an induced abortion or a full-term birth. Similarly, Dr. Michael B. Brachen of Yale University School of Medicine found that babies tended to be of lower birth weight when the time interval between the abortion and the next conception was less than one year. Aside from this, Dr. Brachen, in his 1986 report published in the *American Journal of Epidemiology*, noted no relationship between birth weight in later pregnancies and the abortion technique that was used, the complications that were encountered, or the week of pregnancy in which the abortion was performed.

In contrast to these studies, doctors at Boston's Brigham and Women's Hospital concluded that women who had two or more induced abortions were two to three times more likely to miscarry during subsequent pregnancies. Interestingly, the technique used during the abortions did not appear to be an important contributing factor, in direct conflict with several other studies that stress the importance of the abortion method in determining the success or failure of future pregnancies. Data from the World Health Organization, encompassing the statistics of seven European nations, showed that the use of a sharp curette, rather than the more gentle and modern suction apparatus, increased the likelihood of a future midtrimester spontaneous abortion. Of further interest is that the World Health Organization data suggest that dilatation with an instrument larger than 9 millimeters increases the incidence of incompetent cervix, babies with low birth weight, and premature labor. In 1981, Dr. Susan Harlap and her associates noted that if a woman's cervix was dilated to 12 millimeters or more at the time of an induced abortion, she was more likely to give birth to a premature infant, compared to a woman whose cervical dilatation was 11 millimeters or less. Based on her findings, Dr. Harlap cautioned women to have induced abortions performed as early as possible in order to minimize cervical dilatation and subsequent weakening of the cervix.

Placenta previa, a condition in which the placenta or afterbirth covers the cervix rather than assuming its normal position high in the uterus, may be responsible for severe hemorrhage late in pregnancy. While two small studies have suggested that induced abortion may be a risk factor for a later occurrence of placenta previa, doctors from Grady Memorial Hospital in Atlanta, Georgia, found no such association in their extensive 1984 report that studied more than 29,000 abortions. In her 1985 study of placenta previa, Dr. Patricia McShane and her associates at Harvard Medical School similarly concluded that therapeutic abortion does not predispose to placenta previa.

In a 1979 article published in the *British Medical Journal*, doctors at the Welsh School of Medicine found a higher than normal incidence of spina bifida, a neural tube defect, among children of women with a history of two or more previous abortions. Specifically, the rate was 8.4 per 1,000 births among those studied, versus 2.3 per 1,000 for those who had never undergone abortion. These findings have not been substantiated in subsequent studies on the effects of elective abortion.

Is there any way to decrease the risk of trauma to the cervix during elective abortion?

The three most important determinants in reducing the risk of cervical injury at the time of a first-trimester abortion are an experienced physician, the use of local rather than general anesthesia, and the insertion, prior to the procedure, of cervical dilators such as laminaria digitata, dried seaweed that has been used as a cervical dilator for more than 100 years; Lamicel, a synthetic polyvinyl sponge saturated with alcohol containing magnesium sulfate; Dilapan, a hydrogel polymer rod; or prostaglandins in the form of vaginal and intracervical gels and tablets. Since cervical dilators open the cervix painlessly and atraumatically, it would not be unreasonable for a woman to request and even demand that they be inserted prior to a first-trimester pregnancy termination.

 ABORTION AFTER TWELVE WEEKS

What problems may be encountered by a pregnant woman who has had a previous second-trimester abortion, and how can they be remedied?

Little is known about the effects of a second-trimester abortion on future pregnancies. The limited available information on obstetric outcomes after installation of intraamniotic solutions, such as saline and prostaglandins, suggests no significant increase in the risk of low birth weight or prematurity. However, there is concern that cervical lacerations and fistulas have been linked to the use of prostaglandins.

A cervical fistula, an abnormal opening in the cervix, can result from a rupture or a laceration occurring at the time of a midtrimester abortion. This complication, estimated to occur in 0.5 percent of midtrimester abortions, most often happens to those women who have never carried a previous full-term pregnancy. Prostaglandins, administered either as suppositories or as an intraamniotic injection, are more likely than intraamniotic saline to cause this problem because the uterine muscle contractions produced by the prostaglandins are more forceful and frequent, and adequate time is not allowed for the cervix to gradually efface and dilate.

Fistulas are often difficult to suture, and, even when the surgical repair appears perfect, a woman may still be left with a permanently weakened and incompetent cervix. If you have experienced a cervical fistula from a previous abortion, your doctor may want to place a cerclage suture around your cervix (see page 15). Ideally, this operation is best performed during the fourteenth week of pregnancy, since the risk of early miscarriage has passed and the weight of the uterus is still not great enough to cause excessive pressure on the cervix.

Opinion varies as to the best method of delivery following a successful cerclage operation. Many doctors prefer to leave the suture in place throughout the pregnancy and accomplish delivery via cesarean section. If you request vaginal delivery, the cerclage suture may be cut during the last days of pregnancy, with labor allowed to take place under close supervision. One disadvantage of allowing vaginal delivery is that the pressure of the baby's head during labor may reopen the fistula. A second drawback is that the cerclage operation has to be repeated during each subsequent pregnancy. Occasionally, scarring from the previous surgery makes repeated surgical procedures more difficult.

There is now convincing data to show that dilatation and evacuation (D and E), when performed by an experienced and skilled physician, is the safest way to terminate midtrimester abortions. This method involves use of suction curettage with vacuum cannulas as large as 16 millimeters combined with special forceps and other instruments to remove fetal and placental tissue.

Concern has been expressed in the medical literature that the large 16-millimeter cannulas used for D and E may cause permanent damage to the cervical tissues. It has been theorized that this could lead to cervical incompetence, spontaneous abortion, and premature delivery in subsequent pregnancies. In one study, investigators compared the incidence of low birth weight among children of women who had had cervical dilatation of 16 millimeters for midtrimester abortion with that among babies whose mothers had had previous cervical dilatation of 14 millimeters. They found that mothers in the former group were at a 2.5 times greater risk of delivering a low birth weight infant than were those in the latter group. For this reason, the use of laminaria and other products that slowly and without trauma dilate the cervix prior to D and E are now used extensively in the United States.

 TUBAL STERILIZATION

What is tubal sterilization?

Tubal sterilization refers to any operative procedure on the fallopian tubes which prevents fertilization of the egg by sperm within the tube. Traditional methods have usually involved tying (ligating) combined with cutting out a portion of the tube. Newer techniques have utilized coagulation or burning, as well as the placement of elastic bands and plastic clips around a segment of the tube. This is accomplished through a viewing instrument called a laparoscope, which is placed in the abdominal cavity through the navel. The great advantage of laparoscopy is that it can be performed as a one-day ambulatory procedure. The abdominal cavity may also be entered and the tubes tied through the vagina if a vaginal incision is made behind the cervix.

The highly touted "minilap," or minilaparotomy, is a method of abdominal tubal ligation which is gaining popularity in many countries. In this procedure, an instrument is inserted through the cervix into the uterine cavity in order to push the uterus up against the lower abdominal wall. A 1-inch skin incision is then made directly over the top of the elevated uterus. The tubes are brought up into the operative field and are either tied or cut.

Is pregnancy possible following a tubal ligation, and what effect does the procedure have on the pregnancy?

Yes. Regardless of the method used, there is always the possibility of pregnancy months or even years later, and it may occur in 0.1 to 3 percent of all women who have undergone sterilization procedures. Any future pregnancy has a significant risk of being ectopic. Techniques which destroy a larger section of tube, such as coagulation or burning, lead to a higher ectopic pregnancy rate because these procedures leave fistulas, or openings, from the uterus to the abdominal cavity through which sperm can find their way to the end of the tube and fertilize an egg. The development of a fistula and consequent accidental pregnancy generally take at least two years to develop. Even with impeccable surgical technique, there will be at least 1 pregnancy per 1,000 sterilizations performed. In contrast, a pregnancy that occurs within three months of sterilization is most likely the result of a doctor's inadequate attempt to occlude the tubes at the time of surgery.

Most mechanical methods of sterilization, such as tying, or ligation, of the tubes, elastic rings, and plastic spring clips, are associated with remarkably low ectopic pregnancy rates but are less reliable and associated with higher numbers of intrauterine pregnancies.

 OTHER QUESTIONS

Is a pregnancy which occurs following unsuccessful vasectomy more apt to be abnormal?

Vasectomy means cutting of the vas deferens, the two tubes that carry sperm from each testicle. It is a minor surgical procedure which can be performed with equal ease in hospitals, clinics, or doctors' offices under local anesthesia. Without doubt, vasectomy is the simplest, surest, and safest surgical or medical method known for preventing unwanted pregnancy.

Offspring conceived following unsuccessful vasectomy are at no greater risk of congenital abnormalities.

Can douching immediately after intercourse prevent pregnancy?

Douching with various solutions is an ancient postcoital contraceptive technique that is totally futile. Current research has demonstrated that sperm can move into the endocervix, beyond the reach of a douche solution, within 90 seconds after ejaculation. This does not mean that the ejaculate is not capable of entering the endocervix as soon as 5 seconds later, but only that 90 seconds was the

fastest the researchers were able to collect and examine the postcoital specimens. In addition, recent studies have located sperm in the fallopian tube 10 to 45 minutes following insemination. Even if a douche is used within 10 seconds following ejaculation, it is highly improbable that it could kill all the sperm in the vagina or prevent the ascent of many sperm through the cervical opening.

If pregnancy does occur following unsuccessful douching, is it more likely to be abnormal?

While douching might not decrease a woman's risk of becoming pregnant, there is some evidence that it might increase her chances of an ectopic pregnancy. In an article published in the *American Journal of Obstetrics and Gynecology* in 1986, researchers found that women who douched once or more a week had an average of twice the incidence of ectopic pregnancies as did women who never douched. For unexplainable reasons, those who used a commercial douching preparation were shown to be far more susceptible to ectopic pregnancy than those using water or a noncommercial douching mixture such as water and vinegar.

2

PREPREGNANCY
and
EARLY PREGNANCY

*M*ost couples react to the diagnosis of pregnancy with unequalled joy and excitement. Next comes a torrent of questions and concerns as well as a sobering sense of responsibility and commitment.

It is only in recent years that preconception counseling has emerged as an important adjunct to obstetrical care. Professional evaluation of a couple's medical, genetic, ethnic, occupational, recreational, and nutritional status prior to pregnancy helps to maximize the chances for a successful result as well as pinpoint and correct potential risk factors. In this chapter I discuss the various elements of the preconception consultation and examination, the criteria that couples should use in selecting obstetrical care, and the financial cost of having a baby. Careful planning prior to conception will help to relieve the anxiety of making important decisions haphazardly should an early-pregnancy complication suddenly appear. Questions relating to distressing pregnancy symptoms such as "morning sickness" and potentially more ominous problems, such as vaginal bleeding, require accurate answers and immediate attention.

I also answer some of the more commonly asked questions about conception and early pregnancy. In addition, I present simple methods by which you can diagnose a problem and assess your uterine size and the growth and development of your baby during each pregnancy month.

THE IMPORTANCE OF GOOD HEALTH BEFORE CONCEPTION

What simple measures can a couple take prior to conception in order to improve their chances for a healthy pregnancy?

It is imperative for the health of your baby that you not lose weight or severely restrict your weight gain

during your pregnancy (but also see Chapter 8). Therefore, you should try to get as close as possible to your ideal weight before you become pregnant. If your pregnancy weight is 5 percent or more below the ideal weight for your height, you will be at significantly greater risk of giving birth to an infant of low birth weight, that is, one weighing less than 5½ pounds. It is important that overweight women reach their ideal weight sensibly with a diet low in fat and high in complex carbohydrates; crash diets and rapid loss of weight often result in the impairment of ovulation and infertility.

If you never exercise or exercise infrequently, it is easier and safer to begin before, rather than after, you are pregnant. Exercise will help you achieve your ideal prepregnancy weight faster, improve muscle tone, and give you an important psychological "high" throughout pregnancy, labor, and delivery. Regularly scheduled aerobic activities such as walking, running, cycling, and swimming can usually be continued with slight modifications during pregnancy (see Chapter 3).

It is vital that *all* medications, including over-the-counter products, be evaluated either by your physician or your obstetrician prior to pregnancy. All medications are capable of crossing the placenta and reaching the fetus, and some can cause birth defects and a variety of other serious complications. Often your doctor will discover that a particular medication is no longer necessary or that the dose can be lowered significantly. Sometimes, a drug that is less likely to affect the fetus can be substituted for one you have been taking (see Chapter 9). It is a good idea to have a dental checkup and to complete all dental work before becoming pregnant. Although dental x-rays can be taken and the fetus protected by covering the abdomen with a lead shield, most pregnant women correctly believe that even a single x-ray is one too many.

Alcohol consumption and cigarette smoking are known to cause fetal toxicity. The fetal alcohol syndrome occurs even among moderate drinkers. If you can't make it through a day without an alcoholic drink stronger than a glass of wine or beer, perhaps you should seek counseling before you decide to become pregnant. The chemicals in cigarette smoke cause a host of reproductive problems. Even if you don't smoke, inhalation of so-called passive smoke can be equally detrimental. While evidence implicating marijuana as a fetal toxin continues to mount, data on the dangers of addictive illicit drugs such as cocaine and heroin are well established (see Chapter 5). If you are abusing these or other drugs, you should be seeking professional help for your problem rather than planning a pregnancy.

As more women work throughout their pregnancies, they are understandably concerned about an array of potential occupational hazards. If your job is either physically or emotionally very stressful, it may be in your best interest to find a less demanding vocation or to request a temporary transfer to a less stressful position. Women employed as laboratory technicians, dental assistants, hair dressers, artists, anesthesiologists, and factory workers face unique occupational hazards that should be discussed with an obstetrician; necessary changes should be made prior to pregnancy (see Chapter 10).

 CHOOSING A DOCTOR

How can I select a competent obstetrician to deliver my baby?

Your search for a competent obstetrician should begin before conception, when you will be less apt to make a hasty decision. For the woman living in a rural area served by a small number of doctors, the selection may be limited. Most women, fortunately, can choose from a wide variety of physicians. Despite the options open to her, however, all too often a woman will select a doctor solely on the recommendation of a neighbor or casual acquaintance. Yet "shopping around" and conducting formal interviews to find the best doctor is the right of every pregnant woman—a right that should be exercised.

Of primary importance in the selection process are a doctor's qualifications. Although many family doctors practice obstetrics, you will undoubtedly be in far better hands if you choose someone who has completed a three- to four-year residency program in obstetrics and gynecology. It is also wise to find out if your doctor has been certified by the American Board of Obstetrics and Gynecology. While board certification is no guarantee of excellence, it does mean that the doctor has completed an approved residency and has studied for and passed two rigorous examinations. The American Board of Obstetrics and Gynecology has recently made periodic recertification exams mandatory in order to be sure that its members keep up to date on the latest obstetrical and gynecological advances. Don't be misled by a doctor telling you that he or she is board-eligible. This outdated and confusing term usually means that the doctor has not been in practice for two years, the minimum time required for taking the second part of the board-certification exam. If the doctor has been in practice for longer than two years and is still board-eligible, you can surmise that he or she has failed the exam on one or more occasions or has lacked the ability, ambition, or confidence to study for it.

Obstetricians who are board-certified in the subspeciality of high-risk pregnancy are usually based in large medical centers and are available for patients with problems that are beyond the skills of many local obstetricians. While you may believe that having a high-risk subspecialist as your obstetrician will ensure a successful pregnancy, these doctors do not have the time or the desire to provide routine obstetrical care, and you are more likely to be delivered by one of his or her underlings or residents.

Another indication of a doctor's skill is his or her hospital affiliation. You should be skeptical if the hospital in which the doctor works is not accredited by the Joint Commission on Accreditation of Hospitals. If a hospital has an approved residency program and is affiliated with a medical school, it is more likely to attract highly competent physicians. In fact, many university-affiliated hospitals will not allow family practice physicians to do obstetrics.

The *Directory of Medical Specialists*, published by Marquis Who's Who (200 East Ohio Street, Chicago, Illinois, 60611), is an excellent book, updated every two years, that lists the training, qualifications, and hospital affiliations of all doctors certified by specialty boards in the United States. I have found it to be most helpful when referring patients of mine to new obstetricians in distant cities. The *American Medical Directory*, usually available at large public libraries, is another good source of this information.

One simple and effective way to find a competent obstetrician is to speak to a resident in obstetrics and gynecology at a local hospital. Residents are notoriously critical of their attending physicians, and an enthusiastic endorsement of a particular doctor is a reliable guarantee of competence. If the resident is reluctant to recommend one particular doctor, ask for a list of two or three favorites from which you can make your own choice. Finding out which doctors are most frequently the personal physicians of nurses who work in the obstetrical unit can also be valuable. If you cannot get this information from a resident or an obstetrical nurse, try telephoning a childbirth education group, a local childbirth education instructor, or a branch of La Leche League. All can provide you with lists of highly regarded obstetricians.

Unfortunately, the choice of a competent obstetrician is no assurance that your personal relationship will be harmonious. For this reason, you would be wise to arrange an initial interview with the doctor, preferably with your husband or partner present. At this meeting you should ask the questions about childbirth which most concern you, about nutrition, childbirth preparation classes, "gentle birth," family-centered care, indications for cesarean section, or any other subject (see Chapter 12). Beware of the doctor who appears to be adamant and unyielding over minor points, such as avoiding the enema or the "full perineal prep" (shaving of the pubic hair) on admission to the delivery room. In the event that you require anesthesia, it is nice to know which types are preferred and why. If the doctor appears annoyed by your questions or avoids them with a "leave everything to me" attitude, consider whether you wish to make a commitment to that physician. I would also be suspicious of the doctor who calls you by your first name, unless, of course, you are allowed the same privilege.

Observing the activity in a doctor's waiting room is often a good indication of efficiency. The busiest doctor in town is not necessarily the best. An obstetrician who habitually keeps women waiting for an hour or more is one who has the least concern for patients, is undoubtedly inefficient and disorganized, and is best avoided.

The initial physical examination should be thorough. An examination limited to the breasts and pelvis is inadequate. The doctor must examine your heart, lungs, and abdomen early in pregnancy in order to detect any possible abnormalities. The pelvic examination should be gentle and considerate; there is no excuse for a doctor not using a warmed speculum, and if you have never given birth before, a small speculum should be used. The examination is incomplete without a vaginal, rectal, and recto-vaginal examination (index finger in the vagina, middle finger in the rectum), performed with a well-lubricated glove to minimize discomfort.

Following the examination, you should expect a full discussion of the doctor's findings and all aspects of prenatal care. This should be carried out in the consultation room after you are dressed and feel more comfortable. Having a written list of questions is a good idea for the first visit, as well as for all subsequent visits.

The majority of obstetricians in the United States are in group practices of varying sizes, ranging from as few as two doctors to as many as ten. You should not hesitate to ask what the evening and weekend on-call schedule is; in some groups the senior physician no longer works at these times. It is essential that all members of the group have the same attitudes about childbirth so that promises and assurances given you by one obstetrician are not rejected by another. If you are being cared for by an obstetrical group, it is a good idea to arrange visits on a rotation basis among the doctors so that you familiarize yourself with all of them. You may find one member of a group to be not to your liking. If so, request that another group member be called should you go into labor when the doctor you don't care for is on call. If such an arrangement is not possible, consider finding another doctor or group of doctors. Remember, it is never too late to switch if you are unhappy.

The obstetrician in solo practice is an endangered species. Obviously, continuity of care and a more intimate patient-doctor relationship are of great advantage to a pregnant woman. There are disadvantages to having only one doctor, however, especially if the obstetrical practice is a busy one. The hours these doctors work are often grueling and require sleepless nights. Most women would prefer an alert physician to one struggling to stay awake throughout a complicated labor and delivery.

Efficiency experts have noted that solo practice tends to be far more disorganized than group practice, and canceled office hours and other pertinent inconveniences are more likely to occur. When a solo practitioner takes a vacation or even a weekend off, he or she may refer you to a doctor with whom you are totally unfamiliar. If you choose an obstetrician who is in solo practice, be sure to ask about vacation times, as well as the name of the doctor who will care for you during such absences.

If your family belongs to a health maintenance organization (HMO), expect to be limited in your choice of an obstetrician and hospital, and in the maternity care you receive. The main disadvantage of HMOs is that you are obligated to use only an HMO obstetrician and pediatrician and must give birth at an HMO-designated hospital. One complaint about HMO physicians is that they lack incentive since most are salaried by the HMO. Some of the larger HMOs have hundreds of physicians, and you may see a different doctor during each prenatal visit; it is not unusual for a total stranger to deliver your baby. Preferred providers organizations (PPOs) are groups of independent doctors who individually contract with employers to offer health services at a prearranged fee for each service provided, rather than the fixed monthly or annual rate of the HMO; usually the fee for each service is significantly lower than the doctor would charge other patients. The list of PPO doctors under contract with your employer is likely to be quite limited because many established physicians prefer not to join PPOs. PPO doctor lists are usually a potpourri of young doctors just starting out in practice and older physicians who are willing to live by the dictates of the PPO.

Dealing with HMOs and PPOs can be difficult and frustrating. To maximize the quality and continuity of care you receive in an HMO, try to schedule as many prenatal visits as you can with a physician you prefer. Unfortunately, this bit of personalized care will not extend to your labor and delivery if your doctor is not on call. Participating PPO physicians are listed by specialty in a pamphlet which is updated periodically. Show this list to your family physician or a nurse at your hospital so that they can help you select the most qualified physician.

Discuss the obstetrical fee with each doctor you interview. A good office staff can usually give you an accurate estimate of total hospital costs and tell you which of the laboratory and obstetrical fees will be covered by your particular insurance company. Determine the cost and the number of routine prenatal laboratory tests (see Chapter 11) ordered by one obstetrician as compared to another. Procedures such as ultrasound and nonstress testing, if performed routinely and on more than

one occasion, will raise your obstetrical fee considerably. If you require amniocentesis, be prepared to pay an additional $1,000. Many doctors charge an additional fee if your pregnancy is high-risk, requiring more office visits, greater prenatal surveillance and testing, hospitalization prior to delivery, or cesarean section. Ask about such extras beforehand. Finally, find out how your doctor wishes to be paid. Some doctors require a percentage, usually a third to a half of the total fee, before your due date. Others require full payment by the last month of pregnancy.

What is the approximate cost of having a baby?

The approximate obstetrical, hospital, anesthesia, and pediatric fees listed in Table 2 are based on information gathered from several doctors and hospitals in Connecticut. However, the cost of medical services varies significantly from one area of the United States to another, and even from town to town. Whether or not the range of fees given in the table reflects those you will encounter, the list of activities and procedures constitutes a checklist for your use.

The fees listed in Table 2 do not include additional expenses that can be incurred during a high-risk pregnancy. The highest estimates quoted can be doubled, tripled, or even quadrupled when a pregnancy requires frequent ultrasounds, weekly or biweekly nonstress tests, blood tests, biophysical profiles (see Chapter 11), consultation with medical specialists, hospitalization for control of complications during pregnancy, and intensive care of a sick baby.

The cost of private obstetrical care in the United States makes it virtually impossible for the majority of couples to start a family if they do not have adequate health insurance coverage. Couples must thoroughly familiarize themselves with the benefits and limits of the policies available in order to secure the best possible coverage beforehand. Maternity insurance benefits vary greatly from one company to another. Some policies cover special

TABLE 2

APPROXIMATE COST OF CHILDBIRTH IN CONNECTICUT—1992

	Low	*High*
I. *Obstetrical Fees*		
• Routine delivery (includes prenatal) visits, uncomplicated delivery, and postpartum visit)	$2,000	$3,500
• High-risk pregnancy additional fee (diabetes, hypertension, multiple births, preeclampsia)	0	$1,500
• Additional fee for cesarean section	0	$1,000
• Routine prenatal tests—includes urine, CBC (complete blood count), blood type and Rh and antibody screen, serology (syphilis) test, rubella titre, blood sugar screen, hepatitis B screen	$ 75	$ 120
• Other prenatal tests		
1. Toxoplasmosis titre	$ 35	$ 45
2. AFP blood test	$ 50	$ 75
3. Tay-Sachs, sickle cell, thalassemia screen	$ 35	$ 70
4. Ultrasound (routine)	$ 100	$ 200
5. Amniocentesis with ultrasound guidance	$ 300	$ 500
6. Laboratory fee for chromosomal analysis of amniotic fluid cells and amniotic fluid AFP	$ 500	$ 600
7. Nonstress test	$ 75	$ 125
II. *Hospital Costs*		
• Uncomplicated labor, delivery, and postpartum care with hospital discharge on 3rd morning after delivery	$1,400	$2,200
• C-section with 5 or 6 days in hospital	$5,500	$6,200
• Fee for baby's 3-day stay in well-baby nursery	$1,300	$1,500
III. *Anesthesia Costs (billed directly by the anesthesiologist)*		
• Epidural anesthesia during labor	$ 400	$ 600
• Anesthesia for cesarean section	$ 800	$1,200
IV. *Pediatrician Fees (billed directly by the pediatrician)*		
• Routine baby exams in nursery	$ 75	$ 150
• Circumcision (sometimes performed by obstetrician)	$ 75	$ 150
• Attendance at C-section for routine newborn care	$ 75	$ 150
• Attendance at emergency C-section	$ 100	$ 200
• Routine monthly visits to pediatrician excluding vaccinations	$ 75	$ 120

tests, additional hospital stay, and neonatal intensive care if your baby is sick, while others will pay only a percentage of routine obstetrical costs and none of the pediatric fees. If you belong to a health insurance plan at work, your employer is obligated to pay pregnancy expenses on the same basis as that paid for all other medical expenses. Most couples are shocked when they realize that their health insurance policy does not pay for many of the routine tests performed on their child in the hospital

or in their pediatrician's office. An even more devastating discovery is to learn that your insurance plan does not include major medical insurance in case of a catastrophic, long-term pediatric illness or an injury that requires extensive treatment and months of hospitalization. Although such a major problem is unlikely to occur, if it does major medical coverage can at least relieve you of a severe financial burden.

 ## PREPREGNANCY COUNSELING

What can my obstetrician do to minimize existing medical problems before I conceive?

No obstetrician can guarantee the delivery of a perfect baby, and unfortunately as many as 2 percent of all babies are born with a birth defect. However, evaluation of a couple before pregnancy can help greatly in preventing or minimizing certain fetal and maternal risks. The importance of preconception counseling is based in the fact that organ development begins as early as 17 days following fertilization and is most sensitive to the harmful influences of medications, toxins, and environmental pollutants over the next 40 days. For many women, this important period of time often precedes their first prenatal visit.

During your initial counseling session your doctor should inquire about any illnesses that you or your spouse may have and the medications, including over-the-counter products, that you take. Some medications prescribed routinely for hypertension, lupus, heart disease, arthritis, epilepsy, psychiatric disorders, and acne are potentially harmful to the fetus (see Chapter 9). In many cases the dose can be lowered significantly or discontinued completely, or a safer medication substituted. Since adjustment to a lower dose or a new medication can take weeks or months, your doctor

should advise you on this subject prior to pregnancy.

As medical and obstetrical care has become more sophisticated, growing numbers of chronically and seriously ill women are attempting pregnancy and succeeding at having babies. It is your obstetrician's duty to accurately inform you if pregnancy will adversely affect your disease and how your disease will affect your pregnancy. For example, a woman with asymptomatic heart disease may experience heart failure as a result of the greater circulatory demands on her heart during pregnancy. Similarly, women with hypertension or chronic kidney disease are more likely to give birth to a smaller than normal baby and require frequent monitoring during pregnancy (see Chapter 11). Women with blood pressures on the high side of normal (130/80 to 140/90), those with a strong family history of hypertension, and women who have experienced an elevated blood pressure on the Pill may experience a greater than normal increase in blood pressure and preeclampsia (elevated blood pressure and protein in the urine) toward the end of pregnancy. In contrast, symptoms of rheumatoid arthritis may actually improve during pregnancy.

Women with a strong family history of diabetes and those who have experienced an unexplained stillbirth or the birth of a baby with congenital anomalies should have a glucose tolerance test prior to pregnancy. Even if a woman is found to be only mildly diabetic prior to pregnancy, it is imperative that strict dietary control and insulin be used to reduce her blood sugar level to that of a nondiabetic woman (see Chapter 9). The insulin requirements of diabetic women increase substantially as pregnancy progresses; they return to former levels immediately after delivery. It has been demonstrated that diabetics with good insulin control of their blood sugars have an incidence of miscarriage equal to nondiabetics, but those with poor control experience a higher miscarriage rate. When doctors at the University of California, San Francisco, rigidly controlled the blood sugars of 84 diabetic women prior to conception, only one infant was born with a major congenital anomaly. In contrast, major anomalies occurred at the alarming rate of 12 out of 110 infants born of diabetic mothers who initially received intensive blood sugar control only *after* they had conceived. The dramatic findings of this 1991 report should serve as a stimulus for all diabetic women to seek intensive management and control of their blood sugars prior to contemplating conception.

In addition to maternal diseases, what other areas should be covered during preconception counseling?

A woman's risk of giving birth to a baby with Down syndrome and other chromosomal abnormalities increases progressively with each year after the age of 30. Although the maternal age of 35 has been arbitrarily accepted as an indication for amniocentesis or chorionic villus sampling (CVS; see page 359) in order to diagnose a chromosomal abnormality, all women over 30 should be given information regarding their specific risk (see Table on 32). In my private practice, more and more women are requesting chromosomal analysis. Though paternal age may play a small role in this problem, CVS or amniocentesis need be consid-

ered only when a father is over 50, regardless of the mother's age. A woman who has previously given birth to a baby with a chromosomal defect or has a close family member with such a condition should also undergo chromosomal studies. Most geneticists believe that couples who have experienced two or more consecutive spontaneous abortions should have their blood tested to determine their chromosome pattern, or karyotype, before attempting another pregnancy. If a chromosomal aberration is found, a geneticist can usually predict the likelihood of future pregnancy success or failure and the need for fetal chromosomal studies. A history of previous pregnancies complicated by stillbirth or the birth of a child with anomalies should be explained in detail by a geneticist and plans outlined for diagnosing potential problems in future pregnancies. Inheritance patterns of familial diseases such as hemophilia, muscular dystrophy, and other congenital disorders are often beyond the scope of your obstetrician. Consultation with a geneticist is necessary to determine your exact risk of giving birth to a baby with a similar problem as well as the methods used during pregnancy to determine if your fetus is affected. Confusion surrounding the diagnosis of a familial disease can often be resolved by obtaining medical records from a pediatrician or the record room of the hospital where the birth took place.

Securing previous medical records is also of great value in determining whether or not your mother took DES during her pregnancy with you (see page 13). Often your doctor can determine this at the time of your pelvic exam simply by observing characteristic changes of the cervix and vagina. If you are a so-called DES baby, you should arrange to see your doctor soon after your pregnancy is confirmed and frequently thereafter in order to be certain that the pregnancy is not ectopic and is not complicated by a weakened or incompetent cervix.

All black couples, even those without a family history of a previous problem, should be tested for the gene causing sickle cell anemia. Similarly, Jewish couples require screening for Tay-Sachs disease, while Italian, Greek, and Indian couples should be tested to see if they carry the gene for a blood disease named beta-thalassemia. Asian couples should be screened for a similar disorder called alpha-thalassemia. In all these diseases, both healthy parents must carry the defective trait in order for the disease to appear in the fetus. The odds of two carriers transmitting the disease during each pregnancy are 25 percent. It is especially important that Tay-Sachs testing take place at the time of the preconception examination, prior to pregnancy, since the usual screening test is inaccurate during pregnancy.

An accurate history of drinking and smoking habits is necessary, and the dangers of these two activities both before and during pregnancy need to be emphasized. Likewise, your preconception session will be incomplete if your obstetrician does not review your dietary habits and emphasize the importance of sound nutrition both before you conceive as well as throughout your pregnancy. Several studies from Europe and the United States have concluded that using vitamin supplements rich in folic acid for at least one month prior to conception may decrease a woman's risk of giving birth to a baby with a neural tube defect such as anencephaly or spina bifida (see Chapters 1 and 8). Prescribing such a vitamin during a preconcep-

tion visit makes good sense.

While many women continue to work at the same job throughout most of their pregnancy, some jobs are just too physically and emotionally stressful. Your obstetrician should inquire about work-related problems and determine if it is medically necessary to ask your employer for a change of work assignment during pregnancy. Often a physician's letter can be quite helpful in this regard. If you plan to travel outside the United States either for business or pleasure during pregnancy, ask your obstetrician to find out the specific vaccinations required for the countries you intend to visit (see Chapter 7). Make sure all your immunization records are up to date prior to conception, since some vaccines can't be given during pregnancy and others cause distressing side effects. If you are uncertain whether you have immunity to German measles or rubella, your antibody titre should be tested and rubella vaccine given if you are not immune; you should not conceive for three months after receiving the vaccine. If you are a cat owner, your doctor should determine your toxoplasmosis titre (see Chapter 10). Finally, your doctor should encourage you to have a complete dental checkup before you become pregnant. This will avoid the use of dental x-rays, pain medication, and antibiotics during pregnancy.

 PREGNANCY TESTS

What does a pregnancy test measure?

Although there are a variety of pregnancy tests, they all measure the presence of a pregnancy hormone called human chorionic gonadotropin (hCG). Produced by cells that form the placenta, hCG is detectable in the serum or urine of a pregnant women 8 to 11 days after ovulation, reaching peak levels between the sixtieth and ninetieth day of pregnancy. In the past, levels of hCG were measured in International Units per milliliter. How-

ever, as detection methods have become more sophisticated, concentrations of hCG are now reported in milli International Units (mIU), or amounts equal to 1/1,000th of an IU, per milliliter (ml). At ten days following fertilization, or four days before the expected period, the average hCG concentration is approximately 50 mIU/ml, rising to 200 mIU/ml three to four days later. During a normal pregnancy, hCG will rise at a predictable rate, doubling in amount every 1 to 2 days during the first 30 days after conception. Following peak values that can soar as high as 75,000 to 200,000 mIU/ml between the sixtieth and ninetieth day, concentrations decline to about 5,000 mIU/ml and remain at this level throughout pregnancy.

Though urine and blood tests can both detect the presence of hCG, the newer blood tests are capable of measuring the exact concentration or quantitative amount of a small part of the hCG hormone called the beta-subunit (B-subunit). This incredibly sensitive test can detect as little as 2 to 10 mIU of hCG per milliliter of serum. Even though quantitative hCG B-subunit determinations are more expensive than urine pregnancy tests, doctors gain far more information from them. By reporting B-subunit determinations at 24- to 48-hour intervals, it is possible to follow the progress of an early pregnancy which is in jeopardy. If a woman's hCG values are lower than normal or do not double at 48-hour intervals, impending abortion or ectopic pregnancy should be strongly suspected.

How accurate are the various home pregnancy tests?

Self-administered home urine pregnancy tests, such as e.p.t.-Plus and First Response, may be purchased without prescription at most retail phar-macies for a modest price. These tests vary in sensitivity from 50 to 300 mIU/ml of hCG and may easily be performed within 20 to 60 minutes by anyone who is able to read and follow simple instructions. A home pregnancy test taken one week after a missed period should approach 100 percent accuracy if performed correctly. However, human error in performing the test can be a big "if." In a 1989 letter to the editor of the *New England Journal of Medicine*, researchers from Washington, D.C., reported that they compared the accuracy of the e.p.t.-Plus and ADVANCE home pregnancy tests when performed by experienced technicians versus lay people. While the technicians did both tests with 100 percent accuracy, nontechnical people experienced discrepancies in 9.5 percent of the e.p.t.-Plus tests and 12.5 percent of the ADVANCE tests.

A positive home pregnancy test enables women to seek early obstetrical care, practice sound nutrition, and avoid potentially harmful medications and toxic substances such as alcohol and tobacco. An early decision regarding termination of an unplanned and unwanted pregnancy can also be made. A positive home pregnancy test is a virtual certainty that you are pregnant and, in the absence of complications such as bleeding or pain, rarely requires confirmation by a doctor's in-office test.

 BOY OR GIRL?

Are there any simple methods to predetermine the sex of a child?

The sex of a baby is determined by its father at conception, although women throughout history have been blamed for not giving birth to a child of the desired gender. The adult male has two different sex chromosomes in his body cells, one labeled X and the other Y. Each sperm carries only one of the these chromosomes—an X or a Y. The adult woman possesses two X sex chromosomes in each of her body cells, but no Y chromosomes; therefore her egg always contributes an X to the future offspring. If a sperm carrying a Y chromosome fertilizes the X egg, the result will be an XY male. However, if a sperm cell carrying an X gets there first, the result is an XX female (see Figure 1).

In 1987, scientists at the Whitehead Institute for Biomedical Research in Cambridge, Massachusetts, discovered that it is not the entire Y chromosome but a tiny gene located on the Y chromosome which most determines whether or not an embryo

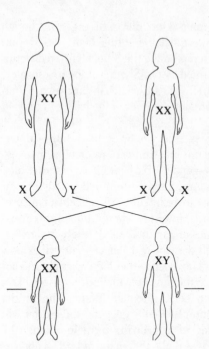

Figure 1

How sex is determined

will grow into a male or a female. This gene, named the testes determining factor (TDF), makes up only 0.2 percent of the Y chromosome but is more important than the other 99.8 percent in determining if testicular development is to occur. The discovery of TDF was aided by the scientific observation that approximately 1 out of every 20,000 men have an XX chromosome pattern, while a similar number of women have an XY. These cases, in which the affected individuals are normal though sterile, are explained by the fact that the tiny TDF gene migrates from the Y to the X chromosome when the father's sperm cells are formed. As a result, the XX male has the TDF gene on his inherited X while the XY female has no TDF on her inherited Y.

Sex preselection received some attention in the 1960s, when Dr. Landrum B. Shettles claimed that he was able to distinguish two types of sperm under a phase contrast microscope: a small, fast-swimming, round-headed, fragile sperm carrying the male-producing Y chromosome and a larger, stronger, slower-swimming, oval-shaped type carrying the female-producing X chromosome. Based on these differences, Dr. Shettle concluded that couples wanting to conceive a boy could improve their chances by timing intercourse as close to the moment of ovulation as possible, douching with baking soda and water immediately before intercourse, using a rear-entry coital position, and encouraging female orgasm. It was his theory that these measures would allow a greater number of weaker, male-producing sperm to be deposited at the cervix. In contrast, to conceive a girl, Dr. Shettles attempted to create a less favorable vaginal environment in which the stronger, female-producing sperm would be more likely to survive. To achieve this, he recommended that intercourse cease two to three days prior to ovulation, that it be preceded by an acid douche of vinegar and water, use of the face-to-face or "missionary position," avoidance of female orgasm, and shallow penetration by the male at the time of his orgasm. Though the public was quick to test this theory, no one has been able to reproduce the 80 percent predictability rates claimed by Dr. Shettles. One investigator, using this method, artificially inseminated 85 patients and predicted the sex of the babies in only 40 instances.

There does seem to be some validity to Dr. Shettles's claim that timing of intercourse may determine the gender of a baby. For reasons which remain obscure, intercourse timed exactly at ovulation seems to result in a 54 percent chance of having a girl. However, when artificial insemination with donor sperm is used, the odds are reversed to 60 percent in favor of males. It is now generally acknowledged that the closer natural coitus occurs to the time of ovulation, the more likely one is to conceive a female infant. The further from ovulation that coitus occurs, the greater will be the odds of conceiving a male infant (the normal ratio of males to females at birth is approximately 106 to 100). Although there are no guarantees, if you time intercourse exactly at ovulation and abstain for at least three days before and after, you may tilt your odds slightly in favor of conceiving a female.

Are there any accurate scientific methods to preselect sex?

Scientists have been trying for years to identify and separate X- and Y-bearing spermatozoa based on differences in their size, weight, speed of movement, and fluorescence patterns under ultraviolet light. Some have claimed success with centrifugation, or spinning of semen specimens at high speeds, allowing the lighter, Y-bearing sperm to stay suspended while the heavier, X-bearing sperm settle to the bottom of the test tube. Others have used electrical separation techniques based on the fact that male-producing sperm normally carry a slight negative charge on their surface while female-producing sperm carry a positive charge. Some scientists have devised special filters and col-

umns of concentrated albumin to achieve sperm cell separation. Of the techniques under development, those utilizing immunologic and DNA probe methods seem most promising. In one laboratory study, when antiserum against Y antigen was placed in the vaginas of female rabbits, there was a shift in the sex ratio of births in favor of females. Special DNA probes specific for either Y or X chromosomes may be used in the future to process spermatozoa and separate out X or Y chromosomes for insemination.

If the quest to isolate X- and-Y-bearing sperm was solely for the purpose of satisfying parental preference for one sex over the other, it would hardly be worthwhile. A far more important goal is to prevent susceptible couples from conceiving a child with a so-called X-linked, or sex-linked, disease. Such diseases are carried on one of a woman's two X chromosomes and appear in the offspring only when the affected chromosome is fertilized by a man's Y chromosome. Usually, only male fetuses inheriting the disease-carrying X will be afflicted with the disease. Those males inheriting the nonaffected X chromosome will be normal. The odds, therefore, of a carrier mother transmitting the disease to her male offspring is 50 percent, but for a female offspring it is zero. Each daughter has a 50 percent chance of being a carrier and transmitting the disease to half of her sons. No male-to-male transmission of X-linked diseases can occur. That is, a father can't pass the disorder on to his son.

Duchenne muscular dystrophy, hemophilia, and 200 other little-known but deadly diseases, with names such as Hunter, Lesch-Nyhan, Menke, and Fabry, are sex-linked diseases. Though progress is being made in diagnosing some of these conditions during pregnancy, at the present time geneticists are often quite limited in their ability to determine with certainty if a male fetus is affected. When it is possible to diagnose one of these diseases during pregnancy, a midtrimester abortion can be offered. More often than not, the diagnosis can't be made, and couples are usually faced with the terrible decision of a mid-trimester abortion of all male fetuses, while allowing females to survive. Sadly this necessitates aborting healthy males 50 percent of the time, but it also prevents the despair of caring for an infant affected with one of these terrible diseases. If a method is ever developed which will allow 100 percent accuracy in separating X- and-Y-bearing sperm, it would be a boon to all couples fearing an X-linked disorder. Women could then be inseminated with pure X-bearing sperm. Unfortunately for couples at risk of X-linked disorders, the methods of sex preselection currently showing the greatest potential are those which isolate Y- rather than X-bearing sperm.

The most popular method of separating X- and Y-bearing sperm was first introduced by Ronald Ericsson, Ph.D., in 1973 and continues to remain popular today. With this method, sperm swim down a viscous solution of human serum albumin and are isolated based on their progressive motility or movement. Since the Y-bearing sperm swim faster than the X-bearing sperm, a sample is obtained with a high concentration of Y-bearing sperm, which are artificially inseminated at ovulation. Ericsson and his licensed followers throughout the world claim a success rate of 75 to 80 percent male offspring, although no large independent studies have confirmed or refuted these claims. While the Ericsson method of sex preselection may help in achieving a greater number of male offspring, the outlook for isolating X-bearing sperm appears bleak. Most authorities would agree that at the present time a totally reliable and accessible sex preselection method will not be available for several years.

How can a baby's sex be discovered during pregnancy without performing amniocentesis?

During the second trimester, a sample of amniotic fluid (the fluid in which the embryo is immersed) may be obtained by placing a needle into the uterine cavity through the lower abdominal wall. This procedure, called amniocentesis, is simple and relatively painless. When the cells of the amniotic fluid are studied in the laboratory, the sex of the fetus may be predicted with an accuracy approaching 100 percent. The disadvantage of amniocentesis is that it can't be offered until at least the fourteenth week of pregnancy, and waiting for the results may take an additional seven to ten days. If an X-linked disease is found and abortion is recommended, it is both medically and emotionally a more difficult procedure at that stage of the pregnancy. Fetal sex can be determined with equal accuracy by using chorionic villus sampling (CVS) as early as the ninth week of pregnancy. CVS is usually accomplished by passing an instrument through the cervix under vaginal ultrasound guidance and obtaining a minute amount of tissue from the chorion (muscular membrane of the early placenta) of the early pregnancy. In 1988, researchers at the Genetics and IVF Institute of Fairfax, Virginia, reported that they were capable of performing CVS as early as the sixth week of pregnancy. This technique, however, is limited to a handful of centers at the present time. (For full discussions of amniocentesis and CVS, see Chapter 11.)

Since both amniocentesis and CVS are associated with a slight risk of fetal loss, the goal of many scientists has been to discover an atraumatic, nonsurgical method of determining fetal sex as early in pregnancy as possible. In one interesting study, Dr. Kurt Loewit and his Austrian colleagues were able to predict the fetal sex with 92 percent accuracy based on a measurement of the urinary excretion of the hormone testosterone. Male fetuses were noted to produce a significantly higher level of this hormone in their mother's urine than did female fetuses.

Researchers in Switzerland have successfully predicted fetal sex by use of a blood test. By isolating those fetal cells that pass into the maternal bloodstream and staining them, the Swiss scientists were correct in predicting fetal sex 86 percent of the time, but they were able to accurately evaluate

after the fourteenth week of preg-
...gators at Stanford University have
discovered fetal cells in the maternal circulation as
early as the twelfth week of pregnancy. (They have
calculated that there may be between 2 million
and 20 million fetal cells of various types which
pass from the fetus to the mother.) It is the aim of
these scientists to develop a blood test which obstetricians could offer to all their patients early in
pregnancy in order to detect both the fetal sex and
a wide range of chromosomal and chemical abnormalities. Successful studies have been carried
out in the People's Republic of China by sampling
cells that are shed into the endocervical canal from
the placenta. The cells are obtained in the same
manner as with a Pap smear, and the accuracy of
sex prediction to date has been 94 percent. Similar
encouraging reports on the use of endocervical
cells for prediction of fetal sex have come from
studies conducted at the University of Alabama
School of Medicine; however, researchers at
Southern Illinois University School of Medicine
were not able to duplicate these results.

As ultrasound technology has improved, it has
become possible to determine fetal gender at earlier stages of gestation. However, it is unlikely that
ultrasound will take the place of amniocentesis in
the diagnosis of X-linked diseases. The fetus develops well-formed genitals at 13 to 14 weeks of
pregnancy, but the gender usually can't be determined with relative certainty until 18 to 20 weeks.
Even then, the position of the fetal back and legs
or the presence of loops of umbilical cord between
the legs makes it impossible to visualize the genitals 20 to 40 percent of the time. These results fall
far short of the accuracy obtained with CVS or
amniocentesis.

A game traditionally played by obstetricians and
midwives is to predict fetal gender based on the
fetal heart rate. The normal rate ranges between
120 and 160 beats per minute, and folklore tells us
that a rate greater than 140 is predictive of a girl,
while one under 140 means that a boy will be
born. In 1986, Dr. Maurice L. Druzin and his
associates at the The New York Hospital—Cornell
Medical Center tested this hypothesis by recording
fetal heart rates at different stages of pregnancy.
Dr. Druzin found that the average fetal heart rate
at 19 to 24 weeks was 143 beats per minute, declining to 132 beats per minute at 36 to 40 weeks.
In addition, there was no discernible difference
between the fetal heart rate of male and female
fetuses at any stage of pregnancy. So much for old
wives' tales!

PREGNANCY AND WOMEN OVER 30

What are my risks of miscarriage if I am over 30?

Statistically, the likelihood of first-trimester bleeding and spontaneous abortion increases progressively with each year over 30.

The overall risk of spontaneous abortion (miscarriage) among women younger than 30 is often
quoted at 10 percent. This escalates to 18 to 20
percent between the ages of 35 and 39. Though
estimates vary, the miscarriage rate for a women
over 40 is at least three times higher than that for
a woman under 30, with some researchers placing
the incidence as high as 40 to 45 percent. Chromosomal abnormalities have been detected in 50
to 60 percent of embryos and early fetuses that are
aborted spontaneously, and the likelihood of this
happening increases in linear fashion with each
year after 20 (see Table 28 on page 403). It is
interesting to note that the spontaneous abortion of
a chromosomally normal fetus is also related to a
woman's age, with a sharp increase in incidence at
the age of 37. Table 3 shows the relationship between maternal age and the risk of spontaneous
abortion, based on a 1986 review of that subject.

TABLE 3

RISK OF SPONTANEOUS ABORTION, BY AGE

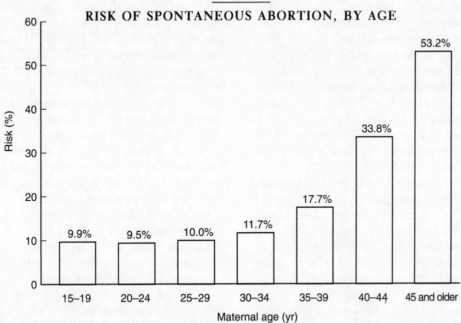

An older woman is also at greater risk of carrying a chromosomally abnormal infant to term (see page 402). At the age of 30 this risk is approximately 1.1 per 1,000 births, increasing significantly to 5.6 per 1,000 at 35, 15.8 per 1,000 at 40, and 53.7 per 1,000 births at 45 years of age. It is comforting for women between the ages of 30 and 39 to know that once a chromosomal abnormality is ruled out they are at no higher risk than other women of giving birth to an abnormal infant. However, the same cannot be said for women over 40. In one study, geneticists found an alarming 200 to 300 percent higher risk of other birth defects such as hydrocephaly, congenital heart disease, and cleft lip and palate among women in this age group.

Aside from a higher miscarriage rate, what are some of the medical and obstetrical problems that a pregnant woman over 30 may encounter?

There have been literally hundreds of articles published in the past five years analyzing potential medical and obstetrical risks associated with childbirth after the age of 30. Though experience confirms that older women are more likely than younger women to encounter a variety of pregnancy complications, the conclusions reached by some researchers are far more optimistic than others. In general, however, all would agree that a healthy women in her 30s or 40s whose pregnancy is managed by modern obstetrical technology can expect an excellent outcome.

An association between stillbirth, neonatal death, and advanced maternal age has been consistently reported in the medical literature. In a 1988 article published in *Obstetrics and Gynecology*, Dr. Andrew Friede and his associates analyzed the relationship between maternal age and infant mortality in the United States. Their conclusions were based on more than 1½ million births, using data from the National Infant Mortality Surveillance. Dr. Friede found that mothers 25 to 29 years of age experienced an incidence of infant mortality nearly identical to that of women

30 to 34 years of age. However, among women 35 to 39 and those 40 to 49 years of age, the infant mortality rates climbed by an astonishing 18 percent and 69 percent, respectively. Most of these deaths were due to low infant birth weights. Among older women, diabetes and hypertension are the two diseases most responsible for pregnancy complications such as fetal distress, prematurity, abnormally high and low infant birth weights, stillbirth, and infant mortality. The incidence of both diabetes and hypertension increases in linear fashion among women in their 30s and 40s.

Maintaining a diabetic woman's blood sugars in the normal range with meticulous dietary control and liberal use of insulin both before and during pregnancy is believed to play a key role in reducing a diabetic woman's risk of spontaneous abortion, fetal anomalies, fetal distress, and stillbirth. Even if a woman's blood sugars are normal prior to pregnancy, if she is over 30, she will be much more likely to develop gestational or pregnancy-related diabetes. This relatively benign condition is easily managed by a diet supplemented with insulin when necessary (see Chapter 9).

Hypertensive women are at two times greater risk for delivering small, growth-retarded babies than are women with normal blood pressure because of a decrease in uterine blood flow, which compromises the oxygen supply to the placenta. Chronic hypertension has been found to occur in as many as one-third of pregnancies in women over 40 and to be linked to two-thirds of all perinatal deaths reported. In one study of more than 36,000 women, the rates of preeclampsia (a disease of unknown cause characterized by an elevation of blood pressure during the last three months of pregnancy) were nearly doubled in women older than 40 when compared to those under 40 years of age. For women having first babies, the risk of preeclampsia was found to increase from 6 percent at 25 to 29 years of age to 10 percent at 35 to 39 and 14 percent at the age of 40 and above.

For reasons which remain obscure, many doctors have observed that the babies of women over 30 are more likely to assume an abnormal position, such as a breech, late in pregnancy and during labor. Poor uterine contractions and delay in dilatation of the cervix and descent of the baby in the birth canal during labor doubles in frequency when a woman is having her first baby after the age of 35. (Women over 30 who have previously given birth do not experience these problems.) Other complications reported in association with childbirth over 30 include abruptio placenta (premature separation of the placenta), placenta previa (low-lying placenta), postpartum hemorrhage, fetal distress, low Apgar scores of the newborn (see page 366), and higher cesarean section rates.

Leiomyomas, also known as fibroids and myomas, are benign tumors of the uterus which are commonly found in women over the age of 30. These tumors tend to grow much larger during pregnancy and then regress in size following delivery. Even if a woman has several large fibroids, they rarely cause abortion. It is the location of these tumors, rather than their size, which determines the risk of early pregnancy complications. Fibroids which lie just under the endometrium, or lining of the uterine cavity, are most likely to create problems. Fortunately, these tumors, known as submucous myomas, account for less than 5 out of every 100 fibroids.

Not all obstetricians are as pessimistic as some of the reports cited above would indicate. In fact, modern obstetric care has made problems such as diabetes, hypertension, and preeclampsia easily manageable (see Chapter 9). One of the most optimistic reports on this subject was written by Dr. William N. Spellacy and his colleagues at the University of Illinois and published in *Obstetrics and Gynecology* in 1986. Dr. Spellacy analyzed 511 pregnancies in women 40 or more years of age at the time of delivery and compared the results with those of an equal number of women 20 to 30 years of age. Although he noted all of the age-related complications found by other researchers, he attributed a good share of these problems to the weight of the mother at the time of delivery. According to Dr. Spellacy, those older women weighing less than 67.5 kilograms (150 pounds) at delivery showed no difference in their incidence of hypertension, babies with abnormal birth weights, low Apgar scores, or fetal deaths when compared to women under 30 years of age. Although these women experienced a higher incidence of diabetes during pregnancy and were more likely to undergo a cesarean section than the younger women, the good news was that the outcome for their infants was the same as that for women under 30. In 1991, researchers at Mt. Sinai Hospital in New York studied the first births of almost 4,000 women and confirmed the findings of previous reports citing higher cesarean section rates in women over 30. Other more frequent complications experienced by older primigravidas included fetal distress, gestational diabetes, pregnancy-induced hypertension, third-trimester bleeding, abruptio placenta, placenta previa, and a second stage of labor lasting longer than two hours. On the positive side, the Mt. Sinai researchers were unable to detect a greater likelihood of preterm labor, low Apgar scores, or perinatal deaths when compared to women in their 20s.

Another reason for optimism is the fact that several epidemiological studies have confirmed that infants born to older women are much less likely to experience sudden infant death syndrome (SIDS), or "crib death." The reasons for this phenomenon remain obscure despite the fact that many theories have been offered.

What effect does paternal age have on pregnancy outcome?

While advanced maternal age is known to be an important contributing cause of Down syndrome and other chromosomal abnormalities, paternal age is believed to play a far less significant role. In a 1981 study reported in *Human Genetics*, researchers concluded that a paternal age greater than 41 significantly increased a couple's risk of Down syndrome. The authors of this report advised amniocentesis solely on the basis of a paternal age over 41, regardless of the age of the mother. Some geneticists now believe that the critical paternal age is 50, others claim it is 55, while some state that paternal age plays no significant role. In one chromosomal study, researchers showed that in 30 percent of Down syndrome cases the extra chromosome was of paternal origin. One mathematical formula used by some to estimate the risk of an elderly man fathering a baby with Down syndrome is to apply the maternal age risk to his age and multiply by one-third. For example, if a 45-year-old woman's risk of giving birth to a baby with Down syndrome is 1 in 30 (see Table 28), the risk for a man of the same age would be 1 in 90.

Recent studies conducted in the United States and France both reached the conclusion that paternal age has little effect on the chromosomal composition of the fetus. However, it is believed that the genes within the sperm cells of fathers in their 40s and 50s may undergo spontaneous random mutations or changes which increase the risk of nonchromosomal abnormalities. These changes are believed to occur in no more than 1 percent of the general population. Since there are literally millions of genes that can undergo spontaneous mutation, a wide variety of defects is possible rather than one specific abnormality. Expert ultrasound monitoring in search of limb, heart, and kidney abnormalities is the best method for evaluating the fetus of an older father.

TEENAGE PREGNANCY

How do teenagers fare in pregnancy?

Several statistical studies have demonstrated that pregnancy outcome is poorest at both ends of the childbearing-age spectrum, namely women over 35 and those under 19. Experts disagree as to whether or not teenage pregnancy complications should be attributed mainly to so-called biological immaturity or to socioeconomic and environmental factors. There is no doubt that teenage mothers in the United States are more likely than older women to be poor, black, underweight, and subjected to poor housing, sanitation, and diets deficient in protein, iron, calcium, and vitamins, especially A and C. Pregnant teenagers are less likely to seek or receive adequate prenatal care, and they are more apt to use and abuse tobacco, alcohol, and a variety of illicit drugs. They are also at greater risk of contracting one or more sexually transmitted diseases.

While many factors contribute to the birth of premature and growth-retarded infants to teenage mothers, none are more important than poor nutrition and inadequate prenatal care. The two most important determinants of a baby's birth weight are its mother's prepregnancy weight and the maternal weight gain during pregnancy. Several studies have demonstrated that if a teenager is provided with closely supervised dietary and vitamin supplementation throughout her pregnancy, she will gain an adequate amount of weight and increase her chances of giving birth to a baby of normal weight. According to one 1987 study, teenagers receiving adequate nutrition gave birth to babies weighing an average of 157 grams more than babies born to teens whose nutritional status was poor. While good nutrition is helpful, it can't completely solve the problem of low birth weights among teenage mothers. The other determinant, namely a woman's prepregnancy weight, especially in girls under 16, is on the average much lower than that of women over 20 years of age. In 1988, doctors from the University of Chicago examined the birth records of more than 180,000 women to determine the influence of maternal age on the incidence of low infant birth weights. Their interesting findings, published in the *American Journal of Obstetrics and Gynecology*, showed that mothers under 17 years of age had a significantly greater risk than older women of delivering a baby of low birth weight. However, when the data were reevaluated after eliminating maternal factors such as race, education, number of previous children, marital status, and adequacy of prenatal care, the surprising result was that teenagers actually had a slightly lower incidence of low-birth-weight babies. Unfortunately, in the real world these basic socioeconomic factors can't be eliminated.

At least three separate reports published in the last eight years have concluded that both major and minor congenital malformations occur with greater frequency in children born to younger teenaged mothers. The association of Down syndrome with advanced maternal age has been well established. Recent data suggest that pregnant teens under the age of 16 may have a risk comparable to that of women over 35.

Since babies of low birth weight, defined as less than 5½ pounds or 2500 grams, have a higher neonatal mortality or death rate, it is not surprising that this unfortunate statistic is higher among teenaged mothers. Death rates for babies weighing more than 2500 grams are also higher when the mother is a teenager, as are infant deaths attributed to accidents, violence, and infections.

LENGTH OF PREGNANCY

How can I accurately calculate my due date?

The chances are only 8 out of 100 that you will give birth on the exact date calculated for you by your obstetrician. The standard method of calculating the expected date of confinement (EDC), or due date, may be roughly determined by a formula called Naegele's rule: count back three months from the first day of your last period, and then add seven days. For example, if your last period began on June 10, subtracting three months give you March, and adding seven days to the tenth gives you March 17 as your due date. This system works relatively well for women who have the classic textbook menstrual cycle of 28 days and who ovulate on day 14. However, women with longer cycles tend to ovulate later, while those with shorter cycles ovulate earlier. The most constant aspect of the menstrual cycle is the fact that ovulation will occur approximately 14 days prior to the next period. Therefore, if your periods come every 38 days, you will most probably ovulate on day 24. Obviously, under such circumstances, Naegele's rule will be inaccurate unless you account for this delay by adding additional days. If you have periods every 38 days, and your last period started on June 10, you have to add ten extra days over the standard 28. Therefore, your EDC would be March 27, or March 17 plus ten days.

Confusion in determining how far along you are in your pregnancy results from the fact that obstetricians traditionally determine your pregnancy length and your uterine size from the first day of your last menstrual period, rather than from the actual onset of pregnancy, which begins with fertilization just after ovulation. Therefore, if your obstetrician says that your uterus is ten-weeks' size, he or she really means that you are 8 weeks from the day of conception. Pregnancy is said to last 40 weeks (280 days) from the last period, provided the start of your period is every 28 days. Actually, the length of pregnancy is closer to 266 days, or 38

weeks. Another source of confusion occurs because an obstetrician thinks of a pregnancy as lasting ten lunar months, each having 28 days, while a patient views it over the usual nine-calendar-month span.

Dr. G. L. Park, an English physician, accurately noted the EDC of 2,100 pregnant women under his care and published his conclusions in 1969. Based on his findings, the long-accepted Naegele's rule may not be totally valid. The important point here is that 68 percent of the women studied went into labor after the fortieth week of pregnancy, with the peak period of births occurring between the end of the forty-first week and the beginning of the forty-second week. If the majority of normal births take place after the fortieth week, it would seem foolish for a doctor to induce labor at the forty-first week from the last menstrual period simply because of the fear that the baby may be postmature (see questions on induced labor and prolonged pregnancy, page 427). It is Dr. Park's practice to consider the forty-first, forty-second, and forty-third weeks of pregnancy as a period of nonintervention unless there is a good medical reason. His very low perinatal mortality figures of 4 per 1,000 attest to the wisdom of this policy. The logical suggestion following this study is that obstetricians should alter Naegele's rule and add 14 days instead of 7 to the first day of the last menstrual period. Support for Dr. Park's conclusions can be found in a 1990 article by Dr. Robert Mittendorf and his colleagues at the Harvard School of Public Health and Tufts University School of Medicine in Boston. They calculated the length of uncomplicated pregnancies in both primigravidas and multiparas and found that the mean duration of pregnancy from the time of presumed ovulation was 274 and 269 days, respectively. Based on these findings, Dr. Mittendorf proposed that Naegle's rule be amended to add 15 days for primigravidas and 10 days for multiparas. Most American obstetricians do not share Dr. Park's and Dr. Mittendorf's optimism about pregnancies that have progressed beyond the forty-second week. Evaluation of fetal well-being in the form of electronic monitoring and sonography are often initiated at or before this time (see Chapter 11).

 FOLLOWING THE PROGRESS OF THE PREGNANCY

How can I follow the growth of the fetus?

The observant woman who has practiced previous self-examination can detect a pronounced softening of the cervix as early as a month after conception. This is one of the earliest signs of pregnancy. If you have a speculum, you may be able to observe a characteristic violet color of the cervix and vagina during the first few weeks of pregnancy. This is due to the increased blood supply, or vascularity, in these areas; when noted in the vagina it is called Chadwick's sign.

You can check your uterine growth as pregnancy progresses by following some very easy rules. Urinate to empty your bladder and then lie on your back on a flat, hard surface. You should be able to touch the top of the uterus starting at the twelfth week from the last menstrual period. At that time, the uterus is palpable just above the symphysis (pu-bic) bone. A second important landmark is your navel, or umbilicus. When the top of the uterus reaches the umbilicus, you should be approximately halfway or 20 weeks from your last period, with another 20 weeks to go until delivery. If the uterus is one finger's breadth below the navel, you are approximately 18 weeks pregnant, while one finger's breadth above the navel means a pregnancy of about 22 weeks. In a pregnancy of 16 weeks the distance is halfway between the pubic bone and the umbilicus. The approximate uterine size with each month of pregnancy is shown in Figure 2.

For greatest accuracy and enjoyment, have your husband or partner keep a record of these measurements throughout pregnancy. If you believe your uterine size is two weeks or more at variance with your dates, tell your doctor. A uterus that is growing at a faster than normal rate may indicate the presence of twins or a very large baby, while a

Figure 2

Height of uterus at various weeks of pregnancy

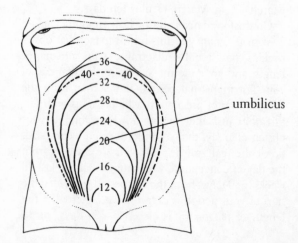

umbilicus

uterus smaller than expected on the dates may mean that there are problems of fetal growth.

For greater accuracy in measuring your uterine height, you can use a tape measure having a centimeter marker. Between the fourteenth and twenty-seventh week of pregnancy you will find that the uterine height above the symphysis, as measured in centimeters, will be approximately equal to the number of weeks that you are pregnant based on the last menstrual period. A good point to remember during the last trimester is that uterine growth will usually progress at an average rate of 3 centimeters per month, with an ultimate height of 28 to 36 centimeters. Don't panic during the last three or four weeks if the uterine height suddenly decreases by a few centimeters; probably your baby's head has dropped into the pelvis.

Can I detect fetal movement and heartbeat in monitoring the progress of my pregnancy?

The detection of fetal movement is an excellent guide for determining how far along in your pregnancy you are. Most women first become aware of a slight fluttering about the eighteenth to twentieth week after the last period. This first fetal movement has been termed "quickening." Among women who have carried previous pregnancies, "quickening" may be noted at the sixteenth or seventeenth week. Fetal movement will increase in intensity as pregnancy progresses, though the number of movements per day varies from one fetus to another. During the last trimester, it is very important to immediately report any sudden increase or decrease of fetal activity from the usual pattern.

If you have a stethoscope or are able to borrow one, you and your husband or partner can detect the fetal heartbeat at about the twentieth week of pregnancy. The rate varies between 120 and 160 beats per minute and should not be confused with the pulsations from your abdominal aorta, which usually are of a frequency of less than 100 beats per minute. The aorta rate is synchronous with the pulse in your wrist. The fetal heartbeat varies from minute to minute throughout pregnancy, with wide variations between 120 and 160 being the usual and healthy pattern. A fetal heart rate below 120 or above 160 may represent a potential problem, and this too should be brought to the attention of your obstetrician.

One final helpful sign for following the progress of your pregnancy is the presence of frequent urination. This is caused by the enlarging uterus, which produces pressure on the urinary bladder, and often begins four to six weeks after the last period. More significantly, it disappears after the twelfth week, when the uterus rises up into the abdomen from its position in the pelvis. Frequency reappears when the baby's head descends into the pelvis days or weeks before the onset of labor.

Is there any way to determine the height and weight of the fetus during each month of pregnancy?

Yes. Thanks to a man named Hasse, the approximate length of the fetus in centimeters can be determined during the first five months by squaring the number of lunar months from the last period; after the fifth lunar month of pregnancy, the fetal length will be equal to the lunar month multiplied by five (see Table 4). It's a fantastic bit of information, and it really works. Table 4 also lists corresponding average weights at the end of each lunar month during pregnancy.

Questions beginning on pages 326 and 370 introduce discussion of the ability of ultrasound techniques to monitor the details of early fetal development.

TABLE 4

AVERAGE FETAL LENGTH AND CORRESPONDING WEIGHT
AT END OF EACH LUNAR MONTH OF PREGNANCY

| End of Lunar Month | Length in Centimeters | WEIGHT | |
		Grams	Pounds and Ounces
2	$2 \times 2 = 4$	1.1	less than 1 oz
3	$3 \times 3 = 9$	14.2	less than 1 oz
4	$4 \times 4 = 16$	100.0	3 oz
5	$5 \times 5 = 25$	300.0	10 oz
6	$6 \times 5 = 30$	600.0	1 lb 5 oz
7	$7 \times 5 = 35$	1,001.0	2 lbs 4 oz
8	$8 \times 5 = 40$	1,675.0	3 lbs 11 oz
9	$9 \times 5 = 45$	2,340.0	5 lbs 2 oz
10	$10 \times 5 = 50$	3,250.0	7 lbs 3 oz

 MORNING SICKNESS

What causes nausea and vomiting during the first three months and what effect does it have on the outcome of pregnancy?

Though its cause is not definitely known, one theory suggests that the nausea and vomiting of pregnancy ("morning sickness") result from the elevated levels of human chorionic gonadotropin (hCG) in the blood. It has also been theorized that it is the ratio between hCG and estrogen and progesterone, rather than the total amount of hCG, which determines whether or not a woman will develop morning sickness. A third hypothesis was introduced by Dr. Goran Samsioe and his colleagues from Gothenburg, Sweden, in 1986. They used ultrasound to locate the corpus luteum, or ovulation site, in 26 women who experienced nausea early in pregnancy and 17 women who did not. The corpus luteum was situated in the right ovary in 17 (65 percent) of the 26 women complaining of nausea. This contrasted with the finding that the corpus luteum was situated in the left ovary in 15

(88 percent) of the 17 women without nausea. Since the right ovarian vein carries hormones from the ovary to the liver in a more direct manner than the left ovarian vein, Dr. Samsioe theorized that ovulation and corpus luteum formation from the right ovary produce hormonal overload to the liver and subsequent morning sickness during pregnancy.

First described by the Egyptians in 2000 B.C., morning sickness affects approximately half of all pregnant women. The most susceptible individuals are primigravidas (women giving birth for the first time), especially if under 20 years of age, women pregnant with twins, those weighing more than 170 pounds, and nonsmokers. Studies have shown that women who do not experience nausea during pregnancy are far more likely to have a pregnancy in jeopardy of miscarriage. Similarly, the sudden disappearance of nausea during the first three months of pregnancy may represent an impending miscarriage.

If you experience nausea and vomiting, symptoms will usually appear at the end of the first month and subside by the end of the twelfth week, or third lunar month, following your last period. However, there are notable exceptions. A 1985 study of over 8,000 women by doctors at the National Institute of Health found that 29 percent of the women interviewed experienced symptoms as late as weeks 13 through 16, as did 20 percent between weeks 17 and 20, and 9 percent after the twentieth week. A second 1986 NIH report was even more discouraging: 25 percent of the women studied had symptoms at the twentieth pregnancy week.

Though morning sickness is often a sign of a healthy pregnancy, it is nonetheless a distressing, unpleasant, and frustrating problem. Though the condition is often more likely to occur in the morning, for many women it may more accurately be described as "all-day sickness."

How can I safely combat morning sickness?

A woman who is suffering from morning sickness during her fifth week of pregnancy finds little consolation in the fact that her symptoms will eventually subside spontaneously. Most drugs that are capable of controlling nausea and vomiting have not been proven safe for the developing fetus, and recent adverse publicity associated with the use of Bendectin (see page 273) has influenced both obstetricians and their patients to seek more conservative remedies.

Certain simple measures may greatly reduce the severity of morning sickness. For example, those beverages and soups which are either very hot or very cold are least likely to elicit nausea. Bouillon, apple juice, grape juice, vegetable juices, ginger ale, and cola beverages are usually the most easily tolerated. Fruit sorbates, ice cream, yogurt, and milk shakes can also be tried. Liquids, including soups, are best handled when taken between meals. For this reason it is best to eat meals without soup or drink and then drink the liquid about 1 hour later. If you find solids easier to keep down than liquids, try to get your liquids in solid form from foods that have high water content, such as fruits and vegetables, particularly lettuce and other greens, melons, and berries. Six or seven light snacks during the day are less likely to cause nausea than two or three large meals. Even if you aren't hungry, it is best that you try to eat, since nausea may become more bothersome when your stomach is empty. Complex carbohydrate foods such as bread, crackers, dry cereal, whole wheat breadsticks, dried fruit, rice cakes, unbuttered popcorn, and baked potatoes are usually tolerated well. Eating dry crackers every 2 hours during the day is an excellent way to combat nausea. Some women wisely carry dry crackers with them during the day and eat one whenever they begin to feel sick. Another good idea is to keep crackers, dry toast, and other nonperishable carbohydrates such as dry cereal, breadsticks, raisins, apricots, and figs next to your bed as a snack immediately upon awakening in the morning. Many women report that protein in the form of hard-boiled eggs and cheese are easy to digest and cause very little nausea, if any. Protein in the form of red meat is usually poorly tolerated; chicken and fish are preferred.

If you discover that certain stimuli, such as particular foods and smells, make you sick, try to avoid them whenever possible. Also stay away from greasy, fried, and highly seasoned foods until the nausea is no longer bothersome. Pepper, chili, and garlic all contribute to nausea. Aromas of coffee, fried fish, or cauliflower occasionally precipitate an attack, so these items are best avoided. To eliminate most kitchen odors, you should cook with the exhaust fan on and the kitchens windows open.

Most prenatal vitamins contain iron supplements, which may irritate the stomach and intestinal lining. In the presence of severe morning sickness it is best to temporarily avoid all iron-containing preparations.

If the above measures fail to bring relief, medications which are both helpful and safe for the developing fetus are available. Emetrol is a pleasant-tasting, mint-flavored liquid which may be purchased without prescription at any pharmacy. It contains balanced amounts of the sugars levulose (fructose) and dextrose (glucose), combined with orthophosphoric acid. An extremely effective and absolutely safe course of action is to take one or two tablespoons of Emetrol at 15-minute intervals until nausea is relieved. Antacids, such as Maalox, Camalox, and Mylanta, may also prove helpful in neutralizing stomach acidity. Vitamin B_6, or pyridoxine, taken orally in a dose of 50 to 100 milligrams twice daily, has been enthusiastically endorsed by some gynecologists as a safe and effective antinauseant. If vomiting prevents ingestion of oral pyridoxine, it can be given as in intramuscular injection. The antihistamine doxylamine is sold without prescription under the trade name Unisom Nighttime Sleep Aid. While formerly a component of Bendectin, doxylamine is not known to cause fetal risks. The 25-milligram dose, taken before bedtime, has been used with some success in the treatment of morning sickness. Other over-the-counter antihistamines considered safe for treatment of nausea and vomiting during pregnancy include meclizine hydrochloride (Antivert, Bonine), hydroxyzine hydrochloride (Atarax, Durax, Orgatrax), buclizine hydrochloride (Bucladin-S, Vibazine), and diphenhydramine (Benadryl, Bendylate). Drowsiness and dry mouth are the only reported side effects of these medications, and there are no known harmful effects to the fetus.

Acupuncture and acupressure (the application of pressure to acupuncture sites) have been proposed as effective methods of treating morning sickness. In a 1988 study from Ireland, doctors instructed a group of morning sickness sufferers to press the P6 acupuncture point on the forearm just below the wrist at hourly intervals each day. Within four days, women complying with these instructions noted significantly fewer symptoms than those given either no instructions or incorrect pressure points.

A very small percentage of women vomit to the point of severe dehydration and weight loss. This condition, known as hyperemesis gravidarum, requires the use of stronger medications such as phenothiazines (see Chapter 9). On rare occasions, hospitalization and intravenous feedings are necessary to control symptoms and restore mineral and chemical balance.

 ## MISCARRIAGE, OR SPONTANEOUS ABORTION

What are the symptoms of impending miscarriage?

The term "miscarriage" describes what doctors call a spontaneous abortion, a natural termination of pregnancy before the fetus is sufficiently developed to survive.

Doctors use the term "threatened abortion" to describe any bloody vaginal discharge or vaginal bleeding which occurs during the first half of pregnancy. This is a fairly common diagnosis, since at least one out of four women experience some bleeding early in pregnancy. Among women who experience bleeding, approximately half actually abort. Doctors prefer to see bleeding of a dark-brown rather than a bright-red color, because the former usually indicates "old blood" from bleeding that has occurred several days before. A threatened abortion may be accompanied by mild cramps or low back pain resembling that of the menstrual period. It has been demonstrated that when bleeding persists for longer than a week, the prognosis for successful pregnancy greatly diminishes.

A threatened abortion becomes an inevitable abortion when uterine contractions become intense, the cervix dilates, bleeding becomes heavy with the passage of clots, or the membranes of the pregnancy sac rupture. The fetus and placenta are usually passed soon thereafter. In early pregnancies of eight weeks duration or less, the fetus and placenta are often expelled together. This occurrence is termed a complete spontaneous abortion. When the placenta, in whole or in part, is retained in the uterus, the event is termed an incomplete abortion. Under such circumstances it is necessary for your doctor to remove the placental fragments retained in the uterus.

In most instances of spontaneous abortion, the fetal demise occurs days and sometimes weeks before the symptoms of heavy bleeding and cramping take place. After the fetus has died but before any symptoms of impending abortion occur, a woman attuned to her bodily reactions will often notice that her breasts are no longer tender, her nausea has subsided, and that she "just doesn't feel pregnant." In the past, the diagnosis of missed abortion, defined in the medical textbooks as a fetal death in utero without actual passage of the fetus for at least eight weeks, was not uncommon. The advent of ultrasound and sensitive blood tests measuring hCG levels has made the classic diagnosis of a missed abortion a highly unlikely event. Doctors are now able to quickly diagnose an early fetal demise and terminate the pregnancy almost immediately after the diagnosis is confirmed.

There is now convincing proof that at least 75 percent of all first-trimester spontaneous abortions occur prior to the eighth week of pregnancy, and a healthy ultrasound examination at eight weeks can be viewed as an optimistic sign for the woman who fears a miscarriage.

Why does first-trimester miscarriage occur?

Although the exact mechanism responsible for a miscarriage or spontaneous abortion is not always apparent, the most common cause appears to be an abnormality in the development of the fertilized egg which makes it incompatible with life. In studying the microscopic chromosomal structure of these so-called abortuses, researches have noted gross chromosomal abnormalities 50 to 60 percent of the time. As previously mentioned, a woman's risk of spontaneous abortion caused by chromosomal defects increases with each year after the age of 30. Even when a woman over 35 is carrying a chromosomally normal fetus, she is still more likely than a younger woman to miscarry. Most chromosomally abnormal fetuses are aborted at or before eight weeks of pregnancy, while chromosomally normal fetuses are more apt to abort at the twelfth or thirteenth pregnancy week. Though estimates vary, the total miscarriage rate for a woman over 40 is at least three times higher than the 10 to 15 percent rate quoted for women under 30 (see Table 3). Less is known about the relationship between paternal age and spontaneous abortion (see page 50), but researchers concur that it plays a far less important role than maternal age. One significant finding is that in 2 to 6 percent of all instances in which a couple experiences two or more consecutive spontaneous abortions, the fault lies with an abnormal chromosome pattern in one of the two normal-appearing parents. The chromosome patterns of such parents should be studied.

Anatomical abnormalities of the uterus existing at birth—two separate uteri connected by a bridge of tissue, for example, or the presence of a wall, or septum, within the uterus—may also be responsible for early miscarriage. The estimated incidence of a uterine anomaly is only 1 or 2 per 1,000 women, but such an abnormality may be responsible for as many as 25 percent of all spontaneous abortions. In most cases, a relatively easy surgical procedure can correct the problem. Occasionally an underdeveloped, or hypoplastic, uterus will be unable to hold a developing pregnancy. This condition is sometimes seen among daughters of women who took DES during pregnancy. Similarly, DES daughters are more likely than other women to have an abnormal T-shaped uterus, which may be responsible for spontaneous abortion during either the first or second trimester (see page 16). When a D and C (dilatation and curettage) is performed in the presence of infection during the postpartum period or after an abortion, scar tissue may form within the uterine lining or endometrium. This may prevent normal implantation and growth of a subsequent pregnancy. Lysis, or breaking the adhesions and preventing their reformation, often results in a successful pregnancy.

Myomas, or fibroids, are commonly found benign tumors of the uterine muscle wall which tend to increase in number and size after the age of 35. Only 5 percent of all fibroids are submucous, meaning that they lie just beneath the endometrium. In this location fibroids can, on rare occasions, distort the shape of the endometrial cavity and cause miscarriage by hindering implantation and normal growth of an early pregnancy. Surgical removal of such fibroids should be considered only after all other possible causes of recurrent spontaneous abortion have been excluded.

Early spontaneous abortion is known to occur when the corpus luteum of the ovary does not produce amounts of progesterone adequate to support an early pregnancy. This condition, termed a luteal phase defect, can be diagnosed prior to pregnancy by determining a woman's serum progesterone level and studying the microscopic appearance of her endometrium on a biopsy taken during the second half of the menstrual cycle. The importance of a luteal phase defect as a cause of recurrent spontaneous abortion is debatable—some doctors claim it is relatively uncommon, while others believe it is responsible for 35 to 40 percent of all spontaneous abortions. In a 1988 report, published in the *American Journal of Obstetrics and Gynecology*, Canadian physicians found that by administering progesterone to women with a history of recurrent spontaneous abortion early in pregnancy they were able to double their successful full-term pregnancy rates. Women who engage in frequent and vigorous exercise following a relatively sedentary existence are more likely to experience a luteal phase defect. For such women, reducing the amount of exercise usually returns the luteal phase to normal.

Endocrine imbalances, such as thyroid dysfunction and poorly controlled diabetes, as well as a wide variety of systemic diseases such as lupus, chronic kidney disease, and congenital heart disease, may also be responsible for recurrent spontaneous abortion (see Chapter 9). Chronic maternal infections have been suspected to cause spontaneous abortion as well. The bacterial organisms cited most often are Brucella, *Mycoplasma hominis*, *Listeria monocytogenes*, and *Ureaplasma urealyticum* (see Chapter 6). The protozoan *Toxoplasma gondii*, the causative organism of toxoplasmosis, has also been implicated (see Chapter 10). Fortunately, all of these diseases respond to appropriate antibiotic treatment.

Although it is often difficult to prove, recreational drugs such as tobacco, alcohol, and cocaine are believed to be toxic to the fetus and are likely to increase a woman's risk of spontaneous abortion. Environmental toxins such as anesthetic gases, lead, formaldehyde, and benzene may also play a role in causing spontaneous abortion (see Chapter 10).

In recent years, scientists have come to learn that immunologic factors may be responsible for causing spontaneous abortion among a small number of susceptible women. So-called antisperm antibodies formed by a woman may cross-react with the dividing embryo and destroy it. A woman may also form antibodies, called autoantibodies, against her own tissues which support the pregnancy at the placental site. This in turn may cause death of the tissues and spontaneous abortion. Finally, a woman may abort repeatedly because her tissues are actually too compatible with those of her fetus. Because she shares the same major antigens or proteins as her fetus, her immune system is not challenged or stimulated to produce the so-called blocking antibodies needed in all normal pregnancies to prevent the body from rejecting the fetus. In the absence of blocking antibodies, the fetus is not protected and abortion ensues.

Despite the many possible etiologies of spontaneous abortion which I have discussed, in at least 30 percent of all cases the cause remains unknown.

Can emotional or physical trauma cause spontaneous abortion during the first three months of pregnancy?

No. Contrary to popular opinion, there is no evidence that emotional or physical trauma is responsible for early spontaneous abortion. In seeking to explain an early miscarriage, parents might associate a particular accident with an abortion that follows soon after. However, in the medical literature there are many examples of severe trauma which failed to interrupt existing pregnancies. Furthermore, most spontaneous abortions occur sometime after the death of the fetus has taken place. If abortion were caused by trauma, it would not be a very recent event but one that had occurred some weeks earlier. Since the height of the uterus is below the pubic symphysis bone until the twelfth week of pregnancy, it would be nearly impossible for physical trauma to the lower abdomen to cause injury to the fetus before this time.

How likely am I to miscarry if I bleed during the first three months of pregnancy?

As many as 22 percent of all women carrying healthy pregnancies may have one or two incidents of light bloody discharge early in pregnancy. Caused by the fertilized egg implanting itself in the lining of the uterus, this is called implantation bleeding. However, you should report any bleeding to your doctor. Often the bleeding is due to an erosion or inflammation of the cervix and is totally unrelated to the developing pregnancy; such bleeding is more apt to occur with penile contact during intercourse and is never a cause of miscarriage. By viewing the bleeding site on your cervix with a speculum your doctor is often able to reassure you that it is innocuous. However, when bleeding comes from within the uterus and not the cervix, it represents a more serious condition, termed a

threatened miscarriage or abortion. It should be noted that an examination at the time of bleeding will not precipitate a miscarriage.

For unknown reasons, bleeding during the first three months of pregnancy seems to be three times more frequent among women with one or more children (multiparous women) than among women having their first baby (primigravidas). Older women and women with a history of a previous miscarriage are also more likely to bleed during the first trimester. There is a widespread belief that pregnancy bleeding may normally occur each month at the time of the expected period. Contrary to this popular misconception, vaginal bleeding at any time during pregnancy should be regarded as abnormal and investigated by your obstetrician.

It is comforting to know that if your bleeding is minimal in amount and soon subsides, your chances of giving birth to a healthy baby are excellent. Several studies, however, have demonstrated that the likelihood of miscarriage increases whenever there is more than one episode of bleeding, when the bleeding persists for longer than seven consecutive days, and when it is moderate to heavy rather than scanty or light.

If I experience bleeding early in pregnancy which then subsides, are my chances of a successful birth equal to those of a woman who has never bled?

Probably not. Studies have demonstrated that women who bleed for several days early in pregnancy are more likely to experience poor fetal and infant outcome even if the course of the pregnancy does not appear to be disturbed at the time of the bleeding. Bleeding problems during the first half of pregnancy have been linked to a host of problems, but the one consistent finding in all studies is a higher incidence of premature labor and the birth of smaller babies. Other complications, such as birth defects, higher stillbirth rates, and the birth of babies with learning disabilities and epilepsy, have been noted in some reports but not confirmed in many others. In 1984, doctors at Harvard Medical School studied the outcome of pregnancy among 523 women who bled prior to the twentieth week of pregnancy. When compared to a control group who did not bleed, women who bled had a significantly higher incidence of premature birth and babies of low birth weight. These babies, however, were not growth-retarded and did not have a higher stillbirth or congenital anomaly rate. The Harvard doctors correctly concluded that a patient who has had vaginal bleeding of any amount in early pregnancy should be followed closely, that preparations should be made for premature delivery, and that measures should be taken to arrest premature labor as needed.

In general, bleeding which persists for seven or more days significantly worsens the prognosis, as does moderate to heavy bleeding rather than light staining. These observations were confirmed in a 1987 article by doctors at New York Medical College. In their study of almost 900 women experiencing threatened abortion, those who bled longer than one week, had several episodes of bleeding, and described their bleeding as moderate to heavy were at a two times greater risk of losing their pregnancies than women who experienced one episode of light bleeding which lasted less than seven days.

Is there anything a woman can do to decrease her risk of a threatened abortion?

There is no convincing evidence that anything you do will change the course of an early threatened abortion. Therefore, it is pointless for an obstetrician to prescribe bedrest. Orgasm may be responsible for uterine contractions and should be avoided for at least two weeks after the bleeding stops. Remember, it is orgasm, not the penile trauma caused by intercourse, that may produce miscarriage in a very small percentage of susceptible women. Orgasm achieved through clitoral stimulation may be equally harmful. As a matter of fact, studies suggest that orgasm achieved through masturbation may produce more intense contractions than those produced through intercourse.

It is unfortunate that so many women attribute the occurrence of a spontaneous abortion to a specific event, strenuous work, or too much physical exercise immediately preceding the pregnancy loss. It is both foolish and inaccurate to experience guilt or to berate oneself, since the loss of the fetus usually precedes the actual symptoms of threatened or spontaneous abortion by days or weeks. Furthermore, early miscarriages usually have specific causes (see page 51), none of which are associated with one's level of stressful physical activity. If an early spontaneous abortion is destined to occur, it will happen whether or not you choose complete bedrest or heavy physical exertion, so you might as well get out of bed and pursue your usual activities.

How should a doctor monitor a woman who is experiencing symptoms of impending abortion?

An examination at the time you are bleeding will not worsen the situation but will help your obstetrician determine if the bleeding is from the uterine cavity or a less serious site, such as an erosion on the surface of your cervix. If bleeding is noted from within the uterus, the diagnosis of a threatened abortion is confirmed. Under these circumstances, sensitive measurements of serum hCG combined with ultrasound should easily determine the condition of your early pregnancy within a week or less following an episode of vaginal bleeding. Doctors who sit back and assume a wait-and-see attitude in the face of first-trimester bleeding are not serving the best interests of their patients. In fact, they are placing their patients at risk by overlooking potentially serious pregnancy complications, such as an ectopic pregnancy (see questions below).

Changes in the levels of the pregnancy hormone human chorionic gonadotropin, or hCG, over a period of two to four days combined with vaginal ultrasound examination should enable your obstetrician to distinguish between a threatened abortion and an ectopic pregnancy. This information is more than academic in view of the fact that ectopic pregnancies account for 5 percent of all maternal deaths. The diagnosis of an ectopic pregnancy requires immediate abdominal surgical intervention and removal of the pregnancy before it reaches a size where it can rupture and cause life-threatening internal hemorrhage, permanent fallopian tube damage, and infertility. While the immediate diagnosis of an impending abortion is not as urgent, it saves women days of anguish and reduces the risk of anemia caused by prolonged bleeding. In addition, extremely low levels of hCG combined with minimal amounts of tissue in the uterus noted on ultrasound can help many women avoid a D and C (dilatation and curettage) for retained tissue fragments.

During a normal pregnancy, the quantitative or numerical concentration of human chorionic gonadotropin, or hCG, in a woman's serum reaches an average level of 200 milli International Units per milliliter (mIU/ml) at two weeks following conception. Today's sensitive pregnancy tests are practically always positive at this level of hCG, which usually corresponds to the first day of the missed period. Two weeks later, or four weeks after conception, hCG levels will climb to an average of 1,000 to 1,200 mIU/ml, followed by a rise to 6,000 mIU/ml two weeks after that. Peak values are

reached at 60 to 90 days of pregnancy. Thereafter the concentration of hCG declines and plateaus at a lower level, which is maintained throughout pregnancy. The normal values of hCG at different weeks of pregnancy serve as important guidelines for doctors since concentrations well below average are often an indication of an abnormal pregnancy. A single quantitative hCG determination is not nearly as useful in predicting fetal health and pregnancy outcome as are two or more tests taken at 48-hour intervals. Under normal circumstances, concentrations of serum hCG will double every two to three days during the first seven weeks of pregnancy. The rate of hCG doubling declines only slightly after this time until peak levels are reached at 60 to 90 days. A rise of less than 50 percent after 48 hours is often a bad omen, while a plateau or decline in the quantitative hCG value provides certainty that either impending abortion or ectopic pregnancy exists.

Ultrasound, or sonography, has revolutionized all aspects of obstetrical care, including the management of first-trimester bleeding (see Chapter 11). Scanning the pelvic anatomy can be accomplished either by applying an ultrasound transducer or probe to the abdomen or by placing a specially designed probe into the vagina (see Figure 3).

Although transvaginal ultrasound has been in

Figure 3

Vaginal Ultrasound

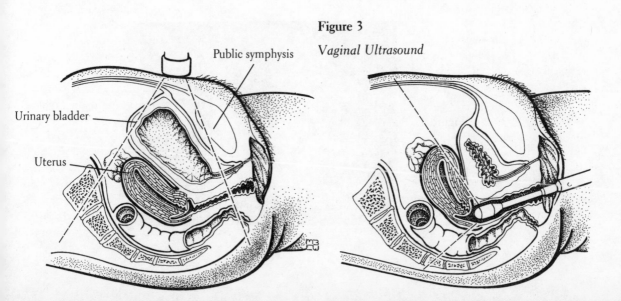

Public symphysis

Urinary bladder

Uterus

existence for a far shorter period of time than the transabdominal method, it is far superior in diagnosing pregnancy complications and visualizing placental and fetal anatomy during the first trimester, because its sound frequency is higher and the endovaginal transducer lies only millimeters away from the pelvic structures. As a result, sound waves have to travel a depth of only 1–2 centimeters, while transabdominal sound waves have to travel a far greater distance and must pass through abdominal fat, bowel gas, and adhesions resulting from previous pelvic surgery or infection. Practically all women report that transvaginal ultrasound is far more comfortable than the transabdominal method because, unlike the transabdominal method, it is not necessary to fill the urinary bladder to capacity to allow visualization of the pelvic anatomy. Though both ultrasound techniques are capable of visualizing normal and abnormal fetal growth patterns early in pregnancy, transvaginal ultrasound can accomplish this an average of seven to ten days earlier than abdominal ultrasound.

The earliest evidence of pregnancy observed on ultrasound is the gestational, or pregnancy, sac, which appears as a small white ring surrounding a fluid-filled center (see Figure 4). The endovaginal ultrasound transducer is capable of identifying the gestational sac at about 4½ to 5 weeks from a woman's last menstrual period, or 16 days following conception. The sac at this time has an average diameter of 3 to 5 millimeters. If a gestational sac can't be visualized with vaginal ultrasound at 6 weeks from the last menstrual period, a problem probably exists. Under normal circumstances a healthy gestational sac will grow at a minimum rate of 1 millimeter per day. Failure of a gestational sac to grow over a period of 3 to 5 days and an irregular configuration of the sac are highly suggestive signs that abortion is likely. These ultrasound findings combined with either a plateauing or decline of quantitative hCG levels is absolute proof that the pregnancy is lost.

Following visualization of the gestational sac, the next key ultrasound landmark is the formation of a yolk sac, an embryological membranous structure that is attached to the embryo until it disappears during the eleventh week of pregnancy. The yolk sac first appears on vaginal ultrasound as a small circle within the gestational sac 5½ weeks after the last menstrual period (see Figure 5). This is followed by a tiny fetal pole, or site, and heartbeat within the gestational sac at 6 to 6½ weeks following the last menstrual period, or 28 to 31 days after conception. These two key vaginal ultrasound landmarks are not seen with abdominal ultrasound until at least one week later. In some

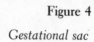

Figure 4

Gestational sac

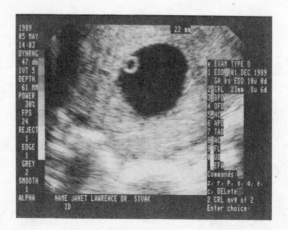

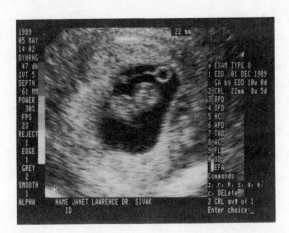

Figure 5

Early gestation with yolk

cases of threatened abortion, one can see an area around the developing fetus suggestive of a hematoma or blood clot. Despite this, if a fetal heartbeat is present, a doctor can responsibly tell a patient that her prognosis for a successful pregnancy remains excellent. In addition to observing the gestational sac, yolk sac, and fetal heartbeat, each successive week during the first trimester brings with it predictable developmental changes which occur with near-clockwork precision (see next question). Any deviation from this anticipated pattern should be regarded as abnormal.

The strong correlation between sonographic findings and quantitative hCG levels is extremely helpful in diagnosing both the condition and location of the pregnancy when a woman experiences first-trimester bleeding. As the gestational sac grows, the average values of hCG should rise proportionately; in situations where hCG levels lag behind gestational sac size or vice versa, the pregnancy is often in jeopardy. The relationship between hCG and ultrasound levels has its greatest application in the early diagnosis of ectopic pregnancy, a potentially dangerous situation in which the pregnancy is located outside the uterine cavity (see questions below). Competent obstetricians immediately suspect an ectopic pregnancy whenever transabdominal ultrasound shows no evidence of a gestational sac within the uterine cavity and quantitative hCG levels of 6,500 mIU/ml or greater. When an endovaginal transducer is used, the magic hCG cutoff number is only 2,000 mIU/ml, and some researchers believe it may be as low as 750 mIU/ml. Consequently, vaginal ultrasound offers a significantly better chance than abdominal ultrasound of detecting ectopic pregnancies before they rupture, and therefore of preventing major hemorrhage as well as preservation of the fallopian tube for future pregnancies when surgery is performed.

When quantitative hCG and ultrasound determinations conclude that an intrauterine pregnancy is lost, termination of the pregnancy by curettage is usually indicated. However, in situations where there appears to be minimal tissue in the uterus as well as very low hCG levels, a conservative approach can be taken and curettage avoided.

After detection of the fetal heartbeat, what are some of the details of early fetal development that can be observed with transvaginal ultrasound during the first trimester?

Except for a distinct heartbeat, early embryos remain essentially featureless for the first 7 weeks, counting from the first day of a woman's last menstrual period. At 7½ weeks, lower limb buds can be seen, though it is practically impossible to see the upper limb buds at this time. Four days later, however, both upper and lower limbs can be seen more clearly. Though a heartbeat is first noted well before this time, the body of the fetus does not move until sometime between the eighth and ninth week. The earliest movement consists of a generalized wiggling of the body. Movement of the arms and legs usually appears after the ninth week. The development of the brain and nervous system can be seen after the eighth week, and by the middle of the ninth week the partitioning between the ventricles in the brain progresses rapidly. At 9 weeks it is possible to see the spine from its uppermost end down to the sacrum, and defects and abnormalities can often be detected at this time. The umbilical cord widens and the intestine can be seen at this time. The measurement of the distance between the two parietal bones on the side of the skull, referred to as the biparietal diameter (BPD), is an important determinant of fetal age; prior to the introduction of vaginal ultrasound, doctors were unable to determine this measurement during the first trimester. We now know that precise determinations of the BPD can begin as early as the ninth week. By the eleventh week, all adult structures of the fetus are formed, and examination can be made of the base of the skull, the facial bones, the ears, the eyes, tissues within the brain, the collarbone, and all five fingers. The upper and lower jaw can first be seen by the end of the tenth week and is fully defined by the twelfth week. Much can be learned about the extremities at eleven weeks. Not only can the digits be counted, but the opposing position of the thumb to other digits can be seen. Based on this information it is possible to diagnose certain types of structural and functional abnormalities. By the end of the eleventh week and the beginning of the twelfth week, complete differentiation of the structures within the brain can be seen, as can the stomach, liver, urinary bladder, and bones of the arms and legs.

After the first trimester, endovaginal ultrasound becomes a less reliable tool because the uterus rises out the pelvis and the distance between the endo-vaginal transducer and the fetus becomes greater. At this point, transabdominal ultrasound becomes a far more reliable diagnostic technique.

Why does spontaneous abortion occur after the first trimester, and how can it be prevented?

An estimated 10 to 20 percent of all spontaneous abortions occur after the twelfth week of pregnancy. Spontaneous abortion occurring beyond the first trimester is more likely to be the result of an anatomic defect rather than a genetic or chromosomal abnormality. A weakening of the cervix, termed an incompetent cervix, has also been implicated in many of these pregnancy losses.

Although the cause of an incompetent cervix is often unknown, a small number of women are born with too little collagen connective tissue in their cervix; this lack results in a weakening and an inability of the cervix to support the weight of a growing pregnancy. However, this congenital cervical incompetence accounts for only 2 percent of all cases reported. More often the weakening of the cervix is secondary to other factors, such as forceful and traumatic dilatation of the cervix at the time of a previous elective abortion, a difficult midforceps delivery with injury to the cervix, in utero exposure to DES, and cauterization, laser, or conization of the cervix as treatment for an abnormal Pap smear. In one recent study from Sweden, doctors found a sevenfold increase in the incidence of late spontaneous abortion following cone biopsy.

Before a woman who has miscarried during the second trimester attempts pregnancy again, several diagnostic tests should be carried out to determine if her cervix is incompetent. One test involves passing either a cervical dilator or a urinary catheter filled with water to a diameter of 6 millimeters through the inner opening of the cervix. Easy passage helps to confirm the diagnosis. Ultrasound determination of the cervical length and shape, and x-rays of the uterus following injection of a contrast dye solution also aid in making the diagnosis.

Treatment of cervical incompetence consists of surgically tying a suture around the cervix. This procedure, known as a cerclage, is best performed at about the fourteenth week of pregnancy, a time when the threat of first-trimester spontaneous abortion has passed but before the weight of the uterus is great enough to prematurely dilate or efface the cervix. At the end of pregnancy, the cerclage suture can be cut and vaginal delivery anticipated. Another option is to leave the suture in place and perform cesarean section. One disadvantage of cutting the suture is that future pregnancies would require a repeat cerclage procedure.

If the diagnosis of cervical incompetence is in doubt, as it often is during the first pregnancy of DES-exposed daughters, most obstetricians believe that it is best not to perform a cerclage. Instead, the cervix should be examined at least once a week after the first trimester with the hope of detecting the earliest signs of cervical dilatation and effacement so that an emergency cerclage can be performed if necessary. Women suspected of having cervical incompetence should be instructed to immediately report vaginal or pelvic heaviness, pressure, or a bloody or watery discharge. The recommendation of some researchers (see page 15) to perform prophylactic cerclage on all DES-exposed daughters has not been widely endorsed.

Developmental anomalies of the uterus are present in approximately 2 out of every 1,000 women giving birth. They are responsible, however, for a spontaneous abortion rate as high as 25 percent. These anomalies may appear either as two separate uterine horns connected by a bridge of tissue, a uterus with a heart-shaped appearance, or as a uterus that appears normal on the outside but is divided by a wall, or septum, within the endometrium. Ironically, although the latter condition leaves the uterus appearing normal from the outside, it is associated with the highest incidence of first- and second-trimester pregnancy loss. Fortunately most of these developmental conditions can be corrected surgically with little difficulty.

Other less common causes of midtrimester abortion include uterine infections, excessive scarring of the endometrial cavity from previous surgical procedures, and the presence of multiple fibroid tumors which distort the endometrial cavity and make it difficult for the placenta to implant and grow normally.

How soon after a spontaneous abortion is it safe to try to become pregnant again?

A couple can safely resume sexual relations two weeks after a spontaneous abortion. Most doctors, however, advise waiting at least two or three regular cycles before attempting another pregnancy, although this advice is based on no scientific evidence. The earlier in pregnancy that a spontaneous abortion occurs, the sooner will a woman resume menstruation, ovulation, and her capability to become pregnant. There is no evidence that pregnancies conceived with the first menstrual cycle after an early pregnancy loss are more apt to fail than those conceived following a delay of two or three months. For many women, this medically prescribed delay is insufferable as well as unnecessary. In fact, Dr. Allen Wilcox and his associates, in their 1988 study, found that 13 of 14 pregnancies conceived in the first cycle after an early pregnancy loss ended with a successful full-term birth.

If I have one spontaneous abortion, am I more likely to have another during my next pregnancy?

Though one's risk of a repeat spontaneous abortion will be influenced by factors such as a woman's age, the presence of uterine defects, and concurrent disease, certain generalizations can be made. Following one first-trimester spontaneous abortion, your risk of recurrent abortion will be greater if the abortus is chromosomally normal rather than abnormal. Moreover, the risk is highest, perhaps 40 to 45 percent, if the chromosomes are normal and the mother has no live-born offspring. The preservation of aborted tissue for chromosomal analysis (see next question) is helpful in determining a woman's prognosis for future pregnancies. Once a woman has successfully given birth, the likelihood of recurrent abortion after one miscarriage is only approximately 25 percent. Even if you experience two consecutive spontaneous abortions, it is comforting to know that your risk of this happening a third time is only slightly above that of the general population.

Habitual abortion is defined as the consecutive occurrence of three or more spontaneous abortions. In the United States, 5 percent of all spontaneous abortions are of the habitual type. Too often obstetricians mistakenly characterize habitual aborters as having little if any chance of achieving a successful pregnancy. On the contrary, recent studies show that following three consecutive abortions a woman's risk of a fourth will be no more than 32 percent, or 17 to 22 percent above the 10 to 15 percent rate usually expected in the general population.

Though the causes of habitual abortion may be varied, they must all be investigated by your obstetrician. Testing the chromosomes of both parents is also mandatory, since approximately 2 to 6 percent of habitual aborters or their husbands or partners demonstrate chromosomal abnormalities, some of which preclude successful pregnancy.

Spina bifida, a congenital abnormality of the spinal cord in which the covering membrane is incomplete, is often associated with hydrocephaly, an abnormal enlargement of the fetal head. Studies have confirmed that this abnormality is significantly more common among women experiencing two or more previous spontaneous abortions.

One cause for concern is a 1989 report published in *Obstetrics and Gynecology* in which doctors from Milan, Italy, found that women with a history of two or more spontaneous abortions experienced four times the frequency of ectopic pregnancy as did women without such history. Although the researchers could not explain why there was an association between these two forms of reproductive failure, they theorized that both conditions may sometimes be the result of delayed ovulation with preovulatory overripeness of an unhealthy egg (see discussion of the rhythm method in Chapter 1).

Until recently, little if any attention has been paid to the details of successful pregnancies which followed three or more previous spontaneous abortions. This subject was addressed in a 1987 article published in the *British Medical Journal*. In this report, doctors in Middlesex, England, reviewed the records of women with this history and found an alarmingly high 27 percent incidence of low birth weights, compared to a usual rate of only 7 percent in England. In addition, perinatal mortality rates were significantly higher in the women with previous miscarriages. Based on this information, it would be wise for doctors to be vigilant in observing for premature labor when there is a history of recurrent spontaneous abortion.

If in miscarrying I pass pregnancy tissue at home, what should I do with it?

Despite the fear and disappointment which spontaneous abortion at home may provoke, it is vital that you collect all pregnancy tissue which is passed and take it to your obstetrician. Tissue may be described as anything that does not look like blood or a blood clot. In the past, the standard advice has been to place the tissue in a glass container and add any type of alcohol to it in order to preserve the specimen. In fact, alcohol is a poor preservative which hardens tissues and makes them difficult to prepare for microscopic analysis and impossible to use for chromosomal study. The best way to insure preservation of the fetal tissues is to save a few fragments in a saline-soaked piece of gauze and then place them in a clean jar. This will allow your obstetrician the option of having the tissues studied for their chromosomal pattern as well as their microscopic appearance. If you will not be seeing your doctor immediately, the jar should be kept in the refrigerator. If your obstetrician sees that you have passed the entire pregnancy sac, a D and C (dilatation and curettage) or suction curet-

tage to remove retained fragments may not be necessary.

 # ABNORMAL PREGNANCIES

What is an ectopic pregnancy, and why does it occur?

An ectopic pregnancy is one which grows outside its normal location in the endometrium. Though ectopic pregnancies have been reported to occur in the abdominal cavity, ovary, and cervix, the fallopian tube is by far the most common site, accounting for 95 percent of all ectopics. It is for this reason that the term "ectopic pregnancy" is often used synonymously with "tubal pregnancy." Rupture of the wall of the tube by an ectopic pregnancy is often a catastrophic medical emergency which can result in severe intraabdominal hemorrhage and even death. Tubal pregnancies may also pass out of the end of the tube and abort into the abdominal cavity. This condition, usually far less dangerous than rupture of the tube, is known as a tubal abortion. In extremely rare circumstances, the fetus implants in the abdominal cavity and continues to grow.

Infection and scarring of the fallopian tubes caused by sexually transmitted infections such as chlamydia and gonorrhea are believed to be most responsible for ectopic pregnancy (see Chapter 6). These infections permanently damage and narrow the tube so that the normal passage of the fertilized egg to the uterus is either impaired or prevented. Convincing data show that the incidence curves for tubal infection and ectopic pregnancy have virtually paralleled each other over the past 15 years. Other conditions which either narrow the tubal opening or alter the speed of tubal transport of the fertilized egg, such as endometriosis, developmental abnormalities of the tubes, in utero exposure to DES (see Chapter 1), previous tubal or pelvic sur-

gery, adhesions or scar tissue from ruptured appendicitis, the use of progestin-only minipills, and IUD-associated infections, may all predispose to ectopic pregnancy. When inadvertent pregnancy follows tubal sterilization, 20 percent prove to be ectopic. The incidence is believed to be highest if tubal cauterization is performed through a laparoscope, with estimates as high as 50 percent. The incidence of ectopic pregnancy also increases with age, although most often no cause is apparent. Although initial reports suggested that a previous induced abortion increased a woman's risk of a subsequent ectopic pregnancy, recent statistical studies have failed to confirm such an association. Regardless of the cause, once a woman has had an ectopic pregnancy, her chances of a second one are at least ten times greater than that of other women. The outlook after two ectopic pregnancies is even more depressing, with the risk of a third ectopic estimated to be 30 to 50 percent. It appears that if a woman begins a reproductive career with an ectopic pregnancy, it is often a portent of bad things to come; more than 50 percent of such women experience subsequent infertility, and only 35 to 40 percent eventually achieve a successful full-term pregnancy.

How do I distinguish between an ectopic pregnancy and a threatened miscarriage?

Cramping, pelvic pain, and vaginal bleeding are symptoms common to both ectopic pregnancy and threatened spontaneous abortion. As a result, an ectopic pregnancy is often mistaken for the more common threatened miscarriage. Inflammation of the tubes, or salpingitis, and pelvic inflammatory disease (PID) may also confuse the diagnosis because they too may also cause lower abdominal pain and menstrual irregularity. Sadly, thousands of women with ectopic pregnancies leave doctors' offices and emergency rooms each year with prescriptions for antibiotics and analgesics when attention should have been paid to the immediate diagnosis and treatment of an ectopic pregnancy.

In this day of sophisticated and advanced obstetrical technology, practically all ectopic pregnancies should be diagnosed prior to rupture and internal hemorrhage, but for this to occur you and your doctor should have a strong suspicion for this diagnosis as well as an awareness of certain differences in the symptoms of ectopic pregnancy and threatened abortion. Though both conditions are characterized by lower abdominal pain, the pain of an impending spontaneous uterine abortion is generally milder, likely to be rhythmic, and located lower in the midline of the abdomen. With a tubal pregnancy the pain may be on the side of the affected tube or it may be generalized, but it is usually far more severe. The external vaginal bleeding noted with an ectopic pregnancy is usually not heavy and is often dark in color, while the bleeding associated with a threatened or incomplete abortion is usually heavier and accompanied by the passage of blood clots. A careful pelvic examination performed by your obstetrician will usually give further clues as to the correct diagnosis.

Characteristically a woman carrying an ectopic pregnancy will experience severe tenderness upon motion of her cervix. Although the uterus, under the influence of pregnancy hormones, may be slightly enlarged when a pregnancy is in the tube, it will tend to be larger and softer when the pregnancy is intrauterine. Occasionally your doctor will be able to feel the enlargement of the tube produced by the ectopic pregnancy, but in most cases this method is unreliable. As mentioned in Chapter 1, if you have an IUD, the above symptoms should be a red flag to your obstetrician that an ectopic gestation is a distinct possibility. Salpingitis and PID both produce tenderness on mo-

tion of the cervix, as does an ectopic pregnancy. However, these conditions are usually associated with a low-grade fever, an elevated white blood cell count and sedimentation rate (see Chapter 6), and, most important, a negative pregnancy test.

Rupture of an ectopic pregnancy is a frightening, life-threatening emergency characterized by sudden, severe lower-abdominal pain often described as sharp, stabbing, or tearing in character. Symptoms of impending shock such as nausea, dizziness, sweating, and fainting soon follow. Treatment at this point must include immediate abdominal surgery, with removal or excision of the pregnancy and control of bleeding from the site of rupture. Often such surgery involves removal of the affected tube, since damage may be so extensive that conservative surgery to salvage the tube and enhance future fertility is no longer possible. Blood transfusions may be required to replace the large amount of blood lost following tubal rupture. Technological advances have allowed doctors to diagnose most ectopic pregnancies before they rupture. These techniques include use of more sensitive quantitative blood tests for pregnancy combined with ultrasound and laparoscopy to locate the site of the pregnancy.

Are pregnancies more likely to be abnormal if they result from artificial insemination?

Offspring conceived following artificial insemination are at no greater risk of being born with congenital abnormalities than are those conceived naturally. One might even argue that if sperm donors are carefully screened before they are selected, the incidence of birth defects may be significantly lower than when fertilization occurs with a natural father having a low sperm count and a high percentage of abnormal spermatozoa.

In recent years, the use of frozen semen obtained from sperm storage banks, or cryobanks, has gained in popularity. The sperm are frozen in liquid nitrogen at $-196°C$ for months or years, then thawed for insemination at the time of ovulation.

Some men undergoing vasectomy have elected first to store several ejaculates should they decide to have children at a later date. Successful pregnancies have been reported with sperm stored for ten or more years. Several researchers have confirmed that pregnancies resulting from thawed sperm may be healthier than those conceived naturally. The reason for this is that freezing may have the effect of killing off weak and unhealthy sperm. In a University of Arkansas study of 1,000 children conceived following insemination with previously frozen sperm it was found that fewer than 1 percent had birth defects, compared to 2 to 3 percent in the general population. In addition, it was noted that the miscarriage rate was less than 6 percent in the inseminated group, compared with the standard 10 to 15 percent which is generally quoted. Several other studies comparing pregnancy outcome following artificial insemination with fresh and frozen sperm have noted no differences in the incidence of spontaneous abortion, fetal or neonatal deaths, prematurity, malformations, or the sex ratio of the infants conceived.

Is the incidence of congenital malformations higher among women who take fertility drugs?

There are many women who in the past were unable to conceive because they do not ovulate. Over the past 20 years, new drugs popularly referred to as fertility drugs have allowed these women to achieve successful pregnancy. These drugs have been incorporated into the new fertility techniques, such as in vitro fertilization (IVF) and others, and their use has been expanded to include women who ovulate but who do so either infrequently or inadequately.

Of all medications used in the treatment of infertility, clomiphene citrate (trade name Clomid) is the most popular. Taken in pill form over a period of five or more days, it is believed to exert its effect by stimulating the hypothalamus to secrete its releasing factors.

Laboratory research has documented that some clomiphene citrate remains in a woman's circulation after conception occurs a week or two following the last pill. Despite this, all experimental and clinical studies have proven clomiphene citrate to be safe for induction of ovulation. There is some evidence, however, that it may adversely affect the developing fetus when it is inadvertently administered after pregnancy is established. One disturbing observation is that the chemical structure of clomiphene citrate is closely related to that of DES. Some studies have found a higher incidence of fetal abnormalities, particularly neural tube defects, when very high doses of clomiphene citrate were given to laboratory animals early in pregnancy. In humans, the beginnings of organ formation and susceptibility to classic birth defects start around 31 days from a woman's last menstrual period, or 3 days after her first missed period. It is not known if damage to a human fetus is more likely to occur when therapeutic doses of clomiphene citrate are inadvertently taken at or after that time. For this reason, it is imperative that you are certain that you are not pregnant before beginning a course of clomiphene citrate treatment.

While clomiphene citrate aids fertility by inducing ovulation, it also has the negative side effect of thickening a woman's cervical mucus, thereby making it impenetrable or hostile to the passage of sperm. To thin the mucus, many infertility experts routinely administer small doses of a natural estrogen named estradiol in the days preceding ovulation. This is innocuous to the fetus since it is a hormone usually found in abundance prior to ovulation and it is stopped prior to conception and organ development. Pure progesterone, in the form of suppositories and intramuscular injections, is helpful in the treatment of infertility caused by inadequate corpus luteum production of progesterone during the second half of the menstrual cycle; correction of this so-called luteal phase defect helps to improve the receptivity of the endometrium to the early embryo. Many fertility programs routinely use progesterone throughout the first six to seven weeks of pregnancy, or until the point is reached when progesterone production is taken over by the placenta. Unlike synthetic progestins (see Chapter 1), natural progesterone is perfectly safe for the fetus since it is found in great abundance during normal pregnancy.

Women who are unable to ovulate with clomiphene citrate and those who have a malfunction of their pituitary gland which prevents ovulation may achieve ovulation and successful pregnancy with the use of human menopausal gonadotropin, or hMG (trade name Pergonal). This very expensive drug consists of the pituitary hormones FSH and LH. It is manufactured from, of all things, the urine of menopausal women, which is rich in these two hormones. When administered as a daily intramuscular injection over a period of one to two weeks, hMG causes follicles to ripen in preparation for ovulation. With use of ultrasound, doctors are now able to retrieve the oocytes within the follicles for use in IVF and similar procedures. Another option is to trigger ovulation or superovulation of several oocytes by injecting the pregnancy hormone hCG following the last hMG injection. Numerous studies have confirmed that pregnancies conceived with this latter regimen are at no greater risk of congenital abnormalities, though the spontaneous abortion rate may be increased slightly. Of greater concern is the risk of multiple pregnancy, which may be as high as 20 percent. Usually this will be a twin pregnancy, although multiple births of three or more children have been reported on many occasions over the last few years. If the dose of hMG is not carefully controlled, a woman taking this medication can encounter significant risks to herself caused by hyperstimulation of her ovaries. For this reason, hMG should be administered only by gynecologists who have extensive experience with this therapy and those who have easy access to vaginal ultrasound and a laboratory which can perform estrogen hormone assays on a daily basis so that the doses of hMG and hCG can be appropriately adjusted and complications avoided.

Some infertile women have extremely high levels of LH and require only pure follicle-stimulating hormone (FSH) to trigger ovulation. This medication (trade name Metrodin) requires the same vigilance in monitoring as does hMG. Research to date seems to confirm that Metrodin is safe for the developing fetus.

The release of the gonadotropins FSH and LH from the pituitary gland is under the influence of a hypothalamus hormone named gonadotropin-releasing hormone (GnRH). Several chemically similar but more potent synthetic GnRH compounds called agonists have been discovered. However, these agents seem to quiet the pituitary gland rather than stimulate LH and FSH release, as was originally expected. Gynecologists have found that by combining GnRH with hMG, stimulation of ovulation can be improved because the inappropriate early release of LH is prevented. The only GnRh agents commercially available in the United States are leuprolide, which is administered either as a daily subcutaneous (below the skin) injection (trade name Lupron) or a monthly intramuscular injection (trade name Lupron Depot), and the nasal spray nafarelin acetate (trade name Synarel). Though research is not extensive, the use of leuprolide and nafarelin during ovulation induction does not appear to have toxic effects on the fetus. Their use during early pregnancy, however, has been associated with a higher incidence of fetal anomalies, deaths, and low birth weights in experimental laboratory animals.

The drug bromocryptine (trade name Parlodel) is useful for patients whose infertility is associated with high levels of the pituitary hormone prolactin. Symptoms of hyperprolactinemia, or high levels of prolactin in the bloodstream, include amenorrhea (absence of menses) and galactorrhea (milk secretion from the nipples). These conditions are due to a malfunction involving the releasing factors of the hypothalamus which are necessary for initiating the process of ovulation. One releasing factor of the hypothalamus, named prolactin-release inhibitory factor (PIF), prevents the pituitary gland from releasing prolactin. Bromocryptine lowers prolactin levels and allows the normal ovulatory mechanism to reestablish itself. Amenorrhea, galactorrhea, and infertility are often caused by tiny, benign, prolactin-secreting tumors of the pituitary gland called microadenomas or prolactinomas. Unlike other tumors which often require surgical removal, microadenomas respond favorably to treatment with bromocryptine. In addition, it has been successfully used to treat postpartum lactation and breast engorgement. The safety of bromocryptine when inadvertently taken early in pregnancy has not been definitely determined. However, evaluation of several hundred pregnancies conceived while women were taking bromocryptine has not demonstrated a higher incidence of spontaneous abortion or congenital abnormalities, nor has extensive research on rats and rabbits shown a relationship between birth defects and the use of this medication. To avoid even a remote risk of taking bromocryptine during pregnancy, some infertility experts limit its use to the first 10 to 11 days of each menstrual cycle. Others are not as cautious and prescribe the drug daily, stopping when the pregnancy test becomes positive.

███ 3 ███

SPORTS
and
PHYSICAL FITNESS

*O*utdated obstetrical textbooks used the term "confinement" to describe the long, quiet days of rest and isolation associated with pregnancy and childbirth. Until recently, most doctors erroneously believed that confinement was preferable to the supposed dangers of fetal and maternal injury which would result from even minimal amounts of exercise. Fortunately, today's pregnant woman is no longer regarded as a delicate flower requiring seclusion until her baby is born.

Unbiased research has yet to be conducted on the long-term effects of intense physical activity on a woman's health or her ability to ovulate and bear children, and important questions concerning the safe limits of exertion during pregnancy remain to be answered. While prenatal exercise has become a popular and profitable business, as evidenced by the number of books and videos flooding the marketplace, too often these commercial enterprises have not been properly researched, have no scientific basis, keep no record of injuries, and are directed by unqualified individuals.

Many of the old myths about the harmful effects of physical activity on pregnancy still exist. Other equally misinformed individuals believe that no limitations should be set on physical activity during pregnancy. The latter advice is far more dangerous. This chapter provides an unbiased review of the latest medical data, practical advice about the positive and negative effects of sports and physical activity on the pregnant woman and her baby, and guidelines for exercise.

 ## SAFE LIMITS

How can I determine my safe limits for exertion during pregnancy?

The appropriate amount of training and physical fitness for a pregnant woman should be determined by her prepregnancy fitness and activity level, her age, and the presence or absence of medical or obstetrical complications. While the physically fit woman can continue most activities at or slightly below her levels prior to pregnancy, it is probably not wise to exceed those levels. Physical fitness prior to pregnancy is best achieved through aerobic exercises, activities which condition the heart and lungs by increasing the efficiency of the body's intake of oxygen. Rhythmic aerobic activities such as walking, jogging, running, swimming, rowing, biking, aerobic dancing, and skipping rope all help to increase the pulse rate as the heart works harder to bring oxygen to the body's various muscle groups. It would be foolish for extremely sedentary women to suddenly initiate a rigorous aerobics program during pregnancy. Such women will benefit from mild and gradually increased exercise, such as walking, water exercises, and kinetics. These are safe and excellent methods of increasing strength and flexibility for all women.

Before you embark on an exercise program during pregnancy it is vital for you to have a complete physical examination and receive medical clearance from your obstetrician. To determine your exercise tolerance, you can undergo a modified stress test on a bicycle ergometer or a treadmill during pregnancy. These studies may be performed in the physical therapy or cardiology departments of most hospitals by an exercise physiologist as well as in some doctors' offices and athletic departments of large universities. Be wary of physical fitness instructors at private health clubs who may claim to be authorities on exercise physiology but in fact know little about the unique fetal and maternal demands which pregnancy imposes.

Even experts on the subject disagree vehemently as to a woman's safe exertional limits during pregnancy. One group claims that if exercise is to have a beneficial effect, it must produce an increase in the heart rate to a minimum of 150 beats per minute over a period of at least 30 minutes, excluding warm-up and cool-down exercises. Workouts to achieve this rate should be carried out at least three times a week, or every other day, but not more than 60 minutes per day or six days per week. Others, including the American College of Obstetricians and Gynecologists, offer more conservative advice, recommending exercise two or three times a week to a degree capable of maintaining the heart rate at about 110 to 120 beats per minute for at least 15 continuous minutes, with the heart rate not to exceed 140 beats per minute. A woman who wants to exercise at levels which increase her heart rate above 140 beats per minute is advised by these experts to seek medical evaluation and clearance.

The pulse rate is simply the rate per minute that your heart beats in transporting oxygen and nutrients throughout your body. You can take your pulse by placing your index and middle fingers on the undersurface of your wrist just above the thumb. The pulse may also be taken over the carotid artery on the outside of the neck, just below the junction of the jaw on one side. (Don't press too hard because you may impede the blood flow and cause dizziness.) By counting the pulsations for 10 seconds and then multiplying by 6, or for 15 seconds and multiplying by 4, you can determine your number of heartbeats per minute.

Is there a method of using my pulse rate to monitor my exertional limits more precisely?

The pulse rate which is taken immediately upon stopping an exercise is appropriately known as your *exercise rate*. Maximum heart rate (MHR) is defined as the highest attainable heart rate recorded during an exercise session. The MHR is directly affected by age, and the older one becomes the lower the MHR should be. It is dangerous and foolish to exert yourself to the point of exhaustion during pregnancy in order to determine your MHR. Instead, the MHR can be calculated through the use of a simple formula: 220 beats per minute minus the number of years of age.

It should not be your goal to achieve your MHR during exercise. Instead, strive for the *target heart rate*, that rate which, when attained, will provide a sufficient level of exercise to efficiently stimulate your cardiac and respiratory systems. Depending on your previous physical condition, this would be between 60 and 85 percent of your MHR. It is ill-advised for a woman in poor physical condition to even attempt to approach a target heart rate above 70 percent. Regardless of your physical condition, if maximum benefit to your cardiovascular system is to be achieved, you should maintain this target heart rate for 30 minutes per exercise session. Table 5 lists the target heart rate you should try to achieve based on your physical condition.

In Table 6 I list the approximate MHR according to age, as well as the corresponding target heart rate for the well-conditioned and poorly conditioned woman.

Many exercise experts believe that the above method of calculating one's target heart rate is not

TABLE 5

TARGET HEART RATE FOR WOMEN BASED ON PHYSICAL CONDITION

Target heart rate (% of MRH)

60%—Women who have not been exercising
70%—Those who have been participating in a cardiovascular program for more than five weeks, twice weekly
80%—Those who have been participating in a cardiovascular program on a regular basis
85%—Those who are well-conditioned athletes

TABLE 6

MAXIMUM HEART RATE AND ESTIMATED TARGET HEART RATE FOR WOMEN BASED ON PHYSICAL FITNESS

Age	MHR/min.	MHR/10 sec.	TARGET HEART RATE	
			Unconditioned (60% MHR for 10 sec.)	*Good Condition* (85% MHR for 10 sec.)
20–25	200	33	20	28
26–30	190	32	19	27
31–35	185	31	18	26
36–40	180	30	18	25
41–45	175	29	17	25
46–50	170	28	17	24

accurate enough because it does not take into account a woman's resting pulse rate, which can vary considerably from person to person. For this reason, the so-called Karvonen method is often preferred. Your *resting pulse* is best determined before getting out of bed in the morning. Take three separate readings and use the average value. The resting pulse is an important measurement of fitness because it tells you how hard your heart is working to keep you alive. While the average resting heart rate for women is between 78 and 84 beats per minute, it is not uncommon for runners and other well-conditioned athletes to have a resting pulse of less than 50 beats per minute. Your resting pulse

may increase by 10 to 20 beats per minute by the end of pregnancy. It is theorized that some hormonal mechanism is responsible for raising the pulse an average of 8 beats per minute as early as the first missed period. The highest pulse is usually achieved by the thirty-second week of pregnancy and remains at this level until delivery at 40 weeks. Your resting pulse may also be higher following a meal, and especially after you drink tea or coffee. Strong emotional responses, fever, certain medications, and recent intercourse also elevate the pulse rate.

To calculate your target heart rate with the Karvonen formula, first find your *heart rate reserve* by subtracting your resting pulse rate from your maximum heart rate, then multiply your heart rate reserve by the percent of desired exercise intensity (60 to 85 percent, as in Table 6), and add this result to your resting pulse rate to yield your target heart rate. For example, a 30-year-old woman with a resting heart rate of 80 beats per minute who wants to work at an intensity of 70 percent of her MHR would calculate her target heart rate in the following manner:

Maximum heart rate = 220 −   30 (age) = 190
Resting heart rate = 80   − 80
Heart rate reserve =   110
Percent desired intensity = 70% =   × .70
                                                          77
Resting pulse rate of 80 added   + 80
Target heart rate =   157

You should not try to rigidly achieve an exact target heart rate; instead try to keep within 10 to 15 beats per minute on either side of your calculated number. Since a woman's resting pulse increases gradually to peak levels at 32 weeks and beyond, you will probably have to recalculate your target heart rate as pregnancy progresses. It is often helpful to monitor your heart rate during the cool-down period immediately following an exercise session. If your pulse returns to normal within 30 seconds after you exercise, the activity was probably not aerobically challenging. An indication of cardiovascular fitness is when your heart rate decreases by 30 or more beats per minute within the first 60 seconds after cessation of maximum exercise sustained for several minutes.

Your ability to exercise usually decreases significantly during the first three months of pregnancy as a result of the nausea, vomiting, breast tenderness, and general discomfort which is so common during the first trimester. Do not be disillusioned, because activity levels can usually increase to near-prepregnancy capacity after the third month. Regardless of your physical condition, it is a good idea to reduce your efforts slightly during the first three months. The relative ease of the second trimester is often followed by severe limitations imposed by the enlarging abdominal girth, pelvic pressure, and generalized discomfort which accompanies the last trimester.

The capacity for exercise during pregnancy varies greatly from one woman to another and from one pregnancy to the next. Some women are able to exercise in relative comfort throughout each trimester; there is even a report in the medical literature of a woman who ran an entire marathon during her last trimester. Provided there are no medical or obstetrical contraindications, such as hypertension, preeclampsia, twins, incompetent cervix, or placenta previa, this positive attitude toward exercise should be encouraged.

 EFFECTS OF EXERCISE ON PREGNANCY

Is it true that physically fit women experience easier pregnancies and labor than women who do not exercise?

Although there has always been a general feeling that women with good physical fitness do better throughout pregnancy and in labor than those who do not exercise, until recently there was little, if any, scientific evidence to substantiate this claim.

Certainly, it is logical to assume that an aerobically fit women will have more stamina and strength to endure a long, difficult labor than an unfit woman, but proving this scientifically is not as easy as it might seem. The other benefits of regular exercise, namely fewer episodes of depression, anxiety, and stress as well as greater self-esteem, self-control, and self-confidence, are even more difficult to validate. These positive emotional effects have been attributed to the body's production of chemicals named endorphins, which are released into the bloodstream during vigorous exercise. Endorphins are believed to play an important role in alleviating stress and reducing one's perception of pain. In a 1989 study published in the *American Journal of Obstetrics and Gynecology*, Italian doctors measured endorphin levels in the plasma of pregnant women who exercised and those who did not. They found significantly higher values throughout pregnancy and labor among the well-conditioned women. To document the analgesic, or pain-relieving, effects of exercise, the doctors interviewed both groups of women during labor to determine their perception of the pain caused by their contractions. Those who exercised perceived the pain as being much milder than the group of women who were sedentary.

In trying to answer the important question of whether or not physically fit women experience shorter labors than women who do not exercise, doctors at the University of Wisconsin, in their 1983 study, found no differences between the two groups. In contrast, researchers from the University of British Columbia, in their 1987 report, noted that physically fit mothers had a shorter second stage of labor than women who did not exercise. The second stage of labor begins with full dilatation of the cervix and ends with the delivery of the baby; this stage, also known as the pushing or bearing-down stage, requires great physical effort. The authors concluded that the shorter second stage for the fit mothers "may be related to their increased cardiorespiratory fitness and ability to postpone fatigue during the active stage of labor." In 1987, when doctors in Grand Rapids, Michigan, compared the speed of labor between exercising women and a control group, they found that exercisers having their first baby (primigravidas) had shorter first and second stages of labor than nonexercising primigravidas. The total length of labor was on average 1.8 hours shorter among the physically fit primigravidas. When multiparous women, or those who have previously given

birth, were analyzed, the researchers found no relationship between physical fitness and the length of labor.

There is some controversy as to whether or not pregnant women should participate in strength training with free weights and fitness machines. Proponents of such programs believe that the resultant increase in muscle strength will ease labor and delivery and make women less susceptible to the muscular aches and pains that are so common throughout pregnancy. Others insist that weight training will only increase susceptibility to muscle and joint injuries. Although there is little scientific research to support either position, a 1987 study from the University of Florida strongly endorsed the value of strength conditioning. In this report, doctors offered either low, medium, or high levels of aerobics and strength conditioning for the legs, arms, abdomen, and back to a group of pregnant women. When compared to a control group of almost 400 women who did not participate in the program, cesarean section rates were found to be 6.7 percent in the high-exercise group, 19 percent in the medium-exercise group, 23 percent in the low-exercise group, and an alarming 28 percent among nonparticipants. While the average length of labor was equal for all of the groups, the average hospital stay was slightly longer for nonparticipants than for those in the three exercise groups.

Can increased body temperature from exercise, hot showers, or saunas cause birth defects?

Animal experimentation and human experience both suggest that prolonged maternal hyperthermia, or increased body temperature, may be associated with a wide variety of spinal cord abnormalities and faulty development of the brain and skull of the fetus. The most likely time for this to occur appears to be the third, fourth, and fifth weeks of pregnancy, although anomalies have been reported following an episode of hyperthermia as late as the fourteenth week. While a person's normal body temperature is 98.6°F (37°C), during pregnancy it will usually rise to between 99°F and 99.2°F as a result of high progesterone levels. Elevations above 102°F (39°C) appear to be associated with fetal anomalies. Intermittent high fevers are not as threatening to the fetus as a sustained temperature rise.

Precise laboratory studies conducted on virtually every animal species have confirmed the harmful effects of hyperthermia on the fetus. At rest, fetal temperatures average approximately 32.9°F (0.5°C) more than that of maternal temperatures. When a pregnant woman exercises vigorously, her temperature initially rises faster than that of her fetus. Following exhaustive exercise, however, maternal temperature drops rapidly, whereas fetal temperatures remain elevated for a considerably longer period of time. The reason for this is that the fetus lacks the ability to dissipate heat through perspiration. In some instances the delay in fetal cooling off following vigorous activity can be an hour or more.

Most studies have shown that under normal conditions the critical maternal temperature rise to 102°F (39°C) will not occur until a woman has exercised at least 45 minutes. However, one study found that only 30 minutes of exercise at 50 percent of maximum heart rate capacity was capable of elevating a pregnant woman's temperature to 102°F. Based on these observations, it would be safe to conclude that the risk of hyperthermia is minimal and probably nonexistent if aerobic exercise sessions are moderate in degree and limited to 30 minutes or less. Your body temperature is certain to be higher if you run in 80 to 90 percent humidity and in temperatures greater than 80°F, so it is best to modify your exercise routine on hot and humid days. To prevent dehydration, it is important that you drink adequate amounts of fluids before, after, and even during your 30-minute workout. If you have fever due to a cold, a sore throat, or the flu, it is best not to exercise. A runner's core, or inner-body, temperature, best measured by taking a rectal temperature, will rise an average of 34.7°F (1.5°C) during a long race.

When interviewed, most long-distance runners claim that they do not feel subjectively hotter while running, thereby negating the old myth that our bodies have a way of letting us know that we are overheated.

If a woman is aerobically fit prior to pregnancy and exercises prudently under climate-controlled conditions, hyperthermia during pregnancy can be avoided. This was demonstrated in a 1985 report by researchers at Pennsylvania State University College of Medicine. They measured body temperatures of four well-conditioned women before, during, and after vigorous treadmill exercises under comfortable and cool conditions throughout pregnancy. Exercise consisted of running three or more miles four or more times per week at a pace of 10 minutes per mile or better. Core temperatures never exceeded 102°F (39°C).

Safe limits of exposure in a hot tub or sauna during pregnancy have not been established. However, one group of doctors has recently determined that a woman can stay in a 39°C (102°F) bath for 15 minutes or a 41°C (106°F) bath for 10 minutes without risk of her body temperature rising above the critical abnormality-causing level of 39°C. Sauna bathing, because it allows for evaporation and convection, requires longer exposure. This may explain the lack of any apparent excess of hyperthermia-associated malformation problems in Finland, where maternal sauna bathing is usually limited to 6 to 12 minutes. The most recent study demonstrating the relationship between maternal hyperthermia in the first trimester and neural tube defects was published in the Journal of the American Medical Association in 1992. In this report, doctors from Boston University School of Medicine and Harvard Medical School studied almost 23,000 women and found that first-trimester use of a hot tub almost tripled a woman's risk of giving birth to a baby with a neural tube defect. Sauna use and fever due to illness played important but less significant roles, while use of an electric blanket was of no consequence.

Until more evidence is available, I would urge

pregnant women not to take very hot baths or showers and to avoid the sauna during the critical period of central nervous system development between the third and fourteenth weeks. The temperature in the sauna is, on the average, 40°C (104°F) to 55°C (131°F) (wet bulb) during use, and the average time in the sauna is 5 to 20 minutes. According to several investigators, a person's rectal temperature rises during a sauna from a normal of 37°C (98.6°F) to between 37.6°C (99.7°F) and 40°C (104°F), depending on the temperature of the sauna and the time spent within the sauna room. In one reported instance of a fetal central nervous system deformity resulting from a sauna, a woman had used it for 45 minutes on four occasions during the fifth week after conception. On one of these occasions the temperature of the sauna rose to 43°C (109.5°F).

Concern has been expressed about the potentially harmful effects of hyperthermia associated with the use of an electric blanket during the first trimester. Fortunately, two separate studies in 1991 and 1992 failed to demonstrate that this is cause for concern.

Aside from hyperthermia, can too much exercise have any adverse effects on the fetus?

There has never been a scientific study to show that exercise or even intense physical activity early in pregnancy is responsible for miscarriage or spontaneous abortion. In a 1989 report, Dr. James E. Clapp III of the University of Vermont College of Medicine studied the pregnancy outcome of serious recreational runners, aerobic dancers, and physically active and fit women who exercised vigorously both before and during pregnancy and found no evidence that exercise increased the risk for either early spontaneous abortion or late pregnancy complications. Dr. Clapp observed that women who continued to exercise throughout pregnancy were more likely to experience shorter labors, lower cesarean section rates, and fewer babies with fetal distress and low Apgar scores than

women who discontinued their regular exercise regimens before the end of the first trimester.

Following an early miscarriage, women are often left with feelings of guilt for having played too much tennis or jogged too many miles or even for having stood or walked for prolonged periods of time. It is a myth that these activities cause early miscarriage. Research on aborted fetuses clearly demonstrates that a very high percentage are abnormally developed or have gross chromosomal defects (see Chapter 2).

It has been found that excessive exercise diverts oxygen-carrying blood away from the uterus to the muscles and skin. The amount of blood rerouted in this fashion depends on the degree of exertion, the environmental temperature, and the length of time spent exercising. Exercise also stimulates the release of body chemicals called catecholamines, such as epinephrine and norepinephrine, which constrict or narrow the blood vessels supplying the uterus with oxygen. Animal research on pregnant sheep and guinea pigs has clearly demonstrated that extreme physical exertion impedes uterine blood flow and causes fetal distress, higher fetal mortality rates, and lower birth weights. Whether or not these physiological changes pose a threat to the human fetus remains unknown at the present time. It is known, however, that women in excellent physical condition demonstrate less of a catecholamine response to a given exercise stress than sedentary individuals. In addition, less blood is diverted away from the uterus during exercise if one is physically fit. Based on these data, it would seem prudent for a woman to condition herself well before the ultimate physical and emotional stress of her life—namely labor and delivery—in order to maximize her chances of adequate blood flow to her baby.

Though the usual fetal heart rate ranges between 120 and 160 beats per minute, rates as high as 180 or as low as 100 are not considered harmful. There is presently no evidence that transitory alterations in the fetal heart rate associated with moderate amounts of exercise are undesirable or pose a danger to the outcome of the pregnancy.

Dr. Marshall W. Carpenter and his associates at Brown University used a special two-dimensional ultrasound technique to accurately record the fetal heart rates of 45 women immediately after maximal and submaximal degrees of exertion on a stationary bicycle. Their important findings, published in the May 27, 1988, issue of the *Journal of the American Medical Association*, were that the normal fetal heart rate of 120 to 160 beats per minute did not change significantly during submaximal exercise, defined as exercise in which the maternal heart rate did not exceed 148 beats per minute. Following submaximal exertion, there was only one episode of bradycardia, or slowing of the fetal heart rate, to less than 110 beats per minute. However, when maternal exertion approached maximum aerobic capacity, fetal bradycardia occurred within 3 minutes in 15 of the 45 women tested. Such episodes were followed by a rapid return of the fetal heart rate to normal, and none of the infants experienced problems during labor or delivery. Despite the optimistic outcome, Dr. Carpenter and his colleagues concluded that pregnant women should limit their vigorous exercise to activities requiring a maternal heart rate of 150 beats per minute or less and should conclude with a gentle and continuous slowing of effort during recovery. This proposed limit is 10 beats higher than the 140 beats per minute recommended by the American College of Obstetricians and Gynecologists.

Although a variety of fetal heart rate changes have been reported to occur in association with maternal exercise, there is no proof that this will result in an adverse obstetrical outcome. In a 1987 study, published in the *American Journal of Obstetrics and Gynecology*, doctors from Grand Rapids, Michigan, followed the obstetrical performance of 85 healthy women enrolled in a program of carefully supervised aerobic activities such as cycling, jogging, walking, and swimming. When compared to a control group of pregnant women not enrolled in the program, no differences could be found in the incidence of obstetrical compli-

cations, birth weights, or health of the newborn.

The Apgar score is a method of grading the condition of a newborn at 1 and 5 minutes of life (see Chapter 11). All studies to date have shown no lowering of Apgar scores among women who exercised regularly, and one 1987 report actually demonstrated higher Apgar scores and birth weights among babies born to women who exercised most vigorously. In contrast to these studies, some researchers have found that pregnant women who reach more sustained and strenuous levels of aerobic exercise are more apt to experience premature uterine contractions, gain less weight during pregnancy, deliver earlier, and give birth to smaller babies. In one report, doctors concluded that women who continued endurance exercise well into the third trimester delivered babies weighing an average of 500 grams (1.1 pounds) less than that of babies whose mothers stopped exercising before the twenty-eighth week.

It is known that a woman's weight gain during pregnancy has a significant effect on her newborn's health and weight. Doctors have expressed concern that excessive caloric expenditure associated with exertional exercise can jeopardize the nutrient supply and growth of the fetus. It is therefore important to carefully adjust and increase your caloric intake during pregnancy in order to compensate for any changes in the frequency or intensity of your aerobic activity. Such adjustments will allow you to maintain a consistent weight gain of 1 to 3 kilograms per month throughout pregnancy and achieve the recommended total weight gain of 24 to 28 pounds. This weight gain is usually far easier to attain than one would imagine, especially since most pregnant women seem to instinctively reduce or totally eliminate extreme exertional activities during the second half of pregnancy.

It has been theorized that exercising in the upright position, as in running, walking, and aerobic dancing, may be more likely to exert pressure on the cervix and stimulate uterine contractions. It would follow that exercising on a stationary bicycle, a non-weight-bearing activity, might have less of a gravitational effect, cause less cervical stimulation, and reduce uterine activity. To test this theory, doctors from the Oregon Health Sciences University instructed women to walk briskly or exercise on a stationary bicycle for 15 minutes during the last eight weeks of pregnancy. They found no changes in uterine activity in the 30 minutes following either exercise method, thereby dispelling the previously held fears about the dangers of gravitationally dependent pursuits.

Much remains to be learned about the effects of maternal exercise on the fetus. Although the findings of various studies are contradictory and somewhat confusing, it is safe to conclude that a healthy pregnant women, free of obstetrical complications, can be reassured that most moderately strenuous activities will not adversely alter fetal health, the incidence of premature birth, birth weights, or Apgar scores of the newborn. This is especially true for women who have participated in aerobic activities prior to conception. If a woman wishes to exercise as close to her exertional limits as possible, she should do so only under careful medical supervision. During the last two months of pregnancy it is probably good advice to significantly reduce your activity level, eliminate most weight-bearing exercises, and take greater rest intervals between activities. Although it is a cliche, the best advice a woman can follow is to "listen" to your body and not push yourself beyond your previously determined exertional limits. If your pregnancy is high-risk, it is best not to exercise unless you are under close medical supervision.

Can the emotional and psychological stress of athletic competition adversely affect my pregnancy?

The emotional stress produced by intense athletic competition may be detrimental to the developing fetus. Under emotional stress due to any cause, body chemicals called catecholamines are secreted in greater amounts; the greater the degree of stress, the higher the catecholamine response. Increased levels of catecholamines, such as epinephrine and norepinephrine, produce a decrease in uterine blood flow, which in turn lowers the amount of oxygen passing to the fetus. In one study of 150 healthy pregnant women having their first baby, the more anxiety-prone mothers gave birth to infants of lower birth weights. British doctors, in a 1979 report, found that 67 percent of women delivering between four and seven weeks prior to their due dates had experienced major psychological stresses which may have precipitated labor. Among women giving birth earlier than this, 84 percent reported experiencing major psychological stress before the onset of labor. In comparison, only 43 percent of women delivering full-term infants had experienced major mental stress before labor. Other investigators have found a positive correlation between anxiety scores and prematurity as well as stillbirth rates. In a sense, some of these studies tend to support the folklore that a pregnant woman who is frightened or subjected to great anxiety may "lose her baby."

Based on these reports, the best advice for the pregnant athlete is to enjoy sports but don't try too hard to win. If you find that competitive encounters make you too anxious, try switching to noncompetitive aerobic activities such as swimming, biking, and walking. These will provide you with greater cardiovascular benefits and actually help to relieve stress and anxiety. However, if competitive sports remain your passion, it is probably advisable for you to learn stress-management techniques such as meditation, visualization, and biofeedback. The relaxation techniques taught in childbirth education classes are not only helpful in labor but may also be applied to other stressful situations such as athletic competition.

Can a blow to the abdomen or a fall cause a miscarriage?

The uterus does not ascend to the level above the pubic symphysis bone until the twelfth week of pregnancy, counting from the last menstrual period (see Figure 2). Until that time it cannot be injured by a blow to the lower abdomen, and vigorous sports, such as gymnastics, competitive skiing, and football, can be played without fear. The implantation of a healthy egg into the uterine lining is very strong; the egg cannot easily be dislodged. This fact can be attested to by the millions of women, who, prior to legalization of abortion, spent hours jumping up and down in attempts to dislodge their unwanted pregnancies.

After the twelfth week of pregnancy, the uterus rises enough to be seen and to be palpated abdominally. At this point, the chance of injury to the uterus by a direct blow increases but is still highly unlikely. Injury to the fetus is even more unlikely, since the amniotic fluid acts as a protective cushion. Nevertheless, it is probably best to avoid contact sports which might involve a direct blow to the abdomen. Many women find training physically uncomfortable after the fifth month because of the increasing size of the uterus and the bouncing inside which occurs while running. This type of movement, however, is not harmful to the baby.

Your risk of injury during athletic endeavors is likely to increase as pregnancy progresses. No matter how agile you are, you will become progressively less nimble with each pregnancy month, and any activity in which there is a danger of falling should be curtailed.

Which medical conditions keep the pregnant woman from active sports participation?

As mentioned previously, you should consult your obstetrician before undertaking any sport or training program during pregnancy. The decision on how active a woman with a particular medical problem, such as diabetes and heart disease, should be is often a difficult one and may require consultation with one or more specialists. For example, exercise in moderation is often beneficial to the diabetic woman, but too much physical activity may result in severe metabolic imbalance. Insulin requirements usually increase significantly during pregnancy, and this, as well as many other factors, must be taken into consideration. Similarly, the treatment of a woman who has a history of heart disease requires frequent consultation with a cardiologist. Often it is more prudent to prescribe rest, rather than exercise, during the critical seventh and eighth months of pregnancy when the cardiac workload reaches its maximum capacity. It is estimated that as many as 10 percent of women have mitral valve prolapse, or "floppiness" of the valve that separates the chambers on the left side of the heart. Most of these individuals are without symptoms and need not limit exercise or alter their lifestyle during pregnancy. However, a small percentage will experience symptoms such as chest pain, fainting, an irregular or rapid heart rate, and fatigue when engaged in activities which are too vigorous or competitive. If such symptoms appear during pregnancy, the precipitating physical activity should either be markedly reduced or eliminated. Women with respiratory diseases, anemia, bleeding disorders, hypertension, and thyroid disease should be meticulously evaluated by both an obstetrician and an internist, and specific exercise guidelines should be outlined as pregnancy progresses. Sickle cell trait is found in 8 percent of the black population. A recently published report in the New England Journal of Medicine suggests that individuals with sickle cell trait face approximately 40 times the risk of dying from extreme physical exercise. Doctors must stress the importance of moderation to women with sickle cell trait. Women who are markedly undernourished and underweight and those suffering from extreme obesity should both be cautioned to limit and in some cases avoid sports and physical fitness endeavors. The symptoms of exercise-induced asthma consist of coughing, chest pressure, shortness of breath, and wheezing precipitated by exercise. Use of a bronchodilator in the form of an inhaler immediately before exercising can often prevent these symptoms and allow women to continue their exercise programs throughout pregnancy.

Even if you have no history of medical problems, it is important that you stop all exercise and consult your doctor if physical activity precipitates chest pain, dizziness, shortness of breath, palpitations, faintness, severe abdominal or pelvic pain, or extreme pain on walking. While a full discussion of the multitude of medical problems is beyond the scope of this chapter, it is important to remember that many diseases are altered in their severity by the hormonal changes of pregnancy. Conditions which have been inactive for many years may suddenly recur with greater severity, while other diseases such as arthritis may dramatically improve, thereby allowing a greater degree of physical activity.

Obstetrical complications may also dictate that physical activity be limited. Women with a history of three or more spontaneous abortions, a previous precipitous delivery, or the birth of a premature infant or one suffering from intrauterine growth retardation (IUGR) should avoid physical activity. Similarly, if the present pregnancy is complicated by premature rupture of the membranes or premature contractions requiring medication, rest is more beneficial than exercise. If a baby is found to be lying in an abnormal position, such as a breech or transverse lie, during the last month of pregnancy, exercise should be curtailed. Vaginal bleeding during the second half of pregnancy may indicate the presence of a low-lying placenta or a premature separation of the placenta. Under these circumstances, physical activity should be severely restricted. Hypertension which specifically occurs during pregnancy is called preeclampsia. Preeclamptic women do best on bedrest and careful medical supervision. Occasionally, the medications used to treat preeclampsia may be associated with dizziness and loss of balance.

Though exercise in the presence of a threatened abortion during the first three months of pregnancy is unlikely to precipitate a spontaneous abortion, this may not be the case after the third month if a woman has an incompetent cervix. Exercise of any type must be avoided both before and after corrective surgery is performed on the cervix. Women carrying twins must curtail their physical activities throughout pregnancy, since the size and excessive weight of the uterus tends to be much greater than that found with singleton births, resulting in a higher incidence of cervical incompetence. Weakening of the ligaments which support the uterus may occasionally cause it to prolapse, or drop. This situation is more likely to occur among women who have carried previous pregnancies. The cervix may actually protrude through the vaginal opening and require a pessary device to reposition it and support the uterus. Women with a significant degree of uterine prolapse should not engage in physical activity during pregnancy.

What effect does exercising have on laboratory tests?

Several important laboratory blood tests may be temporarily altered following vigorous exercise. These abnormal values will usually return to normal within 48 hours. Elevation of three important enzymes in the blood, known as LDH, SGOT, and CPK, are extremely helpful in the diagnosis of a wide variety of diseases. All are extremely high immediately following vigorous exercise. The abundance of circulating progesterone is believed to be responsible for causing pregnant women to breath more rapidly and more deeply. As a result, carbon dioxide levels tend to decline. This effect is enhanced even further when a woman's respiratory rate increases during exercise. Blood glucose, or sugar, values decline even with moderate degrees of exercise. Although the hormonal changes of pregnancy often precipitate abnormal glucose metabolism among certain susceptible women, pregnant women paradoxically experience lower fasting blood glucose levels than nonpregnant women. As a result, exercising on an empty stomach may cause blood glucose levels to drop drastically and cause symptoms of hypoglycemia, or low blood sugar. For this reason it is best that pregnant women eat within 6 hours of exercising in order to maintain adequate amounts of circulating glucose.

Measurements of uric acid in the blood aid in the diagnosis and management of preeclampsia (pregnancy-induced hypertension) during the last trimester of pregnancy. However, intense physical activity can cause uric acid levels to rise. To further confuse the issue, exercise will slightly elevate the systolic (upper) blood pressure reading, a finding also noted in preeclampsia. Another exercise-associated change is a lowering of the hemoglobin, or red blood cell mass. This occurs because there is an increase in the plasma volume in relation to the number of red blood cells. As a result, a doctor may be given a false impression that a pregnant athlete is anemic even though her actual number of red blood cells has not decreased. Testosterone, cortisol, and prolactin are three important hormones which, when measured immediately after running, have been found to be high. When measured after a rest period of 12 hours, however, their levels all return to normal pregnancy limits. The same affect has been observed for serum triglyceride levels.

What is hematuria, and how does it relate to physical exertion?

Hematuria is an abnormal condition in which red blood cells are present in the urine. With many blood cells the urine will turn red. If only a few cells are present, it will remain a clear yellow color, but the red blood cells can still be detected by simple microscopic urinalysis. In addition, rapid urinary screening tests for protein will be positive in the presence of red blood cells. Although doctors are taught in medical school that the presence of red blood cells in the urine often indicates a serious disease of the urinary tract such as stones, infection, or even malignancy, exercise-related hematuria is a frequent and benign condition. If you are a jogger and your urine test is positive for red blood cells or protein shortly after running, ask your obstetrician to retest your urine 48 or more hours later.

 ## *LIMITATIONS AND PRECAUTIONS*

To what types of bone, joint, and muscle injuries is the pregnant athlete most susceptible?

The pregnant athlete experiences the same types of orthopedic injuries as the nonpregnant woman. However, the likelihood of injury is greater because a hormone named relaxin is produced in progressively greater amounts as pregnancy advances. Relaxin does just what its name implies—it relaxes and softens the ligaments in every joint of the body, making them less stable and predisposing joints, muscles, and bones to injury and dislocation. The ligaments most likely to be affected by relaxin are those of the pelvis and the sacroiliac joint of the lower back, but the knee joint is particularly vulnerable to serious injury and dislocation during athletic pursuits. Sports requiring

sudden stops and change in direction, such as squash and racquetball, are most likely to result in knee injuries.

The pubic symphysis bone is actually composed of two separate bones joined together in the midline of the pubic area by a strong ligament. Under the influence of relaxin during pregnancy, this ligament becomes so soft and unstable that the two bones actually separate considerably. This phenomenon has a desirable effect for most women because it increases the dimensions of the bony pelvis and allows more room for the passage of the baby during childbirth. However, a woman with a marked degree of this so-called symphyseal separation will experience severe pain and can actually feel the movement of the two bones when walking or doing any exercise involving movement of the legs. Often the pain is so severe that it limits or eliminates all activity during the last trimester.

Among the many important skeletal and muscular changes that a pregnant woman must adjust to while participating in sports is her constantly changing center of gravity as her weight increases and her abdominal girth enlarges. This in turn alters her stride, posture, and athletic capabilities, creating a predisposition to injuries of the lower back, hips, and knees. Dexterity in sports requiring balance, such as gymnastics and skiing, declines considerably after the fifth month of pregnancy, increasing the likelihood of a fall. When these changes become pronounced it is probably wise to decrease one's activities or switch to nongravitational aerobic pursuits such as swimming and biking.

Lumbar lordosis is a forward curvature of the spine which tends to increase in degree as the uterus enlarges in size. The severity of this condition is often determined by the amount of circulating relaxin. Lordosis often puts excessive strain on a woman's back muscles so that it occasionally becomes necessary for her to reduce all activities requiring sudden forward movement. This strain on posture usually begins at about the fifth month and is always noticeable by the seventh month. Lumbar lordosis is also responsible for causing meralgia, or pain, tingling, and numbness in the area of the outer thigh caused by stretching of a nerve named the external femoral cutaneous nerve. This extremely common and annoying condition usually appears during the second half of pregnancy, is always aggravated by standing, and is relieved by lying flat. Postural changes are also believed responsible for intercostal pain, or pain between the ribs, during pregnancy. Pinpoint pain directly on the rib at a point to either side of the breastbone can usually be attributed to softening of the tissues at the junction where the bone of the rib joins the cartilage.

According to a 1988 study from Sweden, back pain in varying degrees affects approximately one-half of all pregnant women. The cause in two-thirds of these sufferers was found to be dysfunction of the sacroiliac joints in the lower back, often precipitated by strenuous work involving excessive bending or by lifting while turning at the same time. Pain that is present deep in the buttocks rather than in the back is frequently an indication of a low-back ailment known as sciatica, caused by a swelling or displacement of a lower vertebral disc. The diagnosis is a virtual certainty if the pain radiates from the buttocks down to the back of the leg, following the path of the pinched sciatic nerve. Sciatica is likely to occur in association with the postural changes which take place during the second half of pregnancy; symptoms are often precipitated by activities such as running, lifting, and deep bending. Treatment during pregnancy consists of bedrest on a firm to hard surface, analgesics, and anti-inflammatory drugs, some of which must be used with great caution during pregnancy (see Chapter 9). When pain persists despite these measures, a consultation with an orthopedic surgeon is often necessary.

The term "overuse injury" refers to minor areas of inflammation which develop by repetitive motion of a tendon or muscle. Achilles tendinitis and plantar fasciitis cause pain and inflammation to the Achilles tendon and heel of the foot, respectively. Both are the result of exercises that require repetitive pounding or jumping on a hard surface, such as aerobic dancing, running, and jumping rope. These injuries are more likely to occur during pregnancy because of the added weight pressing down on the legs and feet. The ultimate manifestation of an overuse injury is a stress or fatigue fracture caused by repeated insult to the weight-bearing bones, such as the metatarsals of the feet, the pelvis, and the tibia and fibula, the two bones of the lower leg. Stress fractures create a thin break in the bone without separation of the fragments, so that the diagnosis is not always readily apparent on x-ray. Pelvic stress fractures appear to be more common among nonpregnant women runners than male runners. However, there is no scientific evidence to support the belief of most orthopedists that high levels of weight-bearing exercise will increase the likelihood of stress fractures during pregnancy. There is also little if any evidence to support the claim that healing of stress fractures is delayed during pregnancy.

What are some general guidelines that a pregnant woman can follow to decrease her risk of bone and joint injuries during aerobic exercise?

Aerobic exercise such as jogging, running, aerobic dancing, bicycling, swimming, and walking improve cardiovascular fitness and stamina and provide a physiologic energy reserve for the tremendous exertional demands of labor and delivery. To reduce the risk of injury, dislocation, and stress fractures to the ankles, knees, legs, and pelvis associated with impact activities such as aerobic dancing and running it is best that exercise routines involving foot impacts be limited to 30 minutes in duration. In addition, to prevent overuse injuries you should take one day of rest between identical forms of exercise. A non-weight-bearing aerobic activity such as bicycling or swimming would appear to be a far safer alternative during the second half of pregnancy. If you plan to continue impact aerobic activities throughout pregnancy, it is best to do so on a resilient floor, making sure to modify your exercise routine by shortening your stride and keeping your feet close to the floor throughout your exercise program. To reduce the severity of impact shock to the lower extremities, repetitive jumping on the same foot should not exceed four consecutive jumps.

Shoes for running, jogging, and walking should have good cushioning under the heel, since this is the site of greatest impact and the cause of two common injuries known as plantar fasciitis and Achilles tendinitis (see page 78). Shoes specifically designed for walking are different than running shoes in that they are not as stiff in the soles, the sides are not as strongly reinforced, the back of the shoe is not as high, and they require less shock-absorbing padding in the heel. Orthotics and other heel-cushioning and elevating devices inserted into exercise shoes often help provide shock absorption and prevent these injuries. In aerobic dancing, most impact is on the balls of the feet, so shoes for this activity should have good cushioning in that location. Shoes worn for aerobic dancing and calisthenics should have a relatively smooth tread to avoid abrupt halts when the feet strike the floor.

Aerobic exercise should be preceded by a gentle warm-up routine that utilizes the full range of motion of the joints. Muscles that are used repeatedly during aerobic exercises must be carefully stretched before and after each exercise session. Aerobic activity should always be followed by a cool-down period of lighter exercise. Many orthopedic injuries occur among women who exercise faithfully for a time, stop for a while, and then try to restart at their previous level of intensity. When restarting, always begin at a lower level and increase your intensity and length of each session slowly.

For every muscle involved in a physical activity, an antagonistic muscle acts in exactly the opposite manner. Many athletic injuries occur because of an imbalance in strength between antagonistic muscles, with forceful contractions of the stronger one subjecting the weaker muscle to the risk of injury. To prevent this problem, exercise programs should be designed so that no muscle group is strengthened disproportionately to its antagonist. A classic example of two antagonistic muscles is that of the large quadriceps muscle group in the front of the thigh and the hamstrings in the back of the thigh. It is not uncommon for athletes with overly developed and powerful quadriceps to experience painful and incapacitating injuries to their weaker hamstring muscles. Specific exercises to strengthen hamstrings are helpful in preventing this serious injury (see the exercises at the end of this chapter).

To avoid knee problems, don't do exercises that overflex or overextend the knee joint. Deep knee-bends and squatting should be avoided. When using a stationary bicycle, adjust the seat to its proper height. To do this, sit on the bicycle with one leg fully extended. When the height of the seat is correct, your heel should drop approximately 2 inches below the level of the pedal.

Certain relaxin-induced orthopedic changes are inevitable during pregnancy; but if you consciously try to maintain good posture and avoid excessive drooping of the shoulders, you may be able to decrease the severity of symptoms caused by tension on the brachial plexus (see page 97). Similarly, efforts to resist excessive degrees of lumbar lordosis (see page 78) will often be rewarded by fewer symptoms of pain and numbness of the anterior thigh. Often, bedrest is the only treatment that can be offered to women with pain caused by symphyseal separation. Occasionally, use of a tight girdle will limit movement of the bones and relieve the discomfort. Aerobic activities most likely to precipitate sciatica are those that involve rotation of the upper body while standing with your hips and lower spine flexed. The best prevention against sciatic nerve pain is strengthening exercises of the abdominal muscles, which are the antagonists of those which run along the back of the spine.

Aside from orthopedic limitations, how do other bodily changes of pregnancy limit a woman's ability to participate in exercise?

Though physical fitness fanatics are quick to point out that Evonne Goolagong Cawley played tennis professionally through her fourth month, that skier Andrea Mead Laurence won two gold medals in alpine racing at the 1952 Winter Olympics while three months pregnant, and that May Jones successfully ran 13 miles in her ninth month of pregnancy, these events are certainly unusual phenomena that need not be emulated by even the most enthusiastic or skilled pregnant athlete. In fact, interviews with 1984 and 1988 Olympians Evelyn Ashford and Mary Decker Slaney reveal a far more conservative approach to exercise during pregnancy. Ms. Ashford abruptly stopped her usual training program of sprints and road workouts during her fifth month when, as she puts it, "the baby starts letting you know it's in there." Similarly,

Ms. Slaney, whose exercise program was carefully monitored throughout her pregnancy, slowed down markedly during her seventh month when she experienced abdominal pains precipitated by exercise. Physical activity should be a part of every pregnancy, but it is important to understand the natural bodily changes which limit optimal performance. Knowing these physiological changes and adjusting for them in your daily exercise is far more rational than denying their presence while trying to achieve unrealistic and potentially harmful goals.

The most important changes during pregnancy involve the heart and circulation. The amount of work performed by the heart increases during the first trimester. This is reflected in your resting pulse rate, which typically increases about 10 to 15 beats per minute during pregnancy. Take this fact into account when measuring your pulse rate in response to vigorous exercise. Ninety percent of all women develop a slight heart murmur during pregnancy as a result of the greater circulatory load. This is harmless and subsides soon after delivery. During pregnancy, there is a greater tendency for circulating blood to pool or stagnate in small, peripheral blood vessels. As a result, sudden shifts in head position may not allow adequate time for oxygen-carrying blood to reach the brain, and you may experience sudden lightheadedness and dizziness.

It is now firmly established that when a pregnant woman lies on her back during the last four months of pregnancy, the enlarging uterus flops back and compresses the veins that return blood from the lower half of the body. This hindrance of blood return to the heart may result in a dangerous lowering of the blood pressure. Therefore, during the last four months of pregnancy and during labor as well, you should not rest or perform exercises for long periods of time on your back. It is much better to lie on your left side. This position takes the weight from the enlarged uterus off the vena cava, the major vein carrying blood to the heart from the pelvis and lower extremities.

The pressure in the veins of the legs increases at least threefold during pregnancy. The tendency toward stagnation of blood in the lower extremities throughout the latter part of pregnancy is entirely the result of the pressure of the enlarged uterus on the pelvic veins. This is of great importance since it contributes to the ankle edema, or swelling, frequently experienced by a woman as she approaches the end of her pregnancy. It is also responsible for the development of varicose veins in the legs and vulva, as well as enlargement of the hemorrhoidal veins during gestation. Of course, women vary a great deal in their susceptibility to these problems.

Respiratory changes occur early in pregnancy and are often felt as a shortness of breath or increased awareness of a desire to breathe. This increased respiratory effort is believed to result from the stimulation of the respiratory center in the brain by the hormone progesterone. The slight increase in respiratory rate is associated with a greater amount of work performed by the respiratory muscles. During the last two months of pregnancy, breathing may be more difficult because the enlarging uterus, which elevates the diaphragm and limits lung expansion.

The pressure of the enlarging uterus on the urinary bladder may cause involuntary and frequent urination during pregnancy. This is most common during the first 12 weeks of pregnancy. The problem disappears after the third month but then reappears when the fetal head descends into the maternal pelvis during the last month of pregnancy. It is unfortunate that many books dealing with physical fitness and pregnancy rarely mention this embarrassing physiological condition which may deter active sports participation. Wearing a sanitary pad while exercising should make this problem manageable.

Breast tissue is markedly altered by hormonal changes. While the pregnant athlete should take particular care to protect her breasts, the fear of breast trauma generally far exceeds the actual incidence of serious injury. A pregnant woman's breasts are heavier and more glandular, and re-

quire a greater degree of support even during minimal amounts of exercise. Specially designed bras provide the extra support. Irritation of the nipples commonly occurs in runners due to the friction created by a shirt against the nipple. This condition, known as jogger's nipples, may produce redness and bleeding and create a real problem as the nipples enlarge during pregnancy. It may be alleviated by wearing a specially designed runner's bra and adhesive strip bandages or a nursing bra while running. Coating the nipples with petrolatum or lanolin or applying protective dressings and wearing shirts with satin-like finishes, such as those made of synthetic fabrics, should also reduce the irritation.

If you experience uterine or urinary bladder prolapse following childbirth, be assured that it was caused by your beautiful child and not by your activity levels. Whether or not you will develop prolapse is determined by the inherent strength of your connective tissues and muscles which support your uterus and bladder. There are many women with five or more children who have better pelvic support than others who have had only one child. Your genetic inheritance is an important aspect of this condition—if your mother experienced prolapse associated with childbirth, there is a good chance that you will too.

Edema, or swelling of the ankles and the feet, is a normal physiological occurrence of pregnancy created by pressure on the veins of the lower extremities by the enlarging uterus and is more likely to occur during warm weather. Diuretics should rarely be used as treatment for ankle edema during pregnancy and are mentioned only to be discouraged. A guaranteed decrease of ankle edema can be accomplished by lying in bed for 24 hours on the left side with your legs elevated. This has the effect of displacing the uterus from the pelvic veins which carry blood from the legs. This treatment may have to be repeated every few days, but it is far better than taking diuretics.

The combination of excessive exercise and perspiration and intense humidity predisposes the pregnant woman to annoying monilia vaginal infections, which are easily treated with one of many medications. "Jock itch," a rash in the genital area caused by a superficial skin fungus and most likely to occur under conditions favoring an increase in moisture, was formerly believed to occur only in the male athlete. However, gynecologists often see this condition in their physically active patients. The incidence of "jock itch" can be reduced by wearing cotton undergarments and loose-fitting jogging shorts and avoiding exercising under extremely humid conditions. Taking prolonged hot baths also increases moisture in the genital area and should be avoided. Athlete's foot is caused by a superficial skin fungus which invades the skin surface between the toes and causes severe itching, burning, cracking of the skin, and oozing. In order for the fungus to reproduce, the skin must provide a warm and moist environment. The best method of treating athlete's foot is to provide a hostile environment for fungal growth. This is best achieved by keeping the feet cool and dry and avoiding nylon and other synthetics that make you sweat. Most of the many over-the-counter antifungal medications available work remarkably well in both preventing and treating athlete's foot. All can be safely used in the prevention and treatment of athlete's foot during pregnancy without fear of harmful fetal effects.

Although there are no known detrimental effects of cold weather on exercise during pregnancy, high-altitude sports participation may be associated with decreased oxygenation of the fetus and result in the birth of a smaller baby (a discussion of potentially dangerous high-altitude travel and airline trips occurs in Chapter 7 on pages 200–203). A black woman with sickle cell trait may be most in jeopardy at these higher altitudes.

Are there any hazards associated with strength training during pregnancy?

Very few subjects have aroused as much obstetrical controversy in recent years as the advisability of strength training during pregnancy. The prevailing opinion until now has been that strength training is an extremely hazardous form of exercise because it forces women to repeatedly use the Valsalva maneuver in overcoming weight resistance. With this maneuver, air is forceably exhaled in a grunting fashion while the mouth is closed. This has the effect of diverting blood away from the abdominal organs, uterus, and fetus in favor of the working muscles. In contrast to this opinion, Dr. Mona M. Shangold, Director of Sports Gynecology at Georgetown University School of Medicine, firmly believes that these supposed dangers are more imagined than real. She states, "I recommend that pregnant women, regardless of their prior exercise habits, be encouraged to lift weights. Weight lifting strengthens muscles, making women less susceptible to a number of muscular aches and pains that are very common during pregnancy. These aches and pains are probably due to weak muscles that are unable to carry the added weight of pregnancy; especially when affected by the altered center of gravity. Back pain is extremely common among pregnant women. We should encourage women to participate in resistance training programs to strengthen their muscles." Dr. Shangold also believes that the added strength achieved through weight training will help women to more easily endure labor and delivery.

Most experts agree that pregnant women should undertake strength training only under careful supervision, since unsupervised training could cause severe muscle and joint injuries and aggravate lumbar lordosis, disc problems, and other relaxin-induced conditions. Exercises which progressively strengthen the rectus abdominus, the long muscle that passes from the breast bone to the pubic symphysis, will have a positive effect in limiting the degree of pregnancy-induced lordosis and reducing the likelihood of vertebral disc injuries of the lower back. Strengthening of the quadriceps muscle group in the front of the thigh, while also stretching the antagonist hamstrings, can be carried out right through the last trimester, as can exercises which strengthen the lower back.

The American College of Obstetricians and Gynecologists has established some excellent guidelines for strengthening exercises. These general rules would apply to both pregnant and nonpregnant women and should be carefully followed:

- Strengthening exercises should not be performed on the same muscles on consecutive days.
- A general warm-up routine should be performed before muscles are made to work against resistance.
- Muscle strengthening exercises should be preceded and followed by stretching exercises that are specific for the muscles that are made to work against resistance.
- All strengthening exercises should be performed in a slow and controlled manner. Rapid and jerky movements increase the risk of injury.
- The most efficient way to improve strength is to allow brief rest periods between vigorous exercise sessions. Repetitions of a strength exercise should be limited to short sets (ten or less) that are repeated later.
- Weaker antagonist muscles should be strengthened to restore balance around the joint.

What sports should be avoided during pregnancy?

Definite hazards are associated with water skiing, a sport that is best avoided. There are several reports in the medical literature of severe vulvar and vaginal lacerations and hematomas (collections of blood) caused by a direct blow from a water ski. In addition, falling into the water at high speeds while skiing has resulted, on rare occasions, in water rapidly entering through the vagina and cervix and into the uterus and fallopian tubes. Spillage of this water into the pelvis has caused peritonitis or abdominal infection. Furthermore, there is a documented case in the medical literature of an early miscarriage occurring shortly after an involuntary vaginal douche while water skiing. Inadvertent water enemas resulting from a fall while water skiing are fairly common, though this rarely causes more than moderate discomfort. However, perforation of the bowel from this type of accident has been described. The standard swimsuits worn by the majority of water skiers allow water at high pressure to reach the vulva and enter the rectum and vagina. If you plan to water ski despite advice to the contrary, it would be much safer to wear a rubber wet suit or rubber pants rather than a standard swimsuit. The same precautions should be taken for surfing, windsurfing, and high-board diving, all of which can generate high speeds at impact with the water.

Scuba diving has gained great popularity, and many women today are engaged in sport, military, commercial, and scientific diving. However, most experts in the field of diving medicine agree that pregnancy is not the time to learn how to scuba dive. The question as to whether or not it is safe to continue to scuba dive during pregnancy is unanswered at the present time, but one animal study suggests that scuba diving may be potentially hazardous to the fetus and that diving during pregnancy should be avoided. If you insist on diving, avoid depths greater than 60 feet and spend only a short amount of time on the bottom.

Horseback riding is another sport that should probably be avoided throughout pregnancy. There are no objective studies to prove that the bouncing movement of a horse is detrimental to the well-protected fetus, but, aside from the obvious dangers of falling, the pregnant equestrienne may be more prone to tenosynovitis (inflammation of the tendon and joint attachment) of the muscle in the inner thigh called the adductor longus that is attached to the pubic symphysis bone. Symptoms of inflammation are vulvar pain and tenderness. This condition is the most common pelvic complaint among nonpregnant riders. It hurts more during pregnancy because of the increased softening of the ligaments, which causes greater movement of the two halves of the pubic bone. Any activity that involves the Valsalva maneuver (in which air is forceably exhaled in a grunting fashion while the mouth is closed) may divert blood from the abdominal organs to the working muscles and theoretically decrease the amount of oxygen reaching the fetus. It has been said, but never scientifically proven, that English style of riding, which requires forceful muscular contractions of the thigh, may not be as safe in this regard as the more passive and relaxed Western style of riding.

Data collected from the athletic departments of several colleges indicate that of the many sports in which women participate, the greatest number and variety of injuries occur in basketball, followed closely by volleyball and gymnastics. In 1987, the National Athletic Trainers' Association conducted a survey of 400,000 girls playing high school basketball. Amazingly, 23 percent had been injured at least once, and of the 22 injuries requiring surgical repair, 18 were knee-related. The sports which produce the most serious injuries, including major fractures, head injuries, and dislocations, are basketball, field hockey, softball, and gymnastics. Participation in these sports with any degree of intensity would appear to be a foolish endeavor during pregnancy.

As your pregnancy progresses into the last trimester, your increasing weight, diminished coordination, the shift in your center of gravity, and the softening of your joints and ligaments should serve as ample evidence that it's time to switch from weight-bearing endeavors, such as running and jogging, to non-weight-bearing sports such as swimming and cycling. High-impact exercises such as aerobic dancing and jumping rope are especially likely to cause foot, ankle, and knee injuries, and are best abandoned. In addition, racquet sports which incur a risk of lateral movement injuries to the ankles and knees should be stopped during the last trimester. If you play indoor handball, paddleball, or racquetball during the first trimester, be aware of the fact that these courts are rarely well ventilated and pose a threat of hyperthermia (see page 70).

EXERCISES AND SPORTS FOR THE PREGNANT WOMAN

How do specific sports affect a pregnancy?

Cross-country skiing can be an invigorating aerobic exercise for the pregnant woman. If you are an accomplished downhill skier, participate on a slope which is one step below your normal level; in other words, if you are an expert skier, you should ski at an intermediate level or lower. Many accidents occur on icy terrain, so it is best to ski only under optimal conditions. Many skiing accidents result from collisions; try to do most of your skiing on weekdays when the mountain is likely to be less populated. Avoid rapid changes in head position, which may cause dizziness. Because skiing at high altitudes may decrease the oxygen supply to the fetus, stay below 7,000 feet above sea level (see Chapter 7).

Ice skating, roller skating, and roller blading should present no problems if you are an accomplished skater, although changes in your body's center of gravity can hinder your balance. It is a good idea to wear heavy clothing as a buffer against falls. Ankle and foot edema combined with the greater ligament relaxation of pregnancy will make you more susceptible to injuring your ankle or knee. For this reason, it is best not to learn to skate or roller blade during pregnancy.

Bowling, volleyball, and softball are sports which offer little in the way of aerobic benefits. Nevertheless, they are popular and safe activities for the pregnant woman. The continuous jumping in volleyball may precipitate joint and ligament injuries.

Although the walking involved in golf is excellent exercise, don't expect to improve your golf swing during pregnancy. Many pregnant golfers actually have to drastically flatten their swing after the fifth month in order to compensate for their increasing abdominal enlargement. It is important to play golf in loose, comfortable clothing and to avoid playing on very hot and humid days.

The racquet sports of squash and racquetball provide excellent aerobic activity for the pregnant woman. If singles competition is too exhausting, you may want to play squash doubles, paddle tennis, or regular tennis doubles. Singles tennis provides far greater exercise than doubles, but it also requires first-rate physical conditioning. After the fifth month of pregnancy, I advise my patients to limit their tennis to doubles and abandon squash and racquetball because the physiological changes of pregnancy are more apt to precipitate knee, ankle, and foot injuries following lateral movements, sudden stops, and changes in direction.

Contact sports carry a remote risk of uterine trauma and placental separation following a powerful blow to the abdomen. This can happen only after the first trimester, when the uterus rises above the pubic symphysis bone.

Although the maternal and fetal consequences of long-distance and marathon running remain unknown, most sports medicine experts agree that exercise to the point of hyperthermia, or greatly elevated body temperatures, in any sport during the first trimester may cause birth defects (see page 70). Also, strenuous running programs late in pregnancy may lead to a significant shifting of blood from the uterus to the leg muscles. This in turn may decrease the amount of oxygen carried to the placenta. Although such changes are unlikely to affect a healthy baby, they may cause significant distress for a previously compromised infant. Finally, as previously mentioned, a woman's greater weight and joint laxity make running during the last trimester a less than attractive exercise option.

What sports and physical activities provide the best exercise for the pregnant woman?

There is ample evidence to show that the circulatory and respiratory systems are best served by participation in aerobic exercises. Aerobics literally means "with oxygen," and aerobic exercises are those which are most likely to bring in oxygen and deliver it to the muscles and tissue cells, where it is combined with foodstuffs to produce energy. Aerobic exercises benefit your cardiorespiratory system because you're able to take in more air with less effort and your heart becomes stronger because it is able to pump more blood with fewer strokes. It also provides a physiologic reserve for emergencies such as labor and delivery.

Aerobic exercises include walking, jogging, running, cycling, swimming, and cross-country skiing, all sports that utilize the whole body in rhythmic and continuous movement. Swimming and cycling are the best because they are weight-independent, meaning that by performing the exercise you do not have to support your body weight. On the other hand, weight-dependent exercises, such as walking and jogging, require that the body weight be supported and therefore require greater effort to do the same amount of work as pregnancy progresses. Walking on level ground at a comfortable pace will not significantly improve your aerobic fitness. In order to gain significant cardiorespiratory benefits it is necessary to walk at a brisk pace over terrain that has hills and inclines. Carrying a small amount of weight in your hands or in a backpack will also help to develop your aerobic fitness.

Exercise machines specifically designed to improve aerobic fitness have gained great popularity in recent years. Cross-country ski machines exercise virtually every major muscle group, put minimal if any stress on the body, and can be used with safety throughout pregnancy. Stationary bicycles are also very popular, although some women find that their large abdominal girth in the last trimester makes this activity more difficult. Be sure that the bicycle seat is of the proper height. With your leg fully extended, your heel should drop about 2 inches below the level of the pedal. Treadmills offer excellent aerobic exercise because they can be adjusted for walking, jogging, or running, and some can be placed at various angles of incline. Although padding on a treadmill and the wearing of proper shoes will help to reduce injuries caused by repetitive pounding to the knees, ankles, and feet, it is best to allow a day of rest between each treadmill session.

Stair-climbing machines, which have the advantage of enhancing aerobic capacity without causing impact injuries to the feet and ankles, can be used safely and effectively throughout pregnancy. Rowing machines involve many muscle groups, including those of the abdomen, arms, shoulders, lower and upper back, buttocks, and legs. While some experts endorse rowing machines as an excellent form of exercise for the pregnant woman, others have claimed that they are unadaptable for use during the third trimester because a woman's knees and thighs tend to bang into her abdomen. There is also disagreement as to whether or not use of a rowing machine strengthens weak back muscles or increases a woman's susceptibility to back injuries. If you have preexisting back pain, you should not use a rowing machine. To minimize the risk of injury it is important to adjust the rowing machine for correct seating and to position your arms so you aren't leaning too far forward at the beginning of a stroke, thus placing too much strain on your back. The foot rest should be set to avoid overextending the feet and Achilles tendons.

In a 1990 study, researchers from California and New York evaluated the effect of five commercially available aerobic exercise machines on uterine contractions during the third trimester of pregnancy. At equivalent work loads, the stationary bicycle lead to uterine contractions in 50 percent of the exercise sessions, the treadmill in 40 percent, the rowing machine in 10 percent, and the recumbent bicycle and upper arm ergometer in 0 percent. The authors of this study concluded that

the two latter aerobic machines would appear to be safest, especially among individuals at risk for premature labor contractions.

Free weights and multigym equipment, with trade names such as Nautilus, Keiser, Solo-flex, Universal, Polaris, David, and Eagle, are found in most health clubs and some private homes. While all of these machines help to build strength by exercising various muscle groups, they do little to increase aerobic capacity. If you are a novice, it is best to learn the proper use of these machines under the guidance and supervision of a knowledgeable trainer.

Participant sports such as golf, tennis, volleyball, and bowling offer minimal aerobic benefits. Isometrics, weight lifting, and most calisthenics improve strength and flexibility but are aerobically the least beneficial. Many excellent aerobic dancing programs and videotapes have been developed for use during pregnancy. Unfortunately the repeated impact of the balls of the feet against unyielding floor surfaces may predispose the pregnant woman to foot injuries during the second half of pregnancy.

All exercise burns calories. The approximate number of calories expended per hour is often a good indication of the aerobic demands of a particular activity. Table 7 lists the approximate number of calories expended per hour of various activities.

What should I wear in order to be most comfortable and avoid injury while exercising?

Since foot and ankle injuries are more likely to occur while exercising during pregnancy, it is very important to select well-cushioned, properly fitting shoes. Instead of running in an old pair of tennis shoes, buy shoes specifically designed for the activity you intend to pursue.

Properly fitting support stockings and pantyhose are helpful in reducing edema (swelling) of the feet and ankles and in preventing pooling of blood in the varicose veins of the legs. Parke Davis, a drug

TABLE 7

CALORIES EXPENDED PER HOUR FOR VARIOUS ACTIVITIES

Activity	Approximate Number of Calories Used per Hour
Aerobic dancing	660
Jogging	660
Bicycling (13 mph)	660
Bicycling (6 mph)	240
Swimming	300–660
Handball/Squash/Paddle ball	480–600
Tennis singles	500
Tennis doubles	300
Brisk walking (4 mph)	300–360
Slow walking (2 mph)	200–240
Bowling	240
Golf	240
Ballroom dancing	340
Ballet/Disco dancing	420
Downhill skiing	480
Cross-country skiing	660
Jumping rope	660
Rowing	660
Basketball	660
Heavy housework	250

company, sells a variety of good maternity support pantyhose and stockings. These may be purchased either at pharmacies or surgical supply stores, while more fashionable maternity stockings and leotards are available at most department stores. Jobst stockings, which must be fitted to the exact contour of your legs, give better support than any other stocking. They are available in knee-length, thigh-length, and pantyhose styles.

To help prevent "jock itch" caused by a superficial fungus, and vaginitis and vulvitis caused by monilia (see Chapter 6), the physically active woman should wear cotton panties having cotton inserts. To prevent athlete's foot it is best to wear cotton socks while exercising.

Because of the hormonal changes which take place in the breast during pregnancy, a bra with good support is essential. Studies have demonstrated that standard bras are inadequate for the needs of women athletes, especially those who are pregnant. American manufacturers have recently introduced a variety of brands of "sport bras" that provide extra support. Select one that is fairly rigid so that it limits breast motion but does not bind.

What are some of the benefits of walking during pregnancy?

Although we usually don't think of walking as an exercise, it is an excellent way of promoting physical fitness without risking the injuries which may occur with running and jogging. Walking puts far less stress on vulnerable joints. In fact, each running step subjects the joints to a stress three to five times the weight of your body, while the load with walking is only one and one-half times your body weight with each step. As a result, injuries are relatively rare. Studies show that some of the many benefits of walking include a reduction in anxiety and depression, lower cholesterol levels, stronger bones and muscles, and enhanced cardiovascular fitness. Walking is especially suitable for pregnant women who are not athletic, are overweight, or are accustomed to a sedentary lifestyle. When practiced at regular intervals of every other day, it can prevent the gaining of excessive weight during pregnancy. On the average, a 3-mile walk in an hour's time by a 160-pound woman uses up about 285 calories. The same activity by a 120-pound woman uses about 215 calories. For women of average weight, a slow walk of 2 miles per hour will burn approximately 200 to 240 calories, while a brisk walk of 4 miles in an hour will use between 300 and 360 calories. In a 1980 report, doctors at Tel Aviv University Medical School observed a significant improvement in physical fitness within three to four weeks when their patients walked half an hour a day, five days a week, at a pace of 3 miles an hour while carrying a 6½-pound load during their walk.

If you are in less than ideal physical condition and are considering walking as an exercise during pregnancy, be sure to start slowly. You can begin with a 2-mile-an-hour pace for 20 minutes and gradually work your way up to a pace of 3 or 4 miles an hour for at least half an hour at a time. To achieve maximum aerobic benefits, you must walk purposefully, rather than stroll, and you should exert yourself enough to increase your heart rate to at least 130 beats per minute. Walking up and down gentle slopes or tilting a treadmill on a 7 percent incline will further help to challenge your aerobic capacity. It is best, however, to avoid steep grades. Fitness can also be enhanced if you walk with small weights in your hands or if you carry a backpack, shopping bag, or briefcase weighing 6 to 13 pounds.

How can I treat leg cramps which develop during exercise?

During the sixth and seventh months of pregnancy, as many as 30 percent of all women experience leg cramps. A cramp often appears as an acutely painful and visible knot or bulge in a mus-

cle which may last for several seconds or minutes. While intense exercise of an untrained muscle is most likely to precipitate cramps, they may also appear in physically fit individuals and in persons at rest. Women with a history of muscle cramping prior to pregnancy are more prone to experience the condition with greater intensity during pregnancy. For unknown reasons, if muscle cramps remain untreated, they will subside on their own in 50 percent of all cases within four to six weeks of delivery. Any muscle may cramp with exercise, but the calf appears to be the most common site.

The cause of muscle cramps during pregnancy remains unknown, but most researchers blame a relative lack of total serum calcium. The traditional and often successful medical therapy to correct this problem is dietary supplementation with calcium carbonate or calcium gluconate, 1.5 to 2 grams per day. (Quantities of milk in excess of 1 quart per day combined with calcium phosphate as a supplement will actually provoke muscle cramps.) Other remedies for muscle cramps, such as quinine sulfate and phenytoin (trade name Dilantin), are best avoided during pregnancy.

 ## WATER EXERCISES

What advice do you have for participation in water sports during pregnancy?

Regardless of your level of ability, you will derive great benefit from the positive aerobic effects of swimming during pregnancy. In doing laps in a pool, it is important to pace yourself and to do them slowly and without exertion to the point of exhaustion. Several minutes of stretching and toning exercises in the water before swimming laps are thought to provide an excellent treatment for edema (swelling) of the legs, because the pressure of the water forces fluid from the tissues into the veins which carry blood to the heart. Even if you are a nonswimmer or a very poor swimmer, you

can still participate in the prenatal water exercise classes offered by many YMCAs or YWCAs. All these exercises are simple and cause no undue stress to muscles, tendons, or ligaments. In the water, the body's buoyancy makes exercise less difficult than on land. In addition, the body's weight in water is only 10 percent of its true weight. Below is an outline of the prenatal swimming exercise program offered at the Westport, Connecticut, YMCA and other health facilities. A water exercise workout takes 30 to 45 minutes. Although the number of repetitions may vary per exercise, divide your total workout time into the three elements of any good workout: a warm-up, a main set, and a cool-down.

Prenatal Water Exercises

Warm-ups (5 to 10 minutes)

• Jog in chest-deep water in a big circle with both hands on shoulders.

• Stand in chest-deep water. With feet apart and arms stretched out, push water from side to side with both hands. Push water from side to side and reach up into the air. (See Figure 6.)

• Stretch arms out to the sides and make circles, first with your fingers, then with your hands, lower arms, and whole arms. Reverse. Finish by pushing water from side to side again. (See Figure 7.)

• Jog to pool wall.

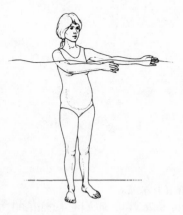

Figure 6 *Warm-ups*

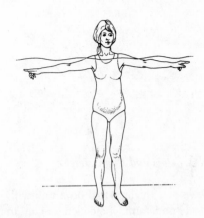

Figure 7 *Warm-ups*

Main Set (20 to 30 minutes)

• Waistline. Stand with feet apart and hold onto pool wall with one hand. Reach the other hand over your head and make ten side bends. Repeat on the other side. (See Figure 8.)

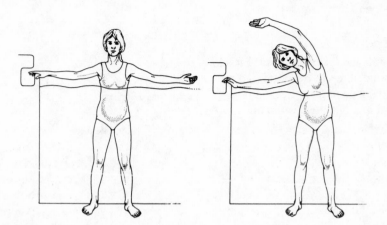

Figure 8 *Waistline exercise*

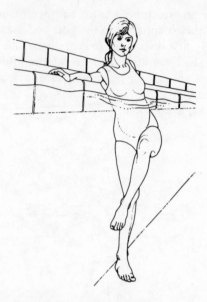
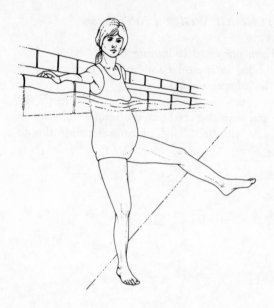

Figure 9 *Pelvis and thigh exercise*

• Pelvis and thighs. Hold onto wall with right hand and underarm, stretch left foot out in front of you so it touches the wall, bring it out to the side, back, down, and up to the wall again ten times. Place same foot on the wall and reach your toes ten times. Turn and repeat exercise with the other foot. (See Figure 9.)
• General stamina. Walk around in a big circle with arms moving in crawl strokes.

Leg muscles and pelvis.

• Hang onto wall and bicycle forward. Bicycle with knee outward. Bicycle backward. To prevent cramps, do not point toes. (See Figure 10.)
• Walk around in a big circle with arms moving in breast strokes.

Abdominal muscles.

• Hang onto wall, back tight against it, then lift up both legs in front of you. Swing your legs apart, together, and down. With back still tight against wall, lift legs up, bend knees, stretch legs out, and lower slowly. Repeat both five times.

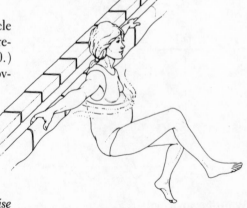

Figure 10 *Leg muscles and pelvis exercise*

• With the legs together, bend the knees and bring them as close to the chest as possible. Then extend the legs again. (See Figure 11.)

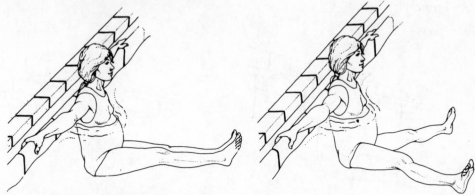

Figure 11 *Abdominal muscle exercise*

• Walk around in a big circle with your arms moving in a butterfly stroke.
• Legs and waistline. Hang onto wall and do crossover bicycling. (See Figure 12.)

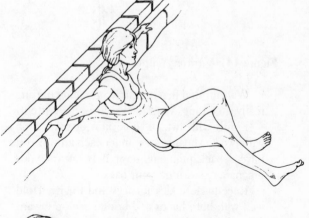

Figure 12 *Legs and waistline exercises*

• Pelvis and inner thighs. Face the wall, hang on with both hands, and walk up the wall with your feet outside your arms; "frog walk". (See Figure 13.)

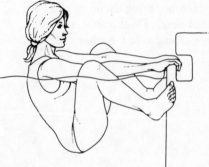

Figure 13 *Pelvis and inner thighs exercise*

Varicose veins.

• Lift one leg, make small circles with foot out in front, sideways to the wall. Repeat with other foot. (See Figure 14.)

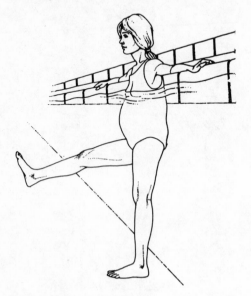

Figure 14   *Varicose vein exercise*

• Walk around in a big circle, grabbing the air, really stretching. Walk back against the current.
• Finish with two or three laps of swimming with two kickboards, one under each arm. If you have a back problem, or if it is late in your pregnancy, swim on your back.
• Knee-to-nose kick for legs and thighs. Hold wall with both hands and bring knee up toward face. Don't point toe. Bring leg down and back up to surface of water. Do this four times with each leg before changing to the other. (See Figure 15.)

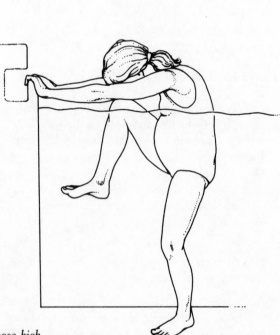

Figure 15   *Knee-to-nose kick*

• Legs and thighs. Leg lifts. Using pull-buoy for resistance, lift one leg at a time to the water's surface, keeping knees locked. Keep legs straight, alternately lifting them as close as possible to the water's surface. (See Figure 16.)

• Arms and wrists. Extend your arms sideward under water and rotate them forward in circles, then backward.

• Upper arms and chest. Water push-ups. Stand with your body facing the wall of the pool and your hands on the pool's edge. Straighten your elbows and lift your body out of the water.

• General fitness and arms. Jumping jacks. Stand with arms down at your sides. Turn your palms upward and bring them to the water's edge as you separate your legs into a "V" position. Return to the starting position by turning your palms downward and bringing them back. (See Figure 17.)

• General stamina, legs, arms. Rope jump. Pretend you are holding the handles of a jump rope with each hand at shoulder level with elbows touching the waist. As arms bring imaginary rope forward, knees bend and legs lift to clear the rope. Continue jumping rope forward, then backward.

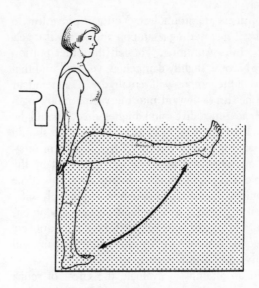

Figure 16 *Leg lifts*

Cool-down (5 minutes)

• Side-hip touch. Stand sideways, an arm's distance away from the pool wall. Keeping your feet together, touch your hip to the wall, then stretch your hip as far as possible from the wall.

• Full body stretch. Face the pool wall and hold on to the edge with hands shoulder-width apart. Place feet against wall in a wide "V" position. Slowly flex and extend arms to and from the wall.

Is it safe to swim or dive in lakes, streams, or the ocean while pregnant?

Women often express fear that water may enter the vagina while swimming and cause infection, especially during the last months of pregnancy.

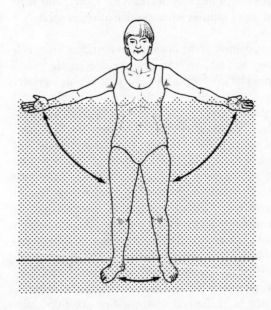

Figure 17 *Jumping jacks*

Such fears are groundless. You can prove this to yourself by inserting a tampon and seeing if it gets wet while swimming. Though the outer portion may become slightly dampened, you will find that most of the tampon will remain dry. Water and air can be thrust upward into the vagina following a high feet-first dive, and higher dives should be avoided; but diving head first into the water should be safe for at least the first three months of pregnancy, when the uterus is well protected by the pubic symphysis bone. Diving after this time should be avoided, although it is probably safe. Even if you accidentally land on your abdomen, injury to you or your baby will be highly unlikely since the amniotic fluid surrounding the baby will easily cushion the impact.

In an attempt to evaluate the effect of scuba diving on human pregnancy, a 1980 report surveyed 208 female divers. The number of fetal anomalies for those who dove during pregnancy did not exceed the range for the general population. However, the data suggested that women who dove during pregnancy, especially if they made deep and decompression dives, tended to have more fetal anomalies than women who did not dive when pregnant. On the basis of these studies, most experts conclude that scuba diving during pregnancy should be avoided. However, if you insist on diving, you should avoid depths of 60 fsw (feet of sea water), and the duration of time spent on the bottom should be one-half the limits established by the United States Navy no-decompression tables.

❧ AN EXERCISE PROGRAM FOR A HEALTHIER PREGNANCY ❧

What exercises can a pregnant woman use to strengthen muscles, increase flexibility, and help to avoid injuries when participating in sports?

In addition to the obvious physical benefits which they achieve, women who exercise regularly and thoughtfully during pregnancy often note a greater sense of emotional well-being and psychological satisfaction. Properly performed strength and flexibility exercises will help to decrease the likelihood of injury to the vulnerable muscles and tendons of the arms, legs, and back. In addition to preventing pain, these exercises can often alleviate pain once it is present. Enhanced physical fitness has its greatest application during labor, especially during a prolonged second, or pushing, stage in which both flexibility and strength are so vital in the Herculean effort to expel the baby. The exercises described below, many of which are learned by women studying the Lamaze method of childbirth, must be performed slowly and purposefully. Vigorous jerking movements should be avoided.

Leg and Thigh Exercises

To prevent what can be a crippling injury to the calf muscles and the Achilles tendon, wall push-ups are extremely helpful. Stand 12 to 15 inches from the wall, facing it. Place your palms on the wall while keeping your heels on the floor, your knees back, and your arms and body straight. Next, bend your elbows and move the upper part of your body toward the wall until your chest presses against it. You should feel a pull in your calf muscles. Hold this position for 10 seconds, slowly push away from the wall, and then return; repeat ten times. This exercise should be performed every morning and night until you no longer feel a pull in your calf muscles. As your muscles become more flexible you can move back a distance of 2 feet from the wall. (See Figure 18.)

Injury to the thigh muscles and tendons can be quite painful and incapacitating. As previously mentioned (see discussion on page 79), the two major antagonistic muscle groups of the thigh are

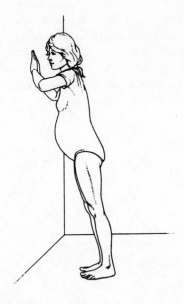

Figure 18 *Wall push-up*

If even the split stretch is too difficult, particularly after the fifth month of pregnancy, place the heel of one foot on a low table or desk, making sure to hold your knee straight with your hand. Then bend the other knee until the leg on the table is resting evenly on the tabletop with the foot pointing up and backward toward your face. Repeat this five times, once a day, on each leg until the tightness in the hamstrings in the back of the thighs is relieved. After you are experienced at this maneuver, you can try leaning over toward your raised foot and holding that position for a count of 10. (See Figure 20.)

the quadriceps in the front and the hamstrings in the back. One simple exercise for increasing flexibility of the thigh muscles is to bend from a standing position and touch the floor with your fingers while keeping your knees straight. Hold this position for 10 seconds, and repeat the exercise four more times per day. If you can't touch the floor with your feet close together, it is permissible to spread your feet apart, provided you don't bend your knees. This is called a split stretch. (See Figure 19.)

Figure 19 *Split stretch*

Figure 20 *Table-top thigh stretch*

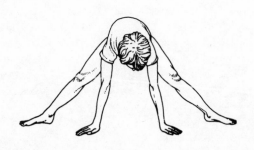

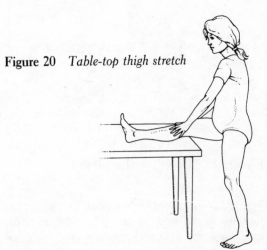

The hurdler's stretch also helps stretch the hamstring muscles along the backs of your legs. This is done by sitting on the floor with one leg outstretched and the other at your side. Lean forward to grasp the foot of your outstretched leg. Hold this position for a count of 10 and then release. Do this a total of five times with each leg once a day. (See Figure 21.)

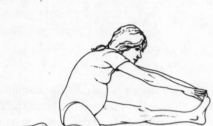

Figure 21   *Hurdler's stretch*

Some women find it easier to perform the hurdler's stretch with the unextended leg tucked inward rather than in the true hurdler position (see Figure 22).

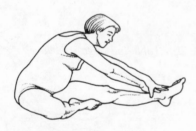

Figure 22   *Modified hurdler's stretch*

Another exercise which benefits the quadriceps muscles in the front of the thigh is named the quadriceps stretch. Stand with one hand resting on a wall or table while grasping your ankle with your

other hand. Pull your foot back until either your heel touches your buttock or you feel a pull in your thigh. This exercise should be repeated five times with each foot, holding each time for a count of 10, once a day, until the pull in the thighs disappears. (See Figure 23.)

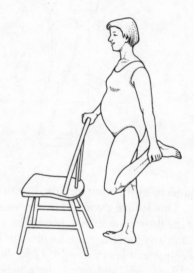

Figure 23   *Quadriceps stretch*

If you can't reach your foot with your hand, you can lie down and loop a towel around your ankle and gently pull on the towel. Do not do this exercise if it hurts your knees. (See Figure 24.)

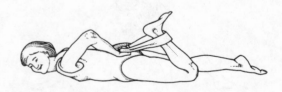

Figure 24   *Modified quadriceps stretch*

Ankle pump exercises are often helpful in reducing ankle edema, relieving leg cramps, and preventing tightness of the Achilles tendons. Sit on a chair with one foot resting across the opposite knee. Point your toes up and down, bending the ankle. Hold the position for a few seconds with the Achilles tendon being stretched. Then rotate your feet in circles in both directions. (See Figure 25.)

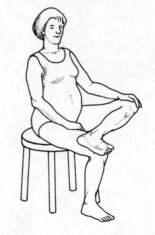

Figure 25   *Ankle pump*

Back Exercises

The accentuated forward curvature of the spine during pregnancy, known as lumbar lordosis, makes the pregnant woman particularly susceptible to low back pain and sports-related back injuries. Though consciously trying to maintain good posture can't be considered an exercise, it will help to reduce abnormal stress on the ligaments and muscles of the back. Good posture consists of keeping your head straight with your chin slightly tucked, your shoulders up and back, the abdomen as far inward as possible, and the knees slightly flexed. (See Figures 26 through 29.)

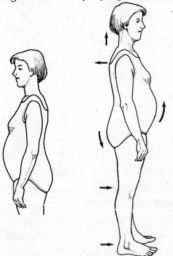

Figures 26 & 27   *Good posture during pregnancy*

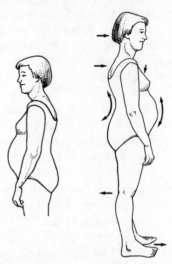

Figures 28 & 29   *Poor posture during pregnancy*

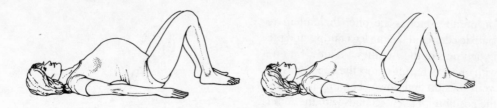

Figure 30   *Pelvis tilt*

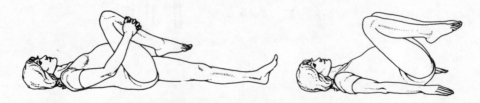

Figure 31   *Knee presser*

The pelvic tilt is helpful in stretching the muscles of the lower back and in relieving back pain. It also helps to strengthen the abdominal muscles. It is performed by lying on your back with your feet on the floor and knees bent. In this position, tighten your buttocks and abdominal muscles, then rotate your pelvis backward, then upward, lifting your hips off the ground. Hold this position for a count of 10, then release and rest for a count of 5. This can be repeated 20 times a day. (See Figure 30.)

One of the best exercises for preventing and relieving low back pain during pregnancy is the knee presser. To perform the knee presser exercise, lie flat on your back and pull one knee up to your chest, holding it in this position with your hand. Hold this stretched position for a count of 5; work each leg a total of five times. After this, bring both legs together five times. Do these exercises slowly, without jerking. (See Figure 31.)

The back raise and the reverse sit-up are excellent exercises for relieving low back pain, though they often become technically too difficult after the

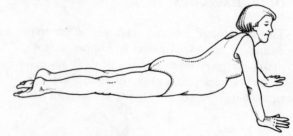

Figure 32   *Back raise*

fifth month of pregnancy. To perform the back raise, place the palms of your hands on the floor in a push-up position. Then raise your upper torso without lifting your legs, and hold the position for 10 seconds. Repeat this exercise four more times in each session. (See Figure 32.)

To perform a reverse sit-up, lie face down on a bench or firm table and extend the upper part of your body beyond the edge and then raise up. Start with three sets of 5 repetitions, working up to three sets of 20. (See Figure 33.)

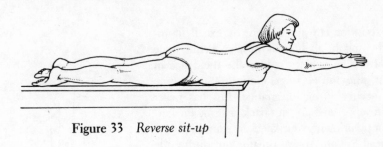

Figure 33   *Reverse sit-up*

Abdominal Exercises

The abdominal muscles are the major antagonistic muscle group to those of the back. As a result, extremely weak abdominal muscles will predispose to a higher incidence of low back pain during pregnancy and a greater number of back-related athletic injuries. Bent-leg sit-ups help to strengthen the abdominal muscles. Bent-leg sit-ups are done in the position shown in Figure 34 and never with the knees straight. Start with 10 per day and gradually work up to 30. Before rising from the supine

position, touch your chin to your chest, then release a deep breath as you begin to sit up. Easier sit-ups may be done with your hands reaching toward your knees. When you have mastered this technique, try sitting with your arms folded across your chest, placing one hand on each shoulder.

A good muscle-relaxing exercise to perform after sit-ups is the hip twister. Lie on your back with your knees bent and slowly move your knees from side to side while turning your head in the opposite direction. Continue this for a period of 30 seconds, gradually increasing to 1 minute. (See Figure 35.)

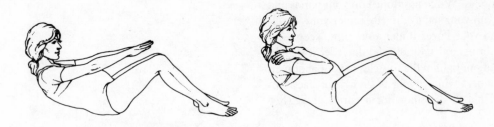

Figure 34   *Bent-leg sit-up*

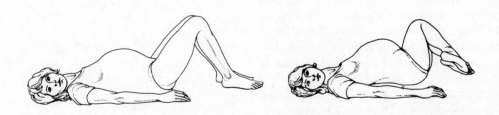

Figure 35   *Hip twister*

The curl or curl-up exercise is excellent for strengthening the abdominal muscles. While some claim it can prevent or reduce the incidence of diastasis, the muscle separation in the midline which occurs during pregnancy, this has never been proven. Lying on your back, assume the curl position by bringing your knees to your chest and your head to your knees. Breathe out during the curl and hold the position for a count of 6. Relax and then repeat the exercise four times. (See Figure 36.)

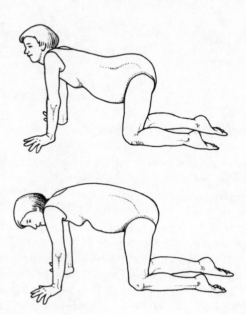

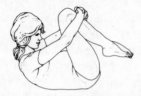

Figure 36 *Curl*

The pelvic rock exercise helps to strengthen the muscles of the lower back and tighten the abdominal muscles. While positioned on your hands and knees with your hands directly under your shoulders and your knees under your hips, keep your back in a neutral position and don't let it sag. In this position, tighten the muscles of your abdomen and buttocks while trying to arch your back upward. Hold this position for a count of 5. (See Figure 37.)

Figure 37   *Pelvic rock*

Shoulder Exercises

A simple apparatus can be used at home to strengthen your shoulder muscles. Hang a pulley on a clothes hook on the wall and run a 6-foot length of rope on a firm cord through the pulley. With hands held together and raised in front of you, grasp an end of cord in each hand, pulling one end toward you while the other arm rises as high as comfort permits. Hold your elbows straight. Pull up and down 20 consecutive times a day. (See Figure 38.)

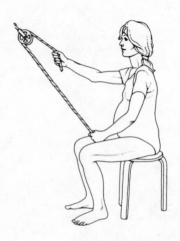

Figure 38   *Shoulder exercise with pulley*

Exercises with Weights

The orthopedic surgeon Dr. James A. Nicholas recommends the use of weights for women who are interested in significantly strengthening their legs. If these exercises are performed carefully, I see no reason why a pregnant woman cannot benefit from them. They are also helpful in strengthening one leg if it is weaker than the other as a result of a previous injury. Expensive equipment is not needed; all that is required is a group of weights, such as whole or half bricks in sizes of 1½ to 5 pounds. Traction weights and metal weights through which a belt can be passed also serve well. Dr. Nicholas recommends an old handbag, a pail, a flour sack, or other receptacle for holding the weights, as well as a belt or strap for attaching the weights to the foot.

To strengthen the thighs, sit on a high desk or table with your legs hanging down. Place a folded towel under the thigh at the edge of the table.

Suspend a comfortable amount of weight from one foot. This should probably be no more than 10 pounds at first. Raise your thigh about 8 inches above the table and hold it there for 1 second; then return to the starting position. (See Figure 39.) Do not persist if you experience pain. If you do not experience pain, do the exercise a total of 10 lifts with each leg. This can be increased gradually to 20 lifts for each leg, and weights may be added gradually. I would not advise lifting more than 15 pounds during pregnancy.

To strengthen the legs, assume the same position. Start with no more than a 10-pound weight. Straighten your leg and hold the extended position for 1 second. Then return to the starting position and hold for 1 second. It is important not to swing the weight up and down. Repeat this exercise six to ten times, depending on your strength, and repeat this group of exercises two more times while taking a 2-minute rest period between each six to ten lifts. (See Figure 40.)

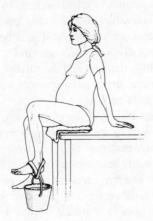

Figure 39 *Thigh exercise with weight*

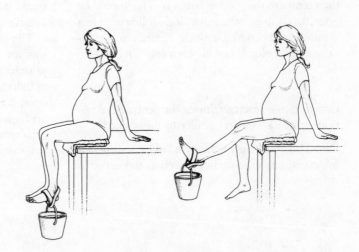

Figure 40 *Leg exercise with weight*

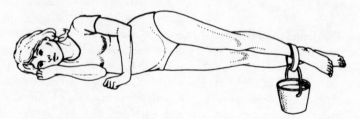

Figure 41   *Side lift with weight*

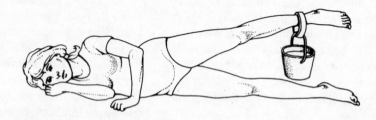

Figure 42   *Side lift with weight*

Side lifts serve the purpose of strengthening the legs and hips but should be done with a weight of 5 pounds or less. (See Figure 41.)

Lift your leg about 12 inches from the top of a bench or low table. Hold it there for 1 second and then return to the starting position. This should be done ten times with each leg, followed by a 2-minute rest period. Gradually increase to a maximum of 30 side lifts with each leg. (See Figure 42.)

Can't vigorous exercise during the postpartum period reduce a woman's ability to breast-feed?

No. This commonly held myth has been dispelled by several scientific studies as well as the personal experience of thousands of active women. In 1990, doctors at the University of California compared the nutritional composition of breast milk between a group of physically active women and another group who were sedentary and found no differences. Surprisingly, the exercising women tended to have higher milk volumes.

Though babies lack fully developed taste buds, they are more likely to reject breast milk in the 90 minutes following maternal exercise. Researchers at Indiana University have attributed this phenomenon to the postexercise accumulation of lactic acid, giving the milk a sour taste. To avoid feeding problems, nurse prior to or at least 90 minutes after you exercise.

4

SEXUALITY DURING PREGNANCY

$\int$ ince the days of Hippocrates, who was the first to suggest that sexual intercourse might bring about a miscarriage, very little has been learned about the medical aspects of sexuality during pregnancy. Even the most up-to-date obstetricial textbooks devote just a few lines to this vital subject, with the result that the majority of obstetricians practicing today know less about sexuality than the women they treat. Few doctors mention anything to their pregnant patients about sexual behavior or alternative coital positions during pregnancy, and rarely are sexual techniques other than intercourse discussed.

Unlike other medical topics presented in this book, many questions about sexuality have no absolute answers. My discussion of what we do know about this important subject is based on the available literature. The medical profession owes a great debt to William H. Masters and Virginia E. Johnson for their pioneering work in the field of human sexuality. As a direct result of their innovative and brilliant research, many taboos and misunderstandings about sexuality in pregnant and nonpregnant women have been dispelled and replaced by a greater open-mindedness between women and their doctors.

 ## THE FEMALE ORGASM AND PREGNANCY

What are the components of the female orgasm and how do they differ for pregnant and nonpregnant women?

Our knowledge of the female orgasm is derived from the extensive research conducted by Masters and Johnson. They were able to divide the female orgasm of both nonpregnant and pregnant women into four distinct and sequential phases: excitement, plateau, orgasm, and resolution. Each phase is characterized by distinct changes in the breasts, external genitals, internal genitals, and vagina.

The Excitement Phase

During the initial stage of sexual response the breasts increase in size because of engorgement, or vasocongestion, of the veins within each breast. The nipples become erect. In the genital area, the clitoris increases in length and width while the labia, or inner lips, increase in size and extend outward. At the same time as these external changes are taking place, the vagina begins to lubricate as well as lengthen and distend. The uterus and cervix elevate higher in the pelvis to make room for the penis.

Vaginal lubrication usually occurs within 10 to 30 seconds after sexual stimulation is initiated. Masters and Johnson demonstrated that vaginal lubrication results from the passage of droplets of fluid from congested and dilated veins surrounding the vaginal walls.

Masters and Johnson studied the excitement phase in six pregnant women, three of whom were having their first baby, who had also been evaluated before they became pregnant. They found that during the excitement phase, the vasocongestive reaction of the breasts and genitals to sexual stimulation is superimposed on the hormonal changes resulting from pregnancy. As a result, the rush of blood to the enlarged breasts can cause tenderness and pain. This was particularly evident in the first trimester, and especially among the women having their first baby (nulliparas, or primigravidas). During the second and third trimesters of pregnancy there was usually a marked reduction in these women's complaints of breast tenderness.

The genitals of the nulliparous woman undergo little change in the excitement phase of sexual arousal during pregnancy. However, for women having a second (primiparas) or later baby (multiparas) there is excessive engorgement and swelling of the labia majora and labia minora. By the third trimester, the external genitals are so swollen by pregnancy that further swelling due to sexual excitation is difficult to detect.

All six women reported a significant increase in the production of vaginal lubrication, beginning at the end of the first trimester and persisting throughout pregnancy. Additional vaginal lubrication in response to sexual excitement also developed more rapidly and extensively during pregnancy.

The Plateau Phase

The bodily changes of the plateau phase in the nonpregnant woman are a continuation and intensification of the excitement phase. The breasts continue to swell. The areola, or pigmented area around the nipple, also enlarges significantly, giving the impression that the nipples are retracted and smaller than they are during the excitement phase. The characteristic change in this phase is that the blood vessels surrounding the outer third of the vagina become markedly congested with blood. This vasocongestion is so pronounced that the outer vaginal opening is reduced in diameter by at least one-third from that noted during the excitation phase. Masters and Johnson named this outer area of congestion the "orgasmic platform."

Another important change occurring during the plateau phase is the retracting of the clitoris under the hood created by the two labia minora. At this point, the clitoris is often difficult to locate and is so tender that efforts to touch it directly may cause discomfort.

At the end of the plateau phase, other muscles in the body begin to tense, the pupils dilate, and a feeling of lightheadedness frequently occurs as orgasm approaches.

The main difference between the plateau phase in pregnant and nonpregnant women is that the vasocongestion of the outer portion of the vagina is far more pronounced during pregnancy. Among the nulliparous women studied, the vaginal opening was noted to be reduced in size by 75 percent. The effect was even more pronounced among multiparous women, where it was noted that vasocongestion occurred to the point that the two lateral or side walls of the vagina were actually touching each other. This condition tended to become more pronounced as pregnancy progressed and explains why some couples complain that "there is no room" or that the vagina is "too tight" when intercourse is attempted.

The Orgasmic Phase

The basic characteristics of the female orgasm are identical in all women and are triggered by direct or indirect stimulation of the clitoris. During orgasm, the congested outer part of the vagina contracts strongly at regular 0.8-second intervals. With each orgasmic experience, the total number of contractions ranges from 3 to 15, while the interval between contractions lengthens after the first 3 to 6. The number of orgasmic platform contractions varies from woman to woman and within the same individual from one orgasmic experience to the next. Usually a mild orgasm consists of 3 to 5 contractions, while there may be 8 to 15 strong contractions in a more intense orgasm.

In addition to the contractions of the orgasmic platform, the uterus also contracts at regular intervals every few seconds. Uterine contractions, unlike orgasmic platform contractions, are less frequent, usually begin 2 to 4 seconds after a woman is aware of the onset of an orgasm, and may last for several minutes following orgasm. Masters and Johnson made the interesting observation that the uterine contractions initiated in response to masturbation were of greater intensity and duration than those induced through orgasm via intercourse.

Other changes which occur during orgasm are a further retraction of the clitoris, a tightening of the anal sphincter, a curling of the toes, and an increase in the heart and respiratory rates. Orgasm rarely lasts longer than 10 to 15 seconds.

Masters and Johnson observed one very important difference between orgasm in the pregnant woman when compared to the nonpregnant woman. During the last trimester of pregnancy, and especially during the last four weeks, instead of normal orgasmic contractions the uterine muscle may go into a spastic and continuous contraction without relaxing. During the last month of pregnancy, some of these contractions have been noted to last as long as 1 minute and to recur as late as a half-hour after orgasm. Masters and Johnson observed that the fetal heart rate slowed during such contractions, but they noted no further evidence of fetal distress. Other investigators have not shared their optimism.

The Resolution Phase

Following orgasm, there is a period of calm and relaxation. In the nonpregnant woman, the blood filling the veins of the breasts and pelvis slowly flows to the other areas of the body, while anatomy and physiology return to normal.

The resolution phase is an uncomfortable experience for the pregnant woman because the intense vasocongestion in the pelvis subsides very slowly following orgasm. According to Masters and Johnson, this condition gets progressively worse as pregnancy advances. During the second trimester, it took 10 to 15 minutes for vasocongestion to subside in the women having their first baby and approximately 30 to 45 minutes for this to occur in the others. During the third trimester, vasocongestion may not be relieved at all following orgasm, and this may result in an increase in sexual stimulation, sexual tension, and frustration for some pregnant women. All six pregnant women who were intensively studied by Masters and Johnson reported no relief of their sexual tension levels during this period despite the fact that three of the women were suddenly able to experience multiple orgasm for the first time.

Declining Sexuality During Pregnancy

Does a woman's interest in sex decline during pregnancy?

Usually, yes. Many men erroneously believe that a woman's increased hormonal levels during the first trimester, as manifested by enlarged breasts and a new voluptuous body contour, produce a heightened sexual desire at this time. Nothing could be further from the truth. Unpleasant physical factors in early pregnancy such as nausea, vomiting, and fatigue tend to significantly reduce coital and noncoital sexual interest for many women. Masters and Johnson interviewed 111 pregnant women in an attempt to learn more about a woman's pattern of sexual interest and response throughout each trimester of pregnancy. They concluded that women having their first baby were more likely to experience a significant reduction in sexual interest and in effectiveness of sexual performance during these early months than women having a second or later baby.

During the second trimester, most women in both groups reported a significant increase in eroticism and effectiveness of sexual performance. Of 101 women studied at this time, 82 noted this positive effect.

Masters and Johnson had difficulty evaluating the sexuality of women during the last trimester of pregnancy, since intercourse was discouraged by their obstetricians during this time. Despite the limitations of this inquiry, the majority of the women studied reported that they gradually lost interest in sexual activity during the last three months.

Other researchers studying patterns of sexuality during pregnancy do not agree with Masters and Johnson. The vast majority of reports demonstrate that most women experience a steady and consistent decline in sexual activity, libido, and satisfaction throughout pregnancy. While some investigators have noted a slight improvement in sexual performance during the second trimester when compared to the first trimester, the level of sexual interest for most women remains far below their prepregnancy levels.

One of the most intensive studies of all aspects of sexuality during pregnancy was performed in 1974 by Drs. Nathaniel N. Wagner and Don A. Solberg of the University of Washington, who interviewed a total of 260 middle-class women. Though coital rates for these women declined progressively throughout pregnancy, the most dramatic changes were noted during the seventh, eighth, and ninth months. Unlike Masters and Johnson, Wagner and Solberg noted no relationship between coital frequency and the number of times a woman had been pregnant. When asked to rate the intensity of their orgasms during pregnancy in comparison to those preceding conception, the majority reported less intense orgasms as their pregnancy continued, particularly in the seventh, eighth, and ninth months.

Wagner and Solberg also studied noncoital methods of achieving orgasm. Although 50 to 60 percent of those women who masturbated to orgasm prior to pregnancy abstained from this practice while pregnant, the frequency of masturbation-induced orgasm in the remaining group was the same as before pregnancy. Similarly, fewer women reported manual stimulation by their partners as a method of attaining orgasm during pregnancy. Of those who continued to use this method, the incidence of achieving orgasm did not vary from their prepregnancy rates. However, in contrast to masturbation and manual stimulation, orgasmic rates achieved by oral-genital stimulation declined significantly during pregnancy. During the prepregnancy period, 16 percent of the women reported no or only rare orgasms from oral-genital stimulation. This number rose to about 60 percent in the ninth month of pregnancy.

What factors are most responsible for a woman's declining sexuality during pregnancy?

Many interrelated physical and psychological changes may adversely alter a woman's sexual response throughout pregnancy. Women asked by Wagner and Solberg to list the factors which were most responsible for their changing sexual behavior during pregnancy mentioned physical discomfort most frequently (46 percent), followed by fear of injuring the baby (27 percent), and physical awkwardness (17 percent). (More than one reason was accepted and recorded.) Approximately one-third of the women interviewed had been told by their physicians to abstain from intercourse at times ranging from two to eight weeks prior to their expected due date. Despite this, only 8 percent of the women cited their doctors' recommendations as a reason for altering their sexual behavior, and only 4 percent cited loss of attractiveness in the eyes of their partners as a reason for diminished sexual intensity.

As previously mentioned, the extensive vascular congestion within the breasts during pregnancy may cause great sensitivity and pain, especially in the nipple and areola. The fact that this previously sensual area is now off limits is often a source of frustration to a couple.

The congestion of the genital tissues during pregnancy may cause a feeling of vaginal discomfort and "tightness" for a woman during coitus. Another rarely discussed deterrent to sexual enjoyment is the greater quantity of vaginal discharge during pregnancy. Many women report that their vaginal secretions have a much stronger aroma, which they often characterize as unpleasant and embarrassing during oral stimulation of the vulva and the vagina, so that they are less likely to enjoy this lovemaking technique. Moniliasis, or "yeast" infection, is a common cause of vaginal and vulvar irritation and discharge during pregnancy. Though this is not a serious condition and is easily treated (see Chapter 6), it can be a source of annoyance for a woman and diminish her sexual interest and participation.

The uterine contractions which follow orgasm during pregnancy may last for half an hour or more in some women. Sometimes these contractions of the so-called postorgasmic syndrome are so painful that a pregnant woman may prefer to avoid sexual intimacy entirely.

Hormonal changes of pregnancy often cause marked alterations in the blood supply to the cervix. Spotting of blood from the cervix following coitus with deep penetration is harmless but can be very frightening to the couple who has not been forewarned by their doctor that this may occur.

What other factors might inhibit a woman's sexuality during pregnancy?

Psychologically, most pregnant women experience a heightened body preoccupation, feelings of insecurity, and a strongly increased need for affectionate rather than sexual touching. Pregnancy seems to have the effect of lowering the erotic component of a woman's sexual functioning while increasing her desire for affection.

The greatest dependency period and time of maximum vulnerability appears to occur during the ten weeks before birth. It is at this time that affection and emotional support are essential to the psychological well-being of most pregnant women. It is sad that many men fail to understand this basic and powerful need.

Many women express resentment against sexually demanding husbands who are unable to understand, appreciate, or accept their decreased inclination for coitus and orgasm. Several surveys have demonstrated that as pregnant women become less interested in sexual contact, they tend to masturbate their husbands more frequently. For some couples this is an acceptable form of lovemaking, but many women object to repeatedly "servicing" their "selfish" husbands.

Ten of the 19 women interviewed by Dr. Celia J. Falicov of the University of Chicago experienced fear, frequently recognized as unrealistic, of harming the fetus or producing miscarriage as a result of coitus. Several reported a "subconscious holding back" from orgasm because of fear of fetal injury. The survey of Wagner and Solberg, as well as many others, confirmed that this fear is quite prevalent and persists throughout the entire pregnancy.

What happens to a man's sexuality during his partner's pregnancy?

Pregnancy is a stressful period for most men. Feelings about their own dependency, masculinity, childhood attachments, and identification with their mothers may surface at this time. For many it represents sudden changes in a previously organized life-style, combined with the need to plan for new economic responsibilities and pressures.

The great majority of surveys clearly demonstrate that most men experience a decreased desire to be sexually intimate with their wives, particularly as pregnancy progresses and the woman appears more visibly pregnant. A man's sexual response is influenced by a variety of factors, the most obvious of which is his wife's sexuality. If she is plagued by discomforting symptoms or is totally preoccupied with her unborn baby, it will adversely affect his enthusiasm and response. Even a mature man may feel somewhat threatened and jealous of this new entity who has suddenly disturbed a previously happy relationship. Under such circumstances, he may prefer not to make demands on his wife. Other men, whose wives stimulate them to orgasm without themselves experiencing sexual gratification, often report feelings of guilt for not being less demanding. While some men note a greater sexual attraction to their wives' larger breasts and more rounded body contours, this interest is usually not reciprocated. Repeated spurning of his sexual advances may be frustrating, and rather than risk repeated rejections a man may simply stop trying. The opposite may also occur: a woman's larger breasts, swollen vaginal tissues, increased vaginal lubrication, and stronger scent during pregnancy may overwhelm some men to the point of creating loss of erection and sexual dysfunction.

The fear of injury to the fetus is often cited as a common reason for a man's declining interest in coitus during pregnancy. This becomes most pronounced after "quickening," the woman's first detection of fetal movement, which occurs at approximately the twentieth week of pregnancy. For many men it is only at this point that the baby as a living human being first becomes a reality. For some immature men, this stated fear of injury may merely reflect an underlying ambivalence about the pregnancy and feelings of hostility toward both the woman and the unborn child.

As strange as it seems, there are reports of men who have avoided coitus because of an irrational fear that the fetus may be watching them or is attempting to grasp or even bite their penis. Although they may recognize such fears as being ridiculous, some men find them impossible to abandon.

Many expectant fathers report that they are frustrated by their wives' extreme breast tenderness, which prohibits manual and oral stimulation. Others state that they avoid oral contact with their wives' genitals (cunnilingus) because of the greater amount of vaginal lubrication and discharge, which most men agree does not have a pleasing flavor or aroma. In addition, as previously mentioned, a couple may note a slight amount of bleeding from the cervix following intercourse. Although this rarely indicates a serious problem, it may further contribute to a man's anxiety and sexual alienation.

Psychiatrists have attributed the sexual dysfunction of some men during pregnancy to what is termed the "Madonna image" or the "mother-mistress" conflict. It is theorized that early teachings cause these men to associate all pregnant women with the purity of the Madonna. Subconsciously, having sex with someone who is so obviously a mother seems akin to incest.

What can a couple do to avoid a sexual crisis during pregnancy?

Problems of sexual adjustment during pregnancy can threaten the stability of the most comfortable and secure relationship. A couple alerted beforehand to the possibility of a woman's diminished libido and sexuality during pregnancy will not be frustrated and disappointed by unrealistic expectations about sexual performance.

In her excellent article published in the journal *The Female Patient* in September 1979, Dr. Elizabeth Wales emphasized the fact that most men do not understand a woman's need for affection in preference to erotic stimulation during pregnancy. A typical sequence of events that often leads to conflict and misunderstanding begins when a woman initiates physical contact merely because she is seeking affection. Her mate may interpret this as a request for intercourse and seek to establish sexual contact leading to orgasm. She in turn may interpret his aggressive behavior as demanding and selfish and may respond by rejecting his advances, leaving him hurt, confused, and angry. A man must be helped to understand that "Not tonight, honey" doesn't mean "I don't love you."

Masters and Johnson introduced the beautiful term "pleasuring" to describe the way a man and woman can think and feel sensuously about each other without any pressure to proceed to orgasm. The end result of all intimate contact, especially during pregnancy, is not necessarily orgasm. There are many ways that a man can communicate his love, and often a hug, a kiss on the cheek, a backrub, or a body massage can be far more meaningful and gratifying to a pregnant woman than an intense orgasm.

The key to averting a sexual crisis during pregnancy is good communication between a couple. If a woman does not desire to have intercourse, she should be able to say so. The man, in turn, should be encouraged to ventilate his feelings and frustrations rather than let them build, to surface angrily at a later date. A couple should experiment with various positions which facilitate comfortable intercourse during the second half of pregnancy. Positions which avoid deep penetration not only add to a woman's comfort, but also help to avoid disturbing bleeding from the superficial capillaries of the cervix. The knowledge that orgasm may bring uncomfortable uterine contractions helps to allay anxieties for most women when this occurs.

Noncoital lovemaking techniques should also be freely discussed. If a man is suddenly turned off by cunnilingus because of his wife's excessive lubrication, he should be comforted in knowing that these feelings are not uncommon and are experienced by most expectant fathers. Some men report that they can still enjoy oral sex by limiting it to the drier clitoral area while using their fingers to stimulate the labia and vagina. A woman who is self-conscious about her increased lubrication and odor can shower or wash the vulva immediately before lovemaking. Another helpful tip is to apply a natural oil, such as coconut or sesame, to the vulva prior to lovemaking. A couple should also realize that self- and mutual masturbation may also increase in frequency as coital interests decline, and that there is no rational basis for the guilt feelings many individuals experience about the natural and harmless act of masturbation.

If your obstetrician instructs you to avoid intercourse at any stage during pregnancy, ask for the reasons for this decision, the length of time that the restrictions are in effect, and whether or not noncoital alternatives leading to orgasm can be safely substituted.

How can unpleasant odors originating in the genital area be avoided?

No society has a greater preoccupation with body odor, and genital odor in particular, than ours. In recent years a variety of perfumes, feminine hygiene sprays, creams, and jellies have appeared on the market, many with a musk, civet, or ambergris base—all of which, ironically, have their origin in animal scent-producing sex glands.

Despite the propaganda of Madison Avenue, soap and water are more effective in promoting genital hygiene and male sexual interest than any of these potentially irritating products. Pregnant and nonpregnant women should be meticulous about personal hygiene, washing the labia and perineum (though no more than once a day) with a mild, nonperfumed, nondeodorant soap. This should be followed by a thorough rinsing and drying. Cleansing the perineum following urination should be done by wiping the labia area first and then continuing the wipe toward the anal region.

Excessive perspiration and odor of the genital area may result from wearing tight-fitting panty girdles, jeans, or slacks. Synthetic fabrics for underwear, panty hose, and panty girdles lack absorbency and therefore retain the moisture of the vaginal excretions, as well as perspiration. This moisture also acts as an irritant to the vulva and perineum, causing chafing and burning. The pregnant woman is extremely susceptible to monilial infections resulting from excessive wetness in the genital area.

 # COITAL POSITIONS

Which coital positions are most satisfying during pregnancy?

While the traditional male-superior (face-to-face or missionary) position is the most commonly used before pregnancy and during the first two trimesters, a woman's increasing abdominal girth in late pregnancy markedly limits the use of this position. The women surveyed by Drs. Wagner and Solberg listed a side-by-side variation of the missionary position as most popular. Rear-entry and female-superior positions also increased in popularity during the last three months but remained less popular than the male-superior position.

The missionary position can be successfully employed if a man lies partly sideways so that most of his weight is off the pregnant uterus. Many couples find that a more comfortable variation of this position is for the man to kneel at the foot or the side of the bed while the woman rests on her back with her buttocks at the edge of the bed and both feet touching the ground. Depending on the height of the bed and the size of the man, adjustments can easily be made by placing one or more pillows under her buttocks or his knees. This variation takes all his weight off her enlarged abdomen and allows him greater freedom to stimulate her breasts and clitoris than does the standard missionary position.

Variations of the side-by-side position are very popular in late pregnancy because they allow for shallow penile penetration. This is especially important during the last month, when the baby's head may be engaged or deep in the pelvis and deep penetration becomes painful.

Many women favor the female-superior (woman-on-top) position in late pregnancy because it puts no weight on the abdomen and allows the woman to control the depth of penile penetration.

Men often find the many variations of the rear-entry position extremely exciting and sexually gratifying. However, during pregnancy several of my patients have stated that they prefer the intimacy of face-to-face contact, which rear-entry position does not provide. The most common variation of the rear-entry position is the "spoon" position in which the couple curls side by side. In this position the male is unable to thrust deeply because he is behind the woman and has little leverage. Another advantage is that it is comfortable while still allowing the woman to enjoy breast and clitoral stimulation during intercourse. For added comfort and a smoother penile entry, the woman may prefer to raise her upper leg with the help of a pillow or two.

Rear entry may be performed with a woman resting on her knees and elbows. While this position is possible and even satisfying for some women late in pregnancy, most find it uncomfortable and difficult to maintain for more than a couple of minutes. Rear entry from a sitting position, with the woman on the man's lap, is far more comfortable and pleasurable. Be sure that the piece of furniture you select to sit on is strong enough to hold the weight of both of you.

The rear-entry standing position has several disadvantages. One major problem is that the man is often taller than the woman order to enter her. The ang is most comfortable if a woma. far as possible, but her ability to do this is limited during the second half of pregnancy. For maximum comfort in this position it helps if the woman can rest her head on a pillow placed on a sturdy table or desk under her.

POSSIBLE HAZARDS OF SEX DURING PREGNANCY

Can male sperm cause miscarriage?

Many body cells, including sperm, contain substances called prostaglandins, which have been synthesized in the laboratory and are used medically to induce abortion by causing intense uterine contractions leading to expulsion of the fetus. It has been suggested that sperm prostaglandins, absorbed through the vaginal wall, may be responsible for recurrent miscarriage and premature labor.

The great majority of researchers refute this theory. Some have actually calculated that in order to deposit enough prostaglandin in the vagina to cause miscarriage and premature labor it would take 15 simultaneous ejaculations of equal volume and potency. Swallowed prostaglandin in an ejaculate are also believed incapable of being absorbed and causing laborlike contractions.

Orgasm itself is much more likely to cause involuntary uterine contractions than is the presence of prostaglandins from an ejaculate, and Masters and Johnson demonstrated that the uterine contractions which accompany orgasm with masturbation are far more intense than those resulting from coital orgasm.

Can orgasmic contractions of the uterus cause miscarriage during the first three months of pregnancy?

There are practically no scientific studies to substantiate the claim that orgasm during the first three months of pregnancy increases the risk of spontaneous abortion. However, in his book, *Spontaneous and Habitual Abortion* (1957), Dr. C. T. Javert stresses the importance for women who have had three or more consecutive spontaneous abortions of eliminating any factor which would stimulate even a mild amount of sexual arousal leading to a uterine contraction.

Current opinion is that it is extremely rare for coital or noncoital orgasm to be a primary cause of spontaneous abortion. However, if a woman has a history of repeated miscarriage, or notes intense and painful uterine contractions following orgasm, abstinence is the best policy for at least the first 12 weeks of pregnancy. If bleeding follows orgasm, and your doctor can demonstrate with a vaginal speculum examination that the blood flow is from the uterus rather than from the capillaries of your cervix, which is harmless, it would be advisable to avoid further orgasm during the first trimester.

Are orgasmic uterine contractions ever responsible for premature labor?

Yes. Each year 200,000 infants are born prematurely, and their prematurity is associated with a significantly higher incidence of severe physical and mental disability. The criteria for prematurity, as defined by most medical researchers, are a gestational age of less than 37 weeks and/or a birth weight of 2,500 grams (5½ pounds) or less.

Dr. Robert C. Goodlin of Stanford University Medical Center, in a letter published in *Lancet* in September 1969, was one of the first physicians to alert the medical profession to the possibility that orgasm during the second and third trimesters might make premature labor more likely. Among 25 women surveyed, 21 reported painful uterine contractions and pains and pressure in the back or pelvis following orgasmic coitus. Of six women who delivered four or more weeks prematurely, four believed that their premature labors probably began with an orgasmic experience, as did three out of five who prematurely ruptured their amniotic membranes prior to the onset of labor. (When this membrane ruptures, an abundant amount of amniotic fluid is released vaginally. Labor often will begin within 24 hours of this event; if it doesn't, medical induction is sometimes necessary to prevent fetal and maternal infection.)

In 1971, Dr. Goodlin and his associates expanded their research by interviewing 200 women. Among this group, a total of 155 (77 percent) were orgasmic during the second and third trimesters of pregnancy. Of these 155 orgasmic women, a surprisingly high number of 127 complained of postorgasmic discomfort in the form of uterine contractions, pelvic pain or pressure, backache, and thigh pain. Whereas the incidence of premature labor prior to the thirty-seventh week of pregnancy is estimated at 10 percent of the general population, it was found to be 21 percent among women who achieved orgasm after the thirty-second week of pregnancy. As part of this same study, Dr. Goodlin noted that coitus in the absence of orgasm had no relationship to premature labor.

As part of another study, Goodlin and his associates asked five women who were seen on vaginal examination to be "ripe" for labor to initiate an orgasm at a specific time. Of the five women, two were admitted to the hospital in labor within three hours and the third within nine hours after orgasm. A fourth woman experienced false labor contractions which soon stopped.

Though Masters and Johnson were unable to document a higher incidence of premature delivery among orgasmic women, they did note that four women who were uninvolved in their study had an experience which was almost identical to that of the five women studied by Goodlin. All four women were within 18 days of their due date, and three began labor immediately after orgasmic intercourse. The fourth woman initiated labor within minutes of a multiorgasmic masturbation.

Support for Dr. Goodlin's orgasm-prematurity relationship was reported in *Fertility and Sterility* in August 1976 by Drs. Nathaniel N. Wagner and Julius C. Butler, who obtained complete sexual histories from 19 mothers of premature infants and compared them to a control group of 19 women who gave birth to full-term infants. During the first trimester, 14 of the 19 mothers of premature babies, or 74 percent, reported experiencing orgasm from three-fourths of the coital times to "always," while only 7, or 37 percent, of the controls noted orgasm this frequently. Although the incidence of orgasm decreased as pregnancy progressed, it remained higher for the mothers of premature infants.

In 1979, Dr. Richard P. Perkins of the University of New Mexico School of Medicine reported detailed sexual and obstetrical data from 155 women who had recently given birth. Based on the responses to his questionnaire, Dr. Perkins concluded that sexual activity, regardless of technique, appeared to have no adverse effects on the incidence of premature rupture of the amniotic membranes, premature labor, and infants of low birth weight. One surprising finding was that orgasmic women, especially those who masturbated to orgasm, had a *lower* incidence of premature infants than women who did not achieve orgasm. This relationship appeared to be true throughout all stages of pregnancy. Furthermore, more women who had sex within 24 hours of labor were admitted with ruptured amniotic membranes if their most recent sexual stimulation was not accompanied by orgasm. These findings led Dr. Perkins to theorize that the sexually unfulfilled individual may be more prone to premature labor than those engaged in regular satisfying sexual relationships. In other words, Dr. Perkins believes that if you're going to be sexual in the third trimester, do it with feeling or don't do it at all. Unlike other researchers, such as Masters and Johnson, Dr. Perkins did not note as strong a relationship between a woman's attainment of orgasm and her perception of uterine contractions. Although women perceived more contractions after coitus with orgasm than with any other type of sexual behavior and response, coitus itself seemed to be as strong a stimulus to uterine contractions as was orgasm.

Support for Dr. Perkins's findings may be found in an article published in *Lancet* in July 1981. In this review of almost 11,000 pregnancies, doctors concluded that coitus during the third trimester did not increase the incidence of premature labor, infants of low birth weight, or perinatal deaths. In 1989, doctors at Albert Einstein College of Medicine in New York City used a home monitoring system (see Chapter 11) to measure uterine contractions associated with sexual intercourse among 15 women previously treated during their current pregnancy with medication to stop premature labor. When compared to a group of 15 low-risk women, those previously treated experienced a significant increase in uterine contractions in the hour following coitus. Though the contractions subsided within 2 to 3 hours, and none of the women went into labor, this small study did show that certain women are more susceptible to postcoital uterine irritability than others. The authors

of this report did not distinguish between orgasmic and nonorgasmic coital encounters.

It is known that women carrying twins are especially susceptible to premature birth. To minimize the risk of premature labor, most obstetricians routinely recommend abstinence during the third trimester. However, a 1989 report published in the *American Journal of Obstetrics and Gynecology* would tend to refute the relationship between coitus and premature twin births. In this study of 126 women carrying twins, interviews on coital activity were conducted periodically throughout pregnancy. Forty percent of the women reported coitus early in the third trimester, with the rate decreasing to 24 percent four weeks before delivery. When compared to women not engaging in coitus during the third trimester, the sexually active individuals showed no higher incidence of premature births. The authors concluded that coitus need not be discouraged in women carrying twins.

In the presence of these contradictory findings, it is difficult to offer specific advice to women about the relationship between intercourse, orgasm, and premature labor. However, there does appear to be a small number of susceptible individuals who will, as a result of their sexual activity, deliver prematurely. If you have previously given birth to a premature infant, avoidance of orgasm during the last three months of pregnancy would appear to be a sound suggestion.

Can orgasmic uterine contractions affect the fetus?

It has been demonstrated that the uterine contractions associated with orgasm may be related to a slight temporary decrease in the amount of oxygen carried to the fetus. This in turn may result in a slowing of the fetal heart rate. However, the opinion of most experts is that this is of little consequence.

In the past there have been scattered unscientific and speculative reports claiming that the lack of oxygen to the fetus during orgasm was responsible for lower IQs in the newborn, as well as severe mental retardation, and some couples reported an increase in fetal activity associated with coital and noncoital orgasm. Few doctors took these claims seriously, until a 1979 letter from St. Bartholomew's Hospital Medical College of England was published in *Lancet* under the heading "Does Sexual Intercourse Cause Fetal Distress?" Of 70 women delivered of their first baby, 30 engaged in coitus during the four weeks before delivery while 40 abstained. The researchers noted that the women who had intercourse showed a higher incidence of fetal distress. While this research involved only a small number of women, I would agree with the authors that there is a clear need for further investigation.

Can the act of intercourse increase a woman's risk of infection during pregnancy?

No obstetrical condition has received more attention in the news than the research on this subject by Dr. Richard L. Naeye of the Pennsylvania State University College of Medicine. Dr. Naeye analyzed 26,886 pregnancies which took place between 1959 and 1966 to determine the relationship between coitus during the second half of pregnancy and the incidence of infection of the amniotic fluid surrounding the baby. Dr. Naeye noted a frequency of 156 infections per 1,000 births when mothers reported intercourse once or more per week during the month before delivery, compared with 117 per 1,000 when no coitus was reported. More significantly, of those infants who contracted infections, 11 percent died when there was a history of coitus, as compared to 2.4 percent of infants whose mothers abstained. Dr. Naeye also found that babies born of mothers who had coitus during the month prior to labor were twice as likely to experience the consequences of prematurity, such as lower Apgar scores, respiratory distress, and jaundice.

It is known that there are powerful antibacterial substances in the amniotic fluid which are capable of destroying a wide variety of bacteria. These substances first appear at the end of the third month, and their strength in combating infection increases progressively until the end of pregnancy. It has been theorized that infection occurs when sperm or enzymes in the sperm facilitate the passage of bacteria through the protective mucus of the cervix and into the amniotic fluid membrane. If too many bacteria enter the amniotic fluid, the protective bacterial-fighting mechanism may be overwhelmed and an infection will spread. Since the concentration of these bacterial-fighting substances increases as pregnancy progresses, their ability to combat greater numbers of bacteria should also increase. Confirmation of this theory was demonstrated microscopically among the women studied by Dr. Naeye. At 20 to 24 weeks of pregnancy, 82 percent of the women with acute inflammation had microscopic evidence of spread. This rate decreased to 78 percent at 25 to 28 weeks and 63 percent at 29 to 38 weeks.

Dr. Naeye also observed a second intercourse-associated increase in the frequency of amniotic fluid infections after the thirty-eighth week of pregnancy. Women who engaged in coitus at least once a week were noted to have a 50 percent greater risk of contracting a serious amniotic fluid infection than women who abstained from intercourse at this time. He theorized that this was probably due to the dilatation and effacement (shortening) of the cervix which normally occurs in the last weeks before the start of labor. These changes of the cervix increase the exposure of the amniotic membrane to semen and bacteria from the vagina and cervix.

Scientists have conducted laboratory studies to determine if the male ejaculate, when it comes in contact with the amniotic membranes, can alter their strength and elasticity and cause them to rupture prematurely. The most recent method of studying this hypothesis was carried out in 1989 by Dr. Yitzhak Romem and his colleagues at the University of Southern California School of Medicine in Los Angeles. In their report, published in *The*

Journal of Reproductive Medicine, they incubated sections of amniotic membranes obtained immediately after delivery with samples of seminal ejaculates. They found that after 1 hour the seminal ejaculate caused the membranes to be stiffer, less elastic, and more likely to rupture, with this effect declining but still present 4 hours later. After 24 hours, membrane elasticity had returned to normal. The scientists surmised that lipids and enzymes in the seminal fluid caused the membranes to stiffen and decreased their ability to dissipate stress. This in turn caused an increased likelihood to rupture prematurely.

From a practical point of view, what decision regarding intercourse should a pregnant woman make during the second half of pregnancy?

Even the most knowledgeable authorities on this subject do not really know what advice to give their patients. Dr. Naeye is currently conducting research to determine if the use of condoms during pregnancy can reduce the frequency of amniotic membrane infections and improve the outcome for babies who become infected. However, one of his concerns is that other complications which these babies experience, such as respiratory distress and jaundice, are not always associated with infection and would not be significantly reduced simply by use of a condom. Following publication of his article, Dr. Naeye said he was not prepared to recommend prolonged sexual abstinence in pregnancy, simply because of the marital discord that it might cause. Whereas many obstetricians recommend abstinence at some point during the last few weeks of pregnancy, Dr. Naeye suggested that it made more sense to abstain in the fourth through seventh months, when the bacterial-fighting substances in the amniotic fluid are in lower concentrations than they are at the end of pregnancy.

Some of Dr. Naeye's research techniques and conclusions have been challenged by several researchers. For example, his criteria for diagnosing an infection was based on finding a small number of white blood cells in the amniotic fluid. This finding, however, is not necessarily indicative of a clinical infection in either a woman or her baby, and some pathologists will not diagnose an amniotic fluid infection unless there is a significant number of white blood cells present. The only definite proof of an infection is a positive bacterial culture, and even Dr. Naeye admits that his diagnosis of infection was not based on this absolute evidence. Another criticism of his widely publicized paper is that there is no mention of the length of labor of the women studied, the presence of complications in labor, or the time elapsed between rupture of the membranes and delivery of the baby. This is unfortunate, since the last of these factors is the most important in determining if an infection will occur. Another challenge to Dr. Naeye's conclusions is a 1981 analysis of 10,477 births in which doctors demonstrated no deleterious effects between coitus in late pregnancy and the development of an amniotic fluid infection. The most emphatic rebuttal of his conclusions appeared in *Lancet* in 1984 and was written by Dr. Mark A. Klebanoff and his associates at the National Institutes of Health in Bethesda, Maryland. In this impressive report, 39,217 women were interviewed, and no relationship could be found between coital frequency during pregnancy and complications such as miscarriage, premature delivery, premature rupture of the amniotic membranes, amniotic fluid infections, or perinatal mortality.

These conflicting findings have created uncertainty and anxiety for couples seeking sound advice about sexual activity during pregnancy. They have also posed vital questions to researchers involved in prenatal health care and human sexuality. Studies by psychologists have confirmed that serious emotional turmoil and tension may result when abstinence is prescribed for prolonged periods of time. On the other hand, a couple who attributes their newborn's infection to their coital activity may face far greater and longer lasting feelings of guilt.

Although further studies are necessary before

definite advice can be given, there are sensible guidelines that women should follow. Those women who have a history of previous reproductive failure and premature labor and those women who, when examined by their obstetricians, are noted to have premature dilatation or effacement of their cervix should avoid orgasm, as well as intercourse, during the last three months of pregnancy. In addition, abstinence is also advised for women whose amniotic membranes have ruptured prematurely. If a woman has previously given birth to one or more healthy, full-term infants despite having experienced both coital and noncoital orgasms throughout her pregnancy, it would appear foolish for a doctor to insist on abstinence for prolonged periods of time during a subsequent pregnancy. In all probability, her current pregnancy will remain normal in either case, and she would be unlikely to heed medical advice which appears contrary to her own personal experience.

How common is anal intercourse, and what are its dangers to the pregnant woman?

Many proctologists believe that repeated anal intercourse may be responsible for aggravating previously existing conditions of the rectum such as colitis and hemorrhoids, although it is an unlikely cause of these disorders. However, the gross enlargement, bleeding, and discomfort of hemorrhoids, which occur in practically all women during pregnancy, is likely to become far worse if anal intercourse is attempted during this time. While stretching of the anal sphincter is uncomfortable and unpleasant to many women, this same sensation is erotic to others. With repeated episodes of anal coitus, the sphincter may become dilated and lose its tone, causing hemorrhoids to protrude more and a small percentage of women to experience involuntary passage of gas, rectal mucus, and fecal soiling of their underwear.

The rectum and anus normally harbor a wide variety of bacteria which are capable of entering a man's urethra during anal intercourse. In addi-

tion, any skin abrasion, cut, or sore on the penis may be a potential site for multiplication of these bacteria. If rectal intercourse immediately precedes vaginal intercourse, bacterial contamination of the vagina, or vaginitis, may occur. Symptoms of this condition are a watery, usually malodorous, and irritating discharge. In the nonpregnant woman this form of vaginitis, though usually not dangerous, requires antibiotic therapy. During pregnancy this type of infection is potentially more serious, since it can spread to the cervix and amniotic membranes. Merely washing the penis with soap and water between vaginal and anal entry is hardly sufficient to remove all bacteria, but it is far better than not washing at all.

When bacteria multiply within a man's urethra they may cause an inflammation, or urethritis, even if he vigorously washes his penis with soap and water. A scant yellowish urethral discharge, frequency of urination, burning on urination, and passage of cloudy urine are signs of this type of urethritis. Occasionally, these symptoms may be accompanied by an elevated temperature and chills. Obviously, passage of the infection to the vagina is more likely to occur with future vaginal intercourse once a man has contracted urethritis. The only adequate precaution to prevent infection requires that a man either wear a condom for the anal portion of coitus or restrict each intercourse to the vagina or to the anus. It is important to remember that similar hygienic precautions must be taken to avoid contamination of the vagina following insertion of a finger into the rectum. At the very least, the finger should be thoroughly washed with soap and water and the nail cleaned with a brush before inserting it into the vagina. Anilingus is the licking of the anus as a means of erotic stimulation. If cunnilingus immediately follows anilingus, bacteria may be transferred to the vagina.

As with vaginal intercourse, anal intercourse should not occur during pregnancy when a woman experiences vaginal bleeding of unknown cause, when ultrasound examination reveals that the placenta is low-lying or even completely covering the cervix (placenta previa), if the membranes have ruptured and fluid is leaking, or if obstetrical history and vaginal examination suggest that the cervix may be effacing and dilating prematurely.

Can erotic stimulation from an enema cause premature labor?

A klismaphiliac is an individual who derives intense erotic pleasure from receiving an enema. Some individuals introduce this practice to their partners and both derive sexual pleasure through mutual enema-giving. Contrary to popular belief, enemas administered during pregnancy will not cause premature onset of labor, and other than aggravating and causing bleeding from enlarged hemorrhoids, they are usually harmless. However, in the presence of obstetrical conditions such as undiagnosed uterine bleeding, a prematurely dilated and effaced cervix, a low-lying placenta, or a placenta previa (placenta covering the cervix), enemas should not be used.

Are there any hazards associated with oral-genital contact during pregnancy?

There are no medical reasons to stop oral-genital contact during pregnancy provided that one bizarre maneuver is avoided. Many deaths have occurred among pregnant women whose lovers have forcibly blown air into their vaginas. When exhaled air is held under pressure by the tight application of the mouth to the vaginal opening of a pregnant woman, the air may enter the circulation via the enlarged and dilated veins of the vagina and cervix, travel to the heart, lungs, and brain, and cause instant death. When air moves through the circulatory system in this fashion it is called an air embolus. As far as I know, there have been no reported deaths from air embolism in nonpregnant women engaged in this form of sexual behavior.

Can air be accidentally introduced in a similar fashion if a woman douches or uses a bidet during pregnancy?

Maternal deaths due to air embolism have been reported in numerous cases where the cause was a douche administered with a bulb syringe. Usually the douche was administered in an attempt to induce an abortion. However, in at least four cases there seems to be clear evidence that the douche was used for hygienic purposes. For this reason, I prohibit douching during pregnancy and explain to my patients that their increase in vaginal discharge is a normal physiological reaction which requires no treatment. If a discharge causes a severe itch and irritation or is malodorous, it is abnormal and does require treatment. However, regardless of the cause, all discharges can be treated adequately during pregnancy without resorting to use of a douche (see discussions of treatment of vaginitis in Chapters 6 and 9).

A bidet is a basin about the size and height of a toilet bowl, usually equipped with fixtures for running water and a built-in spray. With this method of cleansing, the spray of water irrigates only the vulva. Since no air enters the vagina under pressure, use of a bidet is perfectly safe during pregnancy.

Can a woman be allergic to a man's semen?

While it is not a common occurrence, instances of allergy to seminal fluid have been reported regularly, and several women have had this condition start during pregnancy. Allergic reactions never occur with a woman's first exposure to an ejaculate; it takes several contacts before she becomes sensitized. Seminal fluid allergy may be mild and localized to the vulva and vagina, or severe and generalized throughout the body.

Until recently, treatment of seminal fluid allergy consisted of a man wearing a condom during all coital episodes. Another solution to this problem has recently been suggested by researchers at the University of California at San Francisco, who were able to significantly reduce the severity of one woman's generalized allergic reaction with bi-weekly skin injections of dilute samples of her husband's seminal fluid over a period of several months. This form of immunotherapy shows great promise for women with this unfortunate and unusual problem.

Is it safe to use a vibrator as a method of sexual gratification during pregnancy?

There is a wide assortment of battery-powered mechanical devices classified as vibrators. External vibrators are used specifically to stimulate the labia and clitoris. If used too vigorously, they may cause abrasions or a hematoma, a collection of blood below the skin. However, if care is taken, they can safely be used during pregnancy. It is important for a woman to remember that a vibrator-induced orgasm may bring about uterine contractions of greater intensity than those associated with coitus. If these contractions cause great discomfort, or if a woman has a history of premature labor, she should probably abstain from using a vibrator.

Women using intravaginal vibrators are strongly advised to abstain from this practice during pregnancy. If a couple insists on using these devices, it is important that penetration take place slowly and with great care, since the vaginal tissues are more vascular and engorged at this time. If a woman is on top when using an intravaginal vibrator, she will be able to more carefully regulate the pressure and penetration speed and thus avoid abrasions, lacerations, and hematomas of the vaginal wall. Abundant lubrication with K-Y Jelly or Lubrin Lubricating Vaginal Inserts is also helpful in reducing the risk of these injuries.

POSTPARTUM SEXUALITY

How soon after delivery can sexual contact be resumed?

Contrary to what most doctors recommend, there is no scientific evidence to show that a couple must wait the often-advised six weeks before resuming intercourse. Following an uncomplicated vaginal delivery, in which there are no vaginal lacerations and no episiotomy is performed, coitus should be perfectly safe at two weeks postpartum. One good indication of when to resume intercourse is the quantity and character of the postpartum vaginal discharge, or lochia rubra. This soon changes to a paler fluid called lochia serosa. Finally, after 10 to 14 days, it becomes lochia alba, which is white in color and minimal in amount. At this point, the cervix is usually closed, infection is not present, and intercourse may be attempted without fear of introducing infection. However, if the lochia is foul-smelling, infection of the lining of the uterus may be present. A persistent reddish color for more than two weeks often signals the retention of small portions of the placenta or failure of the uterus to contract adequately over the site where the placenta was located. Both conditions may require a dilatation and curettage (D and C). It is best to avoid coitus until these symptoms are evaluated by your obstetrician.

If you have an episiotomy, or a sutured laceration, the stitches will usually be completely dissolved within three weeks. At that time intercourse can be attempted gingerly, and if you do not experience discomfort there is no need to abstain.

Following a cesarean section, the abdominal incision usually takes two weeks to heal; barring unusual medical complications, intercourse should be safe at this time.

As far as noncoital lovemaking techniques are

concerned, I instruct my patients who have delivered vaginally not to engage in cunnilingus too soon postpartum. The mouth contains a variety of potentially harmful bacteria which, when introduced into a periurethral, vaginal, or vulvar laceration resulting from childbirth, are capable of causing an infection. If you are contemplating oral-genital sex earlier than three weeks after delivery, first carefully inspect your vulva and vagina with a hand mirror for evidence of a laceration that has not healed. If you are unable to do this, consult your obstetrician.

Some obstetricians believe that bacteria from a man's mouth can be introduced into the nipple of a nursing mother during lovemaking. When these bacteria multiply, breast inflammation may result. However, babies and mothers usually share the same bacterial flora, and therefore the risk of introducing new and different bacteria during nursing is less than when a man's mouth comes in contact with the nipple.

How does the response to sexual arousal during the postpartum period compare to the prepregnancy response?

The six women previously referred to who were studied intensively during their pregnancies by Masters and Johnson were also evaluated for sexual response between the fourth and sixth postpartum week, between the sixth and eighth postpartum week, and at the end of the third postpartum month.

Although four of the six women reported a return of erotic interest during the first postpartum evaluation, Masters and Johnson found that the sexual target organs responded more slowly and with less intensity when compared to prepregnancy levels. Vasocongestive reactions of the labia, which usually begin in the excitement phase of sexual stimulation, were found to be delayed in development well into the plateau phase. Vaginal lubrication developed slowly, and the quantity was significantly less during the postpartum period. Distention of the

inner two-thirds of the vagina was also noted to be reduced in rapidity of development, as well as in the amount of enlargement that took place during sexual excitation. Although all six women were noted to have a thinning, atrophic appearance of their vaginal walls, this was most pronounced among the three women who were nursing. (The reason why the vagina of a nursing mother resembles that of a postmenopausal woman is because the usual pathway for hormonal stimulation between the hypothalamus and pituitary gland becomes disrupted when a woman is nursing. Prolactin hormone, produced by the pituitary gland, is responsible for milk secretion but also prevents the release of other hormones which are helpful in stimulating estrogen synthesis by the ovary. It is estrogen which thickens the vaginal tissues and gives them a healthy appearance.)

Masters and Johnson also noted a reduction in development of the orgasmic platform during the plateau phase, as well as a marked reduction in the intensity and duration of uterine contractions with orgasm among patients questioned between the fourth and sixth postpartum week.

At the six-to-eight-week postpartum evaluation, the six women studied showed essentially the same physiological responses that they did at four to six weeks. However, at the end of the third postpartum month, the picture changed completely, with all six women showing evidence of full return of estrogen hormone production and prepregnancy sexuality. These beneficial effects included thickening of the vaginal walls, quick vasocongestive response of both labia to sexual stimuli, abundant and rapid development of vaginal lubrication, and full expansion of the vaginal canal. With orgasm, all six women were noted to have a normal intensity and frequency of their orgasmic platform contractions.

Do the breasts undergo physiological changes in response to sexual stimulation during the early postpartum period?

Unlike the vasocongestion of the breasts, which is

intensified by sexual stimulation during pregnancy, little if any physiological change is detected during the postpartum period. If milk production has been suppressed by use of hormones, it may be six months after delivery before any definite vasocongestive reaction can be observed in the breasts in response to sexual stimulation. Similarly, the breasts of nursing women do not demonstrate a consistent increase in size during the excitement phase or during increased levels of sexual tension. For some women there is an uncontrollable spurt of milk from both nipples as soon as they are sexually aroused; for others, this occurs only with orgasm.

How do these postpartum changes influence a woman's subjective evaluation of her sexuality during the postpartum period?

Needless to say, women demonstrate a variety of sexual responses during the postpartum period. Many experience a return of erotic interest within four weeks despite the fact that physiologic research tells us they should not be enjoying themselves that much. The meaning and affection involved in a relationship can increase a woman's subjective rating of the strength and rapidity of the measured physiologic response. For this reason, postpartum women initially resuming intercourse often experience full satisfaction despite the fact that they have not yet returned to prepregnancy levels of functioning.

What factors are most responsible for an early return to prepregnancy sexual enjoyment?

Based on interviews of 101 women in the third month after delivery, Masters and Johnson concluded that female eroticism was not significantly associated with a woman's age or number of children but could be related to whether or not she was breast-feeding. The highest levels of postpartum sexual interest were reported by a group of 24 nursing mothers. Furthermore, the nursing women

who had the longest delay in the return of ovarian function and menstruation reported the highest levels of eroticism. While the group of 24 nursing women stated that suckling by their infants was sexually stimulating, six said they were anxious to resume normal marital relationships with their husbands as quickly as possible in order to relieve guilt feelings about perverted sexual interests. Patients of mine have voiced similar concerns. It should be reassuring to know that it is perfectly normal to experience erotic sensations with nursing, and there is certainly no reason to feel guilty about them.

Unfortunately, some women continue to unconsciously "de-eroticize" themselves by mentally suppressing all normal responses of sexual arousal in the breast. Once a woman denies eroticism, all sex play and lovemaking may become anxiety-provoking. This may surface years later as sexual dysfunction.

Contrary to the findings of Masters and Johnson on the positive effects of breast-feeding on sexuality, doctors from Edinburgh, Scotland, determined that postpartum women who bottle-fed their babies were more likely to resume sexual intercourse sooner and with greater frequency than women who nursed. In trying to explain this phenomenon, the Edinburgh physicians found that concentrations of the hormones testosterone and androstenedione were significantly lower in those women who reported the most severe reduction in sexual interest. While these two hormones are found in great abundance in men, lower levels are also detectable in women. Higher levels of both hormones are known to be associated with heightened sexuality in both men and women.

An interesting finding by Dr. Celia Falicov of the University of Chicago was that most postpartum women, although having intercourse less frequently, were enjoying it more. Similar conclusions have been reached by Masters and Johnson. The reasons for this are varied, but the majority of those interviewed commented that pregnancy, labor, and delivery helped them to shed traces of their timidity in relation to bodily functions, and they found that they were less inhibited following childbirth.

How common is sexual dysfunction during the early postpartum period, and why does it occur?

Sexual dysfunction during the early postpartum period is a far greater problem than is generally realized. For example, of the 101 women interviewed by Masters and Johnson in the beginning of the third month following delivery, 47 described low or essentially negligible levels of sexuality. The reasons given were excessive tension and fatigue in caring for the new baby, pain with attempted intercourse, discomfort related to breast engorgement, persistent vaginal discharge, and fear of pregnancy. Falicov reached similar conclusions in her study of 18 postpartum women.

One should not underestimate the trepidation that most women feel in anticipation of their resumption of intercourse during the postpartum period. If a woman is afraid that her episiotomy is not completely healed, or even if she may know that all her stitches are dissolved, she may still experience a fear, often recognized as irrational, that coitus will be painful. This may lead to vaginismus, or painful spasms of the vagina resulting from contractions of the vaginal walls. If this psychological reaction occurs to a significant degree, the vaginal walls may close completely when intercourse is attempted and penetration may become extremely difficult, if not impossible. Other women express concern that their vaginal tissues have become "too loose" as a result of being stretched while accommodating the birth of the baby.

Few doctors tell their patients that the vaginal tissues of the nursing woman most often resemble those of a postmenopausal woman in that they are thin, atrophic, and lacking in estrogen. The reason for this is the disruption of the usual pathway for hormonal stimulation. Without estrogen the vaginal walls do not thicken, and intercourse may be uncomfortable and even painful.

For many women, breast-feeding is an extremely sensual experience which carries over to their sexual relationship. However, others report marked sensitivity of the breasts and nipples, and a partner's usual caresses may be unwelcome. In addition, as noted earlier, it is not uncommon for nursing women to experience uncontrollable spurts of milk from their nipples during orgasm or as soon as they are sexually aroused. Regardless of when it occurs, the abundant amount of milk released may literally and figuratively dampen a man's sexual response.

Occasionally, the fear and dysfunction associated with coitus may originate with the man, who, having witnessed his partner's labor, episiotomy, and birth, becomes fearful of inflicting further trauma. Under such conditions, it is not uncommon for him to lose his erection during early coital attempts.

What can be done to relieve some of the problems and reduce postpartum sexual dysfunction?

Good communication is a couple's best asset in dealing with the problems of postpartum sexual dysfunction. It is important to talk about these feelings and frustrations, and for men to understand and respect the fact that many women are just not interested in resuming sexual contact during the first eight weeks following delivery. Sex for many postpartum women is more than intercourse; it is touching, pleasuring, massaging, sharing responsibilities, and understanding the reasons why the person you love feels a certain way at a certain time. While fatigue in caring for a new baby often saps a woman's sex drive, some researchers believe that the lack of estrogen and progesterone hormones may also contribute to the postpartum decline in libido experienced by some women. I recommended to all my patients that they set aside a few hours every week to go out alone with their spouse so that they have the opportunity to focus on each other in a quiet, anxiety-free environment.

Some women delay resumption of sex or fail to

reach orgasm because they are afraid of becoming pregnant again. Postpartum contraception should be discussed by the obstetrician before a woman leaves the hospital so that adequate precautions can be taken and fears allayed.

The most common fear of the postpartum woman is that coitus will cause severe pain in the area of the episiotomy. For this reason a man must be extremely gentle during the first few attempts at intercourse. Occasionally, the stitches may actually be too tight, and a doctor can show a woman how to carefully stretch the vaginal opening at home with plastic dilators or a speculum. When apprehension about coital injury is so intense that it causes muscular spasms (vaginismus), an obstetrician should be able to demonstrate to a woman and her partner how to gently overcome this problem, first with fingers, then with increasingly larger dilators.

To minimize discomfort related to the episiotomy, try varying your positions for intercourse. Women with a mediolateral episiotomy, one that goes off to one side, say that it is helpful if their partner leans to the opposite side. Most episiotomies are median (in the midline). This type of incision is far more comfortable and usually heals faster and with less of a scar. Nevertheless, try to choose a position in which the penis presses against the front part of the vagina and clitoris, rather than the tender area in back. Couples should try those positions in which the woman can control the depth of penetration as well as the point of maximum penile pressure. The best in this regard are the side-by-side, woman-on-top, and "spoon" positions.

The lack of vaginal lubrication, caused by a postpartum estrogen deficiency and most pronounced in nursing women, can be easily overcome with liberal use of K-Y Jelly or natural oils such as sesame and coconut. Lubrin Vaginal Lubricating Inserts are unscented, colorless, nonstaining tablets which, when inserted into the vagina 5 to 30 minutes before intercourse, provide continuous lubrication for several hours. Replens is a relatively new

and excellent product which markedly improves the amount of vaginal moisture and increases the thickness and elasticity of the vaginal tissues. Some doctors have advocated the use of estrogen vaginal cream. However, this preparation is absorbed through the vaginal walls and into the circulation. Since this could not only diminish milk production but also pass into the breast milk and be ingested by the baby, I never prescribe vaginal estrogen preparations for a nursing woman.

To alleviate the problem of spurting milk from the nipples during sexual arousement, try wearing a bra or nursing pads that provide enough pressure to stop the flow of milk or at least absorb it. One excellent suggestion is to nurse the baby immediately before lovemaking; this will have the dual advantage of decreasing the amount of milk which leaks and reducing the chances of an interruption from a hungry baby. All these suggestions are helpful, but the best medication for curing postpartum sexual dysfunction is time. Patience, love, understanding, and communication will usually overcome even the most difficult problems.

Do you have any suggestions for couples who continue to experience sexual dysfunction beyond the immediate postpartum period?

It has been my experience that the overwhelming majority of couples who have a good sex life prior to pregnancy will return to their level of enjoyment within a reasonable amount of time. Most sex therapists believe that pregnancy and the immediate six-week postpartum period is not the time to seek help, especially if a couple has had an adequate prepregnancy relationship. Pregnancy introduces many temporary emotional and physical variables which will often subside spontaneously, thereby making therapy unnecessary. During pregnancy and the postpartum period, minor sexual problems may be magnified and appear much more serious than they actually are.

However, a significant number of couples have deep-rooted sexual difficulties which have antedated the pregnancy. Problems among men, such as premature ejaculation, impotence, and inability to maintain an erection, and dysfunction among women in the form of inability to experience sexual interest or orgasm all require treatment. While pregnancy is not the time to seek this type of therapy, there is no reason to delay evaluation later than eight weeks postpartum. Without help, these problems will not suddenly subside spontaneously but will only worsen.

While most family doctors and obstetricians lack the training and expertise needed to deal with these serious problems, many sexual dysfunction clinics have opened throughout the United States. Most reputable sex therapists are accredited by the American Association of Sex Educators, Counselors, and Therapists (AASECT), 600 Maryland Ave., S.W., Washington, D.C. 20021, and the American Society for Sex Therapy and Research (ASSTAR), c/o Oliver Bjorkater, M.D., 171 Ashley Ave., Charleston, South Carolina 29403. Each of these organizations can provide a listing of approved sex therapists in a particular area.

ııı *5* ııı

Bad Habits

The purpose of this chapter is to report the most recent data on pregnancy risks associated with the use of illicit drugs, alcohol, and tobacco. Many of these substances begin to exert their toxic effects during the first few weeks of pregnancy, often prior to a woman's first prenatal visit.

 ## *Tobacco Smoke*

How does cigarette smoking affect pregnancy?

Of the more than 4,800 separate chemicals that have been identified in cigarette smoke, the most harmful are nicotine, carbon monoxide, hydrogen cyanide, tars, resins, and several carcinogens, including such agents as diazobenzopyrene. While all chemicals in tobacco smoke are potentially harmful, nicotine and carbon monoxide are the two which are most detrimental to the outcome of pregnancy. In both animal and human studies, nicotine has been noted to stimulate the release of body substances known as catecholamines, which in turn cause a narrowing of the blood vessels to the uterus. As a result, there is a reduction in the concentration of oxygen in the fetal circulation. This may help to explain why smoking during pregnancy doubles the risk of meconium-stained amniotic fluid, suggestive of fetal distress. Meco-

nium is fecal material that passes from its intestinal tract into the amniotic fluid when the oxygen supply to the fetus is impaired. Researchers now believe that this constriction of blood vessels in the uterus may permanently damage them, affecting the outcome of future pregnancies, and is the most likely reason why smokers give birth to smaller babies. Nicotine can cause a frightening temporary decrease, and even stopping, of fetal movement, along with alterations in the breathing rate, immediately after a woman smokes as little as one cigarette. The higher number of stillbirths and neonatal deaths among infants born of smoking mothers may be attributed, in part, to this phenomenon.

Carbon monoxide is a poison found in significant concentrations in tobacco smoke. It readily crosses the placenta and has been detected in the umbilical cord of infants born of smoking mothers. The danger of carbon monoxide is that it combines with hemoglobin in both the maternal and fetal bloodstreams to form a compound called carboxyhemoglobin, which reduces the blood's oxygen-carrying capacity. One pack of cigarettes smoked per day will raise the maternal blood carboxyhemoglobin level by 4 or 5 percent. Fetal carboxyhemoglobin concentrations are directly related to those of the mother, and under conditions of continuous smoking they may be 10 to 15 percent higher than maternal levels. Scientists fear that the carbon monoxide in cigarette smoke is a more significant cause of permanent and disabling fetal growth retardation than is nicotine or any of the other pollutants.

Regardless of which particular chemical in cigarette smoke is most responsible for a poor fetal outcome, the overwhelming evidence supports the view that smokers are subjecting their unborn infants to cruel and unusual punishment. For example, smokers give birth to babies whose weights are on the average 10 to 15 percent below optimal weight, with smaller head circumferences and body lengths. This difference in weight becomes even greater as the number of cigarettes smoked increases. The smaller size of these tobacco-exposed infants is in part due to the fact that they are born prematurely, but more significant than this is their retarded growth in utero. Such infants are referred to as "small-for-dates." Women who smoke more than one pack of cigarettes a day are almost twice as likely to give birth to a baby weighing less than 5½ pounds than women who smoke less than one pack a day, and nonsmokers are much less likely to experience this complication. Smoking as little as five cigarettes per day is enough to have a negative effect on a baby's birth weight. In 1985, doctors at the Centers for Disease Control coined the term "fetal tobacco syndrome" to describe the condition of a growth-retarded infant weighing less than 5½ pounds at birth and born of a mother who smokes at least five cigarettes per day throughout pregnancy.

The risk of a child's contracting pneumonia and bronchitis during the first year of life is higher if its mother smoked during pregnancy, and the United States Collaborative Perinatal Project found that smoking increases the frequency and severity of Rh disease. An Rh-negative woman, one who is lacking the Rh factor, may form antibodies which destroy the red blood cells of her Rh-positive fetus. The destroyed red blood cells are unable to carry adequate amounts of oxygen to the fetal tissues, and carbon monoxide from inhaled cigarette smoke is believed to further impair this oxygen transport system.

Several studies have concluded that smoking mothers are also more likely than nonsmokers to experience spontaneous abortions and to give birth to infants with lower IQ scores, congenital malformations, hyperactivity, and reading and learning disorders, although whether some of these mental and physical inadequacies are permanent has not been established. The follow-up assessment of the Collaborative Perinatal Research Project demonstrated no differences at age eight in IQ or motor development between offspring of smokers and those of nonsmokers. However, equally impressive studies conclude that the children of smoking mothers do not catch up to the offspring of nonsmokers. In one report, the incidence of children with hyperactive-impulsive behavior at the age of seven was twice as great if their mothers smoked during pregnancy. The hyperactivity rates were also higher in families in which the mother smoked two or more packs of cigarettes than in those in which one pack of cigarettes was smoked daily. Most recently, it has been found that the likelihood of crib death, also known as sudden infant death syndrome (SIDS), is increased by 52 percent among infants born of mothers who smoked.

In a 1980 study published in Lancet, researchers found that the number of cigarettes a woman smokes per day during pregnancy is directly related to the risk of her child developing cancer. Children exposed prenatally to ten or more cigarettes per day had a 50 percent greater risk than children born to nonsmokers. When specific tumor types were considered, the number of cigarettes consumed was found to be directly related to the likelihood of developing acute lymphoblastic leukemia. Doctors at Stanford University, in their report published in the *American Journal of Epidemiology* in 1991, confirmed the relationship between maternal smoking during pregnancy and childhood cancers. In addition, they found that paternal smoking played a significant, but lesser, role as well.

The harmful effects of smoking affect all babies, regardless of their mothers' otherwise normal or above-normal nutrition and weight: A smoker, regardless of her weight, will give birth to smaller infants than a nonsmoker of equal weight. This relationship applies even when the food intake and the pregnancy weight gain are identical between the smoker and the nonsmoker.

In addition to these risks to the fetus, smoking may increase the incidence of serious complications for mothers. In one study, it was found that premature separation of the placenta from the uterine wall (abruptio placenta) occurred with significantly greater frequency in smokers than in nonsmokers. Among moderate smokers, the risk increased by 24 percent, while in heavy smokers it climbed to 68 percent. Placental infarcts are areas of unoxygenated dead tissue in the placenta which are caused by an inadequate supply of oxygen-bearing blood. Researchers have found that placental infarcts occur more frequently among heavy smokers. In 1989, Dr. Michael G. Pinette and his associates at St. Francis Hospital in Hartford and the University of Connecticut Health Center found that the rate of placental maturation and aging, as seen on ultrasound, occurred earlier in the pregnancies of smokers than nonsmokers. Smokers were also more likely to have areas of placental calcification, often an indication of aging, structural defects, and poor placental function.

During the last trimester of pregnancy, the placenta is usually attached to the upper part of the uterine cavity. However, on rare occasions it may attach in an abnormally low position and partially or completely cover the cervix. This condition, called placenta previa, can be responsible for pro-

fuse bleeding during the third trimester. The incidence of placenta previa has been reported to increase by 25 percent in moderate smokers and by 92 percent among heavy smokers.

Are women who smoke more likely to experience an ectopic pregnancy?

A pregnancy located outside its normal location within the uterus is referred to as ectopic (see Chapters 1 and 2). Because the fallopian tubes are by far the most common site for this type of abnormal pregnancy, it is often called a tubal pregnancy. Laboratory research, epidemiologic studies, and clinical experience suggest that cigarette smoking may be a risk factor for tubal pregnancy.

In one laboratory study, researchers found that nicotine-treated rats showed a delay in transfer of the fertilized egg from the fallopian tube to the uterine cavity as well as a delay in the implantation of the egg into the endometrium. Several epidemiologic studies, including one in 1987 which was based on a World Health Organization report on ectopic pregnancy, have concluded that smokers have a two to four times greater risk of tubal pregnancy than nonsmokers. Similarly, doctors in Japan found a higher than normal proportion of smokers among women with a tubal pregnancy than among women undergoing elective abortion. Doctors at Emory University and the University of Washington, in their 1988 study published in *Obstetrics and Gynecology*, found that current cigarette smokers had a twofold increase in risk of tubal pregnancy when compared to women who had never smoked. They also reported that the incidence of tubal pregnancy did not appear to be related to the duration of smoking, the age at which smoking was begun, or the number of cigarettes smoked per day. One surprising, unexplainable, and discouraging finding was that the risk of a tubal pregnancy for a woman who had stopped smoking before conception was still 1.6 times greater than for women who had never smoked. One theory offered to explain this phenomenon was that cigarette smoking may cause reduced immunity in the cells lining the fallopian tubes. This in turn predisposes smokers to tubal infections and pelvic inflammatory disease, two conditions which can inhibit normal tubal passage of the fertilized egg. It should be emphasized that this theory has never been scientifically substantiated.

What are some of the specific effects of cigarette smoking on the fetus?

Some of the most alarming aspects of cigarette smoking are the temporary aberrations of fetal movements, breathing patterns, and fetal heart rates which are noted immediately after a woman smokes. With the help of continuous ultrasound monitoring, doctors at Oxford University in England recorded the fetal breathing patterns of ten pregnant volunteers after they smoked two cigarettes within a period of 15 minutes. Within 5 minutes from the start of smoking, a significant increase in the rate of fetal breathing was noted. This persisted for 60 minutes. The women recorded the number of fetal movements they felt before and after they smoked; the number decreased markedly in the hour after the two cigarettes were smoked. Since fetal activity has become an important method of detecting fetal well-being, this diminution of movement is somewhat disconcerting.

It has long been known that smoking is associated with increases in maternal heart rate and blood pressure as well as a transient elevation in the fetal heart rate caused by the rapid passage of nicotine across the placenta. Using sophisticated Doppler ultrasound (see Chapter 11), doctors at Mt. Sinai Hospital in Toronto, in their 1988 study, were able to measure the velocity of blood flow in the umbilical artery of 15 babies following the smoking of one cigarette by their mothers during the last month of pregnancy. They found that smoking caused a significant increase in the vascular resistance of the placenta on the fetal side, impairing the transfer of oxygen from mother to baby. In a second 1988 study employing the Dop-

pler ultrasound technique, doctors from the University of Lund in Sweden measured the effects of maternal smoking and the chewing of nicotine gum on fetal blood flow in the aorta, umbilical vein, and umbilical artery. They found that fetal blood flow increased significantly in all three vessels immediately following maternal smoking of two cigarettes, and to a lesser degree with the use of two sticks of nicotine gum. However, the Doppler studies also indicated greater resistance to this increased blood flow in the aorta and umbilical arteries of the babies. The author suggested that nicotine impairs uterine blood flow to such an extent that the fetus compensates by increasing its own circulation in direct proportion to the number of cigarettes smoked by its mother.

The nonstress test, or fetal-acceleration determination (FAD), is an important method for assessing fetal status in high-risk pregnancies. In this test, an amplifier is placed on the mother's abdomen and the fetal heart rate is recorded on a strip of monitoring paper. A woman is instructed to immediately push a button, which she holds in her hand, whenever she detects a fetal movement, which is thus recorded on the monitor along with the fetal heart rate. Under normal conditions, most women will experience four or more fetal movements within a 20-minute period, with the heartbeat of the baby accelerating by at least 15 beats per minute in the 15 seconds immediately after the fetal movement is detected. When the fetus responds in this fashion, it is termed a reactive nonstress test, indicating that it is in no distress. However, a nonreactive nonstress test, in which the heart rate does not accelerate adequately, may indicate a compromised infant. In a report published in the *American Journal of Obstetrics and Gynecology* in 1980, a comparison of the nonstress test of 128 smoking and 350 nonsmoking pregnant women with high-risk pregnancies showed, significantly, that 20.8 percent of smokers had nonreactive nonstress tests while only 13.2 percent of nonsmokers experienced this result.

Ultrasonic visualization of the fetal skull

throughout pregnancy enables doctors to determine if growth is being retarded. The distance between the two large parietal bones of the skull, called the biparietal diameter, is the most commonly employed measurement. In one recent study, doctors found that the biparietal growth rate of fetuses of smokers was consistently lower than that of nonsmokers, starting with the twenty-first week of pregnancy.

Thiocyanate is a metabolic byproduct of tobacco smoke. Several studies have found elevated levels of thiocyanate in the umbilical cord blood vessels of newborns whose mothers smoked. Furthermore, a 1984 report by doctors at Lackland Airforce Base in San Antonio, Texas, found that the highest thiocyanate levels in the umbilical cord were associated with the birth of the smallest babies. In addition to thiocyanate, cadmium is one of the more toxic materials found in cigarette smoke, and it is also passed to the fetus. In a 1988 study, published in *The Journal of Reproductive Medicine*, doctors at the University of Medicine and Dentistry of New Jersey found increased cadmium and thiocyanate concentrations in maternal and umbilical cord blood of women who smoked, as well as significant amounts in the amniotic fluid. Since the fetus is continually swallowing and inhaling amniotic fluid, one can only surmise that the effects must be detrimental. Finally, doctors at Karolinska Institute in Sweden, in their 1986 study, found that babies born to women who smoked were more likely to have immunoglobulins E or D in their umbilical cord blood at birth. The presence of these immunoglobulins is often an indication that the infant is more likely than other newborns to develop allergic symptoms in childhood. Paternal smoking played a lesser role in determining the presence of these immunoglobulins.

Are any congenital malformations associated with cigarette smoking during pregnancy?

Despite innumerable studies, it cannot be stated with certainty that a relationship exists between maternal cigarette smoking and congenital malformations. In the largest study to analyze the relationship between maternal smoking and congenital anomalies, published in the *British Medical Journal* in 1979, doctors studied the outcome of 67,609 pregnancies among mothers who were divided into three categories: nonsmokers, light smokers (1 to 9 cigarettes per day), and heavy smokers (more than 20 cigarettes per day). They found that the overall incidence of congenital malformations was about 2.8 percent in both smokers and nonsmokers, and no correlation was found between smoking habits and malformations of the cardiovascular, gastrointestinal, genitourinary, or skeletal systems. A slightly higher incidence of cleft palate, cleft lip, or both was noted in infants of moderate to heavy smokers, although this was not considered to be statistically significant. Only neural tube defects, such as anencephaly and spina bifida, were found to relate significantly to smoking; heavy smokers were the most likely to give birth to infants with these defects. In 1986, one researcher reported that pregnant women who smoked more than two packs of cigarettes per day were more likely to give birth to children with abnormal facial characteristics such as a small lower jaw, a small mouth, and a short upturned nose. These observations have not been substantiated in more recent studies.

In a 1979 report from Sweden, the smoking habits of the mothers of 66 infants with cleft palate and cleft lip and another 66 infants with neural tube defects were studied. While women who gave birth to infants with cleft palate and cleft lip were heavy smokers, no such relationship was noted for neural tube defects.

If a pregnant woman is a nonsmoker, can the health of her baby suffer as a result of breathing the cigarette smoke produced by others?

In 1985, doctors at Yale University School of Medicine found that a pregnant woman exposed to the "secondhand" smoke of others for at least 2 hours per day had double a nonsmoker's risk of having a growth-retarded infant. They concluded that pregnant women should be discouraged from spending long periods of time in smoke-filled places. In 1986, Danish researchers also reported that passive smoking was associated with lower infant birth weights. On average, birth weight was reduced by 120 grams (4 ounces) per pack of cigarettes smoked per day by the father of the baby. In 1988, American physicians found that pregnant women exposed to passive cigarette smoke gave birth to babies weighing an average of 107 grams less than those not exposed. In addition, elevated levels of cotinine, the chief metabolite of nicotine, were found in samples of blood drawn from these women during the second trimester. Other studies, however, published in *Lancet* in 1986 and 1987, failed to demonstrate any differences in infant birth weights between mothers whose partners smoked and those whose partners did not smoke. Thiocyanate is a metabolic byproduct of tobacco smoke. In a 1982 study, reported in the *American Journal of Obstetrics and Gynecology*, doctors found elevated levels of thiocyanate in the umbilical cord blood vessels of newborns whose nonsmoking mothers were exposed to cigarette smoke throughout pregnancy. A subsequent, more optimistic study, published in *Obstetrics and Gynecology* in 1984, has refuted these findings. In this report, doctors found that thiocyanate levels in maternal blood and the baby's umbilical cord blood vessels were virtually identical among passive smokers and those living in a smoke-free environment.

Do ex-smokers have any greater pregnancy risks than women who never smoked?

Based on the 1979 Collaborative Perinatal Project of more than 50,000 pregnancies at 12 United States medical centers, it is now believed that even if a woman gives up smoking before becoming pregnant, her previous habit will increase the risk of certain pregnancy complications. Researchers theorized that smoking before pregnancy may permanently damage small arteries of the uterus of some women. This in turn can result in a higher incidence of spontaneous abortion, placental infarcts (areas of dead and nonfunctioning tissue caused by an inadequate supply of oxygen), placenta previa (low implantation of the placenta), and infant death. These complications are more apt to occur among women who were heavy smokers over a prolonged period of several years.

The conclusions of this study should in no way promote a fatalistic attitude on the part of a woman who is pregnant and still has not given up the habit. It is never too late to quit! Many benefits are realized the moment after the last cigarette is smoked. For example, if you finally stop smoking as late as the early stages of labor, you will still be less likely to transfer measurable amounts of toxic chemicals, such as carbon monoxide and nicotine, to the bloodstream of your baby than if you smoke during this time. In the event of a complicated pregnancy, in which the fetus shows evidence of distress, the cessation of smoking during the last few days may spell the difference between a successful and a tragic pregnancy outcome.

If you can break your habit before the fourth month, you will have the added advantage of giving birth to a baby whose weight is equal to that of a nonsmoker, since the maximum amount of growth retardation associated with maternal smoking takes place during the last six months of pregnancy. Therefore, while it is best that you never start smoking, you will realize positive benefits whenever you break this unwholesome habit.

What are the effects of smoking on breast-feeding?

Reports attempting to determine the relationship between cigarette smoking and the quantity and quality of breast milk have been both inconclusive and contradictory. The two largest studies suggest that smokers have a less adequate milk supply than nonsmokers, although both reports have many scientific deficiencies. One investigator observed a shorter average nursing period for smokers than for nonsmokers among women who nursed for at least two months. Of special note was the fact that mothers who stopped smoking during the last three months of pregnancy nursed as long as nonsmokers. In one experiment, mothers who smoked seven cigarettes in 2 hours noted a marked reduction in milk quantity.

Experiments show most of the chemicals in tobacco smoke are transmitted to the breast milk. When sensitive chemical assays are employed, nicotine can be detected in the milk of all women who smoke. However, deleterious fetal effects are rarely seen. In one case report, an infant whose mother smoked 20 cigarettes per day was noted to have symptoms of a nicotine overdose, characterized by restlessness, vomiting, diarrhea, and a rapid heartbeat. These symptoms subsided spontaneously when the mother stopped smoking.

Although the reasons remain unknown, infants who are nursing from mothers who smoke appear to be at increased risk of gastrointestinal disturbances. In a letter to the editor of the *Journal of the American Medical Association* in 1989, researchers from the University of Oslo, Norway, reported on their studies in which 40 percent of infants breast-fed by smoking mothers were found to have infantile colic. This condition, characterized by excessive crying caused by periodic bouts of abdominal pain, occurred in only 26 percent of the children of nonsmokers. An important finding was that the incidence of colic was not higher among bottle-fed infants even if their mothers smoked. The Norwegian researchers concluded that nicotine and other toxins in the breast milk of smoking mothers predispose their infants to colic.

What medical problems can a newborn encounter if its mother smokes?

Too little attention has been given to the unfortunate baby who lives in an environment in which adults are smoking. Such an infant unwittingly becomes a passive smoker by inhaling tobacco fumes in its environment. This is especially true

for newborns and infants who spend a good deal of their days and nights inside the house. As a result, these babies are at greater risk of contracting respiratory infections, chronic ear infections, bronchitis, and pneumonia during the first year of life. This is especially true if both parents are heavy smokers. In a 1983 study from Harvard Medical School, doctors measured the pulmonary or lung functioning of 1,156 babies exposed to their mothers' cigarette smoke in the home. The frightening conclusion was that the children's pulmonary function was diminished by an average of 11 percent at one year of age if their mothers smoked. At two years of age, the pulmonary function of these children was 9.5 percent below expectation when compared to children of nonsmoking mothers, while at five years of age it was 7 percent below the normal average. In a 1990 study published in the *American Journal of Epidemiology*, doctors found that children living in homes with smokers were more likely than other children to develop a variety of serious illnesses, including digestive system infections. The authors of this report speculated that exposure to tobacco may depress a child's immune system, thereby increasing susceptibility to infection.

Cotinine, the major metabolite of nicotine, can be found in the blood, urine, and saliva of cigarette smokers and those passively exposed to cigarette smoke. Researchers at the University of New Mexico were able to detect high levels of cotinine in children exposed to female smokers in the household.

Are smoking complications of pregnancy less likely with reduced-tar-and-nicotine cigarettes?

It has been demonstrated that the risk of lung cancer may be significantly reduced among women who smoke low-tar-and-nicotine cigarettes. However, there is no evidence that these cigarettes can reduce the complications caused by smoking during pregnancy or that they lower the risk of cardiovascular disease, emphysema, and bronchitis. To replace the flavor lost by cutting tar and nicotine levels, cigarette manufacturers have added such substances as shellac, caramel, and eugenol, some of which produce carcinogens when burned. Some epidemiologists fear that these new additives may eventually prove to be more dangerous than the chemicals they replaced.

While the reduced concentrations of nicotine found in the newer brands of cigarettes should diminish fetal toxicity to a degree, the concentrations of carbon monoxide, the most harmful constituent of cigarette smoke, have remained virtually unchanged. As a result, the amount of carboxyhemoglobin formed in the fetal bloodstream from the low-tar-and-nicotine cigarettes should be equal to that produced by most of the other brands.

In a report published in The *New England Journal of Medicine* in 1986, doctors measured nicotine and carbon monoxide levels in heavy smokers before and after they were asked to restrict the number of cigarettes they smoked each day. It was found that as smokers reduced the number of cigarettes consumed, they were still able to maintain the blood nicotine levels to which they had become dependent simply by smoking each cigarette longer. The same phenomenon has been noted when smokers switch from a standard brand to one with low tar and nicotine.

In recent years, clove cigarettes imported from Indonesia have gained some popularity among young smokers in the United States. These cigarettes contain a mixture of tobacco, cloves, and clove oil, and they smell more like candy than tobacco. This benign scent, however, should not lure pregnant women into believing that they are safe. In fact, clove cigarettes produce as much nicotine and carbon monoxide as domestic cigarettes and significantly more tar. Furthermore, eugenol, a major component of clove oil, may also be responsible for severe lung injuries among individuals who smoke these cigarettes.

Do you recommend nicotine gum or smokeless tobacco as a substitute for cigarettes during pregnancy?

No. Nicotine gum is probably less harmful than cigarette smoking since the inhalation of tars, lead, cadmium, and other substances is avoided. However, nicotine is known to stimulate the release of body substances known as catecholamines, which have the capacity to constrict or narrow the blood vessels to the uterus. This in turn reduces the concentration of oxygen in the fetal circulation. For this reason, pregnant women should not use nicotine gum.

Although nicotine replacement therapy in the form of nicotine patches (trade names Habitrol, Nicoderm, Nicotrol, Proslep, and Cygnus) is currently listed under the serious Category D risk factor for use in pregnancy (see Chapter 9), one expert, Dr. Neal L. Benowitz of the University of California in San Francisco, has recently endorsed its use for women who are unable to break their smoking habit during pregnancy. In his recent 1991 review of this subject in the *Journal of the American Medical Association*, Dr. Benowitz argues that the nicotine patch delivers less nicotine to the system and avoids fetal exposure to carbon monoxide and other toxic elements present in inhaled cigarette smoke.

Nicotine from a skin patch has been shown to readily enter the breast milk, but the concentrations are believed to be much lower than when a nursing mother smokes cigarettes. In addition, the hazards of passively inhaled cigarette fumes are avoided. Nevertheless, manufacturers suggest that patches be administered "cautiously" to women who are nursing their babies.

Smokeless tobacco refers to chewing tobacco, snuff, and the new "smokeless cigarette." Both chewing tobacco and snuff contain tobacco leaves and a variety of sweeteners, flavoring, and scents. In the past decade, snuff use has increased dramatically while that for chewing tobacco has declined slightly. Although there is no danger of smoke inhalation with chewing tobacco or snuff, the nicotine they contain is rapidly absorbed through the inner lining of the cheek and reaches higher levels in the bloodstream than that found with cigarettes. One recent study showed that use of smokeless tobacco for 30 minutes exposed a person to more nicotine than two or three cigarettes. For this reason, smokeless tobacco should not be used as a substitute for cigarettes during pregnancy. In addition, gum recession, bone loss from the jaw, and the development of precancerous and cancerous lesions of the oral cavity caused by smokeless tobacco make these products less than desirable. Although "smokeless cigarettes" reduce a person's exposure to carcinogenic compounds, critics believe that they deliver nicotine in more addicting doses than do ordinary cigarettes.

 # MARIJUANA

How does marijuana use affect pregnancy and nursing?

Although the relationship between a woman's use of marijuana and her likelihood to spontaneously abort has never been proven, research on both rodents and monkeys given marijuana and pure THC (delta g-tetrahydrocannabinal, the drug's chief ingredient) during pregnancy shows a significantly higher incidence of spontaneous abortion, stillbirth, and neonatal death. The mechanism is unknown, but THC appears to pass easily from the maternal to the fetal circulation and to impair normal placental function. Marijuana is fat soluble, so that the amount ingested during one use may take as long as 30 days to be excreted from the body. Thus a single episode of marijuana use will lead to prolonged exposure of the fetus to the drug.

Research on women who smoke pot during pregnancy is quite limited, but Canadian investigators recently noted that those who smoked five or more joints a week during any one trimester of pregnancy were more likely to give birth to an infant with tremors, unusual startle reactions, a high-pitched cry, and abnormal visual and auditory responses. It was also noted that the severity of symptoms in the newborn were directly related to the amount of marijuana smoked by its mother. Of great concern is the fact that the tremors and abnormal startle reactions were still evident at nine days of age, while the visual disturbances persisted for longer than 30 days. Follow-up studies at 12 and 24 months, however, showed that these infants did not have any cognitive or verbal defects. Marijuana was not found to adversely affect the course of pregnancy or delivery, the baby's Apgar score (see page 366), birth weight, length, or head circumference. In a 1982 study from the University of California in Los Angeles, doctors studied the effect of marijuana use on 35 pregnancies. They found that infants born to marijuana users were more likely to pass greenish fecal material, or meconium, into their amniotic fluid, a condition occasionally associated with fetal distress. Users of marijuana also experienced a higher incidence of prolonged and difficult labor than nonusers. This latter finding is in contrast with many other studies showing that marijuana use can hasten childbirth by increasing the strength and frequency of uterine contractions. One investigator reported that precipitate, or rapid and uncontrolled, labor was more common among marijuana users.

The majority of studies have concluded that regular marijuana users have a shorter pregnancy length, are less likely to gain adequate amounts of weight, and are more apt to give birth to smaller infants. After studying almost 4,000 pregnancies, doctors at Yale University Medical School, in their

1986 study published in the *American Journal of Epidemiology*, found that regular marijuana users were more likely to incur premature delivery and the birth of smaller babies. Most recently, doctors from the Boston University School of Medicine, in an article published in the *New England Journal of Medicine* in 1989, interviewed and tested more than 12,000 women attending prenatal clinics at Boston City Hospital. They found that an alarming 27 percent of the women had used marijuana in their pregnancies. Marijuana-exposed infants showed impaired fetal growth, weighed an average of 79 grams less, and were on average 0.5 centimeters shorter than infants born of nonusers. Other investigators at Boston University School of Medicine have noted that women who smoke marijuana are more likely to give birth to infants with anomalies similar to those described with the fetal alcohol syndrome (see section below). The majority of studies, however, have not found an association between marijuana use and specific congenital anomalies. One unexplainable but interesting finding of three separate investigative groups is the significant increase in the ratio of male to female offspring associated with maternal marijuana use.

The anatomic and physiologic response of rhesus monkeys is very similar to that of humans. Ricardo H. Asch, M.D., and Carol G. Smith, Ph.D., have performed extensive research on the effects of THC exposure immediately before and during pregnancy. When THC was administered to female rhesus monkeys immediately before mating, the animals experienced a spontaneous abortion and neonatal death rate four times higher than animals not given THC. If it was given to pregnant monkeys at a dose equivalent to that received by a person smoking two marijuana cigarettes per day, 40 percent of the animals studied experienced reproductive failures which included fetal death, stillbirth, and early infant death. Monkeys not exposed to THC experienced these problems only 11 percent of the time. Although all fetuses and infants of the THC-treated monkeys appeared normal, closer examination of the internal organs revealed developmental abnormalities in the nervous, cardiovascular, or urinary systems.

It has been demonstrated that THC rapidly crosses the placenta, with concentrations in the fetal bloodstream equal to those of its mother within minutes. High concentrations are also found in maternal milk. Suckling male offspring of rodents treated with marijuana for six days postpartum were observed to have both endocrine and behavioral changes. In humans, there are a few unconfirmed reports of drowsiness in nursing infants after their mothers smoked marijuana. While more data are needed, the information available seems sufficiently ominous to discourage women from even occasional marijuana use during pregnancy or the postpartum period if breast-feeding is contemplated.

 ALCOHOL ABUSE

How much alcohol can a woman safely drink during pregnancy?

In 1968, the association between maternal ingestion of alcohol and a variety of developmental abnormalities in the newborn was firmly established. The term "fetal alcohol syndrome" (FAS) was coined in 1973 to describe the gross malformations, prenatal and postpartum growth retardation, and permanent intellectual and psychomotor defects of some infants born of alcoholic mothers. The classic facial appearance noted in FAS is that of a small head circumference (microcephaly), underdevelopment of the jawbone (micrognathia), low-set ears, abnormalities of the eyelids, and underdevelopment of the bridge of the nose. In addition to these distinctive features, bone and joint abnormalities, abnormal creases in the palms, cardiac defects, kidney abnormalities, and female genital anomalies have been reported in more than 50 percent of these children. Infants affected with FAS were found in one study to have an average IQ of 65. As a result, these individuals experience learning and psychological disorders which persist throughout their lifetime. Newborns also exhibit abnormal brain wave recordings which begin as early as three days after birth and persist through adulthood. At birth, alcohol-exposed babies are often irritable, hyperactive, and tremulous, and they exhibit a poor sucking reflex. More recently described abnormalities associated with FAS include dysfunction of the ear's eustachian tube, dental malalignments, eye abnormalities, and impaired eyesight. In addition to FAS, researchers have found that women who drink may also be at significantly greater risk of spontaneous abortion, stillbirth, and the birth of babies with below-normal weights. Alcohol-related defects which are not as severe as those associated with FAS are often referred to as "fetal alcohol effects" (FAE). These include mental retardation, minor congenital anomalies of the skin, heart, urinary tract, and musculoskeletal system, and intrauterine growth retardation (IUGR). The largest study ever conducted on the relationship between alcohol use during pregnancy and IUGR was published in the *Journal of the American Medical Association* in 1984. In this survey of more than 31,000 women, researchers at the National Institutes of Child Health and Human Development found that 5.8 percent of babies born to nondrinkers fell below the tenth percentile for weight. In contrast, women with daily averages of less than one drink, one to two drinks, three to five drinks, and six or more drinks had respective risks for giving birth to a growth-retarded baby of 6.9 percent, 11.6 percent, 16.8 percent, and an alarming 17.7 percent.

Medically speaking, heavy drinkers are defined as those women who consume 3 or more ounces of absolute alcohol per day. This is the amount found in eight beers, 1 pint of whiskey, or one bottle of wine. While most reports have focused on chronic alcoholic women, in whom the risk of fetal abnormalities is estimated at 40 percent or more, it has also been found that sporadic but excessive intake of alcohol at critical stages of pregnancy by nonalcoholic women may lead to a poor pregnancy outcome as well. The most devastating effects occur during the first two months, often before a woman is aware that she is pregnant. However, chronic drinking during the third trimester may hinder fetal growth and contribute to mental retardation.

Even moderate amounts of drinking may be dangerous. Doctors at Columbia University noted a significantly higher rate of spontaneous abortion among women who consumed as little as one drink twice a week. When drinks were broken down according to type of liquor, the investigators found that women who drank wine and spirits ran a greater risk of miscarriage than those who preferred beer. Other studies, however, have shown that beer drinkers are more apt to experience adverse pregnancy outcomes and give birth to smaller babies than wine drinkers. A chemical named thiocyanate, found in beer but not in wine, is suspected as a possible cause of this problem.

The widely held belief that alcohol is harmless if one has an adequate diet is not true. Alcohol is a chemical that is toxic to the fetus, regardless of one's eating habits. There are several reports in the literature of alcoholic women delivering babies with characteristics of FAS despite the fact that they maintained excellent nutrition throughout pregnancy. For this reason, when patients ask me how much they can safely drink during pregnancy, I tell them abstinence is certainly the safest policy. I am in full agreement with the Surgeon General's advisory that pregnant women avoid all alcoholic beverages and food and drugs which contain alcohol. While no safe level of maternal alcohol intake during pregnancy has been established, the United States Food and Drug Administration has concluded that six drinks per day is sufficient to establish a major risk of growth and developmental abnormalities.

In one study, doctors found that the incidence of FAS was 11 percent in mothers who consumed two to three drinks per day, 19 percent for those having four drinks per day, and 32 percent for women consuming more than five drinks daily. One recent analysis of this vital subject was conducted on more than 8,300 women by doctors at Cleveland's Metropolitan General Hospital. Their findings, published in 1987, were that the critical level of prenatal alcohol exposure associated with an increased risk for congenital anomalies is more than four drinks per day. However, the authors were quick to point out that even minimal alcohol consumption during pregnancy should not be condoned, since susceptibility varies from one woman to another, and since subtle anatomic and neurological defects in newborns are often not detected until late in childhood. The Cleveland physicians confirmed previous studies showing that the greatest risk for birth defects due to maternal alcohol abuse was between the second and eighth week after conception, the period when organ formation is most active.

Although alcohol may not cause the obvious and severe intellectual impairments associated with FAS, subtle IQ differences often go undetected until later in childhood. When doctors at the University of Washington School of Medicine conducted IQ tests on children at the age of 4, they found that those born of mothers who averaged three drinks or more a day for the first two months of pregnancy had IQ scores 5 points below the average for babies born of nondrinkers. By their early school years, children of mothers who averaged only one or two drinks a day had slower reaction time and more difficulty paying attention.

FAS has been noted on rare occasions among babies born of previously alcoholic mothers who abstained throughout pregnancy. However, in most cases abstinence or marked reduction of alcohol consumption during pregnancy, including the third trimester, will significantly lower and almost completely eliminate the risk to the fetus.

Based on an evaluation of recent reports, it has been estimated that variations of FAS may occur with an astonishing frequency of 4 to 7 cases per 1,000 live births. The subtle defects known as fetal alcohol effects (FAE) may occur several times more frequently. An estimate from the National Public Health Service suggests that 1,800 to 3,600 babies are born each year with the characteristic signs of FAS, while as many as 36,000 others may be affected by FAE. If these calculations are correct, it would make alcohol consumption the responsible factor for up to 5 percent of all congenital anomalies and the most frequent cause of mental deficiency in the United States.

Does a father's drinking pattern have any adverse affects on the outcome of pregnancy?

Since alcohol is capable of damaging male reproductive organs and causing sperm abnormalities, a man's heavy drinking prior to conception theoretically can result in the birth of abnormal offspring. This theory is supported by laboratory studies in which male animals exposed to high levels of alcohol were found to sire fewer, smaller, and weaker offspring. Most research on human pregnancy has focused on the drinking habits of women before and during pregnancy. However, doctors at the University of Washington and the University of Michigan, in a 1986 study, found that babies whose fathers consumed two drinks daily or at least five drinks in one sitting during the month before conception weighed an average of 6.5 ounces less than those born of fathers who did not drink. The authors of this report suggested that both mothers- and fathers-to-be reduce their alcohol intake for at least a month prior to attempting pregnancy. Further studies are needed before it can be said with certainty that paternal drinking habits prior to conception influence a baby's birth weight.

How does alcohol affect a nursing infant?

During pregnancy, alcohol consumed by a woman crosses the placenta and rapidly reaches levels in the fetal circulation equal to those found in the maternal bloodstream. However, when a woman breast-feeds, only a small fraction of the alcohol she ingests is secreted into her breast milk. Until recently, the commonly held belief has been that alcoholic beverages taken in moderation by a nursing mother appear to have little if any effect on her infant. This view may be altered somewhat as a result of a study published in The *New England Journal of Medicine* in 1989. Dr. Ruth E. Little and her associates at the University of Michigan studied the mental and motor development of more than 400 breast-fed infants at one year of age and found that maternal alcohol consumption had no effect on a baby's mental skills. However, motor skills such as walking, crawling, and coordinated movements were significantly delayed in infants regularly exposed to alcohol in breast milk. Detrimental effects on motor development were noted when women drank as little as one drink daily, and motor skills deteriorated as the number of drinks consumed each day increased. Dr. Little hypothesized that small doses of alcohol received each day by an infant may accumulate in the body and produce these disturbing results. While doctors naturally caution women to avoid alcohol during pregnancy, the results of this study suggest that this taboo should be extended into early childhood if babies are breast-fed. In a second article published in the *New England Journal of Medicine* in 1991, researchers were able to demonstrate that breast milk acquires a distinct odor and flavor which is most pronounced 30 minutes to 1 hour after a woman consumes small amounts of alcohol. Infants were found to consume significantly less milk for up to 3 hours following maternal alcohol use equivalent to one can of beer. The authors of this report theorized that the change in flavor and odor may have deterred the infants from ingesting greater amounts of milk.

There are anecdotal reports in the medical literature in which infants have developed high blood alcohol levels after mothers drank in excess. In one dramatic case, a well-meaning mother said she drank seven beers a day plus other alcoholic beverages in order to increase her milk supply. Her four-month-old daughter became obese, lethargic, and experienced stunted growth. The child improved dramatically when her mother's alcoholic intake was curtailed. In defense of this woman, there is actually a scientific basis for the use of alcohol as a stimulus to breast milk production. Two separate studies have demonstrated that bloodstream levels of prolactin, the pituitary hormone most responsible for lactation, rise within minutes after a woman has a drink. It is also been the anecdotal observation of midwives, doctors, and lactating women that an occasional beer will help to improve milk production. However, too much of a good thing can prove to be troublesome. The second bodily ingredient needed for successful lactation is oxytocin, a hormone secreted by the pituitary gland and used medically to stimulate uterine contractions. Oxytocin is involved in the milk-ejection reflex from the nipples. Alcohol has been shown to inhibit oxytocin release, thereby causing a significant blunting of the milk-ejection reflex when large amounts are consumed. Therefore, the benefits gained by alcohol increasing the concentration of prolactin may be offset by its inhibiting effect on oxytocin release.

COCAINE ABUSE

What effect does cocaine have on the outcome of pregnancy?

It is astonishing that doctors are just beginning to discover the many hazards of cocaine use during pregnancy. Cocaine readily passes across the placenta from the maternal circulation and is detectable in the fetal blood and urine within minutes. It remains longer in the fetus than in the mother because the fetal liver lacks the ability to metabolize and excrete the drug rapidly. Cocaine is converted by the placenta to a more potent form, norcocaine, and remains in the amniotic fluid for as long as five days. By swallowing its amniotic fluid, a fetus takes additional amounts of cocaine into its body. Researchers at Northwestern University Medical School have found that infants whose mothers use cocaine during the 24 hours prior to delivery often show detectable levels of benzoylecgonine, an active metabolite, in their urine for up to 96 hours after birth.

Cocaine constricts or narrows other blood vessels throughout the body; it has the same effect on the uterine arteries supplying oxygen and nutrients to the developing fetus. As a result, early spontaneous abortion, fetal death during the second and third trimesters, and abruptio placenta, or premature separation of the placenta from its attachment to the uterine wall, are much more likely to occur among women who use cocaine. Abruptio placenta is an extremely dangerous obstetrical emergency characterized by hemorrhage, fetal distress, and, on rare occasions, even fetal and maternal death. In a study from Boston City Hospital, 60 percent of all cases of abruptio placenta could be attributed to maternal cocaine use. The hypertension, or elevated blood pressure, associated with cocaine use also contributes to the higher incidence of both abruptio placenta and the development of preeclampsia (pregnancy-induced hypertension). Laboratory studies on sheep confirm that cocaine raises the fetal as well as the maternal blood pressure. Newborns whose mothers have experienced only a single cocaine "hit" during pregnancy have suffered brain-damaging strokes and permanent paralysis, believed to be caused by cocaine's ability to rapidly elevate the fetal blood pressure. While cocaine has been reported to cause an elevation of body temperature, it has not been proven that it can raise the temperature to a level where hyperthermia-induced anomalies are possible.

A woman's craving for cocaine will usually take precedence over good nutrition, and adequate maternal weight gain is usually not achieved. Consequently, fetal intrauterine growth retardation and premature births are the rule rather than the exception. In one study, the average age at birth was 33½ weeks compared to the norm of 40 weeks. In an article published in *Obstetrics and Gynecology* in 1988, doctors at Kings County Hospital in Brooklyn, New York, noted that premature rupture of the amniotic membranes was twice as likely to occur among women using crack. They also found a higher incidence of IUGR and prematurity among crack users. Of greatest concern was the fact that 60 percent of crack-using women received no prenatal care. In a 1991 study, doctors from the University of Miami School of Medicine found that more than 20 percent of crack users have meconium-stained amniotic fluid, suggestive of fetal distress. When doctors at Boston City Hospital recently studied the effects of cocaine use on the outcome of pregnancy, they found that infants of women who used cocaine were an average of 93 grams (3.25 ounces) lighter and 0.7 centimeters (about a quarter of an inch) shorter than infants born of nonusers. The head circumference of the cocaine-exposed newborns was also found to be smaller, suggesting the possibility of retarded brain development. These findings have been confirmed at several other hospitals throughout the country.

Newborn infants born of cocaine-abusing women may demonstrate evidence of addiction at birth since the drug rapidly crosses the placenta. These infants often show signs of permanent central nervous system damage, are less reactive to environmental stimuli, suffer abnormal sleep patterns, tremors, exaggerated muscle tone, and a rapid heart rate. Diarrhea and fever have also been reported. When doctors at Beth Israel Hospital in New York City studied electroencephalograms, or brain wave tracings, of 38 newborns whose mothers used cocaine, they found that more than one-half were abnormal and remained so for the first two weeks of life. Although the long-term effects of in utero cocaine exposure have not been determined, most authorities fear that these infants are bound to suffer permanent mental and psychological defects and learning disabilities. In a 1989 report from San Francisco General Hospital, doctors found that 40 percent of the babies born to cocaine users lacked visual processing ability. This means that, unlike other newborns, they are irritable, withdrawn, and unable to fix or focus and hold their attention on an object, voice, or person. Cocaine-exposed babies are very fragile and respond poorly to attempts at comforting, often crying inconsolably without apparent provocation; the slightest noise or change in position often brings on long crying episodes. These behavior patterns often last for months. In a second California study, doctors at Los Angeles County Hospital found that the incidence of sudden infant death syndrome (SIDS) was ten times higher in infants of cocaine-abusing mothers than in the general population. Some experts quote a SIDS incidence as high as 15 percent in these children.

In a 1988 study, published in *Teratology*, doctors at Northwestern University observed an unusually high incidence of genital and urinary tract malformations in infants of mothers addicted to cocaine. The relationship between cocaine and urinary, but not genital, defects was confirmed in 1989 by doctors at the Centers for Disease Control, who found that the incidence of urinary anomalies

was 7.2 per 1,000 births among women using cocaine during the first trimester. This compared to an incidence of 1.5 per 1,000 in the general population. Included among the urinary abnormalities were kidney malformations which can lead to life-threatening infections. Researchers have also recently described the absence or narrowing of portions of the intestine among babies exposed to cocaine in utero, believed to be caused by the drug's narrowing of the blood vessels carrying oxygen to different areas of the intestine. In a 1989 study, doctors at the University of Texas Southwestern Medical Center in Dallas discovered that maternal cocaine use during the first trimester increased an infant's risk of congenital heart defects to 8 per 100, as compared to 0.8 per 100 births in the general population.

A host of other physical defects and developmental abnormalities associated with in utero cocaine exposure have been reported almost daily over the past five years. These have included limb reduction anomalies and damage to the gastrointestinal tract, brain, and hearing mechanism. The overall incidence of defects was reported at 16 percent in a recent study from Duke University Medical Center, but some experts fear that the true rate may actually be twice as high. Preliminary research reported in 1991 suggests that cocaine use in pregnancy may lead to irreversible chromosomal damage.

Is there a relationship between cocaine use and ectopic pregnancy?

Cocaine is not believed to be responsible for the formation of an ectopic pregnancy, but it may play a role in increasing the likelihood of such pregnancies to rupture and cause potentially catastrophic bleeding. In an article published in *Obstetrics and Gynecology* in 1989, Dr. Samuel S. Thatcher and his associates at Yale University School of Medicine reported the rupture of ectopic pregnancies in two women immediately after they used cocaine. The physicians theorized that cocaine could precipitate rupture by raising a woman's blood pressure, altering the movement of the muscles within the fallopian tube, or constricting the arteries which nourish the tube. The latter theory seems most plausible, since narrowing of the blood vessels reduces the tube's oxygen supply, thereby making it more susceptible to rupture.

Can a cocaine user safely breast-feed her baby?

Probably not. Cocaine passes from a woman's bloodstream to her breast milk and can produce symptoms of cocaine intoxication in breast-fed infants. Studies show that it takes only 30 minutes for cocaine to appear in the breast milk but 60 hours for it to disappear. To be absolutely certain, experts warn cocaine users not to nurse for at least 72 hours after they have had cocaine. Infants who ingest breast milk containing cocaine may experience dilated pupils, irritability, tremulousness, sweating, a rapid heart rate, high blood pressure, and even seizures. In one study, it took 60 hours to clear cocaine from the urinary tract of a baby who ingested the drug while nursing. The most tragic case to date was a 1988 report of a two-week-old infant girl who died shortly after her mother used crack while breast-feeding. The baby was found to

have toxic levels of cocaine in her bloodstream. Similar instances and reports of near-deaths have been published in the medical literature over the past five years.

Just as nicotine from cigarettes can be inhaled by "passive" nonsmokers, cocaine can appear in the bloodstream of individuals who breathe crack-laced air. This can be particularly toxic to infants under one year of age because their undeveloped systems do not produce enough enzymes to metabolize the drug. Epidemiologists believe that several neonatal deaths attributed annually to grand mal seizures or SIDS may in fact be misdiagnosed cases of crack smoke inhalation.

How can a man's use of cocaine effect the outcome of his spouse's pregnancy?

A very important 1991 study by researchers at the Washington University School of Medicine in St. Louis demonstrated that cocaine has the ability to bind or attach itself to spermatozoa. As a result, the cocaine-toting sperm act as a vector in transporting the drug into the ovum at the time of conception. It has been hypothesized that this mechanism may be responsible for many of the cocaine-related complications of pregnancy, even when a woman remains drug-free.

 # *AMPHETAMINES*

What are amphetamines, and how dangerous is their abuse during pregnancy?

Amphetamines are similar to cocaine in that they are psychologically addictive drugs which stimulate the nervous system and produce a feeling of excitation and euphoria. The general term "amphetamine" encompasses three closely related drugs—amphetamine, dextroamphetamine, and methamphetamine, which have a variety of street

names, such as "speed," "uppers," "bennies," "dexies," "crystal," and "white crosses." In pure form, amphetamines are yellowish crystals which are manufactured in tablets or capsules. Some abusers also sniff the pulverized crystals or make them into a solution for intravenous injection. Smokable methamphetamine is the most dangerous technique of abusing amphetamines.

Amphetamines should rarely, if ever, be taken by the nonpregnant woman and never by the pregnant woman. Although limited information exists about the effects of amphetamine abuse during pregnancy, laboratory studies on animals suggest that these drugs may damage and produce abnormalities of the developing fetus. Studies on women who abuse amphetamines during pregnancy have been contradictory. One report claimed an increased incidence of congenital heart disease, while another found faulty bile duct development among exposed fetuses. Three other studies, however, have shown no such association. In a 1988 report published in *Obstetrics and Gynecology*, doctors at the University of Texas Southwestern Medical Center studied the pregnancy outcome of

52 women who used intravenous methamphetamine during pregnancy. When compared to 50 nonusers, methamphetamine abusers gave birth to babies with significantly reduced birth weights, body lengths, and head circumferences. The frequency of congenital anomalies, however, were not significantly greater among the amphetamine abusers.

Substances such as "ecstasy" and "Eve," which contain the hallucinogen mescaline in addition to methamphetamine, add the hazard of fetal chromosomal damage when used during the first trimester of pregnancy.

 NARCOTICS

How does narcotic abuse affect the outcome of pregnancy?

Narcotics are effective in relieving pain, but they also elevate mood, counteract depression, and induce euphoria, sedation, and sleep. Prolonged use produces severe physical and psychological dependence. Drugs in this group are heroin, morphine, methadone (trade name Dolophine), opium, codeine, and meperdidine (best known by its trade name Demerol).

Some investigators have attributed chromosomal abnormalities to narcotic addiction. In a study of 99 methadone- and heroin-addicted pregnant women and their babies, both mothers and offspring were found to have a far greater percentage of chromosomally damaged cells than is usually noted in the general population. Interestingly, the chromosomal changes were unrelated to the dosage or duration of drug use. Similar studies on laboratory animals have confirmed these findings. Equally impressive studies have not found evidence that heroin produces congenital abnormal-

ities or permanent developmental problems in children born to addicted women.

The incidence of obstetrical problems is significantly greater in the pregnant addict. Included among these complications are ectopic pregnancy, low birth weight, premature labor, premature rupture of the membranes, meconium-stained amniotic fluid, IUGR, toxemia, abruptio placenta (premature separation of the placenta), anemia, and multiple births. In a 1989 study published in *Obstetrics and Gynecology*, doctors compared the results of nonstress tests (see Chapter 11) performed during the last trimester on 30 methadone-treated pregnant women before and one hour after receiving their usual methadone dose. Decreases in the frequency of fetal movement and the normally expected acceleration of the fetal heart rate were noted in one-fourth of the patients following methadone ingestion.

One of the most tragic medical conditions is narcotic addiction of the newborn resulting from transmission of drugs via the placenta. Approximately 70 percent of all babies born of addicted mothers show some evidence of withdrawal reaction within a few hours after birth: irritability, tremors, vomiting, high-pitched cry, sneezing, hyperactivity, respiratory distress, and diarrhea. These babies must be treated with the greatest care and skill by medical personnel who are experienced in dealing with this very difficult problem. Even with the best of care, the newborn mortality rate will be approximately 3 to 5 percent. Infants born to mothers who have used narcotics during pregnancy have been found to have a five to ten times greater risk of dying from sudden infant death syndrome.

When pregnant addicts are maintained on low-dose methadone, low birth weight, prematurity, and other obstetrical complications are less frequent. There is a greater risk of convulsive seizures, however, in babies of methadone-maintained mothers, and the frequency, severity,

and length of withdrawal symptoms in these infants are more pronounced when compared to those born to heroin-addicted mothers. The reason for this is that methadone is more fat soluble than heroin. As a result, more will cross the placenta and cause greater adverse effects.

While all narcotics are capable of passing from mother to child in the breast milk, the highest and most unpredictable concentrations occur with heroin. There are cases in the medical literature of infants of heroin-addicted mothers showing withdrawal symptoms when breast-feeding was delayed or discontinued. Nursing mothers on maintenance doses of methadone do not need to discontinue breast-feeding, since the average daily dose received by the infant is minimal. The limited reports available on morphine and codeine also indicate that little if any of these narcotics are present in the breast milk.

 OTHER DRUGS

How do hallucinogens affect the outcome of pregnancy?

Hallucinogens are a group of dangerous drugs, which, although not associated with addiction, physical dependence, or physical withdrawal, may cause permanent emotional damage and psychological dependence. The most notorious drugs in this group include LSD (D-lysergic acid diethylamide), peyote (a mescaline-containing cactus), and PCP (phencyclidine hydrochloride).

LSD is the most potent and potentially the most hazardous. The effects of LSD on the fetus have been studied with more intensity than most other medications, and several investigators have demonstrated significant breaks in the chromosomes of LSD users and their offspring. In one study of 44 women known to have taken LSD before and dur-

ing pregnancy, 6 (13.5 percent) gave birth to infants with serious deformities of both the lower and upper extremities. In addition, 5 of 21 aborted fetuses of LSD users had similar deformities. The usual incidence of these defects in the normal population is only 0.1 percent. It is frightening to note that the damage caused by LSD is random; one cannot predict which infants will be immune from injury and which ones will be deformed. The dose of LSD taken by the mother apparently is not a determining factor.

If a woman has taken LSD at or after the time of conception, therapeutic abortion is recommended. Chorionic villus sampling (CVS, see Chapter 11) performed between the ninth and eleventh weeks of pregnancy can determine if chromosomal damage is present. If pregnancy has progressed beyond the fourteenth week, analysis of fetal chromosomes may be performed by amniocentesis (see Chapter 11). The chromosomes in the fluid may then be studied for abnormalities, but this method of detection is far from foolproof, since not all LSD-deformed infants have broken chromosomes.

Peyote does not cause the chromosomal damage associated with the use of LSD. Members of the Huichol Indian tribe of northern Mexico have a lifelong history and a 1,600-year cultural tradition of peyote ingestion. Researchers from the University of California, in studying these people, were unable to detect chromosomal abnormalities among peyote users or their offspring.

Phencyclidine hydrochloride (PCP), also known as "angel dust," is a hallucinogenic drug that has been responsible for an alarming increase in the number of people treated in hospital emergency rooms for psychological reactions, fatal or near-fatal coma, or respiratory depression following its use. One recent case in the medical literature describes the appearance of an infant born of a woman who used PCP daily throughout her pregnancy. At birth, the baby experienced respiratory depression, lethargy, coarse tremors, poor feeding, and abnormal eye movements. In addition, its face had an unusual triangular shape with pointed chin and abnormal angle to the jaw. While there are no other studies concerning similar infant abnormalities, such effects must be considered a possibility in light of this report. Recent laboratory studies have demonstrated that PCP concentrations in breast milk may be ten times greater than those found in the maternal bloodstream.

Do amyl nitrite users increase their risk of giving birth to a compromised fetus?

Amyl nitrite, probably one of the most popular aphrodisiacs used in this country, comes in small glass ampules and is used as an aphrodisiac by breaking the glass and inhaling the contents just before orgasm. Isobutyl nitrite, also used as an aphrodisiac, is packaged in a small bottle with a screw cap. For this use, the cap is removed and the contents inhaled. Both are classified as vasodilators, which means they open the blood vessels, and amyl nitrite is used medically to relieve the pain of angina. In addition to dilating blood vessels, both drugs lower the blood pressure and speed the heart rate. Sexual sensations are enhanced: orgasms feel more intense and prolonged, and the drugs are effective in relaxing the vaginal and anal openings, thereby permitting easier penetration. Sexual activities which may have seemed repugnant or rejected because of inhibitions often become desirable.

Because amyl nitrite is used in the treatment of heart disease, it has been studied more extensively than isobutyl nitrite. Surprisingly, there are few if any harmful side effects of this drug, and in the medical literature there are no documented deaths or permanent injuries resulting from its recreational use. However, the sudden drop in blood pressure which it is capable of causing could be theoretically dangerous for women with either high or low blood pressure, as well as for individuals with certain heart conditions.

Although there are no reports that I know of which link use of amyl or isobutyl nitrite to congenital anomalies, neither should be used for sexual enhancement during pregnancy. Even a transient drop in blood pressure at any time during pregnancy may be associated with a decrease in the blood flow to the uterus. When this occurs, less oxygen is carried to the fetus, and that deprivation has the potential to cause permanent fetal damage. Recreational use of these drugs is especially dangerous among women with hypertension or pregnancy-induced hypertension (preeclampsia). Among these individuals, the drop in blood pressure is often more dramatic and more likely to compromise the oxygen supply to the fetus.

How do "Ts and Blues" affect pregnancy outcome?

"Ts and Blues" is the street name for the combined use of pentazocine hydrochloride (trade name Talwin) and tripelennamine (trade name Pyribenzamine). Talwin, a narcotic analgesic or pain reliever, is available by prescription but is easy to obtain illegally. Pyribenzamine is an over-the-counter antihistamine sold as a blue tablet. When this combination is mixed with water and then injected intravenously, it gives a quick "rush" similar to that of heroin, followed by a "high" lasting an average of six hours.

In a 1986 report published in the *Journal of Reproductive Medicine*, doctors at Louisiana State University School of Medicine in New Orleans studied 40 pregnant women using intravenous "Ts and Blues" during their pregnancies. Compared to a control group, the "Ts and Blues" abusers had a sixfold increase in fetal intrauterine growth retardation as well as lower 1-minute Apgar scores (see page 366) and lower birth weights. Thirty-five percent of exposed babies showed symptoms of pentazocine withdrawal, including a high-pitched cry, tremors, sweating, increased appetite, diarrhea, vomiting, and irritability. The use of "Ts and Blues" during pregnancy is an extremely dangerous form of child abuse.

Can sedatives and barbiturates be taken with safety during pregnancy?

Minor tranquilizers, such as diazepam (trade name Valium), lorazepam (trade name Ativan), chlorazepate (trade name Tranxene), alprazolam (trade name Xanax), meprobamate (trade names Miltown and Equanil), and chlordiazepoxide (trade name Librium), have the dubious distinction of being the most commonly prescribed category of medicines in the United States. While all these medications help to relieve anxiety, they carry a risk of physical dependency.

None of these drugs should be used during the first trimester of pregnancy because of the possible, though not positively proven, risk of congenital malformations in the fetus. Two earlier studies linked diazepam use to cleft palate and cleft lip, but subsequent reports have not substantiated this finding. Sedatives administered to a woman in labor can be transferred to the fetus via the placenta, causing drowsiness, abnormally low body temperature, poor muscle tone, and respiratory depression in the newborn. In addition, a "floppy baby syndrome," in which an infant demonstrates very poor muscle tone, abnormally low body temperature, and evidence of oxygen deprivation, has been described in newborns born to women using diazepam.

It is very important that a breast-feeding woman be aware that the concentration of Miltown or Equanil will be two to four times greater in her breast milk than in her bloodstream. While Librium and Valium are transmitted to breast milk in lower concentrations, research studies show that infants metabolize Valium more slowly than adults, possibly resulting in accumulations of the drug in a baby's body. Breast-feeding mothers who take diazepam may thus produce drowsiness in their infants.

Barbiturates, also known as "downers," "goofers," and "dolls," act on the central nervous system to produce sedation and sleep. Common trade names are Tuinal, Seconal, Nembutal, and Amytal. Their prolonged use results in both physical and psychological dependence, and withdrawal is more serious and dangerous than from narcotics. Although barbiturates have some very important medical applications (see Chapter 9), it is amazing how many unnecessary prescriptions for barbiturate capsules are written by doctors in this country each year.

In both animal experimentation research and studies of pregnant women, there is strong evidence to suggest that barbiturate use during the first three months of pregnancy increases the likelihood of fetal abnormalities (see Chapter 9). If barbiturates are taken within 8 hours of delivery, the drug can pass through the placenta and cause sleepiness and respiratory depression in the newborn. This type of medical problem is one of the most difficult for neonatologists to treat. Although barbiturates are known to pass into the breast milk, there is only one report in the medical literature of questionable drowsiness of a nursing infant.

Methaqualone, another type of "downer," creates bodily reactions similar to barbiturates, despite being chemically unrelated. It is sold under the trade name of Quaalude, and although it is referred to by devotees as the "love drug," there is no substantial evidence to show that it enhances sexuality. Because of its potency, it should never be taken during pregnancy.

6

SEXUALLY TRANSMITTED DISEASES

*W*hile some sexually transmitted conditions pose little if any threat to the developing fetus or to the baby at the time of birth, others, such as AIDS, hepatitis, herpes, and syphilis, are potentially lethal and require instant detection and therapy. Several of these diseases are totally without symptoms, thereby making the diagnosis particularly difficult. This chapter discusses current methods of diagnosing and treating those sexually transmitted diseases that may affect the pregnant woman and her baby.

 ## AIDS

The word AIDS is an acronym for Acquired Immune Deficiency Syndrome, the most deadly disease known to mankind. It is caused by the human immunodeficiency virus, or HIV.

It is frightening to realize that the 1983 edition of *The Pregnancy Book for Today's Woman* makes no mention of AIDS. First described in 1981, the disease was initially believed to be a rare and isolated condition predominantly confined to homosexual men and intravenous drug users. The first report of probable heterosexual transmission of AIDS occurred in 1983, the same year that AIDS was reported in a pregnant woman. Shortly thereafter, the virus was detected in the amniotic fluid and placenta of a 15-week fetus, confirming that transplacental passage was a real

threat. The enormity of this threat is now known—30 percent of infants born to American women who harbor HIV will develop full-blown AIDS. The rate of maternal-fetal transmission varies in different parts of the world. For example, the rate in Europe is about 14 percent, while the rate in Africa is close to 80 percent. The reasons for these differences remain unknown at the present time.

It is currently estimated that there are about 1 million HIV-infected individuals in the United States, with a cumulative total of over 200,000 cases of fullblown AIDS since the epidemic began. Women comprised almost 13 percent of the total number of AIDS cases reported as of March 31, 1992.

What are the ways in which a woman may contract AIDS?

HIV has been isolated from a variety of body tissues and fluids, including the conjunctiva and cornea of the eye, tears, urine, and saliva, but the low concentrations of the virus in these sites make them almost nonexistent sources of HIV transmission. In contrast, infected blood and semen contain high concentrations of the virus and are the two greatest locations of infection, while cervical mucous, vaginal secretions, and breast milk can transmit the infection to a significant, although lesser, degree. In this era of AIDS paranoia, it is important to remember that HIV is one of the least efficiently transmitted infections; for infection to occur, high numbers of the virus must be directly inoculated into the bloodstream, under the skin, or into a body cavity. Furthermore, the transmission, regardless of one's sexual preferences, is extremely unlikely following a single exposure to HIV-infected body fluids. Coexisting sexually transmitted diseases, such as herpes and syphilis, and other open skin lesions allow the virus easier access to a person's bloodstream. In general, a person with genital ulcerative disease appears to have a threefold to fivefold higher risk of sexually acquiring the HIV virus than someone without such lesions.

While most HIV infections in men are the result of homosexual contact with an infected partner, 51 percent of the cases occurring in women in 1991 were due to intravenous drug use and the sharing of contaminated needles and syringes with other drug users.

Approximately 33 percent of women had become infected via sexual contact with an infected man, compared to only 14 percent in 1983. Another 9 percent had contracted their infections following medical procedures such as the transfusion of blood and blood products, tissue transplantation, and insemination of donor sperm, while a smaller percentage of women had no identifiable risk factors. The number of medically induced HIV infections has been dramatically reduced following the introduction of HIV antibody testing in 1985.

Among the 33 percent of women who acquired HIV via heterosexual contact, the majority became infected as a result of sexual contact with an intravenous drug user. If we add this percent to the 51 percent who contract their disease through use of drugs, we find that almost 85 percent of women with AIDS get it through use of drugs or contact with a sexual partner using drugs. Sex with a bisexual male is responsible for an equal number of AIDS cases as is sex with a pre-1985 male transfusion recipient, especially one with a blood coagulation disorder such as hemophilia or von Willebrand's disease. Women born in countries where heterosexual transmission of AIDS is common, such as Haiti and Zaire, account for the remaining number of heterosexually acquired AIDS infections.

How does the human immunodeficiency virus invade body cells and produce disease?

T-helper lymphocytes are white blood cells which play a primary role in regulating immunity against a variety of infections and rare malignancies. HIV has the ability to invade, reproduce in, and destroy T-helper lymphocytes and other immune system and central nervous system cells which contain antigens known as CD4 or T4 receptors on their surface. When the immune system is not functioning properly the body can fall prey to unusual and severe illnesses, and lower than normal CD4 cell counts are often a good indication of a person's lack of immune competence.

The initial HIV infection may be asymptomatic but more often than not manifests itself as a mononucleosis-like illness two to eight weeks following exposure to the virus. It is characterized by fever, muscle aches, sore throat, joint pain, a diffuse beefy red rash, and occasionally a stiff neck associated with a noninfectious meningitis. These symptoms are transient and often disappear within one to three weeks. An HIV antibody blood test obtained at this time may be negative since it usually takes between six to twelve, and an average of eight weeks, following exposure to turn positive. Scientists define the "window period" as that time period between the initial HIV infection and subsequent detection of the HIV antibody in a person's bloodstream. In some cases, this window period has been reported to be several months and even as long as three years. The spontaneous resolution of the initial infection after one to three weeks is usually followed by a latency period which may last anywhere from six months to ten or more years. During this time symptoms may be nonexistent or minimal, although a person remains infectious.

As T-helper lymphocytes continue to be destroyed by the virus, a person's immune system becomes weaker and is less able to defend itself against the effects of the virus. Most individuals develop early nonspecific symptoms such as low-grade fever, loss of appetite, weight loss, lethargy, chills, night sweats, diarrhea, persistent cough, and, most commonly, a generalized enlargement of the lymph nodes. The lymph nodes most likely to be enlarged are those located in the back of the neck, the underarms, the groin, the elbows, and behind the ears. The term AIDS-related complex (ARC) has been used to describe these nonspecific symptoms in association with a positive HIV antibody titre. By definition, however, these symptoms do not meet the criteria for calling the disease AIDS.

When is a person officially diagnosed as having AIDS?

The progressive destruction of T-helper lymphocytes weakens the immune system and makes an individual susceptible to harmful and potentially fatal infections. These infections are called "opportunistic" because the microscopic organisms that cause them take the opportunity to attack while the body's resistance is low. When a person infected with HIV contracts one of these serious infections or one of several unusual tumors, he or she is said to have the fatal disease known as AIDS. In fact, these infections and tumors are so rare in a healthy person that the diagnosis of AIDS can be made even if the HIV antibody titre is negative. As of 1991, the Centers for Disease Control broadened the definition of AIDS to include any HIV-infected person with a CD4 lymphocyte count of less than 200 cells per cubic millimeter of blood. In a healthy person, the count usually exceeds 1,000 cells per cubic millimeter.

Pneumocystis carinii pneumonia (PCP) is a dangerous parasitic lung infection which is the most common manifestation of AIDS and one of the leading causes of death. This opportunistic infection accounts for more than 50 percent of all initial AIDS diagnoses and affects two-thirds of those suffering from AIDS. PCP is not only difficult to prevent but is often extremely resistant to treatment. Another opportunistic infection is candidiasis or "thrush," the same condition which is usually limited to the genitals of healthy individuals (see page 191). The presence of candidiasis in locations such as the mouth, throat, esophagus, and lungs is characteristic of AIDS. Similarly, the presence of persistent herpesvirus infections in areas distant from the genitals, such as the mouth, throat, gastrointestinal, and pulmonary tract, is also diagnostic of AIDS, regardless of whether the antibody test is positive or negative. Two rare types of cancer—Kaposi's sarcoma and primary non-Hodgkins lymphoma of the central nervous system—are diagnostic of AIDS when found in a person under 60 years of age. Kaposi's sarcoma is characterized by the presence of red or violet lesions on the skin and mucous membranes; although it is a very common finding in male homosexuals with AIDS, it is rare among heterosexuals with the disease. Finally, progressive dementia in a young person, characterized by impaired memory, apathy, inability to pay attention, and psychomotor retardation, is believed to be the result of brain damage caused by the virus attacking the central nervous system. Neurological disease has been reported in 60 percent of AIDS sufferers and is documented at autopsy in 90 percent of those who die of the disease.

There are several other medical conditions which are associated with AIDS less often than the above mentioned diseases. Consequently, each must be accompanied by a positive HIV antibody titre if a person with one of these diseases is to be diagnosed as having AIDS. These include histoplasmosis and coccidiomycosis, fungal infections which cause lung disease; active tuberculosis involving organs other than the lungs; salmonella bacterial infections in the bloodstream; and other bizarre and long-lasting infections. The diagnosis of AIDS is a certainty if an HIV-positive person experiences an unintentional weight loss of 15 pounds or more combined with at least one of the following symptoms for three or four months: an oral temperature greater than 100°F, diarrhea, night sweats, severe malaise, thrush.

How does one's sexual practices influence their likelihood of contracting or transmitting AIDS?

HIV has been isolated from semen, cervical and vaginal secretions, and saliva; however, it is less efficiently transmitted than any other sexually acquired infection. As a result, the risk of contracting HIV following one sexual encounter with an infected person is extremely low, regardless of the nature of the contact. Continued exposure, however, significantly increases the odds of acquiring the infection (see Table 8).

Of all sexual practices, anal-receptive intercourse carries the highest risk because it causes microscopic trauma to the surface tissues and blood vessels of the anus and rectum, thereby providing direct access of HIV-infected semen into the bloodstream. Following one anal-receptive encounter with an HIV-positive male, approximately 1 in 250 women will contract the infection. Condom use by an infected man may decrease the risk somewhat, but it is still dangerous because condoms are

not designed for anal intercourse and are more likely to break or tear when used in this fashion.

Vaginal-receptive intercourse with an infected man is the second riskiest sexual activity, exposing a woman to a 1 in 500 chance of becoming infected after a single encounter. Use of a condom reduces the likelihood to 1 in 5,000. It appears that female-to-male transmission is far less common, probably because the penis is more likely to cause trauma than to be traumatized during coitus. In addition, a woman's tissues are exposed to infected semen for long periods of time following ejaculation, while a man's exposure exists for only as long as the coital act. While fellatio carries some risk for a woman, it is believed to be far less than for anal or vaginal intercourse. There is only one reasonably well documented case in the medical literature of a man who acquired AIDS solely through repeated acts of cunnilingus with an infected prostitute. Female-to-female transmission has been reported only twice. One case resulted from sexual activity during the menses and the other involved significant trauma to the vaginal tissues.

The likelihood of contracting AIDS increases in direct proportion to the number of sexual partners one encounters. Sexual activity in which either partner has open genital skin sores, as occurs with herpes and syphilis, increases the risk for the HIV-negative partner fivefold.

In a 1988 study published in the *Journal of the American Medical Association*, Doctors Norman Hearst and Stephen B. Hulley of the University of California School of Medicine calculated the chances of a person becoming infected with HIV based on the particular risk category of their sexual partner and the number of sexual encounters one has with that partner. This information is presented in Table 8.

Condom use has been shown to reduce the risk of HIV transmission by as much as 90 percent, but Table 8 demonstrates that condoms are far from foolproof and may even provide a person with a false sense of security. While nonuse of condoms for 500 sexual encounters with an HIV-positive

TABLE 8

RISK OF CONTRACTING AIDS BASED ON CATEGORY OF SEXUAL
PARTNER AND NUMBER OF SEXUAL ENCOUNTERS

Risk Category of Partner	*1 sexual encounter*	*500 sexual encounters*
1. HIV blood test unknown, but not in high risk group		
A. Using condoms	1/50,000,000	1/110,000
B. Not using condoms	1/5,000,000	1/16,000
2. High risk group (homosexual and bisexual men, I.V. drug users, heterosexual from country where HIV spread is common, etc.)		
A. Using condoms	1/100,000 to 1/10,000	1/210 to 1/21
B. Not using condoms	1/10,000 to 1/1,000	1/32 to 1/3
3. HIV negative—no history of high risk behavior such as needle sharing or intercourse with member of high risk group		
A. Using condoms	1/5,000,000,000	1/11,000,000
B. Not using condoms	1/500,000,000	1/1,600,000
4. Continuing high risk behavior		
A. Using condoms	1/500,000	1/1,100
B. Not using condoms	1/50,000	1/160
5. HIV blood test positive		
A. Using condoms	1/5,000	1/11
B. Not using condoms	1/500	2/3

person is suicidal, use of a condom still subjects a person to a 1 in 11 risk of contracting the virus. In fact, Table 8 demonstrates that using a condom with an intravenous drug user, bisexual male, or prostitute is far more dangerous than sex without a condom with someone who does not belong to any high-risk group.

The spermicide nonoxynol-9 is found in the contraceptive sponge as well as in a variety of vaginal tablets, foams, gels, and creams. Recently, it has also been incorporated into some of the newer condoms. Laboratory research has demonstrated that nonoxynol-9 is capable of inactivating the AIDS virus. However, there is no proof that it is capable of effectively killing the virus in real-life circumstances, and one should not be lulled into relying on these preparations as a sole disease pre-

ventative. Some individuals are extremely sensitive to nonoxynol-9 and will develop a genital rash or even skin ulcerations which, paradoxically, can increase one's risk of contracting the virus.

Are some condoms better at preventing AIDS than others?

Despite the rising concern about AIDS in our society, the use of condoms has continued to remain low. In a recent survey by the Alan Guttmacher Institute of more than 10,000 sexually active American women 15 to 44 years of age, it was found that only 16 percent regularly used condoms, compared to 12 percent prior to the AIDS epidemic.

A latex condom viewed under an electron microscope appears as a pore-free membrane which will not allow the passage of water, one of the tiniest of molecules. Tests show that an intact latex condom will not allow the passage of the smallest of microbes. In contrast, lamb membrane condoms appear as layers of fibers crisscrossing in various patterns. This latticework allows the passage of an occasional pore measuring an average of 22 nanometers (nn). Since a nanometer is one-billionth of a meter and a sperm cell measures 3,000 nn, the risk of pregnancy is highly unlikely. Similarly, the passage of sexually transmitted organisms such as the gonococcus (2,000 nn), chlamydia (200 to 300 nn), herpes virus (180 to 200 nn), HIV (80 to 120 nn), and hepatitis B virus (42 nn) is highly unlikely, but lamb membrane condoms are not as safe as latex condoms, which are also preferable because they are less likely to slip off during and immediately after intercourse when the penis is withdrawn.

When the FDA tests condoms they use the water-leak method in which the condom is filled with 300 cubic centimeters (cc) of water and then checked for leaks. If water leakage exceeds four condoms per thousand, the manufacturer is ordered to destroy the entire batch. On average, one in ten domestic condoms are rejected as compared to one in five imports; so as far as condoms are concerned, it is a good idea to "buy American." Studies have shown that latex condoms deteriorate rapidly when exposed to heat, light, or oil-based lubricants such as petroleum jelly. For this reason it is important to store them in a cool place out of the sunlight. Latex condoms which appear brittle, sticky, or discolored should not be used.

Female condoms or vaginal pouches made of polyurethane are currently in varying stages of development and show great promise as a method of reducing HIV transmission.

As previously mentioned, anal-receptive intercourse with an HIV-positive male is the riskiest form of sexual activity in transmitting the virus. A recent calculation of condom breakage rates during anal sex is 1 in 105, compared to 1 in 165 for vaginal coitus.

Can a person transmit AIDS through "passionate kissing" or through biting another person?

Concentrations of the human innumodeficiency virus in saliva appear to be low, as evidenced by the fact that there has never been a confirmed report of AIDS transmission solely through kissing. Some researchers believe that saliva may actually inhibit the infectivity of the virus, which may help to explain one case in which an adult AIDS patient bit 30 healthcare workers without one contracting HIV. Similarly, there are several reports of HIV-positive children biting other susceptible children without transmitting the virus to them.

Much has been written in the medical literature about the potential danger of "passionate kissing" in transmitting HIV. One researcher noted microscopic lesions of the lining or mucosa of the mouth as well as the presence of small amounts of blood in the saliva following a prolonged session of deep-tongue kissing. It has been theorized that the virus could enter the bloodstream through these tiny lesions. One interesting observation noted in another survey was that 14 percent of people habitually brush their teeth before kissing. Brushing traumatizes the oral mucosa and often causes gross and microscopic bleeding, which could theoretically increase the risk of disease transmission.

What are some of the myths surrounding the nonsexual transmission of HIV?

AIDS is not an airborne infection and can't be transmitted through sneezing or coughing. In addition, the virus cannot be passed by touching an infected person or by sharing household items such as blankets, sheets, towels, washcloths, clothes, telephones, glasses, dishes, and silverware. Drinking beverages or eating food that an infected person has prepared or touched will not transmit HIV, nor will sharing the use of water fountains, toilet seats, swimming pools, spas, or hot tubs. The AIDS virus is unable to live and reproduce outside the body, so even sharing a toothbrush with someone who is HIV positive, though certainly not recommended, is a highly improbable source of disease transmission.

Regarding the widespread fear of infected mosquitoes, the AIDS virus would have to multiply inside the mosquito to make transmission possible, and studies show that this doesn't happen. Even in mosquito-infected areas of the United States and Africa, children living in the same room as AIDS patients haven't been infected. Other insects such as bedbugs and lice are similarly incapable of transmitting the infection.

What are some of the truths surrounding the non-sexual transmission of AIDS?

A healthcare worker who experiences a needle stick containing contaminated blood faces approximately a 1.3 to 3.9 per 1,000 chance of eventually contracting HIV. One report, however, placed this risk as high as 8 per 1,000. In contrast, approximately 120 to 300 per 1,000 will contract hepatitis B following a needle stick accident. Women have also contracted the disease following artificial insemination with fresh donor sperm. As a result, infertility specialists now favor cryopreserved or frozen sperm, which can be stored for three months to several years so that the donor can be tested and retested for HIV antibodies prior to use of the specimen. Organ donors have also transmitted AIDS and as a result are continually tested for HIV prior to surgery. Recent reports of transmission of HIV from infected dentists to their patients have fueled the debate over whether universal testing of both patients and physicians should be mandated. The risk of such transmission remains unknown at the present time but is considered to be extremely low.

Transfusion of infected blood and blood products, such as platelets, white blood cells, and cry-

oprecipitate, poses the greatest threat to transmitting HIV. Prior to 1985, this risk was significant, but with the advent of antibody screening it is now estimated to range from 1 in 10,000 to 1 in 1,000,000. The incidence of undiagnosed HIV is significantly higher in large inner city areas of New York and San Francisco, where there are a greater number of individuals likely to be incubating the virus but not yet showing a positive HIV antibody titre. In almost 7 percent of carriers, infection cannot be detected by present HIV antibody tests. Nationally, 0.02 percent of all donated blood is HIV-antibody positive, an indication that 2 to 3 units of blood per 1,000,000 are contaminated with the virus without the infection being detectable by current antibody tests. In New York City and San Francisco, the prevalence of HIV is 10 to 15 times the national average. In these cities, 2 to 4 units per 10,000 could be contaminated and go undetected. During a major surgical procedure in which 8 units of blood is transfused, a patient's risk of acquiring AIDS could be 0.2 percent.

As long as the currently available HIV detection methods are not improved upon, people receiving transfusions will continue to experience a very small but significant threat of infection. Since the concentration of a virus is highest in the blood, the unwitting transfusion of one unit of infected blood will result in an HIV-negative individual becoming HIV-positive 90 percent of the time.

Finally, and probably most tragically, HIV-positive pregnant women will transmit a fatal AIDS infection to 30 percent of their offspring.

Since there is a small risk of acquiring HIV with a blood transfusion, doesn't it make sense for a pregnant woman to donate her own blood in the event of an obstetrical hemorrhage?

The donation of one's own, or autologous, blood for possible transfusion at a later date has gained great popularity among several medical and surgical subspecialties. It is somewhat surprising that obstetricians appear to be less enthusiastic than other physicians in utilizing this important method of avoiding transfusion-associated disease, especially since a woman undergoing a cesarean section will lose an average of 800 to 1,000 milliliters of blood, while a routine vaginal delivery is associated with a blood loss of 300 to 400 milliliters, or more than one-half a pint. Further strengthening the argument for donating and receiving one's own blood is the statistic that one in eight blood recipients will experience a complication as a result of a donated blood transfusion. These can run the gamut from mild to severe allergic reactions, antibody formation against the donated red blood cells, and an estimated 5,000 deaths annually due to either AIDS, hepatitis B, or non-A, non-B hepatitis.

In my opinion, autologous blood donations should be offered to pregnant women with a history of either a previous cesarean section or hemorrhage at or immediately after their previous delivery. Women known from previous experience to have multiple red blood cell antibodies and difficulties in finding compatible blood donors should also consider donating their blood. When the present pregnancy is complicated by a placenta previa or low-lying placenta (see Chapter 12), a uterine anomaly, multiple births, or a breech position of the baby in the last month, the odds are greater that blood will be needed. In addition, women giving birth to their fifth or more full-term baby are more likely than other women to experience uterine rupture and postpartum hemorrhage. They, too, should be encouraged to avail themselves of an autologous blood donation.

What are the effects of a maternal HIV infection on the fetus and newborn?

Although babies born to women with HIV may appear healthy at birth, they have a 30 percent likelihood of contracting full-blown AIDS or dying of the disease before their second birthday. Others can take up to five or more years to develop symp-

toms. Usually, however, an average of four months elapses after delivery before the disease first becomes manifested in the newborn. Sadly, AIDS progresses more rapidly and is far more deadly in infants than in adults. Once a woman has given birth to a baby with AIDS, her chances of this happening in a subsequent pregnancy are approximately 65 percent.

At least 95 percent of women harboring HIV are asymptomatic, and their pregnancies and births are usually uneventful. Research has shown that asymptomatic HIV-positive women are at no greater risk of spontaneous abortion, ectopic pregnancy, premature birth, IUGR, birth defects, stillbirths, low Apgar scores, abnormally long duration of labor, or complications at the time of delivery. However, if a woman is suffering from symptoms of AIDS, such as weight loss, diminished appetite, and generalized debilitation, her condition is likely to adversely influence fetal growth and pregnancy outcome. In one study, 33 percent of newborns born to women with full-blown AIDS weighed less than 2,500 grams (about 5½ pounds). In another report, premature rupture of the amniotic membranes occurred in about 60 percent of the pregnant AIDS patients studied.

HIV is most often passed from mother to fetus across the placenta; this has been shown to occur as early as the fifteenth week of pregnancy. Most babies destined to develop AIDS are infected prior to the moment of birth. Studies have shown that few if any newborns become infected with HIV in their passage through the vagina during labor, as evidenced by the finding that the neonatal HIV infection rate is equal for babies delivered vaginally and those born by cesarean section. Other reports, however, have found that many infants do become infected during the birth process. A 1991 article published in *Lancet* studied the incidence of HIV infection among twins and found that 50 percent of first-born twins who were delivered vaginally and 38 percent of first-born twins delivered by cesarean section were infected with HIV. This compared with a 19 percent infection rate of second-born twins delivered by either route. The data suggest that the twin which is lower in the maternal pelvis and exposed to an infected cervix and vagina for a longer period of time is more apt to be exposed to the HIV virus. Although the virus has been isolated from breast milk, epidemiologists are uncertain of how important a role breast-feeding plays in transmitting the disease to a baby.

Infants who contract AIDS are susceptible to many of the opportunistic infections suffered by adults with the disease as well as unique illnesses such as a lung infection known as lymphoid interstitial pneumonitis. Enlargement of the liver and spleen, failure to thrive and gain adequate amounts of weight, and impaired neurological development all appear to be common manifestations of AIDS in a newborn.

What are some the problems associated with diagnosing and treating AIDS in a newborn?

Detecting HIV in an infant is problematic because virtually 100 percent of babies born of HIV-positive women passively acquire their mothers' antibodies before birth and test HIV positive whether they have the disease or not. These so-called IgG antibodies usually disappear from a healthy unaffected newborn's circulation at 15 months of age. However, in rare cases they may persist for as long as two years. Another problem is that an average of four months elapses after delivery before symptoms of the disease become manifest in the newborn. As a result, efforts at diagnosing the disease and initiating early treatment of infected babies are too often thwarted.

If and when an accurate method is devised for distinguishing between healthy and HIV-infected newborns, it will allow doctors to initiate prophylactic therapy with medications such as zidovudine (formerly called AZT, present trade name Retrovir) before symptoms appear. To judge from available research, such treatment will prolong life and delay the time interval until symptoms of the disease first appear. Even in the absence of such an

early test, the 30 percent risk of a baby contracting AIDS from its HIV-positive mother is so great that researchers are establishing protocols for routinely treating all of these babies with zidovudine immediately after birth. The drug is well-tolerated by children and the results to date have been excellent. Alpha interferon has also been tested in several small studies and appears promising in preventing the onset of AIDS in some mothers and babies infected with the virus. In recent studies, doctors have combined low doses of alpha interferon with low doses of zidovudine to delay the onset of AIDS as well as ameliorate the symptoms of the full-blown disease.

Another experimental design being tested is to treat HIV-positive women during pregnancy with zidovudine in order to block passage of the virus across the placenta to the baby. Because of fears that this drug may cause birth defects when administered during the first trimester, treatment is most often initiated during the second half of pregnancy. One encouraging 1992 report published in the *New England Journal of Medicine* found no evidence of birth defects, premature births, or fetal distress among a small number of women when zidovudine therapy was initiated during the first trimester. It is still too early to tell whether zidovudine treatment of HIV-positive mothers will help to diminish the devastation caused by the disease in newborns.

The National Institutes of Health is sponsoring research to see if administering HIV antibodies during the second and third trimesters as well as at the moment of birth to women with the disease can reduce the incidence of maternal-fetal transmission. It is hoped that these antibodies, or immune globulins (HIVIG), will pass across the placenta and destroy the virus before it reaches the fetus.

If I suspect that I have been exposed to AIDS, what should I do?

If you are seeking specific information about AIDS you can call your local or state health department or the National AIDS Hotline at 1-800-342-2437.

Spanish-speaking callers can dial 1-800-344-7432. This service, supervised by the Centers for Disease Control, is open 24 hours a day, 7 days a week. The staff answering calls can tell you where you can get an antibody test locally and whom to contact for counseling, treatment, support groups, and financial assistance. They also answer general questions about AIDS. Questions about AIDS can also be answered by the National Women's Health Network, 202-347-1140; Women's AIDS Project, 213-650-1508; and the Women and AIDS Resource Network, 212-475-6713.

Many private physicians do confidential AIDS counseling and testing. However, some people prefer not to discuss AIDS with their regular physician for fear that a positive test result in their medical record could lead to work, housing, or other forms of discrimination. There are almost 1,000 publicly funded AIDS counseling and testing sites around the country. Many of these centers perform testing and counseling for about $30.00.

There is a tremendous amount of information about AIDS available as leaflets, books, and even videotapes. Some of these are listed in Table 9.

 ## *SYPHILIS*

What causes syphilis, and what are its symptoms?

Syphilis is caused by the bacterium *Treponema pallidum*. The initial syphilis infection may be single or multiple and usually begins as a flat sore on the skin which soon erodes to form a hard, firm-edged, painless ulcer called a chancre (pronounced *shanker*), teeming with millions of highly contagious bacteria. Since it is a painless sore, it often goes unnoticed, although the bacteria are easily spread during coital and noncoital contact. While most chancres appear on the genitalia, they may also be found on the lips, tongue, fingers, nipples, and anus if these areas come in direct contact with areas harboring bacteria. The lymph nodes in the area surrounding a chancre are usually enlarged but are not painful to touch. Syphilis is known as the "great imitator" because it often mimics other diseases such as herpes.

An untreated primary chancre usually heals slowly over a period of three to eight weeks, leaving a thin scar. Its disappearance ends the primary stage of the disease and is often falsely considered as a sign that all is well. However, the secondary stage usually appears within three months after the first stage has healed, although it may be delayed for many months or even years. Its appearance means that the bacteria are now disseminated throughout the body.

Symptoms of secondary-stage syphilis vary, although some form of skin rash, often with a scaly appearance, is usually noted on the trunk, palms, and soles. Occasionally it is most prominent on the moist skin surfaces such as the underarms, the genitals, and the anus. The hair on the head may fall out in patches. The inside of the mouth may show secondary syphilis lesions, known as mucous patches, which have a grayish-white necrotic area surrounded by a dull red border and cause a severe sore throat. All these skin and mucous membrane lesions are extremely infectious. Whereas only the local lymph nodes are enlarged during the primary stage of syphilis, 50 percent of individuals with secondary syphilis experience a generalized lymph node enlargement throughout their bodies: in the groin, under the arms, in the neck, and under the jaw. Since the disease is widespread throughout the body during the secondary stage, it is often accompanied by generalized symptoms such as headache, weakness, loss of appetite, and aching in the long bones, muscles, and joints.

Amazingly, if left untreated, the lesions of

TABLE 9

INFORMATION MATERIALS ON AIDS

Leaflets (Up to 50 free copies)
You can obtain the material below, produced jointly by the PHS.[1] (Public Health Service) and
the American Red Cross, by writing to AIDS, Suite 700, 1555 Wilson Boulevard, Rosslyn, VA
22209.

- *AIDS, Sex and You*
- *Facts about AIDS and Drugs Abuse*
- *AIDS and Your Job—Are There Risks?*
- *Gay and Bisexual Men and AIDS*
- *AIDS and Children*—Information for Parents of School-Age Children
- *AIDS and Children*—Information for Teachers and School Officials
- *Caring for the AIDS Patient at Home*
- *If Your Test for Antibody to the AIDS Virus is Positive* . . .

Additional materials, which were developed by the PHS, are available from the addresses
indicated:

- *Surgeon General's Report on AIDS* (October 1986). Write to AIDS, P.O. Box 14252,
  Washington, D.C. 20044. (Up to 50 free copies) *Facts About AIDS*. Write to AIDS,
  Suite 700, 1555 Wilson Boulevard, Rosslyn, VA 22209. (Up to 50 free copies)

A pamphlet for women entitled *Women and AIDS* is available free of charge from: Women's
Health Research Foundation, 700 Arizona, Santa Monica, CA 90401.
Scriptographic booklets. Write to Office of Public Inquiries, Centers for Disease Control,
Building 1, Room B-63, 1600 Clifton Road, Atlanta, GA 30333. (Up to 25 free copies)

- *What Everyone Should Know About AIDS* (also available in Spanish)
- *Why You Should Be Informed About AIDS* (for healthcare workers)
- *What Gay and Bisexual Men Should Know About AIDS*
- *AIDS and Shooting Drugs*

Videotapes. To purchase tapes ($55 each), write to National Audiovisual Center, 8700
Edgeworth Drive, Capitol Heights, MD 20743-3701. Attn: Customer Service Section; telephone
(301)763-1896. For free loan, write to Modern Talking Picture Service, 5000 Park Street, North,
St. Petersbury, FL 33709, Attn: Film Scheduling, telephone (813)541-5763.

- *AIDS: Fears and Facts* (for the general public)
- *What If the Patient Has AIDS?* (for healthcare workers)
- *AIDS and Your Job* (for policemen, firemen, and other emergency personnel)

Miscellaneous

- A pamphlet entitled *What Is Safe Sex?* contains good information in plain but not
  distasteful language. This pamphlet can be obtained through Justice, Inc., 1537 Central
  Avenue, Indianapolis, IN.
- The March 1989 special issue of *Medical Aspects of Human Sexuality* featured an
  excellent article on sexual guidelines for those at risk for AIDS.
- A self-care manual entitled *Living With AIDS*, published by AIDS Project, Los Angeles,
  contains complete and practical information for the patient who must live with
  full-blown AIDS. Copies are available through AIDS Project, Los Angeles, Inc., 7362
  Santa Monica Blvd., West Hollywood, CA 90046.

A book entitled *Advice for Life: A Woman's Guide to AIDS Risks and Prevention*. Norwood and
Chris (Pantheon), is an excellent reference source.

secondary-stage syphilis also will heal without scarring within two to six weeks. A latent period follows in which there are no signs or symptoms of the disease. During the first two years of this period, known as early latent syphilis, the individual is usually not contagious unless a relapse occurs. After the second year, the disease enters the late latent period, during which time it is not contagious either.

Three to ten years after the primary stage, the earliest lesions of the final stage, called tertiary syphilis, appear. Tertiary syphilis is a devastating disease, capable of causing permanent damage to practically every organ in the body. One characteristic lesion of this stage is a gumma, or localized destructive ulcer, which may vary in size from one millimeter to several centimeters in diameter, or from the size of a pinhead to the size of a silver dollar. Gummas usually occur in groups on any part of the skin or on mucous membranes such as those of the mouth, throat, palate, pharynx, larynx, and nasal septum. They may also occur in the outer lining of the bones, in muscles, in the stomach, intestines, liver, spleen, lungs, and kidneys, and even in the genitals. When gummas involve structures, such as the hard palate and nasal septum, they destroy the supporting bone and cartilage and cause permanent deformities.

About 10 percent of all patients with tertiary syphilis experience permanent damage to the muscles and valves of the heart, as well as the aorta, pulmonary arteries, and vena cava, the three major blood vessels carrying blood to and from the heart. *Treponema pallidum* can also invade the brain and spinal cord, resulting in a wide variety of crippling neurological disturbances and cytological abnormalities.

What are the effects of syphilis on pregnancy?

A fetus is usually well protected from the ravages of syphilis at the beginning by a layer of cells, the Langhans' layer, which is present in the placenta until the eighteenth week of pregnancy. After this point, the Langhans' layer is absorbed, and the infection may then be transmitted from the mother to the fetal bloodstream by the passage of bacteria across the placenta. One recent microscopic finding suggests that the Langhans' layer may not offer as much protection as previously believed, since *Treponema pallidum* was detected in the bodies of fetuses aborted during the first trimester of pregnancy.

The presence of an overwhelming syphilitic infection in the fetus may result in a stillbirth. This is most likely to occur when the mother is in the primary or early secondary stages of infection.

Infection in the newborn is termed "congenital syphilis." Congenital syphilis may be difficult to detect at birth, since physical signs and symptoms do not usually appear for several weeks, and they may not develop until later in childhood, when the manifestations are different from those of infancy. If syphilis is obvious at birth, the infection is usually severe. As many as 30 percent of infants born to mothers with untreated early-stage syphilis die early in life if untreated themselves.

"Early congenital syphilis" is the term used to describe untreated syphilis before the age of two. One of the most frequent signs of this stage is a skin rash similar to that in an adult with the disease. Equally frequent is the presence of "snuffles," a heavy, mucuslike discharge from the nose and throat which makes breathing and sucking difficult and irritates the skin that comes in contact with the discharge. There may also be anemia, inflammation of the long bones of the body, and enlargement of the liver and spleen.

"Late congenital syphilis" is syphilis which has persisted beyond two years of age. While the disease is not contagious at this stage, the effects may be devastating: inflammation of the cornea of the eye, unusual configurations of the teeth, deafness, bone and joint deformities, skin fissures, involvement of the central nervous system, and damage to the valves of the heart.

What should be done to ensure the early diagnosis of syphilis during pregnancy and prevent congenital syphilis?

All pregnant women should have a nontreponemal blood test for syphilis, such as the VDRL or Wassermann, at the time of their first prenatal visit. Since syphilis may be contracted later in pregnancy, when it is most likely to damage the fetus, many authorities now recommend a second nontreponemal blood test for all women during the third trimester. If either of these tests is positive, a more specific evaluation such as the FTA-ABS test should be done immediately to confirm or refute the diagnosis. If the FTA-ABS is also positive, antibiotic treatment must be begun for both the pregnant woman and her sexual partner or partners. (If the man has engaged in intercourse with others, his contacts should be located and treated, too.)

The risk of congenital syphilis in the baby will be minimal if maternal syphilis is adequately treated before delivery. Even in the absence of infection, most healthy newborns still inherit their mother's nontreponemal antibodies, which are passed across the placenta. These so-called 7-S antibodies are responsible for a positive nontreponemal blood test which will become negative within the first year of life.

If the strength or titre of the newborn's nontreponemal antibody test rises above that of its mother, it is a good bet that the baby has active congenital syphilis requiring immediate treatment. Infected infants are frequently without symptoms at birth, and this blood test may be negative if the maternal infection occurred late in pregnancy. Repeated testing, however, will resolve the problem.

Because some treponemal tests are associated with significant false-negative and false-positive results, the diagnosis and follow-up of infants treated with congenital syphilis is best achieved with periodic nontreponemal antibody titres. Infants must be treated with antibiotics if signs or symptoms of the disease are present or recur, if the mother's treatment is inadequate or unknown, if the nontreponemal antibody titre increases or fails to show a significant decrease, or if adequate follow-up of the infant cannot be guaranteed. Many experts prefer to treat all babies with a positive nontreponemal antibody titre immediately with penicillin even if the titre is at or below the level of its mother. With this method many babies will be treated unnecessarily since the titre is usually inherited from the mother and will decline spontaneously over a period of time. However, this aggressive method of treatment avoids the anxiety of repeated blood tests and observation over a period of three to six months.

What is the correct treatment for syphilis?

Penicillin remains the treatment of choice for all stages of syphilis; fortunately, *Treponema pallidum* has never developed resistance to this antibiotic. However, too many people falsely believe that a "shot of penicillin" provides an instant cure. It is not this easy; all penicillins are not the same, and doctors must adhere to the specific treatment recommendations established by the Centers for Disease Control if a cure is to be guaranteed. If you, your partner, or your baby have been diagnosed as having syphilis, be sure your doctor follows the current treatment recommendations. Fortunately, all forms of penicillin are safe to take during pregnancy.

How is syphilis treated if a person is allergic to penicillin?

From 0.3 to 1 percent of the population is allergic to penicillin, with life-threatening reactions occurring 1 to 3 times per 1,000 individuals treated. Tetracycline and erythromycin offer effective alternative treatment for men and nonpregnant women, but tetracycline should never be prescribed for pregnant women or infants because it may cause damage to the bones of the fetus and bluish discoloration of the permanent teeth. Erythromycin has been found to have a cure rate of only

90 percent in nonpregnant women with early syphilis. As a result, many experts now agree that penicillin is the only acceptable therapy. If a penicillin allergy is confirmed by skin testing, an allergist can desensitize a woman by carefully giving her tiny amounts of penicillin over a period of time until her sensitivity to the drug is overcome. When this is achieved, the penicillin can be safely administered in the usual dose.

 GONORRHEA

What causes gonorrhea, and what are its symptoms in a woman?

Gonorrhea is caused by a bacterium called a gonococcus bearing the scientific name *Neisseria gonorrhoeae*. While rapid microscopic identification is made possible with use of a special dye-staining technique called a Gram stain, culturing or growing of the gonococcus in a special medium remains the most accurate method of confirming the diagnosis.

One of the problems in controlling the spread of gonorrhea is the fact that an estimated 30 to 50 percent of men harboring the disease are totally without symptoms, yet these asymptomatic carriers are capable of transmitting the infection to a susceptible woman; and in one study of a group of men with gonorrhea it was found that one-third of the individuals with symptoms of the disease nevertheless denied their presence and continued to transmit their infections. The problem of the asymptomatic carrier is even greater among women: perhaps 80 percent of all those who have contracted the disease. The initial site of infection is practically always the inner lining of the cervix, with the urethra often involved as well. (Interestingly, the vaginal walls are totally resistant to gonorrheal infection.) Symptoms include a purulent discharge from the cervix combined with frequency and discomfort in urination. A yellowish discharge and inflammation may occur in the glands near the urethral opening and those located on either side of the vaginal opening. From its primary location within the cervix, the gonococcus will move along the surface of the endometrium and pass into the fallopian tubes, where it is capable of causing severe inflammation, or salpingitis, followed by permanent damage and distortion of the tubes. Following one episode of salpingitis, a woman will have a 15 to 20 percent risk of permanent infertility. If the infection remains untreated, pus will pass out through the ends of the fallopian tubes and into the abdominal cavity, causing acute pelvic inflammatory disease (PID). Symptoms of PID are fever, chills, cramping or persistent severe abdominal pain, and back pain. In addition, abdominal tenderness with pressing or jarring during exercise or sexual intercourse, pain during bowel movements or urination, and nonmenstrual vaginal bleeding should alert you to the possibility of PID. The presence of upper abdominal pain usually indicates further spread of the infection. Often the tube and ovary will become matted together in an inflammatory mass called a tubo-ovarian abscess. Spontaneous intraabdominal rupture of a tubo-ovarian abscess is a life-threatening medical emergency which usually requires immediate surgical removal.

Following the acute phase of gonorrhea, chronic flare-ups of infection may occur from time to time over a period of years. This stage is called chronic PID. The bacteria involved in these infections are usually not the gonococcus which initiated the problem; instead, they are organisms which thrive in tissues damaged by previous infection. Women suffering from chronic PID are often in pain caused by the presence of adhesions, or abnormal attachments of scar tissue, between the intestines and the pelvic organs. Hysterectomy with removal of the fallopian tubes and ovaries usually offers the only permanent cure.

In healthy women, fertilization normally occurs in the outer third of the fallopian tube. The fertilized egg then passes downward into the endometrium (lining of the uterus) where it attaches and grows. But scarring from gonorrheal infections may completely block the fallopian tubes and cause infertility by preventing fertilization of the egg by the sperm. If the tube is only partially blocked by scarring, the sperm may be able to reach the egg, but the tubal scarring may then prevent the rapid passage of the fertilized egg in its destination to the endometrium. This results in a significantly greater danger of an ectopic pregnancy within the fallopian tube among women with a previous history of gonorrhea.

The gonococcus may also enter the bloodstream and be transported to distant locations. The large joints of the body, such as the knees, ankles, and wrists, are the most common sites for so-called gonococcal arthritis to occur. Symptoms of this condition are tenderness, swelling, and redness of the joint accompanied by fever. In addition, a nonspecific skin rash may develop in any location on the body. In extremely rare cases, gonorrhea has been known to cause inflammation of the heart muscle, of the membrane enclosing the heart, and of the tissue lining the inner surface of the heart. In addition, inflammation of the iris of the eye, and of the membranes surrounding the spinal cord and brain, inflammation around the liver, liver abscesses, kidney inflammation, muscle inflammation, pneumonia, and inflammation of bone have all been reported.

An increasingly recognized form of gonorrhea is sore throat, which occurs two to three days following fellatio with an infected male. The area in the back of the throat, especially around the tonsils, is extremely likely to harbor the gonococcus. Redness of the tonsillar area and enlargement of the

lymph nodes under the jaw may also be noted. Gonorrheal proctitis is an inflammation of the anus and rectum which may occur following anal intercourse with an infected male.

What are the effects of gonorrhea during pregnancy?

A plug of mucus which forms within the inner lining of the cervix, called the endocervix, prevents the ascent of Neisseria gonorrhoeae into the uterine cavity and tubes of pregnant women. This is true for asymptomatic women who harbor the organism in their cervix prior to conception as well as those who are first exposed during pregnancy. For this reason, acute salpingitis and pelvic inflammatory disease caused by gonorrhea are practically unheard of during pregnancy. Instead, the bacteria stay quietly within the endocervix until the time of delivery, when the protective mucus plug is lost. They can then pass through the cervix to infect the tubes. If symptoms of pelvic pain, fever, and a purulent discharge from the vagina occur one week to ten days following delivery, the diagnosis of pelvic infection caused by gonorrhea is a strong possibility.

What is the recommended treatment for gonorrhea during pregnancy?

In the past, one intramuscular injection of 40,000 units of aqueous procaine penicillin G (APPG) was sufficient for curing a gonococcal infection. Today, 4.8 million units, or more than 100 times the original dose, will cure the disease only if the strain being treated is not penicillin-resistant. Infectious disease experts have expressed great concern about the increasing number of Neisseria gonorrhoeae organisms that are resistant to penicillin, ampicillin, amoxicillin, tetracycline, erythromycin, and spectinomycin. The most widespread resistant strain, known as penicillinase-producing Neisseria gonorrhoeae, or PPNG, produces an enzyme named beta-lactamase which attacks and breaks down penicillin and its derivatives. A laboratory can easily identify PPNG strains and this in turn can alert physicians that use of penicillin, amoxicillin, or ampicillin to treat the infection will be a waste of time. While the Centers for Disease Control estimated that 5 percent of individuals with gonorrhea were infected with resistant PPNG strains in 1988, in some clinics that number has been found to be as high as 20 percent. For this reason, treatment strategies for gonorrhea are constantly undergoing change. If your doctor is following an old treatment protocol, the antibiotic and dosage you receive may be less than adequate (see Table 10).

In an attempt to keep a step ahead of the constantly emerging resistant strains, the Centers for Disease Control are no longer recommending penicillin as the first antibiotic of choice for treating gonorrhea. Instead, ceftriaxone sodium (trade name Rocephin), a relatively new antibiotic in the cephalosporin family (see Chapter 9), is now the primary drug for treating gonorrhea. One 250-milligram intramuscular injection will not only cure gonorrhea but also eradicate incubating syphilis that happens to be present. Many researchers believe that half this amount, or 125 milligrams, is probably as effective as the higher dose. Although there are no large and well-controlled studies to prove that ceftriaxone use is safe during pregnancy, experimental laboratory research on animals given 20 times the usual dose has produced no adverse fetal effects. Similarly, while low concentrations of ceftriaxone can be found in breast milk, there is no evidence that it is harmful to the nursing infant. Finally, clinical experience with thousands of pregnant and breast-feeding women who have taken other cephalosporin antibiotics is reassuring evidence of its safety. Cefoxitin (trade name Mefoxin) is an antibiotic similar in structure to ceftriaxone which has also proven effective in treating gonorrhea during pregnancy.

TABLE 10

TREATMENT OF GONORRHEA AND CHLAMYDIA DURING PREGNANCY

Ceftriaxone 250 mgm. intramuscularly on one injection is preferred. Cefoxitin 2 grams intramuscularly in one injection is also effective. The antibiotic options listed below will kill *Neisseria gonorrhoeae* if the organism is PPNG and CMRNG negative:

- Amoxicillin 3 grams and clavulanate with 1 gram of probenecid by mouth
- Probenecid 1 gram orally followed by aqueous procaine penicillin G 4.8 million units intramuscularly divided into two doses and injected in each buttock at one visit
- Ampicillin 3.5 grams or amoxicillin 3 grams, either given with 1 gram of probenecid by mouth
- Spectinomycin hydrochloride 2 grams intramuscularly in one injection if a person had a penicillin or probenecid allergy and is unable to take ceftriaxone

To cover chlamydia infections, all of the above should be followed by either:

- Erythromycin base or stearate 500 mgms. orally for 7 days or erythromycin ethylsuccinate 800 mgms. orally for 7 days

All male sexual partners must be treated in the above fashion except for substituting tetracycline hydrochloride 500 mgms. orally four times daily for 10 to 14 days or doxycycline 100 mgms. orally twice daily for 10 to 14 days for erythromycin. The tetracyclines are not recommended in pregnancy or in nursing women because of potential adverse effects on the fetus, newborn, and the pregnant woman (see Chapter 9).

Although most penicillin-allergic women will easily tolerate ceftriaxone, less than 1 percent with a history of a severe allergic reaction to penicillin could manifest a similar sensitivity to cephalosporins. For those penicillin-allergic women who are unable to take ceftriaxone, an intramuscular injection of 2 grams of spectinomycin hydrochloride (trade names Trobicin and Spectam) is a suitable alternative. Laboratory studies and clinical experience in treating thousands of pregnant and breast-feeding women suggests that this antibiotic is extremely safe. While some doctors have used oral erythromycin instead of spectinomycin to treat gonorrhea in a penicillin-allergic pregnant woman, it is not recommended because investigators have noted a treatment failure rate as high as 25 percent.

If a laboratory determines that a penicillin-resistant strain of *Neisseria gonorrhoeae* is not present, the odds are excellent that treatment with penicillin, ampicillin, or amoxicillin combined with probenecid will eradicate gonorrhea and syphilis and prove safe for both mother and fetus. The use of these medications is identical for both pregnant and nonpregnant women.

To overcome the penicillin-destroying effects of the enzyme beta-lactamase, found in most penicillin-resistant strains of *Neisseria gonorrhoeae*, scientists have combined amoxicillin and clavulanate potassium, a drug that inactivates beta-lactamase. Known by the trade name Augmentin, this combination has proven to be an excellent alternative to ceftriaxone. Newer antibiotics in the quinalone group, such as ciprofloxacin (trade name Cipro) and norfloxacin (trade name Noroxin), and others classified as monobactam antibiotics, such as aztreonan (trade name Azactam), hold promise for controlling antibiotic-resistant strains of gonorrhea in the future.

How should gonorrheal pharyngitis and proctitis be treated?

Gonococcal infections of the pharynx and rectum will respond to the same dose of ceftriaxone that is used for uncomplicated gonococcal infections. No other antibiotic is as successful in eradicating both penicillin-sensitive and penicillin-resistant strains from these two sites. Aqueous procaine penicillin G (APPG), ampicillin, and amoxicillin are less effective than ceftriaxone but will cure these infections provided that a penicillin-resistant strain is not present. Neither erythromycin or spectinomycin are recommended for treating pharyngeal or rectal gonorrhea. If a woman is unable to tolerate ceftriaxone or penicillins, the treatment of pharyngitis and proctitis can be problematical. One solution is the combination of the sulfonamide named sulfamethoxazol and trimethoprim (trade names Septra and Bactrim); a dose of nine tablets (400 milligrams sulfamethoxazol and 80 milligrams trimethoprim in each tablet) daily for five days will cure rectal and pharyngeal gonorrhea even if caused by penicillin-resistant organisms. The use of sulfonamides, however, is contraindicated during the last month of pregnancy and if a woman is breast-feeding, because they readily pass through the placenta and are also excreted in breast milk. Sulfonamides compete with a pigment named bilirubin in the baby's circulation, and this can cause severe jaundice. Little is known about the safety of sulfonamides and trimethoprim during the first trimester, but a small number of reports on women who received the drug at the time of conception or shortly thereafter showed no evidence of congenital abnormalities.

Regardless of the method chosen to treat these two conditions, it is vital to obtain cultures from the pharynx or rectum three to seven days later.

What are the effects of maternal gonorrhea on the newborn?

If gonorrhea is present within the mother's endocervix at the time of delivery, the eyes of the newborn will be exposed to the organism while the baby is passing through the birth canal. This may result in severe inflammation and scarring of the cornea, called ophthalmia neonatorum. If not treated promptly, permanent blindness may result. The early symptoms of gonorrheal eye infection usually appear two to three days following delivery and consist of swelling and inflammation of the eyelids, a cloudy appearance of the cornea, and a yellowish discharge from both eyes. Immediate treatment with ceftriaxone and saline eye irrigations will cure this condition before permanent damage occurs.

A syndrome recently noted among these newborns is an infection of the upper respiratory tract and throat. This is caused by the infant's swallowing infected cervical secretions in its passage through the birth canal during labor. Treatment with ceftriaxone is curative.

Is the routine procedure of giving eyedrops to newborns to prevent gonorrheal eye infections still recommended?

For many years, the most popular form of eye care given to prevent gonorrheal eye infections and the potentially blinding ophthalmia neonatorum (see preceding question) was 1 percent silver nitrate drops applied to the eyes just after birth. In the early 1980s many physicians began to question the benefits of this routine silver nitrate treatment, arguing that it too often causes a chemical irritation on the inner membrane of the eyelid, called chemical conjunctivitis. Another complaint voiced in recent years has been that silver nitrate does not adequately prevent the milder and self-limiting eye infection caused by incubating chlamydia. The onset of this infection, known as inclusion conjunctivitis (see page 164), is delayed until 5 to 19 days following delivery, usually after the baby has left the hospital and is no longer under the close supervision of a pediatrician. Finally, the silver nitrate method is not infallible, since a small percentage of infected babies still develop serious gonorrheal eye infections even after the drops are given.

In order to both treat incubating gonorrheal and chlamydial eye infections and avoid the irritating chemical conjunctivitis caused by silver nitrate, it has become popular throughout the United States to substitute erythromycin or tetracycline eye ointment for silver nitrate drops in newborns. However, the therapeutic benefits of this approach are minimal at best. A 1988 study of almost 3,000 newborns showed that tetracycline was as effective as silver nitrate in preventing gonococcal ophthalmia neonatorum, and other studies have shown equally favorable results with erythromycin eye drops. The problem is that tetracycline prophylaxis still resulted in a 7 percent incidence of chlamydial conjunctivitis, compared to a 10 percent incidence among infants treated with silver nitrate. Dr. Margaret R. Hammerschlog and her associates at the State University of New York Health Science Center in Brooklyn, in their 1989 report published in the *New England Journal of Medicine*, compared the efficacy of erythromycin, tetracycline, and silver nitrate eye treatment in 230 infants whose mothers tested positive for chlamydia. Chlamydial conjunctivitis developed in 20 percent of the infants who received silver nitrate, 14 percent of those given erythromycin, and 11 percent of those treated with tetracycline. Other studies have shown erythromycin to be clearly superior to both silver nitrate and tetracycline in preventing chlamydial conjunctivitis. As a result, it has become the most popular method of newborn eye care in the United States.

Fortunately, chlamydial inclusion conjunctivitis is a very mild, self-limiting inflammation which often subsides without antibiotic treatment. However, respiratory infections and pneumonia caused by *Chlamydia trachomatis* develop later than conjunctivitis and are more serious (see page 164). The source of these infections is the newborn's nasopharynx, an anatomic site out of reach of eye ointment and drops. For this reason, the only way doctors will reduce the incidence of serious chlamydial infections in newborns is through widespread screening for chlamydia and treatment of all pregnant women and their sexual partners prior to delivery.

If an infant is born to a mother with gonorrhea, that baby is at high risk of infection and requires immediate treatment with a single intravenous or intramuscular injection of ceftriaxone in a dose of 125 milligrams. Antibiotic eyedrops can be used, but never as the sole treatment for these infants.

If a newborn contracts a gonorrheal eye infection, immediate isolation is indicated since these infections are highly contagious. Immediate treatment with ceftriaxone for seven days combined with saline eye irrigations should cure this condition. Another antibiotic named cefotaxime is an equally effective alternative. Silver nitrate, tetracycline, or erythromycin eyedrops are of no benefit at this stage of the disease.

What is PGU?

PGU stands for postgonococcal urethritis, the presence of a urethral discharge in a man following successful treatment of his gonorrhea with antibiotics. Cultures taken of this discharge are negative for *Neisseria gonorrhoeae*.

Until recently, doctors could not understand why some men developed PGU and others did not, although it was known that it could be cured with tetracycline. Bacteriologists now believe that men treated for gonorrhea who later develop PGU actually harbor other bacteria in the urethra in addition to those which caused gonorrhea. These bacteria are resistant to penicillin and have the potential to cause urethritis in the absence of gonorrhea. Researchers have determined that the organisms which cause PGU are also responsible for the worldwide epidemic of NGU (see next question).

 # CHLAMYDIA

What is NGU?

NGU stands for nongonococcal urethritis, or urethral inflammation in a man caused by organisms other than *Neisseria gonorrhoeae*. Although many bacteria have been suggested as possible causes of NGU, at the present time only one, *Chlamydia* (pronounced clam-ID-ia) *trachomatis*, has been definitely incriminated. In fact, 20 to 50 percent of individuals with positive cultures for gonorrhea will also have cultures positive for chlamydia. Organisms named *Mycoplasma hominis* and *Ureaplasma urealyticum* have been implicated as other causes of NGU, though the relationship is not as firmly established as it is with chalmydia.

How can a man with chlamydia transmit his infection to his sexual partner?

Although many men harboring chlamydia are asymptomatic, the majority develop symptoms within 7 to 21 days after contact with an infected female. Symptoms of urethral inflammation, or urethritis, include a clear or whitish urethral discharge, burning with urination, and itching at the end of the urethra. This may be accompanied by inflammation of the epididymis, or epididymitis (convoluted tubules that transport sperm from the testes), a condition causing severe pain and swelling of the testicle. Such an infection can cause permanent sterility. It is believed that *Chlamydia trachomatis* is responsible for at least 50 percent of all cases of acute epididymitis.

Chlamydia is easily transmitted from the urethra of a man to the cervix and vagina of a woman during coitus. It is estimated that 50 to 70 percent of women harboring the organism in the vagina and cervix are completely without symptoms. However, more than half the women excreting *Chlamydia trachomatis* in the urethra experience symptoms such as burning on urination, urinary frequency, and urinary urgency.

The cervicitis (inflammation of the cervix) associated with chlamydia is often accompanied by both mucus and pus. Salpingitis and pelvic inflammatory infection caused by *Chlamydia trachomatis* is usually far less dramatic than that caused by *Neisseria gonorrhoeae*. Temperatures are lower and abdominal discomfort is less, but damage and permanent scarring of the fallopian tubes followed by subsequent infertility and higher ectopic pregnancy rates are much more common. Unfortunately, absent or vague symptoms and mild pelvic pain too often delay the initiation of adequate treatment by both patients and doctors. Chlamydial infections can also spread to the Bartholin glands at the vaginal opening as well as to the surface of the intestines and liver. The latter condition, named perihepatitis, is characterized by fever and tenderness on the right side of the upper abdomen.

Once pregnancy is established, it is debatable as to whether or not the presence of *Chlamydia trachomatis* in the cervix plays a role in pregnancy complications such as spontaneous abortion, premature rupture of the amniotic membranes, amniotic fluid infections, premature labor, intrauterine growth retardation (IUGR), or stillbirths. In the overwhelming number of reported cases, contamination occurs during labor and delivery through an infected cervix.

Most research suggests that *Chlamydia trachomatis* can cause postpartum endometritis, or inflammation of the uterine cavity, following childbirth. Postpartum endometritis caused by other bacteria is associated with the onset of symptoms during the first two postpartum days, while chlamydial endometritis can develop anywhere from three days to six weeks following delivery. Symptoms include fever, tenderness over the uterus, and occasionally a foul-smelling vaginal discharge. In one study, doctors isolated *Chalmydia trachomatis* in 25 percent of women with postpartum endometritis. Fortunately, this condition responds rapidly to appropriate antibiotic therapy.

How does chlamydia affect newborn babies?

It has been estimated that 4 to 5 percent of women attending prenatal clinics have cultures which are positive for *Chlamydia trachomatis*. Infants born to women infected with this organism may acquire chlamydia while passing through the birth canal during labor. The symptom most commonly apparent is a relatively harmless eye infection called congenital inclusion conjunctivitis. While the exact risk of an infant's contracting inclusion conjunctivitis from its mother is not known, most authorities believe it is somewhere between 40 and 50 percent. If this is so, more than 74,000 babies contract this disease each year in the United States.

Symptoms of conjunctivitis, such as eye redness and discharge, usually do not appear until 5 to 19 days after birth. (This is unlike the eye infection caused by gonorrhea, which is far more destructive and produces symptoms during the first three days following delivery.) Chlamydial inclusion conjunctivitis responds to treatment with sulfa or tetracycline eye ointment over a period of two to three weeks, although most authorities consider oral erythromycin preferable. Silver nitrate drops, so useful in the prevention of gonorrheal eye infections, are less effective in preventing chlamydial inclusion conjunctivitis (see page 162). Fortunately, this inflammation is both very mild and self-limiting and often subsides without antibiotic treatment. Unlike gonorrheal conjunctivitis, chlamydial inclusion conjunctivitis usually heals without producing residual scarring or blindness.

In addition to conjunctivitis, *Chlamydia trachomatis* may also cause respiratory infections, pneumonia, and infections of the middle ear, nose, throat, and intestine of the newborn. Authorities estimate that approximately one-half of all babies with conjunctivitis, or approximately 37,000 infants per year, will develop chlamydial pneumonia within the first three months of life, most often between the fourth and fourteenth weeks. Epidemiologists have determined that 35 to 50 percent of pneumonias diagnosed in the first six months of life can be attributed to *Chlamydia trachomatis*. Chlamydial pneumonia is a more serious illness than conjunctivitis, although it is rarely fatal and generally resolves even if untreated. In a small minority of cases, however, the pneumonia can be relatively severe and require hospitalization. Infants with chlamydial pneumonia are often without fever and exhibit a characteristically high-pitched "staccato" cough combined with a failure to thrive and gain weight. Long-term consequences such as chronic respiratory disease and abnormal respiratory function tests later in childhood have also been noted. On rare occasions, neonatal chlamydial infections can persist for up to 29 months.

How can chlamydia be diagnosed and treated during pregnancy and in the postpartum period?

At the present time, there is no simple, inexpensive in-office laboratory test that can detect a *Chlamydial trachomatis* infection with 100 percent accuracy. While culture of the cervical secretions has an accuracy approaching 100 percent, the technique is costly, complex, and not widely available; it requires transfer to a laboratory within 24 hours, and results are usually not available for four to seven days. In response to these problems, a variety of other tests which detect the presence of chlamydial antigens in cervical secretions have been developed. Of these, the most popular is a fluorescent antibody staining test in which a sample of cervical secretions mixed with a sample of chlamydial antibodies is studied under a special fluorescent microscope. An ELISA (enzyme-linked immunosorbent assay) test, similar to the one used to diagnose gonorrhea, is also capable of detecting chlamydial antigens but is less accurate.

Selective screening is recommended for those pregnant women who, based on previous experience, are most likely to harbor the organism. Included in this group are unmarried women, those under 20, the economically disadvantaged, substance abusers, women with a mucopurulent discharge from their cervix or a history of other sexually transmitted diseases, and women with more than one sexual partner.

All women diagnosed as having chlamydia during pregnancy should be treated with a full dose of oral erythromycin for one week, or half this dose over a period of two weeks if excessive nausea is experienced with the higher dose (see Table 10). Male sexual partners must be treated simultaneously with either doxycycline, tetracycline, or erythromycin. Oral sulfamethoxazole (trade names Septra and Bactrin) has been used with success to treat chlamydial infections in women who can't tolerate erythromycin. Sulfonamides should not be used during the last month of pregnancy or the first month of life, since they can cause jaundice at these times. At other times, however, they can be used as a safe antibiotic alternative to erythromycin. Amoxicillin, in a dose of 1500 milligrams daily for seven days, appears to be a promising alternative to erythromycin therapy. In a 1990 study, doctors were able to eradicate the organism from 63 of 64 pregnant women (98 percent) with positive chlamydial cultures. In a second 1990 study, the antibiotic clindamycin, in a dose of 1800 milligrams daily for ten days, proved equally effective as erythromycin in treating chlamydia. Both clindamycin and amoxicillin are considered to be relatively safe antibiotics for use during pregnancy (see Chapter 9). Regardless of the antibiotic selected, cervical cultures should be repeated seven days after completion of therapy as well as four to eight weeks later in order to exclude the possibility of a persistent infection requiring retreatment or reinfection by an infected man.

The only way to effectively prevent a chlamydial infection in a newborn is to improve our expertise in diagnosing and treating the infection in its mother and her sexual partner during pregnancy. Prophylactic eye care of a baby at birth with either silver nitrate, erythromycin, or tetracycline is not only inefficient, it also fails to eliminate *Chlamydia trachomatis* from the nose and throat, the two sites responsible for passage of the organism to the respiratory tract. Rather than treat chlamydial conjunctivitis with topical eye care, it is far better to eliminate *Chlamydia trachomatis* from all other sites, such as the middle ear, nasopharynx, lungs, and intestinal tract. To do this, erythromycin can be administered to a newborn in an oral or intravenous dose of 50 milligrams per kilogram of body weight per day in four divided doses over a period of 14 days. Some doctors prefer to extend the treatment period for another week if chlamydial pneumonia is present. The sulfonamide sulfamethoxazol, in an oral or intravenous dose of 100 milligrams per kilogram of body weight daily, may be used as an alternative treatment after the first four weeks of life. Doxycycline and tetracycline, though extremely effective against *Chlamydia trachomatis*, should never be used during the early years.

 # HERPES

What is herpes?

Herpes is one of a group of viruses called DNA viruses which can be transmitted from person to person through sexual and nonsexual contact. Members of this group include the herpes simplex virus Type I (HSV-I); herpes simplex virus Type II (HSV-II); cytomegalovirus (CMV); the Epstein-Barr (EB) virus, which causes infectious mononucleosis, or mono, and a chronic debilitating viral infection; varicella-herpes zoster, which causes chicken pox; and a nonvenereal disease called herpes zoster.

HSV-I, officially named *Herpesvirus hominis*, Type I, is known to cause so-called oral herpes, fever blisters, and canker sores of the mouth and lips. Until recently, researchers believed that HSV-I could be found only "above the waist" and that it was not sexually transmitted because it most commonly occurs in young children. However, ample evidence now suggests that a significant number of sexually active men and women contract HSV-I in the genital or rectal area through oral-genital and oral-anal contact.

HSV-II, or *Herpesvirus hominis*, Type II, is usually transmitted to the genital area through sexual intercourse, but it has frequently been cultured from the mouth, throat, and lips of individuals engaged in oral-genital contact with an infected partner. Genital herpes is a highly contagious, often incurable viral infection; statistically, there is an 80 to 90 percent chance that a previously uninfected woman will contract genital herpes when exposed to a man shedding the virus.

The DNA viruses as a group have been called the "viruses of love." A perfect example of this is the Epstein-Barr virus, the cause of infectious mononucleosis, known also as the "kissing disease," since kissing is believed to be its most usual mode of transmission. CMV is known to be transmitted via sexual intercourse (see page 182), in addition to other methods of spread. While chicken pox and herpes zoster are not transmitted through sexual intercourse, close contact with an infected individual is necessary for transmission of the virus.

What symptoms does a woman experience during her first attack of genital herpes?

Following exposure to an infected male, there is usually an incubation period of two to seven days, although this period may be as short as 24 hours and as long as 12 days. The virus first forms a small, almost undetectable blister on the skin of the external genitals. One of these small blisters may contain millions of viruses which multiply and produce new blisters. Early in the course of this primary infection symptoms are often very mild and a woman may notice only a slight itch or mild irritation. At this stage, it is not uncommon to misdiagnose the condition as monoliasis, or yeast infection (see page 191).

The external genitals soon become covered with extremely painful blistering sores, often accompanied by swelling of the entire genital area. Often these individual sores come together to form larger sores which, after about 24 to 48 hours, break down into open, shallow, painful, grayish ulcers. The disease is now in its most highly contagious stage. Within five days after the ulcers begin to form, the pain finally starts to lessen.

The severity of a primary herpes attack will vary greatly from one individual to another. Symptoms also tend to be relatively mild when the causative organism is HSV-I, while HSV-II attacks are known for their angry course. One notable exception to this rule occurs among individuals who have had an HSV-I infection at any time in their past. Under such circumstances, the antibodies formed against the HSV-I virus tend to offer some protection against a primary HSV-II genital infection. As a result, lesions tend to be less painful and to heal faster.

In addition to its attack on the external genitals, HSV-II often invades the vagina and cervix, where it may produce a profuse, irritating watery discharge. The urethra, or urinary duct, leading to the bladder is particularly vulnerable. The virus produces blisters and ulcers in the urethral lining which cause intense burning on urination. This pain is intensified when urine comes in contact with the sores on the outer vaginal area. Occasionally, the pain on urination is so severe that a woman will retain urine rather than void, requiring a urinary catheter to relieve her discomfort.

The acute stage of the primary attack may be accompanied by chills, low-grade fever, headache, painful enlargement of the lymph nodes of the groin, and a dull aching pain in both legs, along with a general feeling of fatigue. Unlike the relatively mild course of primary herpes infections in men, as many as 4 to 5 percent of women require hospitalization and treatment with antiviral medications to control the disease. Widespread dissemination of the virus through the body, while rare, may result in hepatitis, a dangerously low platelet count, meningitis, encephalitis, and even death. Scratching or touching of the genital lesions can spread the infection to the fingernails, the eyes, and distant areas of the skin.

Spontaneous healing of the skin ulcers usually begins about ten days after the first appearance of the disease and is usually complete without evidence of scarring in three to four weeks. On rare occasions, a secondary bacterial infection at the site of the ulcers not only delays the healing process but may cause permanent scarring.

Scientists have found that a significant number of women experience no symptoms at the time of their primary genital herpes attack. This is especially likely to occur if the blisters are hidden in the upper vagina and cervix.

What determines whether or not herpes will recur following a primary attack?

Antibodies to either HSV-I or HSV-II first appear in a woman's bloodstream seven days following the onset of the primary infection. Peak antibody levels are usually reached in two to three weeks and remain elevated throughout a person's lifetime. Unlike other diseases, the presence of antibodies is no assurance that the disease is cured. For the more fortunate, the primary attack represents their one and only episode of herpes. However, approximately one-third to two-thirds of those who suffer an initial attack experience reappearance of the disease at a later time. The risk of recurrence with primary genital HSV-I is only 15 percent, compared to more than 60 percent with HSV-II. It is theorized that in these unlucky individuals the virus travels from the infected areas on the skin to several of the nerves just below the skin surface and from this location migrates up the nerves to the central nerve cells located near the lower part of the spinal cord, where it remains in a latent state for variable periods of time. When the virus becomes reactivated, it begins to multiply within the nerve cells and retraces its path down the nerve to the genital skin area supplied by that particular nerve. This causes a recurrence of the herpes blisters on the skin surface. Unlike the first infection, which may involve the entire genital area, recurrences usually appear as single blisters or a small group of blisters, although the outbreak is usually in the same location as before, since the virus migrates up and down the same nerves each time.

The first recurrence usually takes place within eight weeks after the primary infection has completely healed, but there have been several reports of the first recurrence taking place as late as two years or more after the primary infection. The frequency of recurrences varies, ranging from as often as every two weeks to as infrequently as every few years. The most usual pattern of recurrences is four to five during the first year, two or three the following year, and spontaneous disappearance of most recurrences during or after the third year, although there are many individuals who suffer from recurrences throughout their lifetime. The blisters of the recurrent attacks heal completely within ten days of their onset.

Recurrent attacks of herpes are often preceded by symptoms such as itching or burning of the skin at the site where the blisters are about to appear. Astute, observant, and considerate men and women attuned to these symptoms can avoid the spread of genital herpes to susceptible sexual partners by avoiding contact at these times. Unfortunately, there are other individuals who will periodically shed the virus without experiencing any symptoms. Shedding by these individuals is one of the main reasons for the genital herpes epidemic in our society.

It is not known what triggers the sudden reactivation of the virus, but it is unrelated to sexual activity. Factors reported capable of triggering recurrences in a susceptible individual include other illnesses, fatigue, lack of sleep, emotional trauma,

fever, change of climate, excessive exposure to sunlight, menstruation, and premenstrual tension. When recurrences do follow sexual intercourse, they are usually the result of direct trauma and irritation to the genital area, as might occur with a penis, douche, or vibrator, rather than the reintroduction of the virus to the skin or tissues by way of one's infected sexual partner.

What is the recommended treatment for herpes?

While there is no known cure for genital herpes infection, the most promising therapy to date has been an antiviral agent named acyclovir (trade name Zovirax). Available as an ointment and oral capsule, acyclovir has been shown to decrease the healing time, duration of viral shedding, and the number of recurrent herpes attacks. Acyclovir works by mimicking another substance that the herpesvirus needs to reproduce. Once the virus is fooled in taking it in, however, acyclovir provides the wrong compound for growth and reproduction of the cells. As a result, the virus is unable to reproduce.

Acyclovir ointment is applied to the affected areas every three hours six times per day for seven days. Best results are obtained if treatment is started within eight hours after the blisters first appear. Acyclovir is far less effective as an ointment than it is as a capsule, since the topical solution applied to the skin blisters is incapable of reaching the viruses living in their inactive state in the nerves deep below the skin surface.

Several studies have shown that when acyclovir treatment is initiated against a primary attack of herpes within six days of the onset of a lesion, it will reduce the time that the virus is shed by three to five days, prevent new lesion formation, reduce the period of painful symptoms, speed the healing process and crusting of the ulcers, and possibly reduce the chances of a recurrence or at least lengthen the time until the first recurrence. Treatment of recurrences, however, offers only modest benefits, since the attacks are rarely painful and the lesions subside spontaneously without treatment in five to ten days. Several recent articles have demonstrated the benefits of taking acyclovir prophylactically on a daily basis for periods as long as one to two years in order to suppress frequent recurrences. Success has been achieved with doses ranging from two to five 200-milligram capsules daily. In two separate studies published in 1988 and 1989, researchers found that women with average genital herpes recurrence rates of 12 episodes per year reduced their frequency of recurrences to an average of only 1.8 per year following treatment with 800 milligrams of oral acyclovir daily. Women given a placebo continued to maintain high annual recurrence rates. Unfortunately, acyclovir does not rid the body of the latent herpes infection, and the virus reactivates when the drug is halted. While the safety of using acyclovir for such a long period of time has been debated, clinical evidence to date suggests that it is an extremely safe, well-tolerated medication.

While limited clinical experience with acyclovir during pregnancy has not been associated with fetal anomalies or adverse pregnancy outcome, experts agree that its use at the present time should be restricted to life-threatening disseminated herpes infections. This recommendation, however, may change in the near future.

Several agents have been tried with mixed results in bringing symptomatic relief and, in some cases, shortening the time that the lesions remain on the skin. Included among these are alcohol and ether applications, betadine, idoxuridine, adenine arabinoside, zinc, 2-deoxy-d-glucose, nonoxynol-9, and adenosine monophosphate. Other purported remedies include the amino acid lysine taken orally and a variety of intramuscular vaccines. Researchers at the National Institutes of Health have been developing a herpes vaccine for several years, although even the most optimistic scientists believe that it will be quite some time before such a vaccine becomes a reality.

When all local remedies for recurrent herpes fail, some doctors recommend surgical removal of

the blisters under local anesthesia. Laser treatment also has its enthusiastic supporters. Aside from acyclovir, none of the methods mentioned here have survived the scrutiny of large-scale clinical trials.

What can a woman do to relieve the intense pain of primary herpes?

Knowing that the acute attack is self-limited is of little consolation to the individual suffering from genital herpes. Mild analgesics such as aspirin and Tylenol are worthless, and if relief of pain is to be achieved, it is best to use narcotic preparations, such as codeine or Demerol. Compresses of cool Burrow's solution in a dilution of 1:40 will relieve discomfort. It is available without prescription at most pharmacies. Cool tap water, either alone or in a 4:1 mixture with white vinegar, is also helpful, as are silver nitrate (0.25 percent), benzalkonium chloride (1:4,000), and boric acid (5 percent) solutions. These should be applied for 15 to 30 minutes three or four times a day, using a soft cotton cloth. Cold applications of potassium permanganate in a dilution of 1:8,000 is an old and effective remedy for relieving symptoms; several applications a day may be used. The one drawback of this treatment is that it permanently soils linens and undergarments. The intense pain on urination can be alleviated if cold water is gently poured on the perineum during urination. Urinating from a standing position is helpful in directing the flow away from the ulcers on the labia. Although many doctors suggest that patients urinate while taking a hot tub bath, I discourage my patients from doing this during the acute state of genital herpes. Prolonged and frequent soaking tends to cause maceration (softening) of the normal skin. In the presence of herpes, it has been demonstrated that new lesions may develop on the macerated area along with local spread of the infection. It is best to avoid soap, since this will cause further irritation and possibly spread the virus.

Ice cubes wrapped in a pack or towel will afford relief when applied continuously to the perineum for 90 minutes at a time. This is an easy home remedy which will relieve symptoms of both primary and recurrent herpes. One researcher even suggests that this form of cryo (cold) therapy also hastens the healing of the blisters.

It is important to keep the sores as clean and as dry as possible in order to prevent a secondary bacterial infection. This can be accomplished by taking a hot sitz bath no more often than twice a day. The sores can be gently washed with a germicidal soap such as Betadine. It is best to dab dry the vulva rather than rub a towel across the skin surface. Use of a hair dryer is a great way to keep the lesions dry without irritating the skin or spreading the infection. Women should wear only clean cotton underwear and avoid nylon underwear or pantyhose, since these tend to trap moisture and prevent air circulation.

Healing of the blisters has been shown to be prolonged if they are covered with creams or ointments. However, if the sores around the urethral opening are irritated by urination, application of a thin layer of Xylocaine anesthetic ointment may be helpful in relieving symptoms.

Are pregnant women more susceptible to genital herpes infections than nonpregnant women?

Probably not. In the past, epidemiologists believed that a pregnant woman was at least three times more susceptible to genital herpes infections than her nonpregnant counterpart. A 1988 review, however, concluded that there is little evidence to suggest that pregnancy increases the frequency or the severity of genital herpes infections.

What effect does a genital herpes attack have on the outcome of pregnancy?

The effects of a primary attack of genital herpes are far more devastating to the outcome of pregnancy than either recurrent infections or chronic shedding of the virus by women with a history of herpes predating the pregnancy.

TORCH is an acronym for a group of diseases—toxoplasmosis, rubella, cytomegalovirus, and herpes—which are capable of causing similar damage to a fetus when its mother is first infected during pregnancy. TORCH organisms have been associated with an increased risk of spontaneous abortion, stillbirth, prematurity, and low birth weight; and the newborn may be affected by lethargy, poor feeding, blood coagulation defects, enlargement of the liver and spleen, calcifications of the liver, jaundice, anemia, pneumonia, skin rash, inflammation of the muscle of the heart, cataracts, inflammation of the retina and surrounding layer in the eye, and nervous system diseases such as encephalitis, microcephaly (abnormally small head), seizures, hydrocephaly (abnormally large head), mental retardation, and complications within the skull. In recent years, epidemiologists have been somewhat relieved to learn that primary genital herpes is less likely to cause these terrible congenital complications than other TORCH-group organisms. Even if a woman contracts a severe primary herpes infection during the first trimester, it is unlikely that it will result in a higher incidence of fetal anomalies or illness, and therapeutic abortion is not warranted.

The greatest danger to a fetus and newborn occurs when its mother contracts the primary disease toward the end of pregnancy. Maternal infections during the last trimester are associated with a 40 percent risk of serious obstetrical and newborn complications including IUGR, premature labor, and neonatal death. Babies exposed to primary genital herpes at this time are in double jeopardy because, in addition to these complications, they are subjected to a greater than 50 percent risk of contracting neonatal herpes as they pass through an infected birth canal during labor. In constrast, less than 5 percent of infants delivered to women with a recurrent herpes genital lesion will develop neonatal herpes.

There are a few documented cases in the medical literature of herpesvirus transmission of a primary infection from a mother to her baby via the placenta during the second half of pregnancy, but this is extremely rare. Infection of the newborn, in practically all cases, occurs when the infant comes in contact with the virus from the mother's cervix, vagina, or vulva during labor. The amniotic membrane provides the baby with great protection. However, if the membrane ruptures before or during labor, the virus can easily ascend through the cervix and infect the unborn infant within four to six hours.

Between 400 and 1,000 babies die each year in the United States as a result of congenital herpes transmitted to them at birth by their infected mothers. If a woman is infected with primary genital herpes at the time of delivery, the risk of a newborn acquiring the virus is about 50 percent. Of those babies who are infected, 60 to 90 percent will either die or develop a severe and permanent disability such as mental retardation, seizures, microcephaly, eye abnormalities, and hypertonicity, or abnormal tensing of various muscle groups. The diagnosis of neonatal herpes is often difficult since infected babies appear normal at birth and are often sent home from the hospital. Nonspecific early signs, such as lethargy, irritability, poor feeding, and breathing problems, develop after the first week, on about the eleventh to sixteenth day of life. This is followed within 24 hours by pneumonia, liver and spleen enlargement, and involvement of the lungs, adrenal glands, and central nervous system. Eighty percent of newborns with central nervous system involvement, as evidenced by seizures, coma, encephalitis, and meningitis, will either die or have permanent neurologic damage. Many newborns with neonatal herpes will not demonstrate characteristic skin blisters, and because of this there is often too long a delay in making the diagnosis and initiating treatment. In one recent report, there was an average delay of 72 hours from the onset of symptoms to rehospitalization of the baby.

HSV-II causes three-fourths of all newborn herpesvirus infections, while HSV-I is responsible for the remaining one-fourth. The severity of the infection in a newborn is equal regardless of which strain the infant contracts. The ability of a doctor to accurately diagnose maternal herpes is complicated by the fact that as many as one-third of infected women have no externally visible lesions and 70 percent of neonatal infections occur without a known history of maternal genital herpesvirus infection.

What measures can be taken to protect babies against the damaging effects of neonatal herpes?

If a pregnant woman has never been infected with herpes, it is imperative that she avoid unprotected intercourse with a man who has even the slightest evidence of a blister suggestive of herpes. Coitus is probably safe if he wears a condom that completely covers the infection site. Cold sores in the oral cavity often go unnoticed, but, if detected in a man, the couple must avoid cunnilingus. Similarly, a woman with herpes of the mouth may become infected in the genital area if she passes it to the mouth or genitals of her lover. Susceptible pregnant women should avoid close contact with children who may have contracted oral herpes. Even if you or your spouse have had herpes many years earlier and never had a recurrence, it is still important to provide your obstetrician with this information during your first prenatal visit.

Many individuals with chronic recurrent genital herpes experience symptoms such as burning, itching, and vulvar pain prior to the eruption of the blisters. Individuals attuned to these body changes should report them to their obstetrician immediately, especially if they occur during the last week of pregnancy, at the onset of labor, or immediately following spontaneous rupture of the amniotic membranes.

The best efforts taken by a couple to prevent neonatal herpes may be thwarted if the infection is passed to their baby by others following delivery. Herpes infection of the hand, face, or lips by people holding or kissing a baby can easily transmit the disease. The herpesvirus can remain alive for several hours outside the body, so avoid sharing towels, washcloths, or toothbrushes if you or someone you live with has herpes. Neonatal herpes is highly contagious, and infants suspected of having the disease must be isolated from other babies in the nursery. It is estimated that as many as 10 percent of herpes infections occurring in newborns are not associated with a maternal genital source of contamination.

A new mother with suspected or active genital herpes should be placed in a private room. Feeding and other contact with her baby should be supervised; the wearing of a cover gown and even gloves is recommended to avoid transmission of the virus. Breast-feeding is usually permissible providing that there are no active lesions on the breast. Blisters at extragenital sites should be covered with occlusive dressings and all maternal bodily secretions should be treated as infections and disposed of properly.

Should weekly genital cultures be performed during the last month of pregnancy to detect women who are asymptomatic herpes carriers?

In order to prevent the 400 to 1,000 cases of neonatal herpes which occur annually in the United States, it became the national standard of care in the 1980s for obstetricians to perform weekly cervical or vaginal cultures during the last four weeks of pregnancy on all women with a previous history of herpes. If the last culture preceding the onset of labor was positive, immediate cesarean section was performed. Sadly, this policy has proved to be a dismal failure, with the incidence of neonatal herpes increasing significantly during this time period, despite a 50 percent cesarean section rate for women entering pregnancy with a history of recurrent genital herpes. The main reason for the increase in neonatal herpes is that at least 70 percent of the mothers of newborns who contract the disease have no previous history of herpes and no genital lesions at the time of delivery. As a result, these women did not meet the criteria for screening during pregnancy. One might argue that this

problem can be solved by performing weekly cultures on all pregnant women during the last month of pregnancy. To do this, however, would cost a staggering 1.8 million dollars for each case of neonatal herpes which is averted.

The lack of a rapid, accurate, and inexpensive test to diagnose the presence of genital herpes at the onset of labor continues to be the main obstacle for obstetricians trying to prevent neonatal herpes. As a result, patient and physician paranoia about the disease have been responsible for thousands of unnecessary cesarean sections being performed each year simply because of widespread and often irrational fear of a baby being infected with a virus during a vaginal delivery.

The current position of the American College of Obstetricians and Gynecologists is that vaginal delivery be encouraged and weekly cultures eliminated in women with a history of genital herpes but no visible lesions during pregnancy. In order to identify potentially exposed infants, a culture should be obtained either from the vagina of the mother during labor or the nose and throat of the newborn. It has recently been proposed that such cultures be done routinely on all women in labor even if there is no history of previous herpes. The yield of positive cultures would be less than 1 percent and the expense considerable, but such a policy would pick up the majority of cases which are now undiagnosed. Culturing either a mother or a baby at the time of birth is an excellent idea because the results are usually available in 24 to 72 hours, while the symptoms of neonatal herpes do not usually appear until the eleventh to sixteenth day of life. This allows ample time to alert a pediatrician and parents so that they can carefully observe susceptible infants and initiate treatment with antiviral agents at the earliest evidence of symptoms.

Can acyclovir be used to treat herpes during pregnancy?

Although limited laboratory and clinical experience with acyclovir during pregnancy has not been associated with fetal toxicity, birth defects, or adverse pregnancy outcome, studies have shown that substantial amounts of the drug do cross the placenta and enter the fetal circulation. Until more is known about its safety, acyclovir use should be restricted to life-threatening disseminated disease in a mother or her newborn, or the rare case in which a baby is exposed to a severe primary maternal infection and is delivered vaginally before a cesarean section can be performed.

When a woman free of symptoms proves to be culture-positive for herpes at the time of delivery, experts do not advise that prophylactic acyclovir be given to suppress the virus. Instead, they recommend that cultures be taken of the baby's nose and throat every four to five days, and antiviral therapy be given only if the cultures become positive or the infant shows early symptoms of neonatal herpes.

Some researchers have suggested that women with a history of either symptomatic or asymptomatic herpes may benefit from prophylactic acyclovir during the last three to four weeks of pregnancy. This would theoretically reduce the likelihood of the virus being shed, eliminate the need for expensive culturing, and lower the number of unnecessary cesarean sections that are performed. Others have recommended acyclovir for all women suffering a primary herpes attack after the tenth week of pregnancy in order to accelerate healing,

decrease the duration of pain, and reduce the number of days that the virus is shed. One fear voiced among scientists is that acyclovir is capable of temporarily delaying the formation of maternal IgG neutralizing antibodies against herpes. As previously stated, these antibodies are passed from the mother to the fetus at the end of pregnancy, and they may play a vital role in protecting most newborns from neonatal herpes. It is theorized that taking away or blunting this important defense mechanism could make an infant more susceptible to the disease.

Is it safe to take acyclovir when breast-feeding?

Nursing women are advised not to use acyclovir. Dr. R. Jane Law and her associates at the University of Utah, in their 1987 study published in *Obstetrics and Gynecology*, collected samples of maternal blood, breast milk, and infant urine following administration of a 200-milligram dose of acyclovir to a small group of nursing women. Acyclovir levels in the breast milk were found to exceed those in the bloodstream, while lower concentrations could be detected in the babies' urine specimens. Dr. Law expressed concern that daily exposure of a nursing infant to such high levels of acyclovir could adversely affect the transfer of protective breast milk antibodies which are passed from a mother to a nursing infant during the first ten weeks of life.

 ## PAPILLOMAVIRUS AND GENITAL WARTS

What is the human papillomavirus?

The human papillomavirus (HPV) is a sexually transmitted virus which is known to cause genital warts, or *Condyloma acuminata*. Only in the last seven to eight years have doctors come to realize the important association between HPV and can-

cer. Convincing evidence now supports the view that most HPV strains, while causing no symptoms and no visible warts, are responsible for a majority of abnormal Pap smears and precancerous and cancerous changes of the cervix and vagina. Researchers have linked HPV infections to vulvar, penile, and rectal cancers as well.

If the majority of HPV infections are without symptoms, what screening tests can be used to detect their presence?

Unlike other viruses such as herpes, there is neither a blood test nor a culture technique that can be used to detect the presence of HPV. When the virus is on the cervix, 80 percent of the time a Pap smear will show characteristic microscopic changes of the cervical cells known as "warty atypia." These changes are often closely associated with precancerous abnormalities of the cervix known as dysplasia and carcinoma in situ.

The detection of the actual HPV virus, rather than the changes it produces in a Pap smear, can be achieved only through specialized DNA technology available in a handful of laboratories. With use of this technology, scientists have identified more than 60 different HPV types. HPV types 6 and 11 are usually associated with benign genital warts which occasionally disappear without treatment, while HPV types 16, 18, 31, 33, 35, and 56 are far more likely to cause precancerous and cancerous disease. Type 18 has been found to be the most virulent and the type most often associated with fast-growing invasive cancers of the cervix. Investigators have shown that HPV infections often involve more than a single viral type; identification of a benign wart on the vulva does not exclude the possibility of a microscopic precancerous lesion of the cervix. It is both interesting and important to note that nearly 95 percent of premalignant and malignant cervical lesions contain HPV nuclear DNA. In one study from the Mayo Clinic, doctors found that women with a previous history of genital warts have a fourfold greater risk of developing carcinoma in situ of the cervix than women without warts. Since a practicing physician does not have the luxury of a laboratory capable of distinguishing one HPV type from another, it is important to perform periodic Pap smears on all women with a current or past HPV infection.

ViraPap is the trade name of a diagnostic kit that can detect the presence of human papillomavirus DNA in cervical secretions. Though this test is unable to distinguish one HPV type from another and costs between $35 and $40, one advantage of the ViraPap is that it can detect HPV infection in women whose initial Pap smear is borderline or equivocal for the presence of HPV. The test will be positive only if types 6, 11, 16, 18, 31, 33, or 35 are present in the cervical cells. Another commercially available test for HPV-DNA is the ViraType. This test is more sensitive than the ViraPap because it differentiates virus types into three groups: types 6/11, 16/18, and 31/33/35. By knowing that a woman is harboring the potentially more dangerous HPV types 16 and 18, a doctor is alerted to perform more frequent Pap smears and colposcopy surveillance (see discussion below). However, the ViraType and ViraPap should never be used in place of the Pap smear or for general HPV screening purposes.

If a Pap smear is abnormal during pregnancy, what is the best method of evaluation and treatment?

Unfortunately, the problem of the abnormal Pap smear during pregnancy is inadequately managed in many areas of the United States. Physicians confronted with this dilemma too often repeat the Pap with the unrealistic hope that it will revert to normal. Until recently, when the repeat smears remained abnormal, a cone biopsy was performed. This technique involves the removal of a large cone-shaped wedge of tissue from the cervix to determine if microscopic precancerous or cancerous changes are present. While the cone biopsy technique has a diagnostic accuracy of at least 95 percent, it may cause serious complications for a pregnant woman, including hemorrhage, accidental rupture of the amniotic membranes with subsequent infection and abortion, and incompetent cervix with premature labor. These potential complications, anesthesia risk, and hospital expense can all be avoided by an office examination of the cervix with a low-powered microscopic called a colposcope. A doctor skilled at this technique can easily and accurately detect abnormal areas on the cervix and obtain tiny biopsy samples without adversely affecting the outcome of pregnancy. A colposcopic-directed biopsy enables a doctor to distinguish between condylomas and the more ominous dysplasias and carcinoma in situ. For this reason, it is vital that you insist on colposcopy, rather than cone biopsy, as the initial method of evaluation if your Pap smear is abnormal at any time during pregnancy.

If a woman is found to have warts on her outer genitals, it is a good idea for her doctor to perform a careful colposcopic examination of the vagina and cervix, since there is a 70 percent chance of finding evidence of HPV in these locations as well. When a 3 to 5 percent solution of acetic acid is applied to the cervix prior to colposcopy, a previously unseen flat wart will turn bright white. More importantly, 30 percent of women with external condylomata will have co-existing more ominous conditions such as dysplasia or carcinoma in situ.

The development of cancer of the cervix evolves slowly over a period of years. Therefore, treatment of asymptomatic HPV infections of the cervix and of precancerous changes such as dysplasia and carcinoma in situ can be delayed until several weeks following delivery. Invasive cancer, although extremely rare, is an ominous disease which requires immediate treatment. It is imperative that a doctor determine with certainty that it is not present during pregnancy, since it spreads rapidly and is life-threatening. Invasive cancer diagnosed during the first six months requires immediate treatment with radical hysterectomy or radiation without regard to the fetus. When invasive cancer is found during the third trimester, consideration should be given to the survival of the fetus. Delivery of the baby in the last two months of pregnancy is best accomplished by cesarean section, as soon as it is deter-

mined that the infant has a reasonable chance of survival. Vaginal delivery of a baby through a cervix with invasive cancer will disseminate the disease and hasten the mother's demise. Radical surgery or radiation for the mother should begin immediately after delivery.

When genital warts are present, what are the symptoms and how are they diagnosed?

The average incubation period from the time of sexual contact with an infected individual to the first appearance of a wart is two to three months, although it may range from six weeks to as long as eight months. In women, the warts most commonly appear on the lower part of the vaginal opening, followed in decreasing frequency by the inner labia minora and clitoris, the outer labia majora, the perineum, anus, vagina, cervix, and urethra. Unlike the lesions of herpes, genital warts cause itching but no pain, and quite often symptoms are nonexistent. Lesions around the anus and within the rectum are far more frequently noted in women who engage in anal intercourse with infected partners.

The number and size of genital warts vary greatly from one person to another, with some individuals experiencing just one pinpoint spot while others suffer with huge cauliflower-like growths which completely cover the external genitals. Diabetic women are especially prone to developing extensive condylomas. The characteristic appearance of genital condylomas usually allows for an easy diagnosis. On rare occasions they may be mistaken for the lesions of secondary syphilis, but this can be resolved by a blood test for syphilis or a biopsy of the wart. Conditions such as sebaceous, or fatty, cysts, a skin disorder named molluscum contagiosum, and vulvar cancer can also be confused with genital warts, but a biopsy will confirm the diagnosis. In rare cases, condylomas of the external genitals can become malignant. For this reason, biopsies are advised when the lesions are extensive, appear extremely resistant to treatment, or rapidly recur after treatment.

How are genital warts treated?

The most widely used treatment approach over the years has been to paint the warts with a 25 percent solution of podophyllin in tincture of benzoin or alcohol. If treatment is successful, the warts should disappear within two weeks. This treatment has the disadvantage of being associated with severe pain at the site of treatment and allergic reactions in a small number of women. Estimates vary, but some doctors report podophyllin cure rates of only 20 percent following one treatment session. Retreatment appears to be the rule rather than the exception. Podofilox (trade name Condylox), formerly known as podophyllotoxin, has recently been approved for use in the United States. It is a chemically pure preparation of the active substance lignin contained in podophyllin resin. Since it contains none of the impurities found in podophyllin, it is associated with few if any toxic local or systemic reactions. In fact, it is so safe that a woman can be easily taught how to apply the solution herself. A typical course of treatment consists of two podofilox applications daily for three days, followed by four days of rest. This weekly schedule may be repeated for up to four cycles. Clinical investigation of the drug has shown that 75 percent of all visible warts are eliminated after one month of treatment, with 40 percent of treated women never developing recurrent lesions. Excellent results have been reported with applications of an 80 to 90 percent solution of trichloracetic acid. This agent is far less damaging to tissues than podophyllin and severe reactions do not occur. Liquid nitrogen has also been used with excellent results.

The application of the anticancer drug 5-fluorouracil, or 5-FU, as a cream once or twice a week has proven to be an effective method of eliminating genital warts. Unfortunately, the severe inflammatory reaction and pain associated with 5-FU discourages many women from completing a course of treatment.

Larger warts and those resistant to treatment can be excised under local anesthesia, cauterized (burned), treated with cryosurgery (frozen), and burned with a high-energy light or laser. Laser treatment of extensive genital warts is often associated with severe postoperative pain and fever. Although some reports claim that permanent cures are higher with laser than with any other treatment modality, other studies refute these findings and show a 30 to 50 percent incidence of a persistent or recurrent HPV infection among those treated. For reasons which remain unknown, laser treatment of condylomata during the last trimester of pregnancy, specifically between the thirtieth and thirty-second weeks, is associated with higher success rates than treatment during the first and second trimesters. The reason for the limited success rates for laser and all other methods is that viral particles present in surrounding normal skin often go unnoticed and untreated.

For difficult cases, experimental vaccines from the substance of the warts have been used with variable success. Promising results have also been achieved with the antiviral and anticancer protein interferon. Interferon (trade names Intron A and Alferon N) can be injected directly into a wart or given as an intramuscular injection. In one study, the injection of genital warts with interferon resulted in a 36 percent complete cure rate, compared to 17 percent among patients treated with a placebo. In another report, marked improvement to total clearing of treated warts was seen in 66 percent of almost 200 patients who were treated. A more impressive statistic was that 81 percent of those cured showed no evidence of recurrence.

Regardless of the method of treatment used, if new condylomas do not appear within three months after treatment, the likelihood of a recurrence is negligible. When warts do recur, they usually do so within two to six weeks after the apparent cure. It is often difficult to tell if these lesions represent a treatment failure or incubating disease that has not yet surfaced. During the treatment period and for at least three months following an apparent cure, it is imperative that condoms be worn during all sexual encounters, although the warts will not be contained if they are on a man's scrotum or other areas not covered by a condom. To achieve a permanent cure, all male sexual partners should be thoroughly examined and treated.

A woman's natural immunity often plays a more important role than a particular method of treatment in determining whether or not her condyloma will worsen or improve. Until recently, gynecologists appeared obsessed with destroying all asymptomatic microscopic infections of the cervix either with laser, cautery, cryosurgery, or surgical excision. Experts now recommend a more conservative, laissez-faire approach if there are no visible warts and there is no microscopic evidence of dysplasia coexisting with the HPV "warty atypia." The reason for this change of attitude is that 50 percent of these asymptomatic microscopic HPV infections recede on their own without treatment within a two-year period; the warts disappear and the Pap smear reverts to normal. In addition, even when extensive and expensive methods are used, it is almost impossible to eradicate the virus from the cervix for very long periods of time. It is for this reason that women with a previous history of "warty atypia" continue to have Pap smears taken at six-month intervals.

What happens to genital warts during pregnancy, and how are they treated at this time?

Genital warts tend to enlarge dramatically in pregnant women and then regress to their prepregnancy size following delivery. Occasionally, they become so massive that they may actually obstruct the birth canal and interfere with a normal vaginal delivery.

One problem encountered in treating genital warts during pregnancy is that the use of podophyllin is ill-advised. There have been several reported cases of absorption of the chemical in the blood-stream, resulting in severe reactions and even fetal and maternal deaths. In addition to podophyllin, 5-fluorouracil (5-FU) is considered too dangerous for use during pregnancy, especially the first trimester. In one recent case, a woman treated with 5-FU cream during pregnancy delivered a baby with a cleft palate. While this one case does not prove cause and effect, 5-FU is still best avoided. Too little is known about the effects of interferon and podofilox to recommend their use during pregnancy.

Fortunately, there are several safe and effective alternative methods of treating genital warts during pregnancy. Tricholoracetic acid does not appear to be harmful to the fetus and is suitable for use. Similarly, cryosurgery, surgical excision, cauterization, and laser surgery are not associated with an adverse pregnancy outcome. Use of laser is especially helpful when the genital warts are extensive. Most warts, regardless of size, do not obstruct the birth canal. If they do, of course, cesarean section is indicated.

In recent years, doctors have become aware that an infant passing through a birth canal harboring *Condyloma acuminata* is in danger of contracting the virus. In fact, this occurs fairly frequently. In a 1989 report from the University of Pennsylvania, Dr. Thomas V. Sedlacek and his associates documented the presence of HPV in the noses and throats of 15 of 45 infants born of mothers with genital condylomas. Most infants apparently rid themselves of the virus without ever experiencing symptoms, but a small number develop benign growths, called laryngeal papillomas, in the larynx or windpipe and vocal cords months and even years following birth.

The precise risk of a newborn acquiring laryngeal papillomas from a mother with genital warts is unknown. However, in a recent review published in *Obstetrics and Gynecology*, doctors estimated this risk at one in "several hundred, and even more than a thousand." Therefore, performing a cesarean section on a woman with genital warts, simply for the purpose of preventing laryngeal papillomas in her newborn, does not seem warranted at the present time.

How should the male sexual partner of an HPV-infected woman be examined and treated?

Research indicates that 85 percent of women with condylomas have been in contact with men harboring the same HPV type. More importantly, doctors in England found that 45 percent of the female sexual contacts of men with penile condylomas developed cervical cancer. In many of these cases, the HPV lesions produced no symptoms in the male carriers. When doctors at the Medical College of Virginia examined the sexual partners of 127 women with precancerous disease of the cervix, they found that 83 men, or 65 percent, had evidence of HPV genital lesions. The majority of men in this 1987 study were also without symp-toms. At least four different investigative groups have observed a higher incidence of cervical cancer in wives of men with penile cancer. These statistics offer adequate evidence that if we are to contain the spread of HPV, all male sexual contacts of infected women must be meticulously screened and treated promptly. This can best be accomplished by urologists, dermatologists, and gynecologists.

The colposcope, used so successfully in diagnosing HPV infections of the cervix and vagina, is also extremely helpful in detecting asymptomatic warts on the skin of the penis, outer urethra, and scrotum of a man. Several studies have observed that between 50 and 80 percent of male partners of women with documented HPV lesions have colposcopic evidence of HPV as well. To perform colposcopy on a man, a generous amount of 5 percent acetic acid is applied to the external genitals, including the penis, scrotum, inner thighs, and skin around the anus. The acetic acid permits easy visualization of previously unseen warts.

The various methods used to treat male genital warts are identical to those used for women. When laser surgery was first introduced, it was believed that it would be the long-awaited panacea for treating general warts. Some reports quoted a treatment failure rate of only 2 percent, but subsequent studies have been far less optimistic. In general, genital warts in men respond better to treatment than they do in women. Recurrence rates also appear to be lower when treatment is begun three to six months after the warts first appeared, rather than before or after this time period. A man should be reexamined one month and three months after treatment of his warts. If none are detected at either follow-up visit, he is most probably cured.

 HEPATITIS

What is hepatitis, and how can it be transmitted sexually?

Hepatitis is an inflammation of the liver often associated with jaundice or yellowing of the skin and the whites of the eyes. Many cases of hepatitis go undetected because jaundice does not occur and symptoms may be minimal or absent. While hepatitis may result from exposure to chemical or environmental agents, most cases are caused by one of four viruses named hepatitis A virus, hepatitis B virus, hepatitis C virus, and hepatitis D, or delta hepatitis, virus. For years hepatitis B, known as serum hepatitis, was believed to occur only in individuals who received blood transfusions from others with the disease or in drug-addicted persons using contaminated needles. As a result of recent studies, epidemiologists now believe that hepatitis B is frequently transmitted sexually. This view is supported by the observation that significant viral shedding has been detected in semen, vaginal secretions, and saliva of infected individuals. In addition, the incidence of the disease is directly related to the number of sexual partners a person encounters. In a 1989 study of 218 patients with hepatitis B, researchers at the Centers for Disease Control found that heterosexual transmission was the source of the disease 23 percent of the time. This report also noted that the recently discovered hepatitis C virus, the cause of non-A, non-B hepatitis (NANB), could be attributed to a sexual source in 11 percent of infected individuals. Delta hepatitis is a rare disease in the United States, but when it does appear it is always in the presence of a hepatitis B infection. It is found in both blood and body fluids, and sexual transmission is believed to be a common method of spread.

In contrast, hepatitis A is rarely transmitted sexually. Instead, it is usually contracted through fecal contamination of food and water, although sexual practices involving oral-anal contact with an infected person can spread the disease.

Hepatitis B has a very long incubation period of 30 to 180 days, and more than 50 percent of all cases are either totally asymptomatic or appear as a mild case of gastroenteritis or fatigue. Only 25 percent of infected individuals become ill with symptoms such as jaundice, fever, extreme lethargy, loss of appetite, nausea, vomiting, and sometimes general body itching and joint pain. When jaundice is present, a person's urine usually appears dark brown in color and the stools light-colored. About 90 percent of those who contract hepatitis B recover within two weeks, but in approximately 2 percent the disease is fatal. Estimates vary, but perhaps one out of ten people who acquire hepatitis B remain chronic long-term carriers capable of transmitting the disease to others. Chronic carriers face an estimated 25 percent risk of dying either from cirrhosis or cancer of the liver.

How does hepatitis B affect pregnancy?

When symptomatic acute hepatitis B is contracted by a woman during pregnancy, she is more likely to experience spontaneous abortion, stillbirth, and premature labor. The virus may also pass from mother to fetus across the placenta during preg-

nancy, and approximately 5 to 10 percent of newborns who contract hepatitis B are believed to do so in this fashion. The overwhelming number of infected infants, however, become infected at or after delivery.

The pregnancy of an asymptomatic hepatitis B carrier does not appear to be associated with a higher incidence of miscarriage, prematurity, or other obstetrical complications. In fact, doctors at Louisiana State University and Tulane University Medical Center, in their 1988 study, found that asymptomatic hepatitis B surface antigen (protein on cell surface indicative of active disease) carriers gave birth to babies weighing an average of 381 grams more than an equal number of antigen-negative women. Of greater concern among epidemiologists is that newborns often acquire the hepatitis B virus from exposure to maternal blood during delivery, with both vaginal and cesarean section births. A mother may also transmit the disease to her baby through kissing and close contact during the immediate postpartum period. It has been demonstrated that 70 to 90 percent of infants born to mothers carrying hepatitis B surface antigen become infected within the first few months of life. Eighty-five to 90 percent of these babies remain chronic carriers and serve as viral reservoirs for spreading the disease to their families and community. Sadly, childhood carriers have a 25 percent chance of dying of cirrhosis or liver cancer during adolescence or adulthood. This represents a far greater threat to society than the 10 percent carrier incidence among adults with hepatitis B. To prevent perinatal hepatitis, a susceptible baby should be treated with hepatitis B immune globulin and hepatitis vaccine immediately after birth. The immune globulin is an antibody substance derived from the blood of persons who have previously had the disease. Marketed as H-BIG and Hep-B-Gammagee, it offers instant protection while the vaccine provides 99 percent assurance that the baby will not eventually contract the disease when placed in a home environment which is known to be infectious. The initial hepatitis B vaccine should be given within 12 hours and no later than seven days after birth, to be followed by booster vaccines one month and six months later.

Whether mothers who are carriers should breast-feed is unknown at the present time. However, recent studies suggest that such women may transmit the antigen to their babies in their milk. Most authorities recommend that all intimate contact between a susceptible baby and a mother with the hepatitis B antigen in her bloodstream be avoided unless the baby is first given hepatitis B immune globulin and the hepatitis B vaccine.

How can a woman avoid contracting hepatitis B during pregnancy?

Ideally, a woman and her sexual partner should be tested before pregnancy to determine if either carries the hepatitis B surface antigen in their bloodstream. If the man has the antigen but the woman doesn't, she should be immunized with the hepatitis B vaccine. This highly effective agent, marketed as Engerix-B and Recombivax HB, is a nonviral, genetically engineered vaccine having the DNA structure of a hepatitis B surface antigen. Following two vaccine injections one month apart and a booster six months later, at least 95 percent of all individuals develop antibodies indicative of disease immunity. Until vaccine immunity is established, a susceptible person should avoid kissing and all intimate contact with anyone testing positive for the hepatitis B surface antigen. Since hepatitis B virus can be found in the semen and vaginal secretions of infected individuals, the wearing of a condom will offer some protection against transmission of the disease to a susceptible person. Many experts emphasize the need to wear latex condoms because the hepatitis B viral particles are capable of passing through condoms made of natural lamb membrane. Use of oil-based lubricants, such as petroleum jelly, may damage condoms and increase the likelihood of contracting hepatitis B.

The American College of Obstetricians and Gy-necologists recommends routine hepatitis B screening for all pregnant women during an early prenatal visit. Through such screening, approximately 16,000 previously undiagnosed chronic hepatitis B carriers will be identified annually and 3,500 infants prevented from becoming carriers. In addition, this policy enables household and intimate contacts to be vaccinated. When a woman tests positive for hepatitis B surface antigen during pregnancy, her obstetrician should perform liver function tests to determine her degree of liver damage. More detailed hepatitis B antigen and antibody studies should also be taken to find out if she has an acute infection or is a chronic carrier.

The hepatitis B vaccine has not been studied extensively in pregnant and nursing women, although it has been given to a small number of such women without negative effect on mother or child. In a 1987 report published in the *International Journal of Gynaecology and Obstetrics*, 72 women who tested negative for hepatitis-B surface antigen were given two intramuscular injections of hepatitis-B vaccine, one month apart, during the third trimester. No adverse effects were noted in either the mothers or their newborns, and 84 percent of the women formed protective antibodies within a month after the second vaccine dose. Passive transfer of antibodies from the maternal to the fetal circulation was noted in 59 percent of the newborns. Immunity passed on to the infants was of short duration and disappeared rapidly after birth. The authors of this report concluded that vaccination of pregnant women with hepatitis B vaccine is safe and may help to prevent the 5 to 10 percent incidence of the disease which occurs via placental passage prior to birth. It may also offer protection to the newborn during the time interval from birth to vaccination immunization. If a woman first becomes aware of hepatitis B exposure during pregnancy, the decision on whether or not to receive the vaccine is often a difficult one. Many infectious disease experts believe that the benefits of the vaccine exceed any possible risks since hepatitis may have serious consequences for a woman and her baby. This is especially true for the woman forced to work or live in an area where the chances of contracting hepatitis B appear likely.

An alternative treatment method for the susceptible woman exposed to hepatitis B during pregnancy is administration of an intramuscular injection of hepatitis B immune globulin (see page 216). Immune globulin prevents the onset of the disease or reduces its severity in more than 80 percent of exposed individuals by providing instant, though admittedly short-lived, antibody protection. However, it does not take the place of the hepatitis B vaccine which provides more certain and lasting immunity.

Isn't there a risk of contracting AIDS from the hepatitis vaccine?

Since the original hepatitis B vaccine, Heptavax-B, was made from the plasma of chronic carriers of hepatitis B, many of whom are also at high risk for AIDS, there has been concern expressed that the vaccine could transmit the AIDS virus. This totally unsubstantiated belief has been so widespread that it has discouraged many healthcare workers and others at risk of contracting hepatitis B from seeking immunization. This discussion is no longer relevant, however, since Heptavax-B has been taken off the market. The Recombivax HB and the Engerix-B vaccines are both genetically engineered vaccines which are not derived from plasma and appear to be more acceptable alternatives for those reluctant to receive a plasma-based vaccine.

How common are non-A, non-B hepatitis (hepatitis C) and delta hepatitis, and how can they be controlled?

Although non-A, non-B hepatitis (NANB) was first identified as a disease in 1975, it was not until 1989 that scientists were able to identify the virus causing most cases of the disease and name it hepatitis C virus. This discovery represents a major breakthrough in the eventual diagnosis and control of non-A, non-B hepatitis.

It is only in recent years that doctors at the Centers for Disease Control have come to realize the significant threat posed by the hepatitis C virus. In their 1989 report, CDC doctors estimated that approximately 3 to 7 percent of our population carries the hepatitis C virus and that approximately 150,000 NANB infections occur each year; of this number, 10 percent (15,000 people) develop chronic hepatitis or cirrhosis. Until now, the diagnosis of the disease was difficult if not impossible since the majority of infected individuals show few if any symptoms. Being asymptomatic, however, is not the equivalent of good health, since 50 percent of all people with NANB hepatitis eventually show evidence of chronic liver disease.

Although NANB hepatitis was once believed to be contracted solely via blood transfusions, recent data from the CDC show that no more than 10 percent of cases occur in this manner. At least 40 percent contract the hepatitis C virus through drug use, while in another 40 percent the source of the infection remains unknown. In the remaining 10 percent, the only identifiable source of infection is heterosexual activity with multiple partners or household or sexual exposure to a contact with this form of hepatitis. Scientific evidence has shown that transmission of the virus from a mother to her baby at the time of birth is a very rare occurrence. This is fortunate since there are presently no medical recommendations for dealing with this problem during pregnancy and no vaccine is available for its prevention. It is not known if giving immunoglobulins, or antibodies, from patients with hepatitis C to a susceptible newborn will offer protection against the infection. To further complicate matters, a second milder form of NANB hepatitis has recently been described. The viral agent responsible for this condition is only transmitted via fecal–oral contamination as is hepatitis A.

In 1989, scientists discovered a new and highly effective blood test capable of detecting antibodies to the hepatitis C virus in a person's bloodstream. Clinical trials to date show an impressive detection rate of more than 80 percent. If these results are confirmed, wide availability of the test to blood banks and practicing physicians will significantly reduce the spread of the insidious hepatitis C virus. Until now, there was no way to limit the damage caused by the hepatitis C virus. Two recent studies have shown that the antiviral protein alpha interferon may have the ability to control the infection and prevent extensive destruction of the liver cells. It may also prove effective against damage caused by the hepatitis B virus and the delta virus.

The delta virus is described by microbiologists as "defective" because it can multiply only in the presence of the hepatitis B virus. Both viruses have been identified in the blood and other body fluids, and both can be transmitted sexually. Although rarely found in the United States, the delta hepatitis virus is endemic to certain areas of the world such as the Mediterranean basin, western Africa, eastern Europe, and the Middle East. Delta hepatitis is often a more serious disease than other hepatitis varieties, with a high mortality rate from the acute disease and an 80 percent risk of cirrhosis when the disease is chronic. Since the delta hepatitis virus is totally dependent on the hepatitis B virus for its survival, a successful worldwide hepatitis B vaccination campaign would prove to be a major step in eliminating the delta virus as a health hazard.

 ## CMV

What is cytomegalovirus (CMV), and how can it affect the outcome of pregnancy?

Cytomegalovirus (CMV) is a member of the group of viruses called DNA viruses. Just as herpes can be transmitted from person to person through sexual and nonsexual contact, so can CMV. The incubation period is one to three months, and most adults, possibly as many as 90 percent who contract CMV, are totally unaware that they harbor the infection. In the United States, 50 to 80 percent of adults have antibodies to CMV in their bloodstream, indicative of a prior infection. When symptoms do occur, they resemble those of infectious mononucleosis and include fatigue, low-grade fever, sore throat, muscular aches and pains, generalized lymph node enlargement, and occasionally a measles-like rash. While few men and women have ever heard of this disease, it is probably the most important infectious cause of birth defects and mental retardation in the United States.

CMV is the most common infection transmitted by blood transfusion. That it may also be transmitted sexually is a relatively new finding. Convincing evidence demonstrates that the incidence of this infection increases after puberty as sexual activity increases. Most recently, doctors at the University of Washington noted a strong correlation between CMV infections and age at first intercourse and the number of sexual partners in one's lifetime. In one study, the virus was found in the cervix of 29 percent of women attending a venereal disease clinic. In addition, CMV has been isolated from the saliva, blood, urine, feces, breast milk, tears, and semen of sexually active individuals. It is probably more easily transmitted than any other venereal organism since men and women who harbor it are without symptoms. Excretion of CMV can sometimes persist for months or years and even disappear for a period of time, only to become reactivated at a later date.

It has been estimated that as many as 10 to 15 percent of all women carry CMV in their cervix during pregnancy, and approximately 30,000 newborns each year excrete the virus at birth. Of these newborns, approximately 10 percent have been found with significant evidence of disease. Abnormalities may not be readily apparent at birth in another 2,500 to 8,000 children who will later develop varying degrees of hearing, learning, and neurological disorders. Some researchers believe that CMV may be the leading cause of hearing loss in children in this country.

It is believed that the greatest risk of congenital birth defects caused by CMV occurs among those mothers who are first exposed to the virus just before conception or during the first four months of pregnancy. Congenital defects caused by cytomegalovirus are more varied and devastating than those produced by other TORCH complex microorganisms. (You will remember that TORCH is an acronym for toxoplasmosis, rubella, cytomegalovirus, and herpes, four diseases which can severely damage the fetus.) Although other diseases have been added to the original TORCH foursome, cytomegalovirus remains the most ubiquitous and most dangerous, and is responsible for 700 infant deaths annually in the United States. Infected babies are often anemic and have a reduced number of platelets in their blood. Many will have purpura, a hemorrhagic skin rash due to a platelet deficiency. Pneumonia and enlargement of the liver and spleen are also commonly seen. The central nervous system appears to be most vulnerable to attack. Among infants showing symptoms at birth, 50 to 75 percent will be left with permanent and severe neurological disease such as microcephaly, seizures, deafness, blindness, and psychomotor disturbances. There is little doubt that many children are born with an infection that goes entirely unnoticed. These children may, however, constitute a proportion of those individuals who later develop perceptual disorders, learning disabilities, behavior problems, and hearing loss. It can be safely predicted that infected infants who do not show evidence of neurological disease at two years of age are not likely to be significantly affected later in life.

The severity of disease in the newborn is dependent upon when in the pregnancy exposure to CMV takes place. While the greatest damage will occur during first-trimester exposure, the more subtle disabilities are likely to occur when the virus attacks during the second trimester. Although a fetus who contracts CMV from its mother during the third trimester may harbor the virus in its body at birth, there are no documented reports of significant damage from primary infections which occur during this time. It is of some consolation to know that the severe damage inflicted by CMV during a mother's primary infection will hardly ever recur in subsequent pregnancies, even though she may still have the virus in her body and transmit it to her baby. Statistically, the incidence of positive CMV cultures among babies born to women with recurrent disease ranges from 0.5 to 1.9 percent.

An infant may also contract CMV while passing through the infected cervix during labor. When a woman has a CMV cervical infection at the time of birth, her infant will have a 40 to 50 percent chance of acquiring the virus during the first three months of life. Although these babies usually do not develop clinical disease, they may shed the virus in their urine and saliva for 12 to 18 months. There are also case reports in which the virus was transmitted to the baby through the breast milk of an infected mother. This is not surprising in view of the fact that 25 to 35 percent of women with CMV excrete it in their breast milk.

If a baby is suspected of having CMV, how can the diagnosis be made with certainty?

The virus is most likely to be isolated from the baby's urine, although the saliva also contains CMV. Since culture samples may take as long as six weeks to show a positive reaction, the test is of no immediate value. A more rapid diagnostic method is to determine if a newborn has produced large IgM antibodies specific against CMV. These antibodies are too large to cross the placenta; therefore, their presence in the newborn's umbilical cord or bloodstream is significant because they are formed by the baby in response to acute infection. Smaller IgG antibodies pass readily across the placenta from the maternal to the fetal circulation. These passively acquired antibodies are found in the newborn's circulation in concentrations equal to those found in its mother. However, if a newborn's IgG antibody level rises significantly in the weeks or months following delivery, it is a good indication that the baby has contracted an acute CMV infection either from its mother or someone else in its environment.

How can CMV be prevented and treated?

There is no known medical treatment for CMV infections, and since the disease in adults is usually totally asymptomatic, there would be little reason for an otherwise healthy woman to suspect its existence. Routine culturing of the cervix for CMV during the first trimester is not recommended because it would be prohibitively expensive and the few laboratories performing the test would be overwhelmed with requests. Furthermore, finding CMV does not necessarily help a doctor determine when a woman's first exposure occurred in relation to the date of conception. Serial IgG and IgM determinations can sometimes help to clarify the situation. If the cervical culture is positive for CMV in the first or second trimester, the only medical treatment that can be offered is a therapeutic abortion, which is most likely to be unnecessary. Recent advances in the use of amniotic fluid cultures, percutaneous umbilical blood sampling (PUBS), and ultrasound appear promising but are far from infallible. If a pregnant woman is among the small minority of individuals who experience a symptomatic CMV infection, an alert physician can make the diagnosis and offer her the option of a therapeutic abortion. Suspicion should be aroused whenever a woman has symptoms of mononucleosis but a negative blood test for the disease.

At least three separate studies have found that a woman's risk of contracting a primary CMV infection increases significantly during the time interval between her first and second pregnancies. The reason for this is believed to be the introduction of the virus into the household by a toddler or infant who contracts the asymptomatic CMV infection from playmates in crowded day-care and pre-kindergarten facilities. In one study, doctors reported that one in five adults acquired the infection from their children. On the positive side, the exposure of so many young children to CMV has lead epidemiologists to predict a sharp decline in the incidence of primary CMV infections of pregnancy over the next 20 to 30 years. The reason for this is that 70 to 80 percent of today's toddlers are being exposed to CMV and are developing antibodies which should protect them from infection during their lifetime.

The treatment of CMV infections has been totally unsuccessful. Acyclovir, which is effective in the treatment of herpes, is of no help in treating CMV infections. Cytomegalovirus immune globulin (CMVIG) has been available in the United States on an investigational basis since 1988; its use is currently restricted to kidney transplant recipients who lack CMV immunity.

Are there any specific vaccines which can be used against CMV?

Not yet. The development of a safe and effective vaccine is the major thrust of current research aimed at preventing CMV infections. Several vaccines made of the weakened virus have provided immunity for varying periods of time. Some scientists fear that use of these live vaccines may activate dormant infections of the same strain, while others have expressed concerns about the cancer-causing potential of the live virus. Work is currently under way to develop a subunit vaccine from noninfectious viral preparations.

LISTERIOSIS

What is *Listeria monocytogenes*, and how does it affect the outcome of pregnancy?

Listeria monocytogenes is a bacterium which, in recent years, has received an increasing amount of attention as a cause of poor pregnancy outcome. In their 1989 report, published in the *Journal of the American Medical Association*, Dr. Bruce G. Gellin and Dr. Claire V. Broome of the Centers for Disease Control estimated that this organism is responsible for at least 450 deaths and 100 stillbirths annually in the United States. Listeriosis is most often transmitted as a food-borne illness via contaminated milk, cheese, raw vegetables, and shellfish. There appear to be other ways in which this organism is transmitted, and there is some evidence to suggest that sexual intercourse may be one of them.

Recent reports suggest that pregnant women, especially those in the second or third trimester, have an increased susceptibility to listeriosis. This is evidenced by the fact that at least half of all listeriosis cases reported occur in pregnant women, fetuses, or newborns. It is estimated that listeriosis complicates one in 20,000 pregnancies. Elderly persons and individuals with poor immunity are also prone to contract this disease. The recent observation of a higher incidence of listeriosis among people with AIDS is not surprising in view of their weakened immunity.

Accurate diagnosis of listeriosis is hindered because there are no specific symptoms which distinguish it from a viral infection or a flu-like illness. Following an incubation period of several weeks, infected women may develop fever, chills, muscle aches, and back pain. Others may experience no symptoms at all.

Maternal listeriosis may severely affect the fetus and newborn infant. An infection in the first trimester has been shown to cause spontaneous abortion, but it remains controversial whether or not listeriosis is responsible for repeated spontaneous abortions. Infected amniotic fluid may lead to premature labor and even fetal death. In one study, French researchers were able to grow *Listeria monocytogenes* from placental and fetal cultures in 1.6 percent of pregnancies that resulted in spontaneous abortions and premature labor. It appears that an infant may contract the disease in utero as well as during its passage through the birth canal during labor. Some babies, considered healthy at birth, begin to show symptoms of fever, irritability, and poor feeding weeks later. Others may experience immediate and severe respiratory difficulty; hypothermia, or lowered body temperature; enlargement of the liver; circulatory disturbances; and occasionally a rash on the skin or an inflammation of the eyes. In rare cases, the infection may lead to meningitis, encephalitis, and death.

How is listeriosis diagnosed and treated?

If doctors do not maintain a high degree of suspicion, the disease is rarely diagnosed. All pregnant women with fever or a flu-like illness, and those with a history of repeated unexplained spontaneous abortion, should have cultures taken from the vagina, cervix, and blood. *Listeria monocytogenes* grows readily in a culture medium and can be identified within 48 hours. Viewing the organism under the microscope, in the absence of cultures, is suggestive but not diagnostic of listeriosis. When the possibility of the disease exists in the newborn, cultures should be taken immediately after the birth from the baby's stomach and pharynx secretions as well as the blood. A variety of blood tests have been devised to diagnose listeriosis, but they are less than accurate because *Listeria monocytogenes* has several antigens that cross-react with other bacterial organisms. A new DNA probe technique that is being developed appears promising.

Listeriosis in both the mother and the newborn is easily treated with a variety of antibiotics, including penicillin, ampicillin, kanamycin, gentamycin, erythromycin, tetracycline, and sulfamethoxazole combined with trimethoprim. Several researchers have demonstrated that aggressive and early antibiotic treatment of a pregnant woman with listeriosis can reduce the risk of spontaneous abortion, stillbirth, premature labor, and neonatal infection. When a baby contracts the infection immediately after birth, it is important to treat it with antibiotics for at least three weeks if a recurrence and the late-onset type of infection is to be prevented.

 # GB-BHS

What is GB-BHS, and how is it related to the outcome of pregnancy?

GB-BHS stands for a bacterium named Group B-beta-hemolytic streptococcus. Although bacteriologists first identified this organism many years ago, it was not until the early 1960s that it was detected in the female urinary and genital tracts. Researchers at that time reported that GB-BHS could be transmitted through sexual intercourse. This is supported by the finding that the organism can be recovered from a male sexual partner at least one-half of the time. Recent studies show that GB-BHS can be isolated from the genital tract of 20 to 30 percent of all pregnant women when special selective culture media are used. The fact that women harboring GB-BHS bacteria are totally asymptomatic is the greatest hindrance to early detection and treatment.

GB-BHS is the cause of approximately 3,000 annual cases of postpartum infection among women undergoing cesarean section. Over the years some researchers have concluded that maternal GB-BHS genital infections are responsible for a higher incidence of spontaneous abortion, stillbirth, prematurity, and premature rupture of the amniotic membranes. However, the majority of studies have noted no such association. All investigators do agree that GB-BHS is a significant cause of death among newborns, and that labor is the time of highest risk for a mother to transmit the infection to her child. Authorities estimate that 12,000 to 15,000 newborns develop GB-BHS infections each year; of these, approximately 50 percent die. These statistics are far more frightening than those associated with herpes, yet the need to protect against and treat these infections has received far less attention in both the medical and lay literature.

There are some very puzzling aspects to GB-BHS infections. For example, although two-thirds of infants born of mothers with positive cultures also have positive cultures, actual infection and illness occur in only 2 per 1,000 live births. Many perfectly healthy infants may harbor the bacterium in their nose and throat for as long as 18 months. It is also interesting to note that the organism, for unknown reasons, disappears from a woman's genital tract without treatment in one-half of all women with positive cultures. GB-BHS is less likely to spontaneously disappear during pregnancy and seems to be especially resistant to treatment at this time. Relapses and reinfection, as evidenced by conversion of genital cultures from negative to positive even after treatment of both partners, is a common phenomenon. It has recently been demonstrated that a woman's intestinal tract may serve as a reservoir for the organism and a likely source of these recurrent vaginal infections. While the infection is usually acquired by the baby at the time of delivery, there are several reported cases of the organism causing infection before the start of labor. This is believed to occur when bacteria enter through the usually protective cervical mucus during coitus or following rupture of the amniotic membranes prior to the onset of labor.

Approximately one-half of the newborns who become seriously ill with a GB-BHS infection do so within the first 24 hours following delivery. These babies often appear sick while still in the delivery room, and over half will show signs of respiratory distress during the first six hours of life. Twenty-four hours following delivery, at least 85 percent will be gravely ill if early treatment has not been initiated. The late-onset form of the disease is usually less ominous, with symptoms sometimes appearing as late as three to five weeks after the baby has been discharged from the hospital.

Delay in diagnosis and treatment is the main reason for the high death rate among newborns infected with GB-BHS. The first sign of infection is usually rapid and labored breathing, which may be mistaken in its similarity to the more common respiratory distress syndrome (see Chapter 11). Within hours, this may progress to an overwhelming and irreversible infection. If the bacteria invade the meninges, or covering of the brain and spinal cord, 50 percent of infected babies will be left with permanent neurological damage.

What factors are most likely to determine if a newborn will contract GB-BHS from its mother?

Although it has not been convincingly demonstrated that a maternal GB-BHS infection causes prematurity, it has been proven that the disease more frequently attacks premature infants, for whom it has a 70 percent likelihood of being fatal. Among extremely premature infants, the fatality rate may be as high as 90 percent, compared to that of less than 20 percent among full-term infants with the infection. The duration of time that the amniotic membranes are ruptured also increases the risk to the newborn. In one study, the

attack rate was 1 per 1,000 live births when membranes were ruptured for less than 12 hours, compared to 5 per 1,000 live births when the time exceeded 12 hours. A third vital determinant is the presence of maternal fever during labor. Women with elevated temperatures have a fivefold greater risk of giving birth to a baby with a serious GB-BHS infection than women with normal temperatures. In one study, when all three of these risk factors were present, the attack rate among newborns was 7.6 per 1,000, compared to only 0.6 per 1,000 if they were absent. The number of bacterial colonies in a woman's vagina and the virulence of the particular GB-BHS strain will also determine the likelihood and severity of her newborn's disease.

How can GB-BHS of the newborn be prevented?

In attempting to eradicate neonatal GB-BHS infections, doctors have employed a variety of treatment strategies, none of which has been completely successful. Some authorities recommend that all pregnant women have cultures taken from the cervix, vagina, and rectum, and that antibiotics be prescribed for all culture-positive individuals and their sexual partners. Others have just the opposite view: that cultures are unnecessary and treatment during pregnancy is incapable of completely eliminating the organism from the genital tract and rectum. Unlike the standardized treatment protocols one finds for other sexually transmitted conditions, there is no consensus of opinion among experts as to the best way of preventing neonatal GB-BHS infections.

The most ambitious plan to eliminate GB-BHS has been to obtain cervical, vaginal, and rectal cultures on all women between the twenty-sixth and twenty-eighth weeks of pregnancy and to initiate intravenous ampicillin treatment at the onset of labor in those women with positive cultures. Some hospitals treat all babies born of culture-positive mothers with ampicillin and gentamycin for an additional 48 hours postpartum. If cultures taken from the baby's gastric fluid, throat, umbilicus, blood, external ear, and rectum at the time of delivery prove negative, antibiotic treatment is discontinued. While this method sounds like a logical treatment strategy, it is extremely expensive to perform GB-BHS cultures on every pregnant woman. In addition, as many as 25 percent of women who are culture-positive at 28 weeks mysteriously become culture-negative without treatment by the time labor begins. As a result, a large number of women are bombarded with high doses of intravenous ampicillin for an infection which is no longer present. Another disadvantage is that a small number of women experience severe adverse reactions to ampicillin. Finally, this treatment protocol overlooks approximately 10 percent of women whose negative cultures at 28 weeks convert to positive cultures during labor because of either reinfection or relapse of a dormant infection.

A more practical treatment approach has been proposed by Dr. Howard Minkoff and his colleagues at the State University of New York–Downstate Medical Center. Instead of routinely culturing all women during pregnancy, Dr. Minkoff obtains cultures on only a select group of high-risk women during labor and simultaneously initiates intravenous ampicillin therapy. Included in this group are women giving birth prematurely, those with prematurely ruptured amniotic membranes for more than 18 hours, and anyone with an elevated temperature during labor. Dr. Minkoff found that he could thus target 90 percent of pregnancies at risk for a serious neonatal GB-BHS infection. With this treatment protocol, even if the cultures taken at the time of birth prove to be negative, fewer women undergo unnecessary treatment than with the more expensive first protocol in which all pregnant women are cultured. On the negative side, however, it overlooks that small percentage of pregnancies in which the mother does not fall into a high-risk group but still has the infection and transmits it to her baby. Women with a GB-BHS infection who are allergic to either ampicillin or penicillin can be treated safely and effectively with either erythromycin, cephalosporins, or clindamycin.

It is obvious from this discussion that none of the currently available treatment protocols are capable of eliminating GB-BHS as a major medical problem of mothers and infants. This will only be achieved through the development of either an effective vaccine to prevent the disease or a rapid, accurate, inexpensive diagnostic test capable of pinpointing those women harboring the bacteria in their genital tract at the onset of labor. Such a test would allow immediate selective treatment of infected women while avoiding overtreatment of those who are not infectious.

Are there any promising methods for preventing and treating GB-BHS infections?

Yes. Vaccines may eventually prove to be the most effective method of preventing GB-BHS infections. Research has demonstrated that mothers of infants suffering from GB-BHS infections are significantly less likely to have high levels of antibodies than mothers with noninfected babies. This fact has led to the development of vaccines which stimulate the formation of high antibody titres among individuals susceptible to GB-BHS. Unlike live vaccines, which are potentially harmful to the fetus, GB-BHS vaccines are extremely safe and contain either protein or polysaccharide antigens. In a multicenter study published in the *New England Journal of Medicine* in 1988, doctors immunized susceptible women during their last trimester with vaccines containing group B streptococcal capsular polysaccharides. Protective IgG antibody levels were induced in 63 percent of the vaccine-treated women. These IgG antibodies were found to cross the placenta and provide passively acquired immunity to the fetus at levels 80 percent of those found in the maternal circulation. Following birth, antibody levels gradually decreased over the next three months. This study demonstrated that protective antibodies can be induced in mothers and their fetuses. If protection for the fetus can be achieved with this method of immunization, it will be a major stride in controlling GB-BHS infections.

VAGINITIS

What causes vaginitis?

Volumes of misinformation have been written about the diagnosis and treatment of vaginitis. As a result, confusion exists as to how a woman contracts different types of vaginitis, what methods should be used to distinguish one type from another, and, most importantly, how each condition should be treated during pregnancy.

Three types of vaginitis may affect the young sexually active woman: trichomoniasis, moniliasis, and bacterial vaginosis, formerly known as nonspecific vaginitis. The organisms are all microscopic. Trichomoniasis is caused by the protozoan *Trichomonas vaginalis*, moniliasis is caused by the yeast-like fungus *Candida albicans*, and bacterial vaginosis may be caused by one of several bacteria, the most common being a bacterium named *Gardnerella vaginalis*, formerly known as *Hemophilus vaginalis*.

How is trichomoniasis transmitted, and what are its symptoms?

Trichomoniasis, although harmless, is truly a sexually transmitted condition which spreads through no other form of lovemaking but intercourse. Also called "trich," it is one of the most common causes of vaginitis, accounting for one-fourth of all cases. An estimated 2.5 to 3 million American women contract trichomoniasis each year.

The incubation period is usually one to three weeks. Symptoms in a woman consist of a malodorous, bubbly, frothy, white, yellow, or green discharge, usually accompanied by irritation, itching, and occasional urinary frequency. The vagina and cervix are often red and inflamed. Men with trichomoniasis are practically always asymptomatic, which contributes greatly to its widespread transmission.

Although the old claim "I caught it on the toilet seat" does not hold true for most sexually transmitted conditions, it may on rare occasions happen with *Trichomonas vaginalis*. The organism is capable of surviving several hours at room temperature, particularly on moist surfaces, and the vulva and vagina can be contaminated with splashing toilet bowl water, teeming with *Trichomonas vaginalis*, at the time of defecation. The suggestion that women flush a public toilet and wipe the seat carefully before use is an excellent one. *Trichomonas vaginalis* has been found to survive on wet towels and bathing suits for as long as 24 hours after they are used by an infected woman. If you know you are infected with trichomoniasis, avoid sharing towels, washcloths, or bathing suits with anyone else.

How is trichomoniasis treated?

Metronidazole, more commonly known by its trade name Flagyl, is the only drug that is effective against *Trichomonas vaginalis*. All sexual partners must be treated simultaneously to prevent reinfection. Ninety-five percent of couples are cured following treatment with either a 250-milligram metronidazole dose three times daily or a 500-milligram dose twice daily for seven days. A cure rate of more than 80 percent can be achieved with a single 2-gram metronidazole dose. Persistent or recurrent trichomoniasis may be due to strains of *Trichomonas vaginalis* which are resistant to metronidazole or to reintroduction of the organism from an untreated or new sexual partner carrying the infection. Epidemiologists have noted a significant increase in the number of metronidazole-resistant organisms in recent years. Individuals not susceptible to treatment can usually be cured by increasing the dose to 2 to 4 grams daily for 5 to 14 days. Metronidazole is not an innocuous drug and should not be casually or routinely prescribed whenever a person becomes reinfected with trichomoniasis. It is capable of decreasing the number of white blood cells which are necessary for fighting infections. Several animal research studies suggest that metronidazole may be carcinogenic, and it should not be taken by those on anticoagulant (blood-thinning) drugs since it can accentuate the effects of these medications and cause bleeding problems. The vast majority of patients tolerate treatment with few if any adverse reactions. If you do not want to take metronidazole, daily douches with an acidic solution, such as two tablespoons of white vinegar in a quart of warm water, are often helpful in temporarily relieving symptoms, since the protozoan survives best when vaginal secretions are less acidic than normal.

Patients may develop moniliasis (see page 191) following successful treatment of their trichomoniasis. This happens because the normal balance between organisms in the vagina may be disrupted when the "trich" is killed. If the foul-smelling, bubbly discharge of trichomoniasis is replaced by a whitish, sticky, and very itchy discharge which is not malodorous, the diagnosis of moniliasis is a certainty.

What are the effects of trichomoniasis on pregnancy, and how is the condition treated at this time?

Trichomoniasis has been reported to occur in 3 to 9 percent of pregnant women, but it is harmless to the developing fetus and does not appear to be associated with an increase in premature rupture of membranes, premature labor, amnionitis, or low Apgar scores. The respiratory tracts of 5 percent of infants become infected with *Trichomonas vaginalis* during the passage through the birth canal. Fortunately, this poses no threat to the health of a newborn. While metronidazole has been taken by hundreds of women during the first three months of pregnancy without evidence of subsequent fetal abnormalities, it passes from the maternal to the fetal circulation in high concentrations and is approved for use only during the second and third trimesters. However, many obstetricians still refrain from prescribing it at any time during pregnancy, since it is not absolutely essential to a woman's health. If you are treated with metronidazole during the second and third trimesters, it is best to use the seven-day regimen rather than the one-day method, since the latter results in higher blood levels reaching the fetal circulation.

Douching is dangerous during pregnancy and should not be used to treat the pregnant woman with trichomoniasis. Creams and vaginal suppositories, such as Vagisec, Sultrin, and AVC, are safe to use but rarely cure the condition or relieve symptoms. Clotrimazole (trade names Gyne-Lotrimin and Mycelex G) is a medication that is useful in the treatment of moniliasis during pregnancy (see page 192). Some preliminary studies have suggested that seven days of therapy with clotrimazole cream or vaginal tablets will cure trichomoniasis 50 percent of the time. MetroGel-Vaginal is the trade name of a new and popular metronidazole vaginal gel. Though its manufacturer recommends its use solely for the treatment of bacterial vaginosis, it is also effective against trichomoniasis and can be safely used after the first trimester. Until recently, Betadine gel was frequently used to treat vaginitis during pregnancy. However, it has been demonstrated that the iodine in this product rapidly passes through the engorged vaginal walls of the pregnant woman and enters her bloodstream. The high maternal iodine blood levels can then suppress fetal thyroid function and cause iodine-induced goiter and hypothyroidism in the fetus. For this reason, any vaginal disinfectant which contains iodine should not be used to treat vaginitis during pregnancy.

How can a nursing mother treat trichomoniasis?

The nursing woman with trichomoniasis can combine vaginal gels with douching. However, she should avoid metronidazole, since it is secreted in the breast milk in high concentrations, and no one has adequately studied the possible deleterious effects of this medication on the nursing infant. If a pregnant woman is known to have trichomoniasis, metronidazole therapy can be delayed until the baby is delivered. If a 2-gram dose of metronidazole is given immediately following birth, practically all of the drug will have disappeared from the breast milk by the time nursing is initiated 12 to 24 hours later. In a 1989 study, nursing women took a single 2-gram dose of metronidazole. Breast milk concentrations of the drug were then measured and found to be highest 2 to 4 hours later, followed by a decline over the next 12 to 24 hours. The authors of this report concluded that a nursing woman could take metronidazole in a single dose if she temporarily stopped nursing for 12 to 24 hours after the drug was taken.

What is moniliasis?

Moniliasis, or "yeast" vaginitis, is an extremely common infection most often caused by a microscopic fungus named *Candida albicans.* This organism, normally found in the vagina of approximately 30 percent of healthy women, causes symptoms of vaginitis only when it overgrows the other microorganisms. *Candida albicans* and other candida species are normal inhabitants of the intestinal tract of both men and women, and many researchers believe that this site serves as a reservoir for reinfection among susceptible individuals. Monilial vaginitis is characterized by a thick, white, creamy discharge, often resembling dried cottage cheese curd, and intense vulva itching, swelling, and redness. Intercourse may be painful because of the accompanying vaginal dryness. Unlike trichomoniasis, the discharge of moniliasis is odorless. A man may harbor candida organisms on the skin of his penis and scrotum as well as in his ejaculate, but symptoms are usually absent.

How can the diagnosis of moniliasis be confirmed?

The diagnosis of moniliasis can easily be accomplished by viewing a sample of a vaginal discharge of the organism under a microscope. Cultures specific for the organism are also diagnostic. A Gram stain and routine Pap smear, although less accurate, are occasionally helpful in confirming the diagnosis.

Is yeast vaginitis frequently transmitted sexually?

Probably not. There seems to be conflicting information on the importance of sexual transmission, but most physicians believe that an individual's susceptibility to the infection is a far more significant factor than one's sexual habits. Some investigators, notably Dr. Benson J. Horowitz and his aassociates at the University of Connecticut School of Medicine, believe that male sexual partners contribute significantly to their mate's repeated vaginal infections. Support for this theory is based on the observation that 25 percent of male sexual partners of symptomatic women are found to have positive genital cultures for the same candida species. However, the role of sexual transmission as a major cause of recurrent yeast vaginitis remains uncertain. To date, there is no proof that treatment of all culture-positive sites of both sexual partners will significantly reduce a woman's susceptibility to recurrent yeast infections.

What are the effects of moniliasis on the fetus and newborn?

Candida albicans in the mother will not affect the developing fetus. However, the baby may contract the infection in its passage through the birth canal during labor. White patches of the organism present in the newborn's mouth are called thrush. The average interval for thrush to develop following birth is approximately eight days. A dermatitis, or inflammation of the skin, of the buttocks may also occur. Both conditions are harmless and easily treated. The rare reported cases of severe overwhelming *Candida albicans* infection and pneumonia in newborn infants occur only in those babies who are already compromised by serious illness or another type of infection.

Is moniliasis common in pregnancy, and what are some of the successful home remedies which a woman can try?

Moniliasis is one of the most common problems seen in pregnancy and is certainly the most common type of vaginitis. In fact, a woman is ten times more likely to experience a symptomatic yeast infection when she is pregnant than when she is not.

The main problem encountered by the woman with genital moniliasis is intense vulvar itching. To relieve this symptom, especially if your pharmacy is closed for the day or you can't immediately reach your doctor, local applications of cool tap water, ice packs, or witch hazel compresses are all helpful. If itching is still not relieved, try a colloid bath: two cups of cornstarch plus one-half cup of baking soda in a tub half-filled with warm water. Equally good is Aveeno colloidal oatmeal added to a half-filled tub of water. This preparation can be purchased without prescription at any pharmacy; it is an excellent idea to keep it in the house for emergencies.

One of the oldest, simplest, and least expensive methods of treating moniliasis is with boric acid capsules and ointment. Capsules containing 600 milligrams of boric acid are placed high in the vagina two times daily for two weeks, and 5 percent boric acid ointment is applied to the irritated areas on the vulva three times daily.

The merits and best methods of using yogurt to prevent and treat yeast vaginitis have been debated in recent years. Yogurt contains *Lactobacilus acidophilus*, the same bacterial organism found in the healthy vagina. Theoretically, a woman who puts yogurt in her vagina will restore the normal bacterial flora and inhibit the overgrowth of *Candida albicans*. Eating yogurt will help to introduce the same bacteria into the intestinal tract, often the source or reservoir of recurrent vaginal yeast infections. Just as candida migrate from the intestinal tract to the vagina, so do the *Lactobacilus acidophilus* bacteria. Unfortunately, the therapeutic usefulness of yogurt is more theoretical than real. One problem is that most commercial yogurts contain few if any *Lactobacilus acidophilus* colonies. As a result, restoration of the bacterial balance and relief of symptoms may take quite a while.

What are some of the more traditional medical methods of treating yeast vaginitis during pregnancy?

There are many excellent medications that can be safely used to treat candidiasis during pregnancy. The newest and most effective of these agents is terconazole. Sold under the trade name Terazol, an applicator of 0.4 percent vaginal cream is inserted daily for a period of one week. A three-day regimen with daily insertion of an 80-milligram suppository is also available. Many women prefer the cream to the suppository because it can be applied to the vulva and perineal skin to soothe irritation and eradicate candida in these locations. Symptomatic relief is rapid, often occurring within 24 to 48 hours. When compared to other antifungal agents, terconazole has been found to have the lowest relapse rate. Though laboratory and clinical testing confirm that terconazole is not associated with harmful fetal effects, the manufacturer still suggests it is best not to use it in the first trimester unless absolutely necessary. It is not known if terconazole is excreted in human milk, and information about its safety in breast-feeding women is too scant to make a sound recommendation. Although miconazole nitrate (trade name Monistat) is somewhat less effective than terconazole, it remains a more popular antifungal medication because it can be purchased without a prescription. Monistat is available as a 2 percent cream and a 200-milligram suppository, prescribed in the same fashion as Terazol. In addition, a 100-milligram vaginal suppository is available for daily use over a period of seven days. In terms of medication strength, a three-day regimen of terconazole is equal to a seven-day course of miconazole nitrate. Pregnancy and breast-feeding precautions are identical for both products. Because recurrences of yeast infections are so common during pregnancy, some obstetricians recommend use of either Monistat or Terazol cream or suppository weekly for the duration of pregnancy.

Another successful agent against *Candida albicans* is clotrimazole, sold without prescription under the trade names Gyne-Lotrimin and Mycelex G. One 100-milligram tablet is inserted daily for seven days. A shorter and equally effective option is to insert two of these tablets daily for three consecutive days. A single-day regimen using one 500-milligram vaginal tablet is faster but not as efficient as the longer course of therapy. Clotrimazole is also available as a 1 percent vaginal cream which may be inserted or applied to the irritated areas of the vulva. In clinical trials, clotrimazole finished third in efficacy to terconazole and miconazole nitrate. One advantage of clotrimazole over other antifungal agents is that it can cure one-half of all cases of trichomoniasis if it, too, is present. Butoconazole nitrate (trade name Femstat) is another vaginal cream which is highly effective against candida. The manufacturers of Gyne-Lotrimin, Mycelex G, and Femstat all recommend that these products not be used during the first trimester.

Then there is nystatin, an antifungal antibiotic sold as a vaginal tablet under the trade names Nystatin, Mycostatin, Nilstat, and O-V Statin. Cure rates, though excellent, are not equal to those of the previously mentioned products. However, nys-

tatin has the advantage of having been used safely for many years without maternal or fetal complications and is considerably less expensive than other products. A tablet is inserted high in the vagina, twice a day, for two weeks. More resistant cases will benefit if treatment is prolonged for one month. Mycostatin ointment and cream are also available for treatment of irritated areas on the outside skin surface of the vulva. If the infection is extensive, or if there is reason to believe that the anus and rectum are a source of reinfection, oral nystatin tablets in a dose of 500,000 International Units per tablet should be taken three times daily for one week. Oral nystatin will eradicate *Candida albicans* from the mouth and intestinal tract; however, since it is not absorbed into the body, it will be of no benefit in treating the vaginal infection. A liquid suspension of nystatin, when administered to each side of the newborn's mouth, four times daily, will cure thrush. While painting of the vulva and vagina with gentian violet preparations is an effective treatment and was quite popular in the past, most doctors now favor newer medications which are less messy to use and not as irritating to the body tissues.

Is the drug ketoconazole effective in treating recurrent and difficult-to-treat candida infections?

Ketoconazole, more commonly known by its trade name Nizoral, is an oral antifungal medication which is extremely effective in treating recurrent yeast infections and those located in difficult-to-treat body sites such as the intestinal tract and the male ejaculate. Ketoconazole treatment has been used for both continuous and intermittent periods of time ranging from as few as two weeks to as long as one year. Unfortunately, the drug is associated with unpleasant side effects such as nausea, headache, itching, and allergic reactions in at least 10 percent of users. Elevation of liver enzymes and hepatitis are rare but serious ketoconazole complications. A man using ketoconazole will experience a decrease in sperm motility within four hours after the drug is taken.

Pregnant women or women planning to conceive should not take ketoconazole. High doses have been associated with embryo toxicity and birth defects. In addition, it can decrease circulating levels of the male hormone testosterone, which is needed for the formation of normal external genitals of the male fetus. Consequently, ketoconazole use during pregnancy may cause feminization of a male fetus.

What is bacterial vaginosis, and how does it affect the outcome of pregnancy?

Bacterial vaginosis, formerly named nonspecific vaginitis, is a type of vaginal inflammation which accounts for 40 to 50 percent of all vaginal discharges and is frequently, but not always, sexually transmitted. It is caused by the bacterium *Gardnerella vaginalis*. The most common symptom of bacterial vaginosis is vaginal malodor, most evident after sexual intercourse, and a yellow-to-gray-green discharge which may be either thick or watery in consistency. Often the discharge is described as having the appearance of a thin paste. Itching or burning of the vagina and pain on urination are reported less frequently. The diagnosis is best made by viewing the characteristic appearance of the bacteria adhering to the superficial vaginal cells under a microscope or by taking a culture from a sample of the vaginal discharge. A characteristic fishy or ammonia odor is elicited by adding a drop of 10 percent potassium hydroxide to the discharge. This test is appropriately named the "whiff" test. Determining the vaginal acidity, or pH, is also helpful, since it will usually be above 4.5 when bacterial vaginosis is present.

Gardnerella vaginalis is a somewhat confusing and mysterious bacterium which has prompted some researchers to express skepticism about its role as a disease-producing organism. One reason for this skepticism is that as many as 40 percent of healthy asymptomatic women harbor *Gardnerella*

vaginalis in their vagina as part of the natural flora. The reason why some women experience symptoms and others do not remains an enigma. In a 1988 report, doctors from the Ohio State University College of Medicine isolated *Gardnerella vaginalis* from the vaginas of 9 of 52 virginal adolescent girls, thereby dispelling the myth that the organism is exclusively transmitted in a sexual manner.

The most successful treatment of bacterial vaginosis is metronidazole (trade name Flagyl), the same medication used to treat trichomoniasis. Treatment, however, involves a much higher dose of 500-milligrams two times daily for seven days. The recent introduction of metronidazole vaginal gel (trade name MetroGel-Vaginal), inserted two times daily for five days, has also proven to be effective therapy. Less favorable results have been obtained with ampicillin, amoxicillin, tetracycline, and cephalosporin antibiotics. Many doctors have combined oral antibiotics with sulfonamide vaginal creams and tablets such as AVC and Sultrin. Recently, use of the antibiotic clindamycin (trade name Cleocin) in the form of a 300-milligram oral dose three times daily for five to seven days, combined with a 2 percent clindamycin vaginal cream, has produced cure rates equal to those of metronidazole. Resistant and recurrent cases have also responded favorably to Augmentin, a combination of amoxicillin and clavulanate potassium. Douching with hydrogen peroxide every other day does not rid a woman of the infection, but it does temporarily abolish symptoms.

Fortunately, bacterial vaginosis is harmless to both the developing fetus and the baby at the moment of birth. If a woman has bacterial vaginosis during her pregnancy, treatment with amoxicillin, ampicillin, or a cephalosporin is recommended; use of oral metronidazole and tetracycline is ill advised, though use of MetroGel after the first trimester is probably a safe alternative.. Not enough is known about the safety of clindamycin to endorse its use in pregnancy, but it is probably safe. Hydrogen peroxide douches, in fact douches of any kind, should not be taken during pregnancy.

CYSTITIS

What is "honeymoon" cystitis, and how is it treated?

"Honeymoon," or postcoital, cystitis is defined as an inflammation of the urinary bladder which occurs approximately 36 hours following intercourse. Although not truly a sexually transmitted disease, cystitis occurs when bacteria from the urethra, vagina, and external rectal area enter the urethra and are "massaged" into the urinary bladder as a result of penile thrusting and oral and manual stimulation to the vagina and clitoris during lovemaking. Once bacteria enter the urinary bladder, they reproduce rapidly, producing symptoms which include frequency of urination, burning with urination, and an urgency to urinate despite the fact that only minimal amounts of urine are passed with each attempt. Hematuria, or the presence of blood in the urine, is commonly observed, and when blood is not present the urine will often have a cloudy appearance. Lower abdominal pain and pain during intercourse are other common symptoms of cystitis.

Cystitis is diagnosed by microscopic examination of the urine and collection of urine for culture, which not only identifies the bacterial organism present but tells the doctor which antibiotic is most likely to eradicate the infection.

The most commonly used antibiotic for the treatment of cystitis is a sulfonamide named sulfisoxazole, more commonly known by its trade name Gantrisin. The combination of the sulfonamide sulfamethoxazole and the antibiotic trimethoprim (trade names Septra and Bactrim) is also very popular. If a woman is sensitive to sulfa, alternative treatment with antibiotics such as ampicillin, amoxicillin, tetracycline, cephalosporins, and nitrofurantoin may be effectively used. To relieve symptoms immediately, a urinary anesthetic is recommended. It is imperative that repeat urine cultures be taken after the full course of antibiotics is administered.

What is the significance of postcoital cystitis during pregnancy?

Pregnancy alters a woman's immune responses in such a way as to make her more likely to develop a urinary tract infection. The hormonal changes of pregnancy cause the smooth muscles of the urinary bladder and ureter to relax, which is bound to result in a greater frequency of bacterial contamination and infection. Compression of urinary structures, such as the bladder and ureters, by the enlarging uterus also predisposes to poor urine flow and infection.

While postcoital cystitis is diagnosed identically in the pregnant and nonpregnant woman, treatment options are more limited during pregnancy, since some antibiotics and urinary anesthetics are not recommended at this time. Sulfonamides, for example, should not be prescribed during the last four weeks because they can cause jaundice in the newborn.

Many women with a significant number of bacteria in their urine are totally without symptoms of cystitis. The diagnosis is made only when a routine urinalysis is performed early in pregnancy or when a dipstick test for bacteria is performed during a prenatal visit. This condition, called asymptomatic bacteriuria, occurs in 3 to 7 percent of all pregnant women. If untreated, bacteria may ascend the ureters and infect the kidneys later in pregnancy or following delivery. It has been estimated that as many as one-third of pregnant women with asymptomatic bacteriuria who are untreated will develop a severe kidney infection, or pyelonephritis, later in pregnancy. Conversely, acute pyelonephritis will develop in less than 5 percent of women with asymptomatic bacteriuria who have been appropriately treated with antibiotics. Pyelonephritis is characterized by high fever, pain in the side of the back in the area over the kidney, nausea, vomiting, and shaking chills. More importantly, it may precipitate premature labor and lead to silent, progressive kidney damage over a period of several years. For these reasons, asymptomatic bacteriuria should be vigorously treated during pregnancy with the goal of eliminating all bacteria from the urinary tract. This is best achieved by hospitalization and high doses of intravenous antibiotics. If bacteriuria recurs, vigorous antibiotic treatment for several weeks and sometimes throughout the remainder of the pregnancy may be necessary. The urine should be constantly recultured for evidence of bacterial organisms.

While asymptomatic bacteriuria in the absence of pyelonephritis is considered to be an innocuous condition, several carefully controlled studies have concluded that women with this condition may be at greater risk for prematurity and stillbirth. One report showed that 10 percent of patients with untreated or inadequately treated bacteriuria developed toxemia. Among a group of women in which cystitis was treated successfully, the incidence of toxemia was only 4 percent.

 # HOW TO GET COUNSELING AND TREATMENT

If I suspect that I have been exposed to a sexually transmitted disease, what should I do?

Most sexually transmitted diseases pose a serious risk to you and your unborn children if they remain untreated for a long time. Therefore, it is imperative to seek immediate medical attention. Most reasonable physicians will treat you with confidentiality even if you are under 18 years of age. If you fear that your family doctor will not do this, seek out another physician. Your county medical society can provide you with a list of competent doctors in your area. There are Planned Parenthood centers in just about every city in the United States where you can be examined for a nominal fee. If you look in the white pages of your telephone directory under your city and county government, there will usually be a listing under the heading of "health departments" or "venereal disease clinics." The American Social Health Association finances a toll-free number called the National STD Hotline: 1-800-227-8922. In addition to answering calls about sexually transmitted diseases, reassuring worried callers, and identifying conveniently located sites where diagnostic tests and treatment may be obtained, the trained volunteers of the STD Hotline are collecting valuable data that document the nature and extent of the sexually transmitted disease problem in this country. Be assured that confidentiality is strictly observed.

7

TRAVEL

*P*regnancy should not stop an otherwise healthy woman from traveling. Unfortunately, many still believe that pregnant women who travel extensively are more prone to premature birth and miscarriage, despite the fact that this has been disproven by as many as five separate studies. In one recent survey of obstetricians in private practice, 80 percent recommended that travel be totally unrestricted during pregnancy or that it be prohibited only during the last month. Women today are traveling more frequently and going greater distances than ever before, both for business and for pleasure. While it is encouraging to note that so many women are not treating their pregnancies as a pathological condition, the pregnant traveler has unique problems to consider. This chapter addresses these concerns and offers some practical tips for traveling during pregnancy.

 ## *TRAVELING IN AUTOMOBILES*

Can I continue to drive a car or travel in one when pregnant?

Barring accidents, automobile travel will not harm your pregnancy. In one study of almost 2,000 pregnant drivers, spontaneous abortion and premature labor actually occurred less often than is usually found in the general population. While many women find that their coordination and muscular control are decreased during pregnancy, statistics show that the risk of an automobile accident is the same, whether you are pregnant or not.

What are the most common automobile injuries, and how do they affect pregnancy?

Although the uterus seems extremely vulnerable during pregnancy, the greatest numbers of deaths resulting from automobile accidents are from blows to the head or injuries to the chest, spleen, liver, kidneys, and intestines. Among survivors, the most severe injuries are multiple fractures, including fractures of the pelvis, followed by single extremity fractures. The enlarged amniotic-fluid-filled uterus actually provides good protection for the baby within, as well as the organs that lie behind it, by absorbing blows to the abdominal wall.

However, when the uterus is damaged, the results may be devastating for both the pregnant woman and her baby. Until the end of the twelfth week, the uterus is well protected by the pubic symphysis bone, and rupture or injury as a result of an automobile accident during this time has never been reported. Spontaneous abortion caused by an automobile accident during the first trimester is an unlikely event. In one large study of women less than 13 weeks pregnant, the spontaneous abortion rate following a severe collision was 10 percent, an incidence actually less than that of women in the general population.

Beyond the twelfth week, premature separation of the placenta from its uterine attachment, known as abruptio placenta, is the most common injury, and the degree of maternal hemorrhage and survival of the infant is determined by how much of the placenta becomes detached. Even when less than 25 percent of the placenta is involved, a woman is still at an increased risk of premature labor; and if more than 50 percent of the placenta is separated, the fetus usually dies. In one study, abruptio placenta was found in 29 percent of women severely injured in automobile collisions and accounted for 21 percent of the fetal deaths reported.

A rupture, or breaking apart, of the muscle of the pregnant uterus is an extremely rare but hazardous situation which may result in death to both a mother and her fetus. Although studies have demonstrated that the uterus may rupture on impact, with or without a seat belt, rupture is far more likely to occur when a belt is not worn or is worn improperly. Use of a lap belt without a shoulder restraint will also increase a pregnant woman's risk of a ruptured uterus. The leading cause of fetal death in a motor vehicle accident is maternal death, while the extent and severity of fetal injuries are directly related to those incurred by its mother. Maternal shock from loss of blood is another potential mechanism of fetal death, because reduc-

tion in uterine blood flow decreases the amount of oxygen reaching the fetal circulation.

Trauma to the uterus at the time of a serious accident may be responsible for a greater number of premature births hours, days, or weeks later. However, the causal relationship between the collision and the unfortunate pregnancy outcome is often difficult to prove. In a 1990 study of 84 pregnant women whose pregnancies were complicated by major blunt abdominal trauma in the third trimester, preterm labor occurred in a surprisingly high 28 percent.

What are the risks and benefits of using a seat belt if I am pregnant?

Automobiles manufactured in the United States after 1990 are required to have both shoulder restraints and lap belts on all front and rear seats of the vehicles. In addition, air bags are being installed in new cars to comply with Federal safety guidelines. While air bags provide extra protection in some head-on collisions, they are a poor substitute for a seat belt.

If one must ride in an older car containing only lap belts, using them is still preferable to using no belt at all. The lap seat belt reduces the chances of injury to a woman's head and extremities by keeping her from striking the steering wheel and dashboard or being thrown from the vehicle. But a far greater amount of force is directed toward the pregnant uterus when the mother jackknifes over the belt during a sudden stop, so her uterus, fetus, and placenta are more likely to be injured than if she did not wear the belt. Lap belts when worn alone can also induce severe injury or death by crushing vertebrae, the spinal cord, and internal organs. Dr. Warren Crosby, a pioneer in the field of maternal auto safety, found an equal occurrence of abruptio placenta in belted and nonbelted pregnant drivers. However, it is still advisable for a pregnant woman to use a lap seat belt rather than nothing at all, since the belt will keep her from being thrown from the vehicle and protect against head injuries that are often associated with the highest death rates.

The addition of a shoulder harness to the lap belt has significantly reduced the frequency of severe maternal and fetal injuries by distributing the body force more evenly and by preventing jack-knifing of the upper body during a crash. As a result, both fetal and maternal risks of death are reduced by approximately 50 percent as are injuries to the head and chest from striking the steering wheel, dashboard, or windshield. The shoulder harness, however, when used without the seat belt is totally unsatisfactory, since a person will slip under the restraints and expose the legs and pelvis to a significant risk of fracture.

How should a pregnant woman wear her seat belt for maximum safety?

Proper placement of the lap seat belt is of the utmost importance. Too often it is deliberately worn loosely in the mistaken belief that tightening it may harm the uterus or fetus. On the contrary, the belt should be fastened snugly in order to decrease forward motion and injury to the uterus at the moment of impact. Position it at a level as far below the uterine bulge as possible and against your upper thigh. Separate it from the abdominal wall by a small pillow or cushion, which helps distribute the force of the automobile's acceleration. Keep the buckle on the lap belt to one side, rather than centrally located; this positioning will cause less trauma to the uterus at the moment of impact. Be sure to sit up straight, as slouching can cause the belt to slide up on the abdomen.

As with seat belts, shoulder restraints should be as tight as possible. They should be positioned between the breasts and should cross the shoulder without chafing the neck.

 # AIRPLANE TRAVEL

How does airplane travel affect the pregnant woman and her fetus?

Federal aviation regulations mandate that modern aircraft maintain a cabin oxygen pressure corresponding to an altitude of no greater than 8,000 feet above sea level. At actual flight cruising levels of 30,000 to 40,000 feet above sea level, even at the 50,000 to 80,000 feet where the Concorde flies, these requirements will be easily met in all but the most unusual of circumstances, such as extreme weather conditions or other aircraft in the vicinity of the flight plan. Flights at these altitudes do result in a slight decrease in the amount of oxygen carried in the circulation of a healthy mother to the bloodstream of her baby via the placenta. Most authorities agree that this oxygen reduction is insignificant. On the other hand, travel at altitudes higher than 8,000 feet in nonpressur-

ized aircraft such as private planes, cargo planes, propeller-driven airplanes, and "executive jets" may present a real hazard to the oxygen supply of the developing fetus and are best avoided.

In 1986, Doctor Renate Huch and her associates at the University Hospital in Zurich, Switzerland, first measured the physiological changes associated with air travel during pregnancy in a study of ten healthy women between 32 and 38 weeks of pregnancy. Respiratory rates were noted to increase briefly before and during takeoffs and landings, but they returned to normal throughout the rest of a flight. These changes were attributed to the greater emotional stress we all experience at these times. The reduced oxygen concentrations in the cabin at higher altitudes is reflected in lower oxygen levels in all jet passengers. Although the pregnant women in this study had reduced oxygen concentrations, they remained asymptomatic and clearly tolerated this change. Maternal carbon dioxide concentrations remained unchanged throughout the flights, uterine contractions were absent, and the fetal heart rates remained normal. Available evidence suggests that the low levels of noise and vibration found in modern commercial aircraft are harmless. Dr. Huch and her associates concluded that routine commercial jet travel posed no hazards to the healthy mother and fetus. The potential dangers of high-altitude work schedules among pregnant stewardesses needs to be addressed in future research.

Few people are aware that the humidity in jet aircraft is only about 8 percent, causing passengers to experience a small but significant body water loss. Pregnant women should compensate by drinking lots of water on long flights and avoid use of diuretics, or "water pills," which unfortunately some doctors still prescribe to healthy pregnant women.

Edema, or swelling, of the ankles may be accentuated during any trip in which the legs are below the body for prolonged periods of time. You can prevent edema by taking frequent walks or elevating your legs on an adjacent seat if one is available. If it is possible to stretch out across two seats, the best position for rest is to lie on your left side. This position takes the weight from the enlarged uterus off the vena cava, the major vein carrying blood to the heart from the pelvis and lower extremities. Carry a pair of loose-fitting shoes or slippers aboard the plane, since edema of the ankles and feet may be so pronounced at the end of the flight that your original pair of shoes may no longer fit.

Sitting for prolonged periods of time may slow the blood flow in the veins of the legs and pelvis, which in turn may cause clotting or thrombus formation in the veins (phlebs), accompanied by inflammation (itis). Thrombophlebitis involving the superficial or the deep veins of the legs is more common during pregnancy. Thrombophlebitis of the veins deep in the legs and pelvis often presents a real threat to a woman's life and can occur without any warning symptoms. When one of these deep clots becomes dislodged from the wall of the vein, it trav-

els through the circulatory system and is called an embolus. If the embolus reaches the lung, it is then called a pulmonary embolus. There, it may block the opening of a large oxygen-carrying blood vessel, causing instant death. To prevent this condition, walk about the cabin at least every 45 minutes for a period of no less than 10 minutes.

Motion sickness is common among pregnant women during air travel, and any existing morning sickness usually is aggravated. To minimize this problem, pregnant women should reserve seats in the middle of the plane near a window, recline slightly during the flight, and fly at night if possible. If you have been suffering from morning sickness, you may want to ask your obstetrician for medication in the event that it worsens during the flight (see page 224). If you experience motion sickness, lie as flat as available space allows with your eyes shut in order to reduce sensory stimulation.

Is it safe for pregnant women to be exposed to airport x-ray security machines?

The security machines currently in use in most airports throughout the world emit either low levels of nonionizing radiation or ultrasound waves, rather than the more dangerous ionizing radiation found in x-rays. Both hand-held security scanners and the walk-through machines employ nonionizing radiation techniques which, while infinitely safer than ionizing radiation, are not totally innocuous (see Chapter 10). It is my belief that a pregnant woman should not have to expose her baby even to this minimal amount of unnecessary radiation. If necessary you can request a search by a female security guard instead of passing through the machines.

Are there any radiation hazards which may be encountered inside the aircraft?

A person in an aircraft flying above the earth's atmosphere is exposed to high-energy cosmic radiation given off by the stars and sun as well as oc-casional bursts of radiation that accompany sunspots. It is only very recently that scientists have learned that these natural sources of radiation are exposing some commercial air carrier crew members, frequent travelers, and pregnant women to far greater doses of radiation than previously recognized.

The amount of radiation one receives during a flight depends on the plane's altitude and geographic location as well as the length of the flight. With the economic incentive of saving fuel, most commercial jets cruise at altitudes above 30,000 feet, while the Concorde often reaches altitudes between 50,000 and 80,000 feet. The protection afforded by the earth's atmosphere in screening out cosmic radiation is lost at these altitudes. Secondly, the earth's magnetic fields tend to concentrate radiation at both polar regions, so that flights following these routes expose passengers and crew members to higher radiation levels. More planes than ever before are now flying between North America and Asia or Europe over the North Pole, a route on which radiation levels are four times greater than flights passing over the Equator. While scientists state that these radiation doses are far too low to cause acute illness even for crews flying the most vulnerable routes, the doses accumulated by some airline crews exceed the government guidelines that call for employers to warn workers of a potential hazard. For the pregnant traveler, and especially the pregnant flight attendant, any dose of radiation is too much, and repeated trips over high radiation routes should be avoided.

According to the Environmental Protection Agency and the Nuclear Regulatory Commission, exposure to radiation should not exceed 500 millirems (mrem) annually for people in non-nuclear fields. On average, the cumulative amount one receives in a year is between 200 and 300 mrems. Government guidelines for pregnant women limit exposure to no more than 50 mrems for any month of pregnancy. Exposure to natural background radiation varies with altitude, climate, soil, and occupation, but the average American receives about 96 mrems a year from cosmic and ground radiation and about 25 mrems from water and food. In addition, exposure to non-natural background radiation occurs in the form of medical and dental x-rays, with the exposure from one chest x-ray averaging 10 mrems. Other non-natural sources include small amounts of radiation from nuclear power plants and even smaller amounts from electron microscopes, television sets, and airport security machines.

An average 5,000-mile flight above the protective layer of the earth's atmosphere exposes a passenger to about 4 mrems of cosmic radiation, although this can vary significantly depending upon the route traveled. A flight altitude of 40,000 feet passing over the North Pole will expose you to approximately 1.4 mrems/hour. A similar flight across the northern United States will incur an exposure of 0.6 mrems/hour, while one across the Equator averages approximately 0.4 mrems/hour. One variable and unpredictable source of radiation is the presence of solar storms linked to sunspots. These release streams of subatomic particles that can produce radiation doses thousands of times above normal exposure levels. For example, on September 29, 1989, one such storm briefly produced a dose of 110 mrems/hour at 65,000 feet near the poles, more than doubling the pregnant woman's monthly exposure limit.

In June 1989, the Federal Aviation Administration issued a belated warning to pregnant flight attendants that even one long, high-altitude flight over polar regions could expose a fetus to more radiation than the Federal government currently recommends. A minority of experts have gone so far as to extend this warning to all pregnant travelers, advising that they avoid flights to Europe during the eighth through the fifteenth weeks of pregnancy when the fetus is most susceptible to radiation-induced abnormalities. Such flights always pass over the North Pole, where exposure is greatest.

If a pregnant traveler has a specific disease, how may it be affected by a long-distance flight?

Few patients and physicians are aware of the fact that the dosage of certain medications should be altered on trips in which several time zones are crossed. For example, the insulin needed by a diabetic woman will vary according to the direction in which she is traveling. Eastward travel of five to seven time zones may require a 15 percent decrease to account for the shorter day of travel, while westward travel often necessitates an increase in dosage. In addition to insulin, many other vital drugs such as cortisone, digitalis and other medications for heart disease, thyroid medications, anticonvulsives, and medications used for gastrointestinal ulcer therapy all follow similar principles. It is important for pregnant women who use any of these medications to consult with a knowledgeable physician before departure so that appropriate changes in doses and scheduling may be planned.

Are there any medical conditions which rule out high-altitude flying for pregnant women?

Pregnant women with a history of heart disease, respiratory problems, or blood disorders are advised to avoid flights on aircraft that may attain cruising altitudes between 30,000 and 50,000 feet, heights often reached during long-distance flights. Although Federal law mandates that modern aircraft be pressurized to correspond to a maximum of 8,000 feet above sea level, for some women this slight but significant reduction in oxygen saturation within the arteries carrying blood from the heart is often enough to precipitate a cardiac, respiratory, or hematologic crisis. Anemic women are also more likely to be adversely affected by mild reductions in oxygen within the cabin of the aircraft. If a woman who is unable to tolerate a cabin altitude of 8,000 feet must fly in the event of an emergency, supplemental oxygen can be administered by face mask throughout the flight. This equipment is maintained and certified by the airline and rents for 35 to 50 dollars per flight.

Pregnant women often suffer from intestinal gas, which may be intensified by air travel since gases expand when barometric pressure decreases, as it does in modern commercial aircraft flying at high altitudes. To alleviate the symptoms of intestinal gas somewhat, it is best to not eat too quickly or too much before or during a flight, to avoid eating legumes and other gas-forming foods for one or two days before departure, and to avoid drinking large quantities of fluid, especially carbonated drinks and beer. It is also best not to chew gum as the plane ascends because when chewing gum you may swallow a great deal of air.

Is it dangerous for some black women to fly during pregnancy?

A black woman with sickle cell trait may experience severe pain in the upper left quadrant of the abdomen or blood in the urine following a flight as short as 1 hour. Fortunately, symptoms usually subside spontaneously without permanent damage within two to three days. Since individuals with sickle cell trait may become quite ill at high altitudes, it is advisable that all blacks be tested for this condition before vacationing at altitudes above 5,000 feet. Even flying in pressurized aircraft at altitudes below 10,000 feet may occasionally precipitate problems. If susceptible women must fly, it is a good idea for them to breathe supplemental oxygen by mask when altitudes exceed 5,000 feet above sea level.

Sickle cell anemia, on the other hand, is a very serious disease among a small number of blacks. Since pregnancy usually exacerbates this disease, air travel or vacationing at high altitudes by pregnant women with sickle cell anemia is ill-advised.

What specific obstetrical complications make airplane travel hazardous to the fetus?

Although the fetus is much more able to cope with reduced oxygen than the adult, conditions such as chronic hypertension, preeclampsia and toxemia (elevated blood pressure after the twenty-eighth week of pregnancy), diabetes, multiple pregnancy, and intrauterine growth retardation (IUGR) may result in a significant reduction of the oxygen supply delivered to the fetus. When these complications exist, the added insult of even a slight reduction of oxygen caused by high-altitude flying may be all that is needed to further distress the developing fetus. There are no specific rules or guidelines to follow, but I personally believe that women with any of these complications should not fly in pressurized aircraft above 7,000 feet in the last trimester.

Women with a history of repeated miscarriages, incompetent cervix, in utero DES exposure, premature births, and multiple births are at a greater risk of an unpredictable premature labor and are best advised to stay close to home. Individuals on tocolytic drugs for the prevention of premature labor should not fly because there is always the possibility that labor will start suddenly and without warning. In addition, tocolytics increase a wom-

an's risk of hypoxia, or reduced oxygen, because of the drug's potential to interfere with the body's compensatory mechanism for maintaining uterine blood flow during times of reduced oxygen levels.

What regulations govern airline travel by pregnant women?

The International Air Transport Association allows women to fly up to the thirty-sixth week of pregnancy on domestic flights and up to the thirty-fifth week on overseas trips. A physician's permission is required for air travel after these cutoff dates. Most airline personnel couldn't tell the difference between a six- and nine-month pregnancy. In addition, many women appear much larger than their due date would indicate. It is a good idea to carry a signed letter from your obstetrician when traveling by air during the last four months of pregnancy, giving your due date, an accurate assessment of your health, and a list of all pertinent medical and obstetrical information.

 # SEA VOYAGES

Do cruise ships have regulations that govern travel by pregnant women?

Cruise lines vary in the restrictions they place on pregnant travelers. Most will carry pregnant women up to the seventh month, and then they require a letter releasing them from responsibility in the event of a problem. Check the requirements with the cruise line you plan to use.

Cruise lines usually have elaborate hospital facilities and a well-stocked pharmacy, and all are required to have a physician aboard. Some even have nurses trained in midwifery and emergency obstetrical care. It is a good idea to investigate these arrangements when making your reservations. All ships have ship-to-shore communications so that,

in the event of an emergency, a woman can contact her obstetrician or pharmacist for advice about medications.

Are there any suggestions that I should follow when traveling by sea?

The hormonal changes of pregnancy, which increase the likelihood of nausea and vomiting, also bring about a greater susceptibility to motion sickness. Try to plan sea travel for a time of year when storms and rough seas are least likely to occur. A large seaworthy ship with modern stabilizers has less side-to-side roll. Cabin selection is also important; a midship cabin offers the greatest stability and least amount of movement in rough seas, and although many individuals prefer a cabin location high above the main deck, the best cabins for avoiding motion sickness are on the lower middle deck. Dimenhydrenate (trade name Dramimine) is an over-the-counter antihistamine which can be safely used during pregnancy to provide some relief from motion sickness. Emetrol, another over-the-counter product, will help to alleviate nausea. Promethazine (trade name Phenergan) is a prescription antihistamine which has proven to be effective against motion sickness. It has been used by millions of pregnant women over the years without untoward maternal or fetal effects. For best results, all of these medications should be taken several hours before departure and the dosage repeated every 4 to 6 hours during the trip. Long-lasting relief for up to three days can be obtained with use of a transdermal scopalamine disc placed behind the ear (trade name Transderm Scop). This drug, when studied on experimental pregnant laboratory animals, produced no adverse fetal effects, but too little is known about its use during pregnancy to unequivocally guarantee its safety.

It is a good idea to wear low-heeled, slip-proof shoes when walking on deck, since the compromised balance one experiences during pregnancy combined with an unexpected roll of the ship can cause a potentially serious accident.

What restrictions do bus lines place on the pregnant traveler?

Neither Greyhound nor Trailways imposes rules or regulations on pregnant women, whether they are traveling short distances or taking cross-country tours. Although there are occasional stories of babies born aboard a bus, remember that drivers have no training in childbirth or first aid, so it is not advisable to plan an extensive trip during the ninth month of pregnancy.

 # SUNBATHING

Does sunbathing intensify the "mask of pregnancy"?

Yes. Exposure to sunlight intensifies chloasma, the name for what is commonly called "the mask of pregnancy," the presence of dark-brown pigmented areas on the face. The effect of sunlight on chloasma can be reduced to some degree by using a sunscreen. If the chloasma is well established, the pigmentation can be safely lightened with Eldoquin bleach products. Another product, RV Paque, is recommended for women who have lightened their hyperpigmentation but still need protection from the sun.

LIVING, WORKING, OR VACATIONING AT HIGH ALTITUDES

What effect does high altitude have on pregnancy?

Several studies have demonstrated that the chronic lack of oxygen (hypoxia) and the reduced maternal plasma volume at high altitudes is responsible for significantly lower infant birth weights. It is known that many placental alterations, such as a greater size and vascularity and a higher incidence of infarcts, or bloodless areas of dead tissue, are more common at higher altitudes. These placental changes occasionally play a role in producing a poor pregnancy outcome.

What is acute mountain sickness and how is it treated?

Acute mountain sickness (AMS) is a potentially serious illness which generally has its onset 6 or more hours after a susceptible person ascends to altitudes greater than 9,800 feet (3,000 meters). It is characterized by headache, loss of appetite, nausea, vomiting, insomnia, extreme lassitude, flatulence, psychological changes, incoordination, shortness of breath, and a diminished urinary output. In more serious cases, AMS may progress to a life-threatening medical emergency characterized by a rapid heart and respiratory rate as well as an accumulation of fluid in the lungs (pulmonary edema) and brain (cerebral edema). In most cases, however, AMS runs a fairly benign course, with symptoms abating in three to seven days as one becomes acclimatized. Although the exact cause of AMS remains obscure, its incidence increases at the highest altitudes and when ascent to these altitudes is rapid rather than gradual. It also appears to be more prevalent in individuals with anemia, acute and chronic illnesses, or respiratory and cardiac disease; in men, those participating in activities requiring a high level of exertion; and heavy smokers.

Abrupt exposure to altitudes higher than Mount Rainier's 14,000 feet (4,000 meters) may cause varying degrees of AMS in as many as 60 to 75 percent of exposed individuals, while the incidence decreases to approximately 30 percent at an altitude of 9,800 feet (3,000 meters). It was not until 1989 that doctors realized that AMS may even appear at moderate altitudes of 2,000 meters. In a report published in the *Journal of the American Medical Association* in 1989, doctors found that 25 percent of individuals vacationing at Steamboat Springs, Colorado (2,100 meters), experienced three or more cardinal symptoms of AMS.

To reduce the incidence and severity of AMS, experts recommend a graded, staged ascent to higher altitudes. Staging is the process of remaining at an intermediate altitude of 2,000 to 3,000 meters (6,600 to 9,800 feet) for a few days before attaining the highest planned altitude. This allows acclimatization, as does a slow and steady ascent without stopping. Approximately two to five days of staging, or a rate of ascent of less than 3,000 meters (1,000 feet) per day above 3,000 meters, helps to prevent AMS. For those venturing above 14,000 feet (4,200 meters), a rest of two days is recommended for each 1,000 feet ascended.

A high carbohydrate diet and the avoidance of alcohol prior to departure is recommended for preventing symptoms from developing. Once symptoms appear, however, immediate administration of oxygen and descent to a lower altitude is the fastest and most successful method of curing AMS. A variety of medications have been used to both prevent and treat this condition. Of these, the diuretic acetazolamide (trade name Diamox) may be used only if absolutely necessary during pregnancy and preferably never in the first trimester. Recent studies suggest that the potent synthetic steroid dexamethasone may be more effective than acetazolamide in preventing AMS, and combining dexamethasone and acetalozamide appears to be a promising treatment option. Though prednisone and other cortisone derivatives have been used extensively and safely for a variety of medical and obstetrical problems during pregnancy, they are potent drugs which must be prescribed with great caution.

In a preliminary report published in the *New England Journal of Medicine* in 1991, Swiss investigators administered the antihypertensive nifedipine (trade names Procardia and Adalat) to ten mountaineers prior to and during a climb to higher altitudes. Though all had a previous history of acute mountain sickness complicated by accumulation of fluid in their lungs, symptoms developed in only one of the ten individuals treated. In contrast, seven of eleven individuals given a placebo developed symptoms. It is believed that nifedipine may exert its effect by lowering the pressure in the pulmonary artery of a susceptible individual (see Chapter 9).

What advice can you offer to pregnant women living or vacationing at higher altitudes?

Although pregnant women already living at high altitudes have been studied extensively, little is known about the acute effects on pregnant visitors to a high-altitude location. Some experts believe that temporary exposure may be more detrimental to the fetus than long-term high-altitude residence because a fetus lacks the time to make compensatory physiologic adjustments, such as increasing red blood cell production to maintain tissue oxygen transport. The fetus of a mother vacationing in Aspen or a similar high-altitude location may suffer from hypoxia since maternal arterial oxygen saturations at 8,000 feet are only 60 percent of that at sea level. Skiing or hiking above 10,000 feet, where maternal arterial oxygen saturations are half those found at sea level, will only further compound the potential for fetal anoxia, severe hypoxia that can result in permanent damage. Based on all available data, it would appear to be best for pregnant women not to live at altitudes 7,000 feet or more above sea level. Furthermore, I try to discourage pregnant patients from skiing, hiking, or vacationing in, or traveling to, these areas.

Women who, despite the above warning, still choose to travel to mountainous areas during the last trimester should be monitored carefully. Some experts have even suggested that a nonstress test be performed on arrival and be repeated daily for two days and then twice weekly (see Chapter 11). A nonreactive test, a subjective decrease in fetal movement, or the development of acute mountain sickness should be treated with oxygen and prompt removal to a lower altitude.

 LYME DISEASE

What is Lyme disease?

Lyme disease was first identified in Lyme, Connecticut, in 1975 and since then has been reported in 43 states and all six continents. In this country it is predominantly found in the coastal Northeast, upper Midwest, and parts of California and Oregon. While Lyme disease may occur at any time between the months of March and October, it is most prevalent during July.

A pinhead-sized deer tick with the scientific name of *Ixodes dammini* is responsible for transmitting Lyme disease, but the causative organism is a spiral-shaped bacterium or spirochete named *Borrelia burgdorferi*. The adult tick feeds exclusively on deer and does not transmit Lyme disease to humans. However, a smaller immature stage of the tick, known as a nymph, has less discriminating taste and will feed on the blood of a variety of hosts, including white-tailed deer, white-footed mice, migratory birds, squirrels, raccoons, possums, house pets, and humans.

A tick does not actually bite, but buries its head into the skin of its host and siphons the blood from the capillaries beneath the skin surface. The salivary gland of an infected nymph contains many *Borrelia burgdorferi* spirochetes, which are injected into the host's bloodstream during the feeding process. Ticks do not fly or jump, but they have an uncanny ability to attach themselves to the clothing or body surface of an unsuspecting person or animal that brushes up against them. Wooded areas and high grass are especially popular habitats for *Ixodes dammini*. From such locations they can easily be carried to a manicured lawn by a squirrel, bird, field mouse, or raccoon, while a pet dog or cat can bring the tick into the household.

Fortunately, of the thousands of individuals known to have contracted the disease, the majority have not become seriously ill and have recovered rapidly following treatment. For others, however, Lyme disease has caused devastating, long-lasting, and sometimes crippling complications. Most of these unfortunate outcomes can be attributed to either a delay in making the diagnosis or in initiating appropriate antibiotic treatment.

What are the symptoms of Lyme disease?

It is unknown how long a tick must remain attached to a human host before injecting the *Borrelia burgdorferi* spirochete, but experimental studies suggest that it may be 24 hours or more. Since only one-third of infected individuals recall the usually painless tick bite, the disease may progress unnoticed and cause severe disability and bodily damage over a period of months and even years. Although symptoms are sometimes variable and unpredictable and often mimic other diseases, more often than not Lyme disease occurs in three distinct clinical stages.

The first and mildest stage is characterized by an expanding circular rash at the site of the tick bite as early as 2 days and as late as 30 days later. This distinctive red rash, known as erythema chronicum migrans (ECM), spreads out from the tick bite like a ripple wave produced by a pebble dropped in a pond. The term "bull's eye" rash is also used to describe ECM. In roughly one case in five, additional rashes appear at sites distant from the tick bite, presumably because the spirochete can spread through the bloodstream. The rash is painless, clears from the center outward, and fades completely within three to four weeks even in untreated individuals. It is estimated that 25 to 40 percent of infected individuals either never develop ECM or never notice it, often making the diagnosis of Lyme disease extremely difficult. Other

symptoms which may be present in the first stage include profound fatigue, low-grade fever, flu-like symptoms, chills, loss of appetite, sore throat, swollen lymph nodes, joint pain, and muscle aches. A small number of infected individuals note symptoms resembling meningitis or encephalitis, such as stiff neck, headache, or visual disturbances. Others experience hepatitis, an enlarged liver and spleen, or a cough.

The second stage of Lyme disease, seen in only 15 to 20 percent of those infected, may start anywhere from two weeks to three months following the primary stage. Symptoms of this stage include arthritic pain that moves from one joint to another but most often involves the knees. Debilitating neurological complications such as temporary paralysis of the facial nerve (Bell's palsy), visual disturbances, emotional instability and memory defects, and movement difficulties may also accompany the arthritic symptoms. Serious but reversible cardiac symptoms may develop in 5 percent of sufferers during the second stage.

The third and chronic stage of Lyme disease may appear months to years following the initial infection. Arthritic symptoms, especially those of the knee joints, worsen and are often mistaken for rheumatoid arthritis. Severe neurological symptoms, mimicking those of multiple sclerosis, may also occur. Inflammation of the heart can damage the nerves that control the beat, producing irregular rhythms which on rare occasions can be fatal without the aid of a pacemaker.

How can Lyme disease affect the outcome of pregnancy?

Laboratory tests show that approximately 1 percent of pregnant women have antibodies to the Lyme disease spirochete, indicative of previous exposure at some point in their lives. Approximately half of these women have no recollection of having had the disease. The recorded experience of Lyme disease during pregnancy is too limited to permit firm conclusions. Nevertheless, transplacental passage of the *Borrelia burgdorferi* spirochete has been documented, and the organism has been isolated from several fetal organs following a maternal infection. In one report of 11 women who contracted Lyme disease at the time of conception or in the first trimester, one woman aborted spontaneously and two gave birth to infants with congenital heart disease. In another report, a woman became ill with Lyme disease during the twenty-seventh week of pregnancy and, despite prompt treatment with antibiotics, gave birth to an infant with blindness and delayed development. In two other studies, a small number of women who were treated immediately failed to demonstrate adverse fetal outcomes. The Centers for Disease Control have conducted two studies on the effects of Lyme disease on pregnancy. In the first report of 19 women, five of the pregnancies had adverse outcomes including prematurity and developmental delay as well as one intrauterine fetal death in the second trimester. None of these complications, however, could be linked directly to the disease. The most recent study by the Centers for Disease Control in 1987 followed the outcome of the pregnancies of 17 women who acquired Lyme disease during pregnancy, all of whom received antibiotic treatment. Fifteen delivered normal infants with no evidence of infection. One woman spontaneously aborted at 13 weeks, after having acquired the disease after the fourth week of her pregnancy. Another woman who acquired the disease at seven weeks delivered a baby with syndactaly, or fusion and webbing of two or more digits.

Although data are limited, the conclusion of infectious disease experts is that if Lyme disease is diagnosed and treated promptly during pregnancy, it will most often result in a normal fetal and maternal outcome.

What can a person do to prevent Lyme disease?

Preventing Lyme disease by avoiding contact with a spirochete-infected tick is far easier than treating the disease after it is established. If you live in an area where the disease is endemic, it is important to remember that your risk of encountering the infection may be as close as your own lawn and not necessarily in the typically described wooded areas, brush, and high grass. The ubiquitous white-footed field mouse is capable of depositing the tick in your flower beds, wood piles, bushes, and rock walls, while your pet cat and dog can introduce the hardy tick into your home. For this reason it is best not to walk barefoot on your lawn or in your garden. In addition, when walking in likely tick habitats, such as high grass and brush, wear long pants tucked into your socks. A hat and long-sleeved shirt with tight cuffs and collar are also protective. Light-colored clothing makes the pepper-colored tick nymph easier to detect and remove. If you intend to walk or work in an area where ticks may be prevalent, it is a good idea to apply a DEET (diethyltoluamide)-containing insect repellent to your clothing, especially around the ankles, although pregnant women should not apply DEET directly to their skin since its potential for toxicity is unknown. DEET has been associated with convulsions in children who have had it applied repeatedly to their skin. Allergic reactions to DEET have also been reported in adults who used it on the skin in high and frequent doses. Unfortunately, products containing less than a 38 percent DEET concentration are unlikely to repel the deer tick. Permanone (permethrin 0.5 percent) sprayed on the skin and clothing is also effective in reducing the number of adherent ticks. This product is poorly absorbed from the skin and is therefore safer than DEET.

Upon returning home, brush off your clothing before entering the house. Once inside, remove your clothes, shower using a washcloth, and then inspect your body for ticks. This inspection must be meticulous since the nymph is as tiny as a speck of pepper and can easily be overlooked. Look especially around the groin, hairline, scalp, underarms, navel, and behind and in your ears.

Pets should be checked for ticks and combed or brushed daily, preferably over a light-colored cloth. To ward off ticks, pets should be fitted with a flea-and-tick collar. One containing Dursban, available through veterinarians, is considered safe and effective. Pyrethrin applied to a pet's fur is also effective.

Unattached ticks can be easily removed with your fingers. Those that have already buried their mouths into your flesh should be removed slowly but firmly with needle-point tweezers held as close to the skin as possible. Apply the tweezers to the head, not the body, so you don't leave feeding parts behind. Pull the tick straight out without twisting and do not squeeze it or try to kill it with heat or nail polish before removing it, since this may force infected fluid into your bloodstream. One good trick for removing a stubborn tick which refuses to loosen its grip is to smother it in a blob of petrolatum. This cuts off its oxygen supply and it will loosen its grip. The Tick Solution is a stainless steel instrument that looks like tweezers but contains a spring-loaded pinching mechanism specifically designed for clasping a tick's body and removing it from the skin. The device is designed to loose its grip if the tick remains embedded in the skin and there is a risk that the head and body may detach. The Tick Solution, which comes with a magnifying glass to help in finding ticks on the skin, is manufactured and distributed nationally by Instruments of Sweden, based in Stamford, Connecticut. It is available for $12.95 from Instruments of Sweden Department FS, P. O. Box 10810, Waterbury, Connecticut 06726. You can also order by calling 800-955-TICK.

After removing a tick, wash your hands with soap and water and cleanse the area with an antiseptic. Save the tick in a covered jar and label it with the date, time, and area of the body from which it was removed. The tick should be inspected by a physician or another knowledgeable person to be sure that it is a deer tick rather than a harmless dog tick. If it is a deer tick, you should closely observe the bite site for the next 32 days for evidence of the characteristic bulls-eye rash or symptoms resembling Lyme disease.

How can the diagnosis of Lyme disease be confirmed?

The diagnosis of Lyme disease is certain to be missed unless you and your doctor maintain a high index of suspicion. Medical decisions based on a carefully taken history, the characteristic rash, and the presence of arthritic, neurological, or cardiac symptoms are far more important than the information obtained from the currently available antibody tests for the disease. Lyme disease is renowned for mimicking other diseases such as rheumatoid arthritis, infectious mononucleosis, and multiple sclerosis, and the diagnosis is often made only by carefully testing for and excluding these other diseases. The importance of saving any tick you remove from your skin and having it identified by an expert cannot be over-emphasized.

On rare occasions the spirochete can be visualized under a special microscope and the diagnosis confirmed. Usually, however, this is not possible. Culturing the spirochete has also proven to be difficult and unreliable. All antibody tests have serious shortcomings, but the main disadvantage is that *Borellia burgdorferi* can't be detected until a person has had Lyme disease for at least four weeks. In addition, a positive blood test may simply mean that one was exposed to the disease in the past and currently has no active infection. Finally, false-positive Lyme disease test results have been found in individuals with a history of syphilis since the antibodies to the *Treponema pallidim* spirochete can cross-react with those of the *Borrelia burgdorferi* spirochete. Other conditions which may give false-positive Lyme disease antibody readings are neurologic disorders, autoimmune diseases, and a previous history of Rocky Mountain spotted fever. Results of antibody tests may vary significantly from one testing facility to another and are often inconclusive.

How is Lyme disease treated?

Since an association between the onset of Lyme disease during pregnancy and fetal malformations has been suggested, and since transplacental infection is postulated to occur very soon after the infection is contracted, it is appropriate to treat pregnant women earlier, more aggressively, and with less confirmatory testing than nonpregnant individuals. If a tick nymph is removed from the skin of a pregnant woman and is identified as being *Ixodes dammini*, there is no place for watchful waiting and no reason for an obstetrician to become overly scientific and withhold treatment until a rash or other Lyme disease symptoms appear. Instead, treatment with either amoxicillin, penicillin, or ceftriaxone should be initiated immediately. It is also not unreasonable for an obstetrician to prescribe antibiotic therapy for any pregnant woman who says she has been bitten by an unidentified tick, even if it is not documented by capture of the tick. An antibiotic regimen is also effective in treating the first stage of Lyme disease while a woman is nursing. Ironically, it is not uncommon for symptoms to temporarily worsen shortly after antibiotic treatment is started; this is believed to be due to the release of proteins from the dead spirochetes. Of all forms of oral penicillins, penicillin G is the most unsuitable for use in treating Lyme disease during pregnancy because oral doses are absorbed erratically. For pregnant women who are allergic to penicillin and its derivatives, erythromycin has proven to be an adequate though slightly less effective substitute.

If Lyme disease strikes during the first trimester, a doctor should perform periodic ultrasound examinations of the fetal heart structures since a few scattered reports have linked the disease to fetal cardiac defects. The placenta should be carefully examined in a bacteriology laboratory after delivery to determine if the *Borrellia burgdorferi* spirochete can be seen microscopically. All newborns should be checked for abnormalities and a specimen obtained from the umbilical cord and tested for IgM antibodies to *Borrellia burgdorferi*. The presence of these large IgM antibodies is usually indicative of active infection in the infant rather than transplacental transfer of antibodies from its mother.

Whether or not to treat the newborn of a woman with Lyme disease depends on the case's circumstances and the pediatrician's assessment of them. If there is any suggestion that the mother was not given adequate therapy, and especially if the infant shows any clinical signs of infection, intravenous penicillin should be administered.

Questions and concerns about Lyme disease can be answered by contacting the Lyme Borreliosis Foundation, Box 462, Tolland, Connecticut 06084; telephone (203) 871-2900. The foundation, which has chapters throughout the country, has established the Lyme Disease and Pregnancy Registry to follow the progress of women who contract the disease during pregnancy, make available information regarding the treatment protocols that have shown the most promise, and provide various testing options for both mother and child.

 FINDING A DOCTOR ABROAD

What should I do if I need medical attention in a foreign city?

A variety of private medical assistance organizations, insurance agencies, and credit card companies have entered the potentially lucrative but overcrowded business of providing health services to travelers. These services run the gamut from a simple telephone conversation to medical evacuation via an air ambulance.

Many medical assistance organizations employ multilingual individuals who are able to translate to a healthcare worker at the scene, give directions to the nearest hospital, and even arrange for a medical evacuation if required. Most companies give their clients one or more toll-free 800 numbers that can be dialed from the United States or from overseas, and the person answering the phone usually has access to other interpreters as well as medical specialists capable of evaluating the emergency and coordinating the logistics of evacuation and hospitalization.

A potential buyer of a travel insurance policy should ask specifically about reimbursement polices, the company's definition of preexisting medical conditions, specific obstetrical emergencies covered, and exclusions of the policy. For example, injuries incurred in downhill skiing or mountain climbing may not be covered in some policies. It is possible that you may not need travel insurance since most regular Blue Cross and Blue Shield plans and most private insurance coverage will reimburse you for overseas medical expenses if you have the patience to fill out the necessary forms. Medicare, however, does not cover foreign hospitalization.

IAMAT (417 Center Street, Lewiston, New York 14092; telephone (716) 754-4883) stands for International Association for Medical Assistance to Travelers. For either no fee or a minimal contribution of your choice, you will receive a directory listing IAMAT centers in 450 cities and 120 countries throughout the world. The centers furnish the names of English-speaking physicians, a world immunization and malaria risk chart, and a personal clinical record form on which your physician can note any important medical data.

NEAR Services (450 Prairie Avenue, Suite 101, Calumut City, Illinois 60409; telephone (800) 654-6700 or (708) 868-6700) is an acronym for Nationwide/Worldwide Emergency Ambulance Return. This organization provides medical services and evacuation in the United States and throughout the world. For a fee of $3.00 per person per day, NEAR will cover up to $100,000 in medical expenses, including hospitalization, doctors fees, and medical evacuation costs.

Another source of help is International SOS Assistance (1 Neshaminy Interplex, Trevose, Pennsylvania 19047; telephone (800) 523-6586 or (215) 245-4707). For either a fixed fee or one based on the number of days that you plan to travel, SOS assists in finding local English-speaking physicians and provides emergency evacuation to the closest adequate medical facility. One major limitation of SOS services for the pregnant traveler is that emergencies occurring beyond the first six months of pregnancy are not covered.

Access America (600 Third Avenue, Box 807, New York, New York 10163; telephone (800) 851-2800) is a medical insurance subsidiary of Blue Cross/Blue Shield which offers coverage for travel in North America and overseas for periods ranging from one day to several weeks. Medical transportation approved by Access America assistance experts is fully covered.

In their efforts to attract new members and expand services for present cardholders, most credit card companies offer medical assistance plans for travelers in the form of phone consultations and other medical options. One assistance company named Europ Assistance provides medical assistance services for American Express members, while Citicorp Diners Club works with a company named Inter-Claim to provide similar services. Travelers Insurance of Hartford, Hartford Insurance Company, Arm Coverage, Cigna, and several other insurance companies sell a variety of travel medical insurance policies directly to clients or through a variety of subsidiary companies with ever-changing and all-encompassing names such as HealthCare Abroad, Healthcare Global, Med Help Worldwide, and WorldCare Travel Assistance International. BankAmerica offers a medical assistance program to its traveler's check customers in which they guarantee a $1,000.00 deposit, which most foreign hospitals and some American hospitals demand. In addition, BankAmerica provides a 24-hour referral service to English-speaking doctors and translators.

Lacking these sources of information, the pregnant traveler with a medical problem can probably receive a competent referral from a local United States or British Embassy or Consulate. During non-business hours, the duty officer can provide the names of physicians in the area. The nearest medical school or university hospital will also be able to refer you to an English-speaking physician.

Travelers with medical illnesses such as severe allergies, diabetes, heart disease, epilepsy, and other potentially emergency-producing conditions, can register with the Medical Alert Foundation (P.O. Box 1009, Turlock, California 95380; telephone (209) 668-3333). Members of this worldwide organization receive either a bracelet or a necklace bearing a red Medic Alert emblem. This emblem lists the wearer's identification number and gives a brief description of his or her medical problem along with a 24-hour "hotline" number. This service accepts collect calls from physicians or public health officials from all over the world, providing them with a person's full medical history within seconds.

One of the most complete guides to preparing for a healthful trip is a paperback book, *Traveling Well: A Comprehensive Guide to Your Health Abroad*, by W. Scott Harkonen, M.D. (Dodd Mead, 1984, $11.95). *Health Information for International Travel* is a yearly publication of the United States Public Health Service. It gives health warnings and information about the prevalence of almost every disease in every country of the world. It also provides maps and tables as well as an index listed both by country and by specific disease. This book can be ordered from the Superintendent of Documents, Washington, D.C. 20402, and costs $4.75.

What medications and first-aid supplies would you recommend for the pregnant traveler?

It is an excellent idea for any traveler to carry a small medical kit for use in an emergency.

If you are taking essential medications such as insulin or cortisone, be sure to have a sufficient supply from your doctor, with full instructions for using the medication, its proper storage, and how to protect it from damage and deterioration. Ask your physician or pharmacist for the generic names of all prescription and nonprescription drugs that you may need, since brand names differ in other countries. It is a good idea to take along extra doses of all medication you use regularly, and don't forget those which you may only use sporadically but may need during an emergency. If you require syringes, be sure you have an adequate number and a letter from your doctor indicating to immigration officials that they are necessary for your medical condition. Some areas of travel require special precautions such as insect repellents, special eye ointments, electric immersion heaters for boiling water, and water purification tablets. Prepare for these situations before departure. Purification tablets containing iodides should not be used by pregnant women since they can impair fetal thyroid function. If you are planning a trip to a malaria-ridden area, you should start weekly preventive medication two weeks before you leave and take enough pills to carry you through your entire stay and for several weeks after your return (see page 223). All items should be packed carefully to avoid breakage. It is best to carry the medical kit with you rather than subject it to the beating inflicted on most luggage. If there is room in the kit, and your trip is scheduled to take you to an underdeveloped country, pack a roll or two of toilet paper and a bar of soap since these items may be in short supply in some countries.

For the items I consider most important for the pregnant traveler, see the Pregnant Traveler's Medical Kit following. All recommended medications have been shown to be safe for both mother and fetus. The safety of using a DEET-containing insect repellent during pregnancy is unproven, however. Products containing less than 38 percent DEET will not repel the deer tick responsible for causing Lyme disease. If Lyme disease is not a concern, most other insects can be repelled for up to 2 hours with Skintastic, a white lotion made with aloe and a 7 percent concentration of DEET. Permethrin-containing repellents for use as clothing sprays may be more acceptable for most pregnant women. Another alternative is Avon Skin-So-Soft Bath Oil, which is completely safe, although its effectiveness lasts only 10 to 30 minutes.

Though the transdermal scopalamine disc (trade name Transderm Scop) for treating motion sickness has not been associated with adverse fetal effects, too little is known about its use during the first trimester to unequivocally guarantee its safety. Therefore, the other medications listed should be tried first.

 Pregnant Traveler's Medical Kit

First-Aid Kit

Gauze pads, gauze roll, adhesive tape, ace bandage, scissors, tweezers, thermometer, band-aids of various sizes, small amount of sterile cotton, antiseptic cream or powder.

Medications for Specific Problems

1 *Headache*—Acetaminophen (trade names Tylenol or Datril) for mild pain, codeine or acetaminophen with codeine for more severe pain.
2 *Constipation*—Milk of magnesia.
3 *Diarrhea and abdominal cramps*—Attapulgite (trade name Kaopectate) chewable tablets or liquid, paregoric liquid, diphenoxylate hydrochloride (trade name Lomotil) liquid or tablets, loperamide hydrochloride (trade name Imodium A.D.) capsules.
4 *Indigestion and heartburn, hyperacidity*—Maalox liquid or tablets, Mylanta liquid or tablets.
5 *Nausea and vomiting*—Emetrol liquid for mild cases, proemthazine hydrochloride (trade name Phenergan) tablets or syrup for more severe cases.
6 *Motion sickness*—Dimenhydrinate (trade name Dramamine) liquid or chewable tablets, ginger capsules, scopalomine adhesive disc behind the ear (trade name Transderm Scop), diphenhydramine hydrochloride (trade name Benadryl) liquid or tablets, promethazine hydrochloride (trade name Phenergan) tablets or syrup for more severe cases.
7 *Eye irritation*—Visine.
8 *Ear inflammation or pain*—Auralgan otic solution.
9 *Painful or bleeding hemorrhoids*—Preparation H for mild cases, Anusol-HC suppositories for more severe problems.
10 *Varicose veins*—Any brand of support hose, Jobst elastic stockings, or leotards for more severe cases.
11 *Sore throat*—Chloraseptic or Cepacol lozenges (antibiotics not recommended unless first evaluated by doctor).
12 *Cough*—Robitussin or Phenergan for mild cough, add codeine for more severe cough (Phenergan with codeine or Robitussin A–C).
13 *Insect bites*—Insect repellent with concentrations of DEET greater than 38 percent, permethrin-containing repellents, Avon Skin-So-Soft bath oil, sleeping net, Calamine lotion for applications to bites.
14 *Sprains*—An instant (squeezable) ice pack and elastic bandage.

15 *Sunburn prevention*—Suntan lotion with sunscreen protection containing PABA (para-amino benzoic acid), SPF (sun protection factor) of 15 or greater. If you will be in the water, choose a waterproof sunscreen.

16 *Toothache*—Oil of cloves.

17 *Hives, allergic reactions*—Benadryl liquid or tablets, Phenergan syrup or tablets, epinephrine only if history suggests near-fatal reactions to insect bites.

18 *Cuts and scrapes*—Bacitracin ointment.

19 *Skin irritation*—A and D ointment, anesthetic aerosol such as Americaine.

20 *Superficial fungus infections of skin*—Lotrimin cream, lotion, or solution, Monistat-Derm cream or lotion.

21 *Dermatitis or skin rash from contact with plants such as poison ivy*—Ointment or cream containing hydrocortisone applied two to three times daily (concentrations of 0.5 percent hydrocortisone or less may be purchased without prescription).

22 *Dry skin*—Ointment or cream containing hydrocortisone.

23 *Vaginitis accompanied by itching*—Monistat or Terazol cream.

24 *Cold, nasal congestion, sneezing, upper respiratory allergies*—Actifed syrup, tablets, or capsules, Sudafed liquid or tablets, Phenergan, Afrin nasal spray.

25 *Insomnia and nervous tension*—Count sheep during the first trimester since all medications are potentially dangerous. After this time, on rare occasions a barbiturate such as Seconal may be used. Phenergan is also excellent for reducing tension and inducing light sleep.

 IMMUNIZATIONS

Can a pregnant woman be safely vaccinated?

Ideally, if you are planning to travel to a foreign country, you should receive all recommended immunizations at least three months before becoming pregnant. Certain vaccines administered after this time may present hazards to the developing fetus.

A vaccine enables an individual to form immunity against an infectious agent without experiencing significant illness. Protective antibodies in the pregnant woman, whether induced by prior routine immunization or through exposure to a disease, are transferred across the placenta to the fetus and transiently protect the newborn from a variety of infections during the first few months of life. There are five categories of vaccines: toxoids, killed or inactivated bacterial vaccines, killed or inactivated viral vaccines, live viral vaccines, and the new genetically engineered DNA vaccines made from inert yeast rather than a bacterial or viral source.

Toxoids are preparations of chemically altered toxins, or poisons, produced by certain bacteria. The combined tetanus and diphtheria vaccine is one example. There is no evidence to show that the fetus is at risk when this preparation is administered during pregnancy. Nevertheless, when a toxoid is to be given during pregnancy it is best to wait until the second or third trimester to eliminate any concern about causing fetal anomalies. Giving tetanus toxoid to women who were never vaccinated or have not had a booster dose for more than 10 years should be viewed as part of good prenatal care, especially if extended travel to a developing country is contemplated during pregnancy.

Killed or inactivated bacterial vaccines, such as cholera, plague, typhoid, meningococcus, and pneumococcus, contain heat-killed or chemically altered microorganisms. Although much remains to be learned about the effects of these vaccines on the fetus, in most cases they are probably harmless. However, in reaction to killed vaccines, a few individuals run a high fever which may jeopardize the pregnancy. For this reason, killed vaccines are best avoided by pregnant women unless there is a substantial risk of contracting one of these serious diseases in the anticipated area of travel.

Vaccines comprised of killed or inactivated viruses include influenza, rabies, and the inactivated poliomyelitis vaccine (IPV) of Salk. There is no evidence to suggest that immunization with these vaccines poses any risk to a mother or her fetus, and public health officials recommend that doctors use the same criteria for vaccinating pregnant and nonpregnant individuals. The inactivated influenza vaccine varies each year according to which two or three viral strains experts predict will be most prevalent. These vaccines are comprised of protein or antigens from viruses and have been shown to be safe for use during pregnancy. However, since one has the option of prophylactically administering the vaccine over several months prior to the winter flu season, it is probably best to give it after the first trimester in order to remove even the slightest theoretical risk to the developing fetus. The inactivated poliovirus vaccine (IPV), may be safely given as a booster during pregnancy to someone who has previously been immunized several years earlier. There are no incidences of adverse pregnancy outcome following use of this vaccine. Similarly, the use of killed rabies vaccine for postexposure prophylaxis following an animal bite has proven to be safe for mother and fetus.

Live viruses used for vaccination are either viral strains which are altered in the laboratory or those which are inherently weaker than the virulent wild virus. Live vaccines, such as those for mumps, measles (rubeola), German measles (rubella), smallpox, polio (oral vaccine, Sabin), and yellow fever, theoretically pose the greatest risk to pregnancy because the organisms which they contain may occasionally cross the placenta and infect the fetus. As a result, these vaccines should not be given during pregnancy or in the three months before a contemplated conception. However, if they are given, it is comforting to know that the risks associated with their use are more theoretical than real.

Although specific information is not available on adverse effects of yellow fever vaccine on the developing fetus, it is prudent on theoretical grounds to avoid vaccinating pregnant women and to advise that they postpone travel to areas where yellow fever occurs until after delivery. Pregnant women who must travel to areas where the risk of yellow fever is high should be vaccinated since, under these circumstances, the risk of a yellow fever infection far outweighs the small theoretical risk to the fetus from vaccination. However, if international travel regulations constitute the only reason to vaccinate a pregnant woman who will never set foot outside her air-conditioned hotel, efforts should be made to obtain a letter of waiver from a physician.

Although the live oral polio vaccine (OPV) of Sabin is theoretically riskier for the fetus than the inactivated vaccine of Salk (IPV), it has been given during pregnancy without apparent ill effects and is preferred to the inactivated vaccine for the susceptible pregnant woman needing rapid immunization prior to departing for an area which is endemic for poliomyelitis. Since polio has been found to cause maternal paralysis far more frequently when contracted during pregnancy, the remote risk of using the vaccine is far outweighed by the dangers of contracting the disease.

The original hepatitis B vaccine has been replaced by a new, genetically engineered DNA vaccine (trade names Recombivax HB and Engerix-B) derived from inert yeast. Pregnancy is not a contraindication to use of this vaccine, and viral hepatitis B may result in a severe and chronic infection for a woman and her newborn, so vaccination should be encouraged for all pregnant women at significant risk of contracting the infection.

Can gamma globulins be safely taken by a pregnant woman to prevent disease, and when should they be taken?

Gamma globulins are antibodies which may be detected in a person's bloodstream following exposure to an infectious disease. Although gamma globulin injections are not truly vaccines, they supply antibodies or immune globulins which the person lacks, providing temporary immunity. Unfortunately, they are misused by many physicians for treating colds, allergies, and many other conditions for which they are of no benefit.

There are two types of gamma globulins: standard human immune serum globulin (HISG) and special human immune serum globulin. Both may be used with complete safety during pregnancy. An intramuscular injection of HISG administered to a susceptible woman within six days of exposure to measles effectively presents or modifies the disease symptoms. This is particularly important since measles has been reported to cause spontaneous abortion in up to 50 percent of infected pregnant woman and is also associated with an increased rate of congenital malformations and premature labor. While HISG will effectively prevent or modify disease symptoms among women exposed to measles, it is far less likely to be effective in preventing rubella and mumps after exposure and is only recommended following rubella exposure for pregnant women who would not consider therapeutic abortion should they contract the disease in the first trimester.

HISG should also be given to all pregnant women exposed to hepatitis A, and pregnant travelers planning to visit parts of the world where hepatitis A is prevalent, such as Africa, Asia, Central America, rural Mexico, the Philippine Islands, the South Pacific Islands, and South America, are advised to receive HISG prior to departure. If you plan an extended stay in an area that is off the normal tourist route, the injection should be repeated every three to six months.

The second category of gamma globulins, known as special human immune serum globulins, has a variety of uses. They are given the name "special globulins" because each contains high antibody titres against one specific virus. The immune globulins in this group include hepatitis B immune globulin (HBIG), varicella-zoster immune globulin (VZIG), rabies immune globulin (RIG), and tetanus immune globulin (TIG). While the hepatitis B vaccine will provide permanent immunity against the virus, HBIG is used to give immediate temporary antibody protection to a susceptible person following exposure. A pregnant woman can be safely treated simultaneously with hepatitis B vaccine and HBIG immediately following exposure, regardless of the month of pregnancy when this occurs. Although hepatitis B is not classically considered a disease of travelers, researchers believe that in some areas of the world aberrant modes of transmission of the hepatitis B virus may take place. In the tropics, for example, HBV infection is said to increase in frequency late in, or shortly after, the rainy season, adding credibility to the suspicion that hepatitis B can be transmitted by a mosquito.

Varicella-zoster immune globulin (VZIG) can prevent or ameliorate chicken pox if given within 72 hours, and no later than 96 hours, following exposure. A person who has never had chicken pox faces a 95 percent risk of contracting the disease if not treated with VZIG. Although VZIG will ameliorate or eliminate the disease in approximately 60 to 80 percent of individuals treated, it is unknown if it will prevent fetal infection as well. Since chicken pox in a newborn may be life-threatening, VZIG should be given immediately following birth to offspring of women who contract the disease within five days before or two days after delivery. Even when VZIG is given, as many as 5 percent of newborns will still develop full-blown chicken pox five to ten days following delivery.

RIG and TIG are abbreviations for rabies immune globulin and tetanus immune globulin. Both are effective and safe preparations for use in conjunction with vaccines as well as for postexposure prophylaxis.

Information about immunization during pregnancy is summarized in Table 11.

If a pregnant traveler contracts one of the common childhood illnesses, how will it affect the outcome of pregnancy?

In most countries, childhood viral diseases such as measles, mumps, rubella, and chicken pox remain uncontrolled. Therefore, the risk of a susceptible woman contracting one of these illnesses while traveling abroad is greater than that incurred within the United States. Women travelers of childbearing age should know their immune status and receive all necessary vaccinations prior to pregnancy. A woman who is immune to all childhood diseases, as evidenced by high levels of specific circulating gamma globulins, performs a great service for her baby. Transplacental passage of these maternal antibodies begins during the first trimester and increases markedly throughout the final two months. A premature infant born at 32 weeks of pregnancy has gamma globulin levels approximately half that of a full-term baby, whose levels equal or exceed those of its mother. This deficiency of gamma globulins in premature infants partially explains their greater susceptibility to infections during the first few months of life.

Measles is one of the most contagious viral diseases, characterized by a rash, fever, red eyes, and cough. When a woman who has never had measles contracts the disease during pregnancy she faces a greater likelihood of spontaneous abortion, premature labor, and a low infant birth weight. Although cases of congenital malformations following measles infection during pregnancy have been reported, no consistent pattern has been demonstrated. Pregnant women who lack proof of measles immunization are best advised to defer travel abroad during the course of their pregnancies. Susceptible women should be treated with gamma globulin within six days of exposure. Measles vaccine must never be given

during pregnancy but should be administered to all susceptible women in the immediate postpartum period.

Exposure of a susceptible pregnant woman to mumps during the first trimester may be associated with a slightly higher risk of spontaneous abortion. In addition, isolated cases of fetal malformations, most notably a disease of the heart called fibroelastosis, have been reported. However, there is no conclusive evidence linking mumps with specific congenital malformations. Administering gamma globulin following exposure to mumps during pregnancy is of no therapeutic benefit.

Rubella, or German measles, is a far milder illness in adults than either measles or mumps, but the associated fetal hazards are far more devastating. If a pregnant woman contracts rubella during the first trimester, she faces a 40 percent risk of spontaneous abortion. Eighty to 90 percent of surviving fetuses will acquire the virus and almost 40 percent will suffer the effects of the congenital rubella syndrome. Rubella, along with toxoplasmosis, cytomegalovirus, and herpes, make up the so-called TORCH complex of disease organisms (see page 170). Newborn abnormalities which they produce include low birth weight, lethargy, poor feeding, blood coagulation defects, enlargement of the liver and spleen, calcifications of the liver, jaundice, anemia, pneumonia, skin rash, myocarditis (inflammation of the muscle of the heart), cataracts, chorioretinitis (inflammation of the retina and surrounding layer in the eye), and nervous system diseases such as encephalitis, microcephaly (abnormally small head), hydrocephaly (abnormally large head), mental retardation, and calcifications within the skull.

When a rubella-susceptible pregnant woman is exposed to the disease, her rubella antibody titre should be tested immediately, and the test should be repeated three weeks later. A fourfold or greater rise in titre confirms the diagnosis of maternal rubella. In questionable cases, the detection of rubella-specific immunoglobulins (IGMs), indicative of recent or current infection, will establish

TABLE 11

IMMUNIZATION DURING PREGNANCY

Immunobiologic Agent	Risk from Disease to Pregnant Female	Risk from Disease to Fetus or Neonate	Type of Immunizing Agent	Risk from Immunizing Agent to Fetus	Indications for Immunization During Pregnancy	Dose Schedule[a]	Comments
Live Virus Vaccines							
Measles	Significant morbidity, low mortality; not altered by pregnancy	Significant increase in abortion rate: may cause malformations	Live, attenuated virus vaccine	None confirmed	Contraindicated (see immune globulins)	Single dose SC, preferably as measles—mumps—rubella[a]	Vaccination of susceptible women should be part of postpartum care
Mumps	Low morbidity and mortality; not altered by pregnancy	Probable increased rate of abortion in 1st trimester.	Live attenuated virus vaccine	None confirmed	Contraindicated	Single dose SC, preferably as measles—mumps—rubella	Vaccination of susceptible women should be part of postpartum care
Poliomyelitis	No increased incidence in pregnancy, but may be more severe if it does occur	Anoxic fetal damage reported; 50% mortality in neonatal disease	Live attenuated virus (oral polio vaccine [OPV]) and enhanced-potency inactivated virus (e-IPV) vaccine[b]	None confirmed	Not routinely recommended for women in U.S., except persons at increased risk of exposure	Primary: 2 doses of e-IPV SC at 4–8-week intervals and a 3rd dose 6–12 months after the 2nd dose. Immediate protection: 1 dose OPV orally (in outbreak setting)	Vaccine indicated for susceptible pregnant women traveling in endemic areas or in other high-risk situations
Rubella	Low morbidity and mortality; not altered by pregnancy	High rate of abortion and congenital rubella syndrome	Live attenuated virus vaccine	None confirmed	Contraindicated	Single dose SC, preferably as measles—mumps—rubella	Teratogenicity of vaccine is theoretic, not confirmed to date; vaccination of susceptible women should be part of postpartum care
Yellow fever	Significant morbidity and mortality; not altered by pregnancy	Unknown	Live attenuated virus vaccine	Unknown	Contraindicated except if exposure unavoidable	Single dose SC	Postponement of travel preferable to vaccination, if possible
Inactivated Virus Vaccines							
Influenza	Possible increase in morbidity and mortality during epidemic of new antigenic strain	Possible increased abortion rate; no malformations confirmed	Inactivated virus vaccine	None confirmed	Women with serious underlying diseases; public health authorities to be consulted for current recommendation	One dose IM every year	
Rabies	Near 100% fatality; not altered by pregnancy	Determined by maternal disease	Killed virus vaccine	Unknown	Indications for prophylaxis not altered by pregnancy; each case considered individually	Public health authorities to be consulted for indications, dosage, and route of administration	
Hepatitis B	Possible increased severity during 3rd trimester	Possible increase in abortion rate and prematurity; neonatal hepatitis can occur; high risk of newborn carrier state	Recombinant vaccine	None reported	Pre- and post-exposure for women at risk of infection	Three- or four-dose series IM	Used with hepatitis B immune globulin for some exposures; exposed newborn needs vaccination as soon as possible

Inactivated Bacteria Vaccines

Cholera	Significant morbidity and mortality; more severe during 3rd trimester	Increased risk of fetal death during 3rd trimester maternal illness	Killed bacterial vaccine	None confirmed	Indications not altered by pregnancy; vaccination recommended only in unusual outbreak situations	Single dose SC or IM, depending on manufacturer's recommendations when indicated
Plague	Significant morbidity and mortality; not altered by pregnancy	Determined by maternal disease	Killed bacteria vaccine	None reported	Selected vaccination of exposed persons	Public health authorities to be consulted for indications, dosage, and route of administration
Pneumococcus	No increased risk during pregnancy; no increase in severity of disease	Unknown	Polyvalent polysaccharide vaccine	No data available on use during pregnancy	Indications not altered by pregnancy; vaccine used only for high-risk individuals	In adults 1 SC or IM dose only; consider repeat dose in 6 years for high-risk individuals
Typhoid	Significant morbidity and mortality; not altered by pregnancy	Unknown	Killed or live attenuated oral bacterial vaccine	None confirmed	Not recommended routinely except for close, continued exposure or travel to endemic areas	*Killed:* Primary: 2 injections SC at least 4 weeks apart. *Booster:* single dose SC or ID (depending on type of product used) every 3 years. *Oral:* Primary: 4 doses on alternate days. Booster: Schedule not yet determined.

Toxoids

Tetanus-Diphtheria	Severe morbidity; tetanus mortality 30%, diphtheria mortality 10%; unaltered by pregnancy	Neonatal tetanus mortality 60%	Combined tetanus-diphtheria toxoids preferred; adult tetanus-diphtheria formulation	None confirmed	Lack of primary series, or no booster within past 10 years	*Primary:* 2 doses IM at 1- to 2-month interval with a 3rd dose 6-12 months after the second. *Booster:* single dose every 10 years, after completion of the primary series	Updating of immune status should be part of antepartum care

Specific Immune Globulins

Hepatitis B	Possible increased severity during 3rd trimester	Possible increase in abortion rate and prematurity; neonatal hepatitis can occur; high risk of carriage in newborn	Hepatitis B immune globulin (HBIG)	None reported	Postexposure prophylaxis	Depends on exposure; consult Immunization Practices Advisory Committee recommendations (IM)	Usually given with HBV vaccine; exposed newborn needs immediate postexposure prophylaxis
Rabies	Near 100% fatality; not altered by pregnancy	Determined by maternal disease	Rabies immune globulin (RIG)	None reported	Postexposure prophylaxis	Half dose at injury site; half dose in deltoid	Used in conjunction with rabies killed virus vaccine
Tetanus	Severe morbidity; mortality 21%	Neonatal tetanus mortality 60%	Tetanus immune globulin	None reported	Postexposure prophylaxis	One dose IM	Used in conjunction with tetanus toxoid

TABLE 11

IMMUNIZATION DURING PREGNANCY (Continued)

Immunobiologic Agent	Risk from Disease to Pregnant Female	Risk from Disease to Fetus or Neonate	Type of Immunizing Agent	Risk from Immunizing Agent to Fetus	Indications for Immunization During Pregnancy	Dose Schedule[a]	Comments
Varicella	Possible increase in severe varicella pneumonia	Can cause congenital varicella with increased mortality in neonatal period; very rarely causes congenital defects	Varicella-zoster immune globulin (obtained from the American Red Cross)	None reported	Can be considered for healthy pregnant women exposed to varicella to protect against maternal, not congenital, infection	One dose IM within 96 hours of exposure	Indicated also for newborns of mothers who developed varicella within 4 days prior to delivery or 2 days following delivery. Approximately 90%–95% of adults are immune to varicella; not indicated for prevention of congenital varicella
Standard Immune Globulins							
Hepatitis A	Possible increased severity during 3rd trimester	Probable increase in abortion rate and prematurity; possible transmission to neonate at delivery if mother is incubating the virus or is acutely ill at that time	Standard immune globulin	None reported	Postexposure prophylaxis	0.02 ml/kg IM in 1 dose of immune globulin	Immune globulin should be given as soon as possible and within 2 weeks of exposure; infants born to mothers who are incubating the virus or are acutely ill at delivery should receive one dose of 0.5 ml as soon as possible after birth
Measles	Significant morbidity, low mortality; not altered by pregnancy	Significant increase in abortion rate; may cause malformations	Standard immune globulin	None reported	Postexposure prophylaxis	0.25 ml/kg in 1 dose of immune globulin, up to 15 ml	Unclear if it prevents abortion; must be given within 6 days of exposure

[*]ABBREVIATIONS: SC = subcutaneously; PO = orally; IM = intramuscularly; ID = intradermally.

[a] Two doses necessary for adequate vaccination of students entering institutions of higher education, newly hired medical personnel and international travelers.

[b] Inactivated polio vaccine recommended for nonimmunized adults at increased risk.

REPRODUCED FROM: American College of Obstetricians and Gynecologists, Immunization during pregnancy (ACOG Technical Bulletin #160). Washington, D.C. ACOG, October 1991. The Appendix, Immunization During Pregnancy, describes methods and techniques of clinical practice that are currently acceptable and used by recognized authorities. However, it does not represent official policy or recommendations of the American College of Obstetricians and Gynecologists. Its publication should not be construed as excluding other acceptable methods of handling similar problems. IPV recommended for unimmunized adults at increased risk.

the diagnosis of an active maternal illness. Since the risk of acquiring rubella while traveling outside the United States is greater than the risk incurred within the United States, all women travelers, especially those of childbearing age, should be immunized before leaving the United States and before contemplating pregnancy. Susceptible pregnant women should defer their travel plans until after delivery.

If a susceptible pregnant woman is exposed to someone in her household who has chicken pox, there is a 95 percent chance that she will contract the disease within 10 to 20 days. Though chicken pox is often viewed as an annoying but harmless skin rash, the risk of life-threatening complications such as encephalitis and pneumonia is 25 times greater for adults than for children. Furthermore, chicken pox pneumonia may be more severe when contracted during pregnancy.

Epidemiologists have determined that women who contract chicken pox during the first 14 weeks of pregnancy face a 5 to 10 percent risk of giving birth to a child with a characteristic varicella syndrome consisting of gastrointestinal, genitourinary, skeletal, and neurological anomalies in addition to scarring of the skin and low birth weight. Beyond the fourteenth week, the fetus will practically always escape injury to its various organ systems, though it may on rare occasions exhibit scarring of the skin at birth. There is no evidence to show that chicken pox is responsible for a higher incidence of spontaneous abortion or premature birth. A baby is in greatest jeopardy when its mother contracts chicken pox within five days before or two days after delivery. When this occurs, there is a one in three chance that the newborn will be infected. In such cases, 30 percent of infected infants die. These babies must be treated immediately with varicella-zoster immune globulin (VZIG) in order to prevent or moderate disease symptoms.

If a woman is exposed to chicken pox during pregnancy and is unsure as to whether or not she has had the disease in the past, an immediate antibody titre should be obtained. If she is suscepti-ble, as evidenced by an absence of varicella antibodies, the administration of VZIG within 96 hours of exposure can help to prevent or moderate the clinical disease in more than one-half the women treated.

How can I find out about the immunization requirements of a particular country?

This information is available from most state and local health departments, but the Centers for Disease Control, Bureau of Epidemiology, Quarantine Division, Atlanta, Georgia 30333, telephone (404) 639-3311, is the best national and international resource for information on changing epidemiologic factors and immunization practices.

Specifically, which immunizations are usually required for travel abroad?

Immunizations are rarely required by law for entrance into most countries. The areas most frequented by Americans—Europe, Canada, Mexico, and the Caribbean—do not require vaccinations.

Of all currently available immunizations, only yellow fever and cholera vaccines are required by the local health departments of various countries in order to prevent the introduction and spread of these potentially epidemic diseases. Several African countries require a certificate of yellow fever vaccination from all entering travelers, while other countries in Africa, South America, and Asia require evidence of vaccination from travelers coming from infected or endemic areas. Although other vaccines are recommended for the personal protection and well-being of the traveler, they are not required. For fear of discouraging tourism, many tropical countries where yellow fever is present do not require vaccination as a condition for entry, but you may be stopped when you leave such a country and try to enter another which is free of yellow fever. Countries currently reporting yellow fever and cholera are identified biweekly in the *Summary of Health Information for International Travel*, and information on known or probably infected areas is published annually in *Health Information for International Travel*, which also lists specific requirements for cholera and yellow fever vaccinations for each country. Most state, county, and city health departments receive both publications, which are published by the United States Public Health Service.

Yellow fever and cholera vaccinations are not recommended during pregnancy, although both are probably harmless to the fetus. Nevertheless, in most instances vaccination is unnecessary since rigid international travel regulations, rather than a real threat of a disease, constitute the only reason for vaccination. While some countries may not enforce these regulations if risks are minimal, other nations regularly and periodically enforce them. The arriving traveler who does not meet the immunization requirements of a country may, under World Health Organization authority, be subject to quarantine and even vaccination. Fortunately, you can avert these problems because most countries accept a written statement from a personal physician confirming that you are pregnant and that the vaccine in question should not be given. This letter must be dated, signed, and written on stationery bearing the physician's letterhead. It is a good idea to check at a local embassy or consulate office beforehand to see if such a letter would be accepted. Although a doctor's letter allows you to avoid vaccination, it may not be enough to prevent your isolation or quarantine at the time of an epidemic.

Any immunization against cholera and yellow fever you have received before pregnancy should be recorded on an International Certificate of Vaccination form by your doctor and validated by a city, county, or state health department. Without properly validated certificates, you may encounter serious difficulties and delays later in your travels. Vaccination certificates for cholera are valid for a period of six months before revaccination is necessary, while yellow fever immunization is valid for a period of ten years.

Do you recommend the influenza vaccine for pregnant women?

The influenza vaccine currently in use is a trivalent preparation comprised of proteins or antigens from three prevalent viruses which have been killed or inactivated. The two main influenza strains—the A virus and the B virus—change their antigenic characteristics frequently, and the formulation for each year's vaccine is determined by which viral strains the experts predict will be most prevalent. When the vaccine is correctly matched to the prevalent flu strain, it is about 80 to 90 percent effective in preventing or lessening the severity of the disease. Immunity lasts only for the duration of one flu season.

There is no evidence to suggest that influenza immunization of pregnant women presents any risk to mother or fetus, and public health officials recommend that doctors use the same criteria for vaccination of both pregnant and nonpregnant individuals. However, since the influenza vaccine may be administered at any time over a period of several weeks prior to the flu season, it is probably best to wait until after the first trimester in order to eliminate even the slightest concern about its effects on fetal development. Women who have experienced severe allergic reactions to eggs in the past should not be given the flu vaccine since it is prepared in an egg media.

While most obstetricians do not routinely recommend the vaccine to their healthy prenatal patients, this policy may soon change. Everyone agrees that it should be given to pregnant women at high risk for serious illness if they contract influenza. If you suffer from heart disease, chronic anemia, diabetes, kidney disease, and pulmonary or lung diseases, such as asthma and chronic bronchitis, you should be vaccinated. The vaccine should also be given if there are many cases in your area, or if you plan to travel to a place which is experiencing an epidemic. Recently, some experts have been recommending the influenza vaccine for all pregnant women, especially those who will be in their last three months of pregnancy during the winter. These doctors believe that pregnant women face a significantly greater risk of complications from the flu than nonpregnant individuals, and that the risks of an untoward reaction to the vaccine are outweighed by its benefits.

Tell your obstetrician not to panic if you test positive for AIDS or non-A non-B hepatitis soon after you receive your influenza vaccine. These false-positive reactions have been reported in a number of healthy individuals who, upon further and more sophisticated testing, prove to be free of these diseases. The cause of this bizarre phenomenon remains unknown at the present time.

Do today's travelers risk contracting malaria, and how does malaria affect pregnancy?

In recent years, there has been a staggering increase in the worldwide incidence of malaria. It is hard to convince people that malaria occurs not only in exotic, far-off lands but may be found in places commonly visited by tourists, such as the Dominican Republic, Mexico, Central America, and South America.

The disease is transmitted by the bite of a female Anopheles mosquito that is infected with the Plasmodium protozoan, the causative microbe. The incubation period for all strains of malaria, defined as the time from the mosquito bite to the appearance of symptoms of chills and fever, varies from eight days to as long as several months after departure from a malarious area. The symptoms recur every few days over a period of four to six weeks. After this time, the organisms reside in the liver and cause unpredictable periodic relapses, anemia, and enlargement of the liver and spleen. The deadly strain of the disease, *Plasmodium falciparum,* may attack blood vessels in the brain and other internal organs. Symptoms may include severe headache, coma, convulsions, profuse vomiting and diarrhea, severe anemia, jaundice, and circulatory failure.

The acute attack of malaria is likely to be more severe for the pregnant woman. In addition, the stress of pregnancy and labor is more likely to activate a quiet or latent case of malaria. There are several reports in the medical literature in which fatal collapse occurred immediately following delivery. The fetus may also be jeopardized by extremely high maternal fevers during the first trimester, and a higher spontaneous abortion rate has been reported. During the second and third trimesters, malaria causes placental swelling and hemorrhage, which are often responsible for a significantly greater incidence of prematurity, stillbirths, and newborn deaths. In 2 to 4 percent of infected pregnancies the organism may migrate to the fetus. Symptoms of congenital malaria appear in the newborn two to three days after birth and include fever, vomiting, convulsions, jaundice, and enlargement of the liver and spleen; death may occur from respiratory failure. Congenital malaria is most likely to be contracted by the fetus during the mother's first attack of the disease, not when it is in its chronic form.

How can malaria be prevented and treated?

Since there is no vaccine against malaria, the only sure preventive is to avoid travel to areas where the disease is prevalent. There are a host of antimalarial drugs that are recommended for travelers to such areas. These drugs suppress the multiplication of Plasmodium in a person's red blood cells but do not prevent entry of the organism into the body. With continued use of these medications, the organism is eventually eliminated from the body and symptoms of malaria are prevented. Unfortunately, most antimalarial preparations are not recommended during pregnancy because they may be responsible for causing birth defects. The one exception is chloroquine, which has been proven safe in pregnancy. If you must travel to an area of the world where the malaria risk is significant, chloroquine should be taken at weekly intervals, starting one week before arriving and continuing for at least four weeks after departure, in order to completely eliminate the organism from the bloodstream. This course of suppressant therapy is also essential for a short visit of only a few hours in an airport or harbor in a malarious region. This is especially true if the visit is likely to occur between sunset and dawn, when the mosquito is most apt to bite. Side effects of chloroquine include nausea, diarrhea, headache, and blurring of vision. Chloroquine is deposited in high concentrations in the liver and white blood cells and should be used with caution in persons having liver disease and blood disorders.

Chloroquine-resistant strains of *Plasmodium falciparum* have tripled in number since 1980 and are posing serious and ever increasing hazards to travelers throughout the world. These organisms have now been found in most of the countries where chloroquine-sensitive falciparum strains are known to exist, and epidemiologists believe it is just a matter of time before they appear in many new locations. Because there is no universally applicable regimen for preventing and treating malaria caused by these resistant strains, recommendations vary among and within countries and change frequently. Prospective travelers and doctors treating malaria can receive updated information by calling the Centers for Disease Control Malaria Hotline at (404) 332-4555.

Treating chloroquine-resistant *Plasmodium falciparum* infections during pregnancy is not without risk. Fansidar is the trade name of a drug containing the combination of pyrimethamine and the sulfonamide named sulfadoxine. Though it is capable of eliminating most chloroquine-resistant *Plasmodium falciparum* strains, a growing number are developing resistance to Fansidar. The safety of pyrimethamine during pregnancy has not been established, and sulfadoxine, should not be taken during the last month of pregnancy since it can cause jaundice in the newborn. Unfortunately, questions have been raised about the safety during pregnancy of mefloquine hydrochloride (trade name Lariam) and another promising drug named Halofantrine (trade name Halfan). Emerging resistance to mefloquine hydrochloride has been recently reported. Some experts recommend primaquine phosphate, but its effect on the fetus during the first three months has not been adequately studied; and primaquine can cause severe hemolytic anemia in certain susceptible newborns when it is given during the last trimester. The tetracycline doxycycline (trade name Vibramycin) is also effective against most strains of chloroquine-resistant *Plasmodium falciparum* but, like all tetracyclines, it should not be taken during pregnancy. Older remedies such as quinine, quinidine, and an ancient Chinese herb named artemisinin, are actually quite effective against resistant organisms, but they can cause severe maternal and fetal toxicity and are not advised for use during pregnancy. Women who are pregnant, or likely to become pregnant, should avoid travel to areas where chloroquine-resistant *Plasmodium falciparum* organisms are known to exist.

 MOTION SICKNESS

Are anti-motion sickness medications safely taken during pregnancy?

While I share the concern of pregnant women that medication be taken only when absolutely necessary, it is also true that the persistent vomiting associated with motion sickness can result in severe dehydration, acidosis, and electrolyte or chemical imbalance, consequences far more detrimental to the developing fetus than those caused by careful use of drugs to relieve the symptoms.

Dimenhydrinate (trade name Dramamine), one

of the most popular drugs prescribed for motion sickness, is an over-the-counter antihistamine. It has been studied intensively and found to be safe for use during pregnancy. Emetrol, an over-the-counter liquid solution, may be safely used during pregnancy to relieve nausea. It contains balanced amounts of the sugars fructose and dextrose, combined with orthophosphoric acid. Take this medication with you on your travels and have it available in the event of an emergency. Meclizine hydrochloride (trade name Bonine), a popular nonprescription preparation, is also frequently recommended, but it has been associated with congenital abnormalities in laboratory animals and so should not be used during pregnancy. For the same reason, I do not prescribe cyclizine lactate (trade name Marezine) during pregnancy.

Promethazine (trade name Phenergan) is an excellent prescription medication for combating motion sickness. Although its safety during pregnancy has not been firmly established, it has been used millions of times without any known deleterious effects on the fetus. Doctors often use Phenergan interchangeably with another drug, hydroxyzine hydrochloride (trade name Vistaril). This is an unfortunate error since experiments on pregnant rodents indicate that Vistaril may be associated with a significant incidence of fetal abnormalities. Chlorpromazine (trade name Thorazine) is another popular and effective drug used for relieving nausea and vomiting. However, its use by pregnant women should be discouraged; there are reported instances of jaundice and neurological abnormalities among newborn infants whose mothers have received this drug. A similar drug, triethylperazine (trade name Torecan), is also inadvisable during pregnancy. Tri-

methobenzamide hydrochloride (trade name Tigan), another member of this group of drugs, is excellent in controlling nausea and vomiting, although its safety during pregnancy has not been firmly established.

Diphenydramine hydrochloride is more commonly known by its trade name Benadryl. This antihistamine is excellent for relieving motion sickness. Reproductive studies on rats and rabbits in doses five times the human dose have found no evidence of impaired fertility or harm to the fetus. The manufacturer warns, however, that it should not be used by nursing women.

Motion sickness relief for up to three days can be obtained with the use of a transdermal scopalamine disc placed behind the ear (trade name Transderm Scop). This drug, when studied on experimental pregnant laboratory animals, produced no adverse fetal effects, but too little is known about its use during the first trimester to unequivocally guarantee its safety.

In one study, doctors found that the old-fashioned herbal remedy ginger root was twice as effective as Dramamine in preventing and treating motion sickness. Ginger root capsules may be purchased at most health-food stores, and as many as 10 to 12 capsules can be taken hourly without any ill effects. Larger doses, however, can cause stomach and intestinal irritability. Unlike Dramamine and other similar medications, the ginger root produces no sedation or other reactions on the central nervous system because it acts entirely on the gastrointestinal tract, absorbing toxins and restoring normal gastric activity. The researchers also found that ginger root was effective in relieving the diarrhea and vomiting associated with a variety of intestinal disorders.

TRAVELER'S DIARRHEA

How does traveler's diarrhea affect the pregnant woman?

Diarrhea, or "turista," complicates the travel plans of about 50 percent of all persons visiting foreign countries. It is usually caused by bacteria, viruses, or parasites which contaminate food and water supplies and is most commonly experienced by tourists from temperate, industrialized countries who visit more tropical, less developed areas. Turista is characterized by the sudden onset of watery diarrhea, abdominal cramps, weakness, nausea, loss of appetite, chills, and headache. Vomiting is infrequent, occurring in less than 10 percent of all persons afflicted. Symptoms usually begin within 14 days and last for less than 5 days. If a pregnant woman experiences symptoms for longer than 5 days, she should seek medical assistance in order to be certain that she is not the victim of a virus. Diarrheal fluid loss may be particularly hazardous for pregnant women suffering from underlying chronic intestinal diseases, diabetes, heart disease, and kidney disorders.

What preventive measures can a pregnant woman take to decrease her risk of contracting traveler's diarrhea?

Travelers to areas where turista is prevalent are advised to drink only purified or processed bottled water and to avoid ice or iced drinks. Wash and brush your teeth with purified rather than tap water. Before drinking water from the tap, be sure to boil it for 15 minutes. Never drink stored water on trains, buses, and planes. Bottled beverages such as cola and beer are always safe, as are coffee and tea, provided that you personally observe the water being boiled immediately before serving. Carbonated beverages are safe to drink because the carbonation kills off the bacteria by making the water too acidic for them to survive. In some countries, water is disinfected by the addition of iodine (Globaline) or chlorine (Halazone). Chlorine is preferred during pregnancy, since iodine may cross the placenta and adversely reduce fetal thyroid function after the first trimester.

Dairy products such as cheese, butter, ice cream, custards, and yogurt may be teeming with bacteria and must be avoided. Pasteurization kills many harmful bacteria in milk, but in many countries this precaution is not observed. If the label on the milk bottle or container does not specify that the milk is pasteurized, boil it for 10 minutes immediately before you drink it. Since milk is a necessary ingredient of your diet during pregnancy, take along a few cans of evaporated or condensed milk which can be added to bottled or boiled water. Powdered dry skim milk takes up less room in a suitcase and can be added to coffee or tea or reconstituted with bottled water.

Fresh tropical fruits and vegetables often look inviting but, with the exception of fruits that you can peel immediately before eating, avoid them. Avoid salads, mayonnaise, cold buffets, and frozen desserts. Eat only well-cooked vegetables that are served when hot. Many people have the mistaken impression that eggs in the shell and cooked vegetables that are not eaten do not need immediate refrigeration. Do not eat uncooked oysters, shrimp, mussels, and fish, and be sure that all meats are well cooked. Be wary of foods prepared well in advance of a meal, since bacteria may be incubating and multiplying in them. And remember to wash your hands thoroughly just before eating.

How can traveler's diarrhea be treated?

Doxycycline hyclate (trade name Vibramycin) is an antibiotic which has gained popularity as a preventive for traveler's diarrhea, but since it is a type of tetracycline it should not be taken during pregnancy. Other antibiotics such as ampicillin, trimethoprim combined with sulfamethoxazole (trade names Bactrim and Septra), trimethoprim alone, and a new class of antibiotics known as quinolones have also been recommended for this purpose. Most infectious disease experts, however, discourage use of antibiotics in this fashion since they may actually increase a person's susceptibility to more serious intestinal ailments by killing off protective bacteria in the intestine. In addition, by upsetting the normal bacterial flora of the intestine, antibiotic therapy may actually cause diarrhea. Finally, even the safest of antibiotics may occasionally cause potentially serious allergic reactions. Such a serious complication would be difficult to justify in view of the fact that the disorder being prevented is rarely life-threatening. A small number of authorities believe that the use of prophylactic antibiotics is warranted since it will prevent 90 percent of all cases. For the pregnant woman, the use of antibiotics poses additional concerns about fetal safety. For example, rats and rabbits given trimethoprim in doses many times those given to humans experienced a higher incidence of fetal abnormalities. While there are no large, well-controlled studies on the use of trimethoprim in pregnant women, and while limited experience has shown no adverse fetal effects, trimethoprim is known to interfere with folic acid metabolism and may eventually prove to be associated with birth defects (see page 260). Sulfonamides should not be used during the last trimester and especially during the last month because they can cause serious neonatal jaundice. Because the safety of the newer quinolone antibiotics is as yet unknown, their use cannot be endorsed.

Iodochlorhydroxyquin (trade names Diodoquin and Enterovioform) is a drug which was widely used in the past to prevent and treat traveler's diarrhea. This is an extremely dangerous medication which is no longer available in the United States. However, it is sold over the counter in many countries, such as Mexico. Chloramphenicol, another potentially lethal drug rarely used in this country,

is also sold without prescription as a preventive against traveler's diarrhea.

When turista strikes, the natural tendency is to prescribe medications which will control the symptoms. Until recently, standard treatment consisted of nonspecific antidiarrheal agents such as Lomotil (diphenoxylate hydrochloride and atropine sulfate), Kaopectate (kaolin and pectin), Imodium A.D. (loperamide), and paregoric. While these medications have the capacity to decrease cramps and diarrhea, many doctors now believe that they may produce more harm than good, since diarrhea is the body's way of ridding the intestine of harmful bacteria and toxins. Antidiarrheal agents, by slowing the movement of the intestine, actually prolong the time that these poisons remain in the body. However, another viewpoint is that these products are helpful, because by controlling diarrhea they reduce loss of fluids and electrolytes and prevent dehydration. Combining antidiarrheal agents with antibiotics in the treatment of traveler's diarrhea also has its advocates.

The most promising and least toxic method of preventing and treating traveler's diarrhea is with bismuth subsalicylate, better known by its familiar trade name Pepto-Bismol. In a 1980 study published in the *Journal of the American Medical Association*, researchers at the University of Texas confirmed their earlier observations that Pepto-Bismol in doses of 2 ounces taken every 6 hours will prevent diarrhea at least 75 percent of the time. For the person suffering with traveler's diarrhea, a dose of 1 to 2 ounces every 30 minutes for eight doses will significantly reduce the episodes of diarrhea and bring subjective relief from abdominal cramps within 24 hours. One serious concern about the use of Pepto-Bismol is that it contains a form of salicylate, the same compound found in aspirin. The recommended daily dose of Pepto-Bismol for the treatment of traveler's diarrhea is equivalent to about eight aspirin tablets. Aspirin ingestion in pregnancy, especially during the last month, may be associated with fetal complications (see Chapter 9). It has been theorized that prolonged ingestion of bismuth in Pepto-Bismol may cause neurological toxicity, but to date there are no known reports of such an occurrence. Bismuth, however, is known to cause birth defects in sheep.

Regardless of the cause of diarrhea, the most important rule in treating it is to replace the water, sodium, chloride, potassium, and bicarbonate that is lost in the stool. In mild and moderately severe cases, rehydration with broths, carbonated drinks, or preparations such as Gatorade usually suffice. Reconstituted oral hydration packets are excellent for this purpose. A solution, sold in many countries under the brand names ORS and Oralyte, is also recommended. For more severe diarrhea, fluids should contain sugar, which helps in the ab-

sorption of sodium and chloride from the intestine into the bloodstream.

Both the Centers for Disease Control and the World Health Organization have established formulas for fluid replacement in the treatment of moderately severe diarrhea. These solutions, presented in Table 12, can be made up readily with materials found in even the most remote markets or stores. If either of these treatment schedules is followed, intravenous fluid replacement will rarely be required.

The pregnant woman must be especially careful in taking antibiotics for acute traveler's diarrhea. *Escherichia coli*, the most common cause of traveler's diarrhea, rarely requires antibiotic therapy.

TABLE 12

FORMULAS FOR TREATMENT OF DIARRHEAL DISEASE

Very mild

Any convenient source of drinkable water, Gatorade if available.

Moderate

World Health Organization regimen:
    Sodium chloride (table salt), 3.5g (4 tsp.)
    Sodium bicarbonate (baking soda), 2.5g (3 tsp.)
    Potassium chloride, 1.5g
    Glucose, 20g, or sucrose, 40g

Instructions: Dissolve in 1 liter drinkable water. Drink 2 to 5 liters per day

Centers for Disease Control regimen:
Prepare one glass each of the following:

Glass No. 1	*Glass No. 2*
8 oz. apple, orange, or pineapple juice	8 oz. boiled or carbonated water
½ tsp. honey or corn syrup	½ tsp. baking soda
1 pinch table salt	

Instructions: Drink alternately from each glass and supplement with carbonated beverages or water and tea made with boiled or carbonated water as desired. Avoid solid foods and milk until recovery occurs.

Severe

Hospitalization and intravenous fluids recommended.

However, in those severe and persistent cases in which the organism invades the intestinal wall, ampicillin has been found to be safe during pregnancy provided there is no history of penicillin allergy. Ampicillin is also helpful in the treatment of *Shigella* and *Salmonella*, the two other major bacterial causes of turista. As previously mentioned, the combination of trimethoprim and sulfamethoxazole (trade names Bactrim and Septra) is excellent for treating traveler's diarrhea, but it must be used with caution and should be avoided during the last month. *Campylobacter jejuni*, another bacterial organism that causes traveler's diarrhea, appears to be growing increasingly resistant to treatment with trimethoprim and sulfamethoxazole but is easily treated with the new class of antibiotics known as the quinolones. The safety of the quinolones in pregnancy remains unknown, and they should only be used when absolutely necessary.

Giardiasis is a gastrointestinal disorder caused by a microscopic protozoan named *Giardia lamblia*. The vast majority of people with giardiasis have no symptoms or only mild diarrhea and often require no therapy. However, when it is characterized by severe nausea, vomiting, diarrhea, and weight loss, immediate treatment is mandatory. Metronidazole (trade names Flagyl and Protostat) or quinicrine (trade name Atabrine) are equally effective in the treatment of giardiasis. Of the two, quinacrine is preferred for use during pregnancy, especially during the first trimester. Furazolidone (Furoxone) is another giardiasis treatment alternative, but it should not be used toward the end of pregnancy because it may cause hemolytic anemia in certain susceptible infants. Paromycin, an antibiotic once considered a promising cure for giardiasis, has not proven to be an effective treatment alternative. Since giardiasis often causes minimal if any symptoms, treatment can usually be delayed until after delivery. In contrast, amebiasis (see next question) is a potentially more serious disease which necessitates more aggressive treatment. Despite the theoretical fetal risks, oral and even intravenous metronidazole should be used whenever necessary. Paromycin has also been found to be an effective treatment alternative for amebiasis, but emetine is too potent to be recommended for pregnant women.

How does amebiasis affect the outcome of pregnancy?

Entamoeba histalyticum is the scientific name for the protozoan responsible for causing amebiasis or amebic dysentery. It is contracted through the ingestion of fecal-contaminated food and water, as is the protozoan which causes giardiasis; but amebiasis is potentially a far more serious disease, accounting for 40,000 to 100,000 annual deaths worldwide.

When *Entamoeba histalyticum* cysts are accidentally ingested, they are able to resist destruction by acids in the stomach and pass directly to the large intestine, where they invade the surface cells or mucosa. A person may remain asymptomatic for days or months, but eventually another stage of the parasite's life cycle, known as a trophozoite, enters the blood vessels below the mucosa. From there, the organism may be carried to the liver and, on rare occasions, even to the lungs and brain where they form abscesses.

An acute attack of amebiasis can complicate the outcome of pregnancy. Severe colitis, dehydration, anemia, fever, and weight loss are often associated with a higher incidence of intrauterine growth retardation (IUGR) and premature labor. Though *Entamoeba histolyticum* does not cross the placenta or infect the fetus, a mother can transmit the disease to her newborn at the time of delivery or in the postpartum period.

Regardless of the potential fetal risk, treatment for all but the mildest cases of amebiasis should be initiated with high doses of either oral or intravenous metronidazole and paromycin. Intramuscular dehydrometine is an alternative medication for treating severe cases of amebiasis.

8

NUTRITION

*I*n a survey conducted in 1987, researchers found that as many as 40 percent of American women between the ages of 18 and 34 take some form of nonprescription vitamin or mineral supplement, most often without proper medical guidance. In addition, more than 4,000 cases of vitamin poisoning occur in the United States each year. Misinformed but well-intentioned women often ingest dangerous megadoses of vitamins, minerals, and "pseudovitamins," even after learning that they are pregnant. Unfortunately, when it comes to nutritional supplements, too much of a good thing is often as detrimental to the outcome of pregnancy as is a deficiency of these elements.

A clear understanding of nutritional requirements is essential if a woman is to maximize her chances for a healthy pregnancy and childbirth experience.

 ## *WEIGHT*

How much weight should I gain during pregnancy?

Animal experimentation and studies of human gestation clearly demonstrate that the weight of a baby at birth is directly related to two independent factors: the mother's weight before pregnancy and her weight gain during pregnancy. The growth of the fetus requires energy, and this can come about only through adequate intake of calories by the mother.

Until 1990, the standard advice offered by most nutritionists and obstetricians was that a woman's optimum weight gain during pregnancy was between 24 and 28 pounds. This approach, however, is far too simplistic and does not account for variations in a woman's prepregnancy height, nutritional status, age, ethnic background, and socioeconomic status. In response, the Institute of Medicine of the National Academy of Sciences formed several committees comprised of experts on nutrition to review the world's scientific literature on the subject and to formulate more precise recommendations for desirable weight gain and nutritional supplementation during pregnancy and lactation. The results of this monumental effort were published in a 1990 report entitled *Nutrition During Pregnancy*. The findings and suggestions which follow will undoubtedly become the standard adopted by obstetricians and their patients during the next decade.

In order to target the pregnancy weight gain that is best for you, first determine your prepregnancy weight for height, expressed as your body mass index (BMI). The BMI has been found to be a far more accurate indicator of a person's nutritional status than is weight alone. It can easily be determined by the following formula:

$$BMI = \frac{\text{Weight (in kilograms)}}{\text{Height}^2 \text{ (in meters)}}$$

As an example, if you weigh 70 kilograms (154 pounds) and are 157 centimeters tall (1.57 meters = 62 inches = 52), your prepregnancy BMI is calculated as follows:

$$BMI = \frac{70}{1.57 \times 1.57} = \frac{70}{2.46}$$

$$BMI = 28$$

This BMI would place you in an overweight category (see Table 13), and your targeted weight gain should range between 15 and 25 pounds, with a recommended average weight gain of 0.66 pounds per week during the second and third trimesters.

The Institute of Medicine nutritionists further recommend that young teenagers and black women, two groups that have low-birth-weight babies, try to gain weight at the upper end of their weight-height target range. Conversely, shorter women, especially those less than 52 inches (1.57 meters) in height, should try to stay at the lower end of their target range. The reason for this is that a very high weight gain will increase the baby's birth weight and the risk of disproportion in size between the fetus and the baby, forceps delivery, birth trauma, and cesarean section. Women carrying twins require a greater total weight gain in order to adequately nourish both infants; a weight gain between 16 and 20.5 kilograms (35 to 45 pounds) would appear to be most appropriate.

How concerned should I be if I fail to meet my targeted weight gain?

It is unrealistic for you to expect that your weight increase will follow the ideal textbook pattern. More often than not, the number of pounds gained varies significantly from one prenatal visit to the

TABLE 13

RECOMMENDED WEIGHT GAIN RANGES FOR PREGNANT WOMEN BASED ON PREPREGNANCY BODY MASS INDEX (BMI)

Weight-for-Height-Category	Recommended Total Weight Gain Kg	lbs	Amount of Weight Gain per Week during 2ND & 3RD Trimesters
1) Underweight (BMI <19.8)	12.5–18	28–40	At least 0.5 Kg or slightly more than 1 lb.
2) Normal (BMI 19.8–26)	11.5–16	25–30	0.4 Kg or 1 lb per week
3) Overweight (BMI 26–29)	7–11.5	15–25	0.3 Kg or 0.66 lb.
4) Obese (BMI >29)	6.8 (lower limit)	15	Determine on an individual basis

next, and a total weight gain greater than 40 pounds is not necessarily harmful and may even be beneficial for some underweight women. Similarly, there is no convincing evidence to show that a weight gain of less than 15 pounds by an extremely obese woman is harmful. Remember, wide variations in weight gain still manage to produce overwhelming numbers of healthy babies. However, total disregard for sensible eating habits and the abandonment of all dietary restraints should not be encouraged.

Most of the weight gain for the baby takes place during the last three months, while that for the mother is more evenly distributed throughout pregnancy. The effect of first-trimester weight loss on fetal growth and development is unclear, but some studies have suggested that it may have permanent effects on the embryo through a reduction in the number of its body cells. For this reason, persistent vomiting and weight loss should be viewed with concern and steps taken to remedy the situation (see page 50).

It is unwise for your doctor to strictly preset the maximum amount of weight that you may gain during pregnancy since you may reach your limit well before your expected due date. In such a case, intentional weight control may be harmful to the fetus. It has been estimated that a baby gains 1 ounce a day and its brain develops most rapidly during the last eight weeks of pregnancy; more calories and nutrients are required during this time than at any other, and restricting the mother's caloric intake may compromise fetal growth and brain cell development.

Of great concern is the woman who gains little weight or loses weight during the third trimester despite an adequate caloric intake. This may signify a poorly functioning placenta and a distressed infant. Equally disconcerting is the woman who has a sudden and marked weight gain over a short period of time during the last trimester. This may be an early indication of impending preeclampsia (pregnancy-induced hypertension). For this rea-son, weigh yourself at weekly intervals and report significant deviations from your normal pattern of weight gain to your doctor.

Assuming that the ideal prepregnancy caloric intake is about 2,000 calories per day for most adult women and 2,300 calories for growing teenagers, the recommended intake necessary to achieve an adequate weight gain should be increased by at least 300 calories per day to 2,300 and 2,600 calories, respectively. This adds up to a caloric cost of pregnancy equal to approximately 84,000 calories (300 × 280 days). Many authorities believe that the minimum daily caloric intake for all women during the last trimester should be at least 2,600 calories.

Often a woman's greatest concern about gaining weight during pregnancy is that she will be unable to shed her excess pounds following delivery. In actuality, however, the weight is quickly lost. Approximately 12 to 14 pounds disappear at the moment of delivery if one adds the average weight of the baby, placenta, and amniotic fluid. Over the next six weeks, reduction in the size of the uterus (involution) is accompanied by the loss of excessive body fluids and body fat. Several studies have found that breast-feeding women tend to lose their pregnancy fat at a faster rate than women who do not nurse their babies. The most pleasant surprise for many women at their six-week postpartum visit is that they have no more than 5 to 10 pounds to lose in order to achieve their normal prepregnancy weight.

What are some of the problems encountered by underweight and malnourished women during pregnancy, and how can they be remedied?

When a woman's prepregnancy weight is 5 percent or more below the ideal weight for her given height, she will be at significantly greater risk of giving birth to an infant of low birth weight, one weighing less than 5½ pounds. Infants who are growth retarded, or small for their gestational age, are at greater risk during the neonatal period and may suffer from long-term and permanent difficulties such as reduced intellectual and physical development. Such babies are also at greater risk of dying during the neonatal period.

Sadly, the consequences of being born to a mother who is underweight may never be reversed. Therefore, a woman who enters pregnancy with a BMI of less than 19.8 must gain a total of 28 to 40 pounds, at a rate of at least 1 pound per week after the first trimester. If by the twentieth week of pregnancy a gain of at least 11 pounds has not occurred, a woman must be strongly urged to eat more and even seek dietary counseling.

How much weight can an obese woman safely gain during pregnancy?

In contrast to underweight women and those of normal weight, the birth weight of babies born of overweight and obese women is not significantly influenced by maternal weight gain during pregnancy. A far more important determinant is an obese woman's prepregnancy weight.

While it would seem logical that an obese woman would naturally gain more weight during pregnancy than a woman of normal weight, several studies have shown the opposite is true. It is estimated that between 10 and 30 percent of obese pregnant women actually lose weight or gain less than 5.4 kilograms (12 pounds) during pregnancy. Despite this low weight gain, about one out of three full-term infants born of obese women weigh more than 4,000 grams (9 pounds), compared to a rate of less than 10 percent for women of lower weights. The average birth weight of full-term infants of obese women who lose weight during pregnancy is greater than that of normal-weight women who gain 9 to 13.5 kilograms. Researchers have now come to realize that lower weight gains for overweight women may be appropriate, and limited weight gains may even be beneficial in reducing the number of abnormally large babies born of obese women.

Most nutritionists believe overweight women should not lose weight during pregnancy, but few have suggested an ideal amount of weight that these individuals should gain. Strict diets which result in significant weight loss can deprive the baby of an adequate supply of protein and other essential nutrients which could impair development of its brain and body. Furthermore, when a person loses weight, fat is metabolized to toxic chemicals called ketone bodies. Accumulations of ketone bodies in the maternal blood and urine are harmful to the developing fetus.

The suggestions offered by the Institute of Medicine in its 1990 report are a welcome guideline to obstetricians treating obese women. If your prepregnancy BMI is between 26 and 29 (see Table 13), a weight gain of 15 to 25 pounds would appear appropriate. For obese women with BMIs greater than 29, the nutritionists set 15 pounds (6.8 kilograms) as the lower limit of weight gain during pregnancy, while recognizing the fact that many obese women with good pregnancy outcomes gain even less weight. The best advice one can offer an obese woman contemplating pregnancy is that she diligently strive to lower her weight to levels that are more appropriate for her height. Though there are no absolute upper limits of weight gain for obese women during pregnancy, gains in excess of 25 to 30 pounds would appear to be excessive.

What are some of the medical and obstetrical complications associated with obesity?

Overweight women have a greater likelihood of pregnancy-related diabetes, hypertension, and preeclampsia (pregnancy-induced hypertension) as well as an increased risk of difficult labor and the birth of an abnormally large infant. In 1987, when doctors at the University of Iowa examined the risk of maternal obesity in 588 pregnant women weighing at least 250 pounds, they found a higher incidence of labor induction for medical indications, a prolonged second stage of labor, birth trauma, shoulder dystocia, or inability to deliver the shoulders at delivery, and operative or anesthetic complications associated with cesarean section such as hemorrhage, postoperative infection, and deep vein thrombophlebitis.

While obese women are less likely than women of normal weight to give birth to premature and growth-retarded infants, when they do give birth to a small baby it does not fare as well. In a report published in the *British Medical Journal* in 1988, doctors found that the risk of death for premature

infants weighing 1,800 grams (4 pounds) or less during the first 18 months of life was four times higher for obese women than for women of normal body weight.

Since obese women are eight times more likely than other women to develop gestational diabetes (0.8 percent versus 6.5 percent), screening for glucose intolerance should be performed early in pregnancy and repeated at 28 weeks if the initial test is normal. Seven percent of obese women begin pregnancy with chronic hypertension, compared to 1 percent in the general population. During pregnancy the obese woman is four to eight times more likely to develop preeclampsia.

 PROTEIN INTAKE

How much protein is necessary during pregnancy, and which foods are protein-rich?

Protein forms the basic structure of every cell in the body and is vital to normal development of the fetus and placenta. An increase in the intake of protein is required during pregnancy to provide for fetal needs and to allow for the necessary maternal bodily changes such as an expansion of blood volume, growth of the breasts, and enlargement of the uterus. While the recommended daily protein intake for a nonpregnant woman is 45 grams, the minimum daily amount needed during pregnancy is 75 grams. Some women, especially those in their teens, will fare better with 100 grams of protein daily. If a woman elects to breast-feed, she will usually require 20 grams of protein above her pregnancy total of 45 grams. Since protein is abundant in most American diets, these requirements are easily attained by practically all pregnant women. Routine use of specially formulated high-protein supplements, protein powders, or formulated high-protein beverages are not only unnecessary but are potentially harmful.

Proteins are made up of small elements called essential amino acids. During pregnancy there appears to be an active transfer of amino acids across the placenta to accommodate fetal protein synthesis. Amino acids are found in greatest abundance and in the most ideal proportions in animal proteins such as meat, fish, milk, cheese, and eggs. For this reason, foods from animal sources are called complete proteins. Animal proteins also supply iron, phosphorus, zinc, iodine, vitamin E, and B vitamins, such as riboflavin, niacin, vitamin B_6, and vitamin B_{12}. About two-thirds of the protein consumed during pregnancy should be of this high biologic quality. Vegetables contain significantly less protein than meat, but they are valuable because they supply the pregnant woman with iron, thiamin, folic acid, vitamin B_6, vitamin E, phosphorus, magnesium, and zinc.

Because foods from vegetable sources lack one or more of the nine essential amino acids, they are called incomplete proteins. Vegetables with the most abundant sources of protein are lima beans, kidney beans, lentils, tofu or soy bean curd, soy beans, and other dried beans, nuts, and sunflower seeds. Vegetable protein is enhanced in nutritional value when it is served at the same meal as animal protein.

What are the effects of maternal protein deprivation on the fetus?

It has been demonstrated that a reduced protein intake during pregnancy decreases the availability of amino acids for the fetus, which may affect its mental and motor development. Animal experimentation and human experience have shown that protein restriction adversely affects fetal and placental size. Litter sizes among protein-starved animals are often significantly reduced, while protein-deficient women are more likely to give birth to shorter babies with reduced birth weights.

Doctors are usually able to clinically recognize several different types of growth-retarded babies. When the cause of the problem is a poorly func-

tioning placenta, the babies will characteristically have a reduction in size of all their organs except the brain, which will maintain a normal number of cells. If, however, the cause of fetal growth retardation is protein malnutrition, the number of brain cells will be diminished by at least 15 percent. Following childbirth, protein deprivation in the newborn will lead to a 20 percent reduction in the number of brain cells. When a combined prenatal and postpartum protein restriction occurs, the reduction in the number of brain cells will be approximately 60 percent.

Preeclampsia is a condition characterized by an elevation of blood pressure during the last three months of pregnancy. When preeclampsia becomes severe it may be associated with convulsions or coma; it is then called eclampsia or toxemia. The incidence of preeclampsia is far greater among indigent women and those who eat practically no protein during pregnancy.

SALT

Should I limit my salt intake?

I always seem to encounter a look of skepticism when I tell my prenatal patients that they need not restrict their dietary salt intake. Until the early 1980s, obstetricians preached that sodium was the cause of toxemia (see discussion above), but this theory has been totally discredited. It is now known that sodium is essential for the normal expansion of the pregnant woman's tissues and blood volume. If anything, restriction of dietary salt may actually hasten the onset of toxemia by decreasing the volume of fluid in the circulatory system, thereby causing a greater concentration of blood cells in relation to plasma. While we often use the words "salt" and "sodium" interchangeably, the salt we add to our food contains 40% sodium and a variety of other chemicals. It is important that

you use only iodized or sea salt, since this will prevent goiter or abnormal enlargement of the thyroid gland caused by a lack of iodine.

A regimen of restricting sodium and taking diuretics, or water pills, serves only to compound the circulatory problems that could lead to toxemia. It is generally agreed that diuretic therapy in pregnancy is of no benefit; instead it entails multiple risks. If you are receiving prenatal care from a doctor who believes in the implementation of a low salt diet and the use of diuretics, please find another obstetrician. If you experience swelling of the hands and legs, bedrest on your left side for 24 hours at a time will prove remarkably effective in alleviating the problem. There is some controversy as to whether salt should be restricted once a woman has developed preeclampsia (see page 42). Most authorities now believe that salt restriction is of little if any benefit in the treatment of this disease and that use of salt will not precipitate a toxemic crisis.

For some unexplained physiological reason, women tend to crave and digest more salt during pregnancy. In a 1986 study published in the *American Journal of Clinical Nutrition*, researchers at the University of Minnesota presented pregnant and nonpregnant women with five salt solutions of varied concentrations. The women were asked to rank them as best they could by order of strength. Each was also asked to identify the solution she most preferred. Pregnant women were far less likely than nonpregnant women to rank the solutions in their true order of strength. In addition, they pre-

ferred the taste of the solutions with the greatest salt concentrations.

A common treatment for nonpregnant women with chronic hypertension is sodium restriction and long-term diuretic therapy. Whether these women should continue this treatment during pregnancy is controversial, but there is some evidence that kidney and uterine blood flow may be affected with such treatment. Instead, a more logical approach would be to discontinue the diuretic and use specific antihypertensive drugs (see Chapter 9) only if they are absolutely necessary. While it may not be essential to totally eliminate salt from the diet of a chronic hypertensive during pregnancy, foods with a high salt content should be used sparingly.

      # CAFFEINE

How dangerous is caffeine consumption for the pregnant woman and her fetus?

Research linking high doses of caffeine with a variety of birth defects in rats, mice, and rabbits received much publicity in recent years. However, what these reports failed to stress was that the amounts of caffeine needed to produce these defects are the equivalent of a woman drinking 24 to 70 cups of coffee daily throughout her pregnancy. Despite extensive research, there is absolutely no evidence linking birth defects to coffee consumption in humans. However, it can have other effects.

Caffeine stays in a woman's circulation two to four times longer when she is pregnant. It rapidly crosses the placental barrier and is distributed to all fetal tissues. The ability of the fetus to clear or remove caffeine from its bloodstream is far less efficient than that of its mother. Studies have clearly demonstrated that the caffeine levels in the umbilical cord blood of the baby at birth are al-

most twice as high as those detected in the mother's bloodstream. Furthermore, caffeine stays in the bloodstream of the fetus and newborn almost 15 times longer because of a lack of enzymes necessary to metabolize it. These enzymes often do not appear until several days and sometimes up to nine months after birth. The accumulation of caffeine in a newborn's blood circulation is especially pronounced among premature infants.

In a 1978 study from the University of Washington, researchers tested hundreds of newborns for behavioral and physical condition on the first day of life. They found that heavy maternal caffeine use during the first five months of pregnancy was responsible for the birth of babies with the lowest scores. In 1986, doctors at Yale University School of Medicine followed more than 3,000 pregnant women and evaluated the association between their caffeine consumption and the likelihood of miscarriage. Those consuming more than 151 milligrams of caffeine, or the maximum amount usually contained in one cup of strong brewed coffee (see Table 14), were almost twice as likely to experience a late first- or second-trimester spontaneous abortion than nonusers. Those classified as light coffee drinkers (less than 151 milligrams per day) had an increased risk of spontaneous abortion only if they had an abortion in a previous pregnancy. No other studies have confirmed these findings, and the Yale researchers correctly cautioned that "additional studies are needed before the association of caffeine with spontaneous abortion can be more definitely evaluated".

In 1989, Doctors Herminia S. Salvador and Brian J. Koos of Loma Linda University School of Medicine used ultrasound to view fetal activity following consumption of either 450 milligrams of caffeinated coffee or 12 milligrams of decaffeinated coffee by eight women who were 32 to 36 weeks pregnant. Maternal ingestion of regular coffee was associated with a twofold increase in the incidence of fetal activity and a fall in the baseline fetal heart rate by an average of 12 beats per minute within 1 hour. Decaffeinated coffee increased fetal breathing activity and lowered the fetal heart rate to a lesser degree.

Based on available information, most authorities would conclude that ingestion of two cups of coffee or a caffeine-containing drink per day should cause no harm to the developing fetus. However, I do not feel confident in recommending amounts greater than this. Because caffeine lowers iron absorption, women should be cautioned not to take prenatal vitamins or iron supplements with their morning cup of coffee. In 1988, researchers at the University of California found that coffee drinkers were more likely to give birth to babies with reduced hematocrit and hemoglobin levels indicative of anemia. Coffee may also decrease the availability of calcium and zinc.

The approximate amounts of caffeine present in various products are listed in Table 14.

If caffeine is added to a product, it must be listed on the label. Carefully read the labels of all beverages during pregnancy. Decaffeinated coffee is a logical and safe alternative coffee substitute, since each cup is estimated to contain only 1 to 6 milligrams of caffeine.

How much caffeine is secreted in breast milk?

Doctors at the Washington University School of Medicine have shown that caffeine rapidly enters the breast milk and achieves peak levels 60 minutes later. The caffeine level in breast milk is only 1 percent of that found in the mother's plasma, an amount that is safe for the nursing infant. With repeated maternal caffeine ingestion the risk of caf-

TABLE 14

APPROXIMATE CAFFEINE CONTENT OF COMMONLY USED PRODUCTS

Cola	15 to 30 milligrams per 8-ounce cup
Cocoa or hot chocolate	Up to 50 milligrams per 5-ounce cup
Chocolate bar	25 milligrams (6 milligrams per ounce) of solid milk chocolate
One cup brewed coffee	80 to 120 milligrams
One cup of instant coffee	66 to 100 milligrams
One cup of leaf tea	30 to 75 milligrams
One cup of bagged tea	42 to 100 milligrams
One cup of instant tea	30 to 60 milligrams
One cup of freeze dried coffee	66 milligrams
One cup of decaffeinated coffee	1 to 6 milligrams

feine accumulation in the infant depends upon a variety of factors, such as the volume of breast milk ingested, the infant's clearance rate for caffeine, and the average concentration of the drug in a woman's serum and breast milk. There have been reports of restless, wakeful babies after the ingestion of more than 600 milligrams of caffeine by breast-feeding mothers. No ill effects in infants were observed, however, with maternal intakes of 200 to 350 milligrams.

Are there any caffeine-containing medications which the pregnant and nursing woman should avoid?

Yes. Caffeine is present in a variety of over-the-counter analgesics, diet pills, decongestants, cold preparations, and medications used as stimulants for maintaining mental alertness. For a more detailed list, see Table 15. As stated in Chapter 9, it is best to avoid these and all other medications during pregnancy and nursing unless they are absolutely necessary.

Can a nursing mother drink herbal teas or cocoa?

Herbal teas should be used judiciously by nursing mothers. Many herbal teas contain active in-gredients that a woman may secrete in her milk in sufficient amounts to affect her infant. Cathartics, such as buckthorn bark and senna, when present in herbal teas may cause cramps and watery diarrhea. Chamomile tea can cause an allergic reaction in someone who is sensitive to ragweed pollen. Herbal tea manufacturers are not required to list the ingredients of their products on labels, so nursing mothers must be cautious about the possible side effects of the use of these teas. Recent studies show that a chemical found in cocoa passes freely into human milk; it may cause a number of adverse reactions such as diarrhea, constipation, eczema, irritability, and sleeplessness.

Besides its caffeine content, are there other problems associated with drinking tea?

Drinking tea with meals may contribute to iron-deficiency anemia during pregnancy. The tannins in tea inhibit the absorption of iron from the intestinal tract; this is especially likely to occur if the diet is rich in vegetables. However, iron absorption is not affected when meat is regularly eaten.

 VITAMINS

Why is folic acid necessary during pregnancy, and what is its recommended dietary allowance each day?

Folic acid, also referred to as folate and folacin, is a B vitamin which is essential in the synthesis of a vital cellular protein named deoxyribonucleic acid (DNA). DNA is found in the nucleus of all cells of the body, especially those undergoing rapid division. For this reason, the fetus, placenta, and maternal bone marrow would all be primarily affected by a folic acid deficiency. Folic acid also enables red blood cells to carry oxygen to cells of the body which require it.

The daily Recommended Dietary Allowance (RDA) for folate in an adult is 400 micrograms, and many authorities believe that this amount should be doubled during pregnancy. While one would assume that a well-nourished woman would easily meet these requirements in her daily diet, there is some evidence to show that the average dietary intake by pregnant women is less than the

TABLE 15

CAFFEINE-CONTAINING DRUGS

Nonprescription Brand	Use	Milligrams Caffeine per Tablet	Comments
Anacin Analgesic Tablets, Maximum Strength Anacin	Pain relief	32.0	Avoid if possible since Anacin contains aspirin.
Aqua-Ban	Diuretic (medication to relieve fluid retention)	100.0	Do not use during pregnancy.
Bio Slim T	Aid in weight reduction	140.0	Dieting not recommended during pregnancy and nursing.
Cope	Pain relief	32.0	Avoid if possible, since it contains aspirin.
Excedrin Extra-Strength	Relief of pain of headache, sinusitis, muscular aches, minor pain	65.0	Contains aspirin-like medication, which is best avoided.
Stanback Analgesic Powders	Relief of headache, musular aches, other pain, control of fever	15 (Per dose)	Avoid if possible since it contains aspirin.
Vanquish Analgesic caplets	Relief of headache, muscular aches, other pain, control of fever	33.0	Avoid if possible since it contains aspirin.
No Doz	Stimulant to maintain alertness and prevent sleep	100.0	Avoid if possible.
Vivarin Stimulant Tablets	Stimulant to maintain alertness and prevent sleep	200.0	Avoid if possible.

Prescription Drugs

Cafergot Tablets and Suppositories	Relief of migraine headache	100.0	Contains ergotamine tartrate which may cause dangerous uterine constriction of blood vessels.

TABLE 15

CAFFEINE-CONTAINING DRUGS (Continued)

Nonprescription Brand	Use	Milligrams Caffeine per Tablet	Comments
Esgic Tablics and Capsules	Sedative and pain reliever	40.0	Avoid because it contains barbiturate.
Darvon Compound	Relief of mild to moderate pain	32.4	Contains propoxyphene hydrochloride which has not been proved safe in pregnancy and withdrawal symptoms in newborns have been reported.
Fiorinal	Pain reliever, especially for tension headaches	40.0	Avoid because it contains aspirin and a barbiturate.
Fioricet	Pain reliever, especially for tension headaches	40.0	Barbiturate.
Migralam	Relief of vascular and tension headaches	100.0	Contains isometheptene mucate, which may cause dangerous uterine contractions and constrict blood vessels.
Damason-P	Relief of moderately severe pain	32.0	Avoid if possible since it contains aspirin.
Norgesic and Norgesic Forte	Relief of mild to moderately severe pain of acute musuclo-skeletal disorders	30.0, 60.0	Avoid if possible since it contains aspirin.
Synalgos-DC Capsules	Relief of moderate to severe pain	30.0	Avoid if possible since it contains a narcotic and aspirin.

RDA. For this reason and the fact that there are no known harmful consequences resulting from an excess of folic acid during pregnancy, most obstetricians in the United States routinely prescribe prenatal vitamins containing between 500 and 1,000 micrograms of folic acid. This view contrasts sharply with that of the nutritionists at the Institute of Medicine who, in their monumental 1990 report entitled *Nutrition During Pregnancy*, concluded that folate supplementation need not be given routinely during pregnancy. Instead, they recommend supplementation with 300 micrograms of folate daily only if a woman's diet is suspected to be inadequate.

Folic acid is abundant in many foods, especially liver, kidney, green leafy vegetables, broccoli, asparagus, peanuts, mung bean sprouts, cow peas, wheat germ, fruit, wheat bran, kidney beans, peas, lima beans, soybeans, and garbanzo beans. Surprisingly, chocolate is a fairly good source of folic acid.

Aside from individuals with dietary inadequacies, which women should be carefully observed for folate deficiencies during pregnancy?

Excessive vomiting during pregnancy is probably the most common reason for poor folate absorption. A small number of otherwise healthy women are incapable of absorbing folic acid during pregnancy and require intramuscular supplements in order to maintain their normal blood levels of this vitamin. Several rare intestinal diseases, known as malabsorption syndromes, also cause a decrease in folate absorption; celiac disease is an example. Phenytoin (trade name Dilantin), a drug which is commonly prescribed in the treatment of epilepsy, also interferes with folate absorption into the body from the intestinal tract. Other anticonvulsants, such as phenobarbital and primidone, may have a similar effect, as does the urinary antibiotic trimethoprim. Alcoholic women, too, are more likely to experience a folic acid deficiency, as a result of their inadequate food consumption. It has been demonstrated that women on strict vegetarian diets and those on birth control pills for long periods of time may have lower folic acid levels than other women.

Various blood disorders characterized by premature destruction, or hemolysis, of red blood cells create a greater demand for folic acid; examples are chronic hemolytic anemias, sickle cell disease, G6PD deficiency, and thalassemia. All these disorders require a supplement of at least 1 milligram of folic acid daily during pregnancy.

Women with two or more pregnancies in rapid succession have less time to replenish their folate stores. Similarly, women experiencing a multiple birth deplete more of their folic acid in meeting the greater fetal and placental demands.

What are the symptoms of a folic acid deficiency, and how is it diagnosed?

Although folic acid deficiency during pregnancy is uncommon, it may develop slowly, and most women with this condition are without symptoms. Overt disease, characterized by severe anemia and bone marrow abnormalities, is extremely rare and apparent only if the deficiency is long neglected.

When a person with a previously adequate diet is suddenly deprived of folic acid, it takes approximately three weeks for the serum folate levels to reflect this decline. While the serum folate test is the earliest method of detecting a folic acid deficiency, it is never routinely performed during pregnancy.

At seven weeks following folate deprivation, a type of circulating white blood cell, called a neutrophil, will demonstrate a greater number of segments in the lobes of its nucleus. These characteristic changes can easily be viewed under the microscope and represent a simple and highly specific test for diagnosing a folic acid deficiency. A good laboratory technician should be able to make the diagnosis while performing the routine prenatal blood count. However, if the diagnosis is missed at this point, it will take 14 weeks of folate deprivation for a urine test to detect the disease.

The severe and symptomatic stages of folic acid deficiency occur approximately 18 to 20 weeks following its removal from the diet. These include bone marrow abnormalities, severe anemia characterized by abnormally large and bizarre red blood cells, and a pronounced platelet deficiency (thrombocytopenia).

How will a folic acid deficiency affect pregnancy?

In the rare event that a folic acid deficiency is neglected to the point of anemia and thrombocytopenia, the pregnancy will be adversely affected.

Severe anemia is associated with a higher incidence of fetal loss, premature birth, and perinatal complications, while a low platelet count may cause life-threatening maternal hemorrhage during pregnancy, labor, and the postpartum period. Both situations can be treated and prevented by adequate supplements of folic acid. Studies which have attempted to correlate folic acid deficiency with recurrent spontaneous abortion and congenital abnormalities have come to conflicting conclusions.

As previously mentioned (see Chapter 6) a folic acid deficiency may be associated with a falsely abnormal Pap smear suggestive of cervical cancer. By providing folic acid supplements rather than surgery, the astute obstetrician can cure this condition without unnecessary surgical intervention.

What is the relationship between the use of folic acid supplements and the incidence of neural tube defects?

It was first theorized in 1966 that a relationship existed between folate deficiency and the presence of severe fetal neural tube defects such as anencephaly and spina bifida. Although the chances of giving birth to a baby with a neural tube defect are quite small, once this misfortune occurs a woman will be at a 2 to 5 percent risk of its happening again. For unknown reasons, women in the United Kingdom and Ireland are more likely to give birth to infants with these abnormalities than women living in the United States. In this country, the overall incidence of neural tube defects has been most often reported as occurring in less than 1 per 1,000 births, though other estimates place it at 2 per 1,000. This translates to 3,000 to 5,000 births annually.

The prevalence of neural tube defects is dependent upon many demographic factors, including a woman's socioeconomic status, family history, race, nutritional status, and geographic location. As a result, periconceptual use of folic acid will not completely eliminate this condition. Nevertheless,

researchers in Great Britain and the United States have demonstrated that a woman can significantly reduce her risk of giving birth to an infant with a neural tube defect if she takes a daily 400 microgram (0.4 milligrams) folic acid supplement for at least a month prior to conception. In a 1989 study of almost 23,000 pregnancies, Dr. Aubrey Milunsky and his colleagues at the Center for Human Genetics at Boston University School of Medicine found a prevalence of neural tube defects equal to 3.6 per 1,000 among women who had not taken a folic acid supplement prior to or during the first trimester. This compared to an incidence of only 0.9 per 1,000 for women who had taken supplements. This difference was even more striking among women with a family history of neural tube defects—13 per 1,000 versus 3.5 per 1,000 respectively. Since anencephaly and spinal bifida defects are usually present in the fourth week of conception, the research of Dr. Milunsky emphasized the importance of taking folic acid supplements prior to this time.

Doctors at the Centers for Disease Control currently recommend a daily 400 microgram folic acid supplement in the four weeks prior to conception and throughout the first trimester for all women who have previously given birth to an infant with a neural tube defect. On September 14, 1992, the United States Public Health Service took the unprecedented step of recommending a daily 400 microgram folic acid supplement to all fertile women of childbearing age.

Aside from folic acid, how essential are other B vitamin supplements during pregnancy?

Contrary to what the pharmaceutical companies may tell you, the requirements for all vitamins are easily met through the normal diet. Despite this knowledge, it is customary in the United States for doctors to prescribe prenatal vitamins to practically all pregnant women. Although these vitamin supplements do not cause harm when taken in the normal dosage, the fact is that they are most often unnecessary. Furthermore, too many women mistakenly rely on vitamins as a quick and easy substitute for good nutrition and proper dietary habits.

The B vitamins are numbered 1 through 12. In general, the requirements for all B vitamins may be met with adequate servings of milk, meat, poultry, eggs, fish, whole grain bread and cereal, wheat germ, and brewer's yeast.

According to the Institute of Medicine's 1990 report, even when a pregnant woman's nutritional intake is inadequate, the only B vitamin supplementation she is likely to need is folic acid and vitamin B_6 daily. Those most likely to require supplementation include women carrying more than one fetus, heavy cigarette smokers, vegetarians, and alcohol or drug abusers. To promote the absorption of all supplemental vitamins, it is best to take them between meals or at bedtime.

Thiamine, or vitamin B_1, is essential for a healthy appetite, normal digestion, and good muscular tone of the gastrointestinal tract. While it is needed for bodily growth and lactation, a maternal deficiency will not necessarily be harmful to the fetus. In one report, a thiamine deficiency was noted in 30 percent of pregnant women studied, but selective transport of this vitamin across the placenta was proven by the fact that all the newborn infants had normal thiamine levels. Especially good sources of thiamine are pork and pork products, liver, heart, kidney, peas, beans, and wheat germ. Since this vitamin is not stored in the body, it is important that pregnant women maintain an adequate diet each day in order to prevent its depletion.

Riboflavin, or vitamin B_2, is necessary for the normal growth and development of the fetus. A deficiency of this vitamin may be manifested by skin dryness, cracking of the lips and corners of the mouth, inflammation of the tongue, and eye problems such as burning, itching, poor vision, and light sensitivity. A good source of riboflavin is milk, and four cups of milk or milk products a day will meet all of the pregnant woman's requirements. Beef and calf liver also contain large amounts of

riboflavin. Since marginal amounts of riboflavin are present in total vegetarian diets, pregnant vegetarians should be encouraged to consume large amounts of green leafy vegetables, legumes, and whole-grain foods which supply a fair amount of riboflavin. Several studies have shown that women who use birth control pills are more likely to be deficient in riboflavin. For this reason, a woman who conceives shortly after stopping the Pill should be made aware of the importance of adequate riboflavin intake.

The United States RDA for riboflavin is 1.3 milligrams. It has been suggested that an additional 0.3 milligram be added during pregnancy and 0.5 milligram for nursing. A study from Cornell University found that women who engage in regular, vigorous physical exercise may need more riboflavin than the current recommended RDA. For the woman who remains active during pregnancy, this would indicate a greater need than that currently advised.

Niacin is an important B vitamin found in abundance in peanuts and brewer's yeast and also in canned tuna, beef, and pork. It is vital in the building of brain cells and prevents infection and bleeding of the gums. Early signs of a niacin deficiency are loss of appetite, nausea, vomiting, abdominal pain, headache, dizziness, and burning, numbness, and weakness of the hands and feet. As with riboflavin, women who use birth control pills prior to conception are more likely to be deficient in niacin.

The RDA for niacin is approximately 15 milligrams for women 15 to 18 years of age and 13 milligrams among those in the 18- to 35-year age group. Suggested increases for pregnant and nursing women are 2 and 5 milligrams, respectively.

Pyridoxine, or vitamin B_6, is essential for the metabolism of fat and fatty acids and for the production of antibodies. Labels on food packages and supplements may list B_6 as pyridoxine, pyridoxal, or pyridoxamine, names that may be thought of as being identical. Symptoms of a vitamin B_6 deficiency are mental depression, lethargy, fatigue, impaired glucose and insulin metabolism, numbness and tingling of the arms and legs, loss of balance, and anemia. A pyridoxine deficiency during pregnancy has been implicated as the cause of depression which some women experience at this time. Milk, cereals, yeast, liver, and wheat germ contain abundant amounts of pyridoxine. Other sources are grains, beans, nuts, and dried fruits. If a woman restricts her intake of high carbohydrate foods, she may not take in enough vitamin B_6 in her diet.

Researchers from Purdue University have expressed concern that some pregnant women may need significantly more vitamin B_6 than the daily 2.5 milligrams currently recommended. They concluded that vitamin B_6 levels be checked at the fifth month of pregnancy and that additional supplements be given if necessary.

Although a 0.5-milligram increase in the RDA for pyridoxine is currently recommended during lactation as well as pregnancy, there has been great controversy as to the wisdom of this policy. A minority of researchers have claimed that pyridoxine will reduce the quantity of a woman's breast milk. From the available reports, I would surmise that pyridoxine, in the currently recommended amount of 2.5 milligrams daily, would be an unlikely cause of inhibited or faulty lactation.

Vitamin B_{12}, also known as cobalamin and cyanocobalamin, is essential for the normal development of red blood cells. The RDA for vitamin B_{12} has been set at 3 milligrams, with increased increments of 1 milligram recommended for pregnancy and lactation, respectively.

Biotin is a B vitamin which is found in an infinite number of foods. While milk, egg yolk, meats, cereals, legumes, and nuts are especially rich in this vitamin, it is also produced in the human intestine by microorganisms. A naturally occurring isolated biotin deficiency has never been reported. The RDA for biotin is set a 0.3 milligram, though this is probably twice the amount that is actually needed. Pregnancy and lactation do not alter the body's need for biotin.

Pantothenic acid is a B vitamin found in just about all foods. Especially good sources of pantothenic acid are liver, kidney, eggs, peanuts, and wheat bran, although even poor diets usually contain adequate amounts of this vitamin. As with biotin, a pure pantothenic acid deficiency has been created only under experimental conditions. The RDA for pantothenic acid is 15 milligrams. Since the bodily requirements for this vitamin are unchanged during pregnancy and lactation, it would be difficult to justify the use of pantothenic supplements during these times.

What are the recommended dietary allowances for vitamin A during pregnancy?

Vitamin A, or retinol, a form of vitamin A usually found in supplements, plays an important role in building resistance to infection. It is also necessary for normal formation of tooth enamel, hair, and fingernails and is responsible for functioning of the thyroid gland. Vitamin A greatly contributes to the development of fetal eyes, skin, and glands. Claims have been made that vitamin A will relieve skin diseases, warts, sinusitis, ulcers, and stretch marks, but there is no scientific justification for these supposed benefits.

The usual recommended dietary allowance (RDA) of vitamin A for nonpregnant women is 5,000 International Units (IU). This need not be increased in pregnancy or during lactation. Some nutritionists measure vitamin A requirements in retinol equivalents (RE), with 800 RE, suggested for nonpregnant, pregnant, and lactating women, respectively. A woman's serum levels of vitamin A will usually decline in early pregnancy and then begin to rise between the thirteenth and sixteenth weeks. At 36 weeks, vitamin A levels reach an average of 1½ times normal. The reason for this is that vitamin A, as well as other fat-soluble vitamins such as D, E, and K, is stored and accumulates in the body. As a result, the likelihood of maternal and fetal toxicity is increased.

Several experimental animal studies and a small

number of case reports of human pregnancies have confirmed that very large overdoses of vitamin A, in the range of five to ten times the RDA, may be associated with greater risks of characteristic abnormalities in the fetus, including kidney malformations, skull and facial defects, thymic dysfunction and cardiac anomalies. The potential for birth defects with amounts of vitamin A less than five times the RDA is extremely unlikely, but a supplemental dose of 8,000 IU per day should not be exceeded during pregnancy. A supplement of 5,000 IU is perfectly adequate and theoretically even safer.

Much has been written about the hazards associated with the use of isotretinoin (trade name Acutane), a synthetic derivative of vitamin A, to treat acne in women during pregnancy. In one series of 36 women who continued their pregnancies after receiving isotretinoin, 8 (22 percent) experienced spontaneous abortions, 23 (64 percent) gave birth to normal infants, and 5 (14 percent) delivered babies with malformations characteristic of a vitamin A overdose. Concern has been expressed about the use of products which contain beta carotene, a vitamin A precursor. However, beta carotene has been found not to produce vitamin A toxicity.

Animal studies have shown that both a deficiency of vitamin A as well as an excess may be associated with fetal abnormalities. It is believed that several factors, one of which is a deficiency of vitamin A, may be linked in some way to the development of cancers of the colon, stomach, esophagus, breast, liver, and uterus. One study showed that premature babies had lower levels of vitamin A than full-term infants, although the significance of this has not been evaluated.

Fortified whole milk, cream, ice cream, fortified margarine, butter, egg yolks, fish, liver oils, liver, kidney, green leafy and yellow vegetables, such as green or red peppers, kale, pumpkins, spinach, sweet potatoes, and carrots, and cantaloupe are all excellent sources of vitamin A. Good sources of vitamin A include apricots, broccoli, tomatoes, watermelons, and winter squash.

What are the vitamin C requirements during pregnancy and lactation?

Vitamin C, or ascorbic acid, has very important functions. In addition to helping in the formation of body connective tissues and hemoglobin, it also plays a role in the metabolism of folic acid, the strengthening of capillary and cell walls, improving resistance to infection, the removal of body toxins or poisons, the absorption of iron from the intestine, the acidification of the urine, wound healing, and the repair of fractures. A severe vitamin C deficiency will result in a rare and serious disease called scurvy, and a lesser deficiency may manifest itself as swollen, reddened gums, which readily bleed, bruise easily, and have a greater susceptibility to infection.

Unfortunately, the public has been too ready to accept as fact the supposed benefits of vitamin C megadoses. According to a 1990 survey conducted by the National Center for Health Statistics, vitamin C is the most commonly used single vitamin supplement in the United States. Of the many who have taken up the fad of using vitamin C in this manner, few are aware of its potential dangers. It is known, for example, that large doses of vitamin C can cause diarrhea, excessively acid urine, kidney stones, interference with the germ-fighting ability of the body's white blood cells, high blood cholesterol levels in rats and some humans, and the blockage of the activity of certain drugs.

Doses of vitamin C in excess of one gram (1,000 milligrams) daily may also be harmful to the fetus. Vitamin C readily crosses the placenta from the maternal circulation, and fetal levels are often twice as high as maternal levels. Unlike its mother, the fetus is unable to rid its environment of the excess ascorbic acid. As a result, it swallows and recycles vitamin C byproducts in the amniotic fluid. When a woman ingests excessive vitamin C during pregnancy, it stimulates the enzyme system of her fetus to metabolize this overload. Following birth, normal amounts of vitamin C may be insufficient to satisfy the overly stimulated enzyme system of the newborn. As a result, these babies may paradoxically experience a severe vitamin C deficiency and even scurvy.

The RDA for vitamin C is 60 milligrams for the nonpregnant woman, though many knowledgeable nutritionists are convinced that one-half to two-thirds of this amount is more than adequate. In 1989, the National Research Council of the National Academy of Sciences raised the RDA for vitamin C to 100 milligrams daily for smokers. It has been suggested that an additional 20 milligrams should be added for pregnancy and 40 milligrams during lactation. These modest increases can be readily provided in the diet, and the traditional practice of incorporating supplements of approximately 90 milligrams of vitamin C in most prenatal vitamins would appear to be both excessive and unnecessary. The best natural source of vitamin C is citrus fruits, although spinach, cantaloupes, strawberries, broccoli, green and red peppers, kale, tomatoes, white and sweet potatoes, cauliflower, parsley, watermelon, brussels sprouts, cabbage, turnips, asparagus, okra, green beans, and lima beans are all sources of this vitamin.

What specific obstetrical benefits have been attributed to vitamin C?

As a result of several nonscientific anecdotal claims made by vitamin C enthusiasts, there is a widely held belief that megadoses of this vitamin can improve many aspects of pregnancy and childbirth. Supposed benefits of using 10,000 or more milligrams of vitamin C daily include a lower rate of miscarriage and bleeding, shorter and less painful labor, a marked reduction in the incidence of lacerations and tearing during delivery, fewer stretch marks (striae), a lower number of complications such as postpartum hemorrhage and retention of placental tissue, and a quicker maternal recovery following delivery. Vitamin C enthusiasts have also claimed that babies born of megadose-treated women have higher Apgar scores (see Chapter 11), are healthier during the first few weeks of life, and are less likely to experience sudden death in childhood.

Although all these superlatives attributed to vitamin C sound impressive, they are not supported by substantial scientific data. In fact, there is more evidence to show that megadoses in excess of 1,000 milligrams daily are more likely to harm the fetus than help it.

How much vitamin D is required during pregnancy?

Vitamin D is essential in the metabolism and deposition of calcium and phosphorus in teeth and bones. The vitamin crosses the placenta freely, and its concentrations in the fetus are directly dependent on maternal levels. A vitamin D deficiency in late pregnancy may be associated with low calcium levels (hypocalcemia) in the newborn's circulation. More severe maternal deprivation can cause enamel defects of the teeth and irreversible deformities of the fetal skeleton. Premature infants born of mothers with little or no prenatal care are far more likely to have a vitamin D deficiency and hypocalcemia.

At the opposite extreme, too much vitamin D may also be harmful. Of all vitamins, D is probably the easiest to take inadvertently in toxic excess. High doses of vitamin D raise blood levels of calcium and phosphorus by enhancing their intestinal absorption, removal from the bones, and retention by the kidneys. This in turn can cause damage to muscles and bones, gastrointestinal disturbances, kidney stones, and lymphatic, lung, and pancreatic disease. Studies suggest a possible association between excess maternal vitamin D and severe infantile hypercalcemia, skull and facial abnormalities, and narrowing of the aorta and pulmonary artery of the newborn. For this reason, I discourage all women from indiscriminately taking vitamin D supplements during pregnancy.

There are two sources of vitamin D: ingested food and sunlight. Most nutritionists concur that the RDA for vitamin D during pregnancy and lactation should remain unchanged from the 400 International Units (IU), or 10 micrograms, per day suggested for nonpregnant women. However, half this number is probably more than adequate in meeting fetal and maternal needs. Total vegetarians and others with low intakes of vitamin D are especially likely to benefit from vitamin D supplements during pregnancy.

In addition to vitamin D-fortified milk, other good sources are fish, liver oils, mackerel, salmon, tuna, sardines, and herring. Curiously, this vitamin is very scarce in most other foods. When the ultraviolet light of the sun comes in contact with the skin's surface, a chemical reaction takes place and vitamin D is formed. A woman can receive her entire daily allowance of vitamin D in this fashion depending, obviously, on the amount of skin surface exposed to the sun.

Several studies, including one conducted in 1980, clearly demonstrate that breast-fed infants have lower vitamin D concentrations than bottle-fed babies. As a result, many nutritionists now recommend that breast-fed newborns be given a supplement of vitamin D.

What is the function of vitamin E?

Contrary to the claims, vitamin E supplementation of the ordinary diet will not cure ignorance, impotence, frigidity, sterility, heart disease, skin disorders, wrinkles, or ulcers. It will not prevent spontaneous abortion, alleviate burns or minimize their scars, increase resistance to infection, delay the aging process, or prevent crib death in infants. The known and accepted functions of vitamin E are its ability to aid in the metabolism of vitamin A, promote healing, and develop healthy red blood cells. Vitamin E is also a potent antioxidant. This means that it helps govern the amount of oxygen the body uses and prevents oxygen from combining with and prematurely breaking down important substances in body cells.

Vitamin E is found in essentially every food. Its wide distribution in vegetable oils, wheat germ,

margarine, cereal grains, corn, peanuts, eggs, and animal fats makes a deficiency of vitamin E in humans extremely unlikely. Notable exceptions are premature babies with low vitamin E stores and little if any body fat, and women with cystic fibrosis and other intestinal fat-absorption diseases. Vitamin E is a fat-soluble vitamin, along with vitamins A, D, and K. All may be deficient in the presence of one of these rare diseases.

Scientists have learned that premature infants may be the greatest beneficiaries of vitamin E supplementation. In 1987, doctors from Manchester, England, reported that vitamin E helped to decrease the incidence of periventricular brain hemorrhage among infants born eight or more weeks prematurely. Other studies have found that vitamin E supplementation may help to prevent anemia in premature newborns. In addition, the risk of severe eye damage and blindness caused by giving oxygen to premature infants can be eliminated or significantly reduced by first administering vitamin E to these babies.

The RDA for vitamin E has been set at 8 milligrams for nonpregnant women, 10 milligrams during pregnancy, and 13 milligrams during lactation, although one-half of these amounts easily satisfies a person's nutritional requirements. Although vitamin E enthusiasts have endorsed amounts as high as 30 times the RDA, there is absolutely no evidence that these high doses are of any benefit. While it is commonly stated that there are no known harmful consequences associated with vitamin E megadoses, some animal studies do not support this claim. Physicians have reported that large doses in humans may be associated with dangerous coagulation disorders, thrombophlebitis (clots and inflammation in the veins), hypertension, fatigue, headache, dizziness, nausea, diarrhea, intestinal cramps, muscle weakness, and a variety of other problems. The long-term effects of vitamin E supplementation have never been adequately tested, and until more is known its use should be discouraged. Even less is known about the safety of using megadoses of vitamin E during the first trimester, but two reports have suggested that it may cause birth defects.

Topical application of vitamin E in oil, expressed from capsules, has become a popular treatment for sore nipples early in the course of breastfeeding. In 1985, researchers from Brigham and Women's Hospital and the Massachusetts College of Pharmacy found elevated, although not dangerous, levels of vitamin E in the bloodstream of infants who were breast-fed by these women.

What are the vitamin K requirements of pregnancy?

Vitamin K is vital for normal coagulation of the blood. It is synthesized in the intestinal tract by bacteria and does not come from a specific food source.

A baby born with a deficiency of vitamin K-dependent clotting factors is at a great risk of serious and even fatal hemorrhage. This complication is far more common than is currently realized and is especially likely to occur when maternal convulsions such as those of epilepsy are treated with phenytoin (trade name Dilantin). Neonatal hemorrhage in susceptible newborns can be prevented by treating them with an intramuscular injection of vitamin K. Oral anticoagulants such as warfarin (Coumadin) and bishydroxycoumarin (Dicumarol) are known to cross the placenta and inhibit vitamin K and clotting factors dependent on vitamin K. As a result, fetal and neonatal hemorrhage may occur. For this reason, oral anticoagulants are not recommended for use during pregnancy.

What are pseudovitamins, and which ones are recommended during pregnancy?

By definition, a vitamin is an essential nutrient that cannot be synthesized by the body, while so-called pseudovitamins are produced by the body in sufficient quantities. Proponents of pseudovitamins claim that they are capable of preventing and curing a variety of ailments, but scientific studies have confirmed that they are unnecessary and are best avoided. Included among the pseudovitamins are bioflavonoids ("vitamin" P), carnitine ("vitamin" Bt), pangamic acid ("vitamin" B15), inositol, lecithin, choline, para-amino benzoic acid (PABA), and "vitamins" Q and U. These preparations are mentioned with the hope that both pregnant and nonpregnant women will avoid their use.

 MINERALS

How essential are iron supplements during pregnancy?

The body's requirements for iron increase tremendously during pregnancy, and there is no doubt that supplemental iron is essential. Without iron, a woman is unable to make red blood cells, which are vital to the transfer of oxygen to both maternal and fetal body cells. Unfortunately, the nonpregnant woman stores an average of only 300 milligrams of iron in her bone marrow. This amount is totally inadequate in meeting the great demands imposed by pregnancy. In addition, previous pregnancies, poor nutrition, multiple fetuses, vegetarian diets, and menstrual blood loss only tend to further reduce and even deplete iron stores.

As the pregnant woman's plasma volume increases, her red blood cell count will also expand, but at a much slower pace. It has been calculated that a total of 500 milligrams of iron is needed during pregnancy to satisfy the expanded maternal blood volume. The development of the fetus and placenta requires an additional 300 milligrams of iron, for a total iron requirement for pregnancy of about 800 milligrams. If the iron obtained is all at the expense of the pregnant woman's limited reserves, she may easily become anemic. It is estimated that as many as one-half of all pregnant women who do not receive supplemental iron will be anemic at the time of delivery.

In their 1990 review of nutritional supplements during pregnancy, researchers at the Institute of Medicine concluded that iron is the only known nutrient for which requirements cannot be met reasonably by diet alone, and that a low-dose supplement of 30 milligrams of ferrous iron daily can provide that which is needed. In the case of iron supplements, more isn't necessarily better, and dosages well above this amount may interfere with the absorption of other essential nutrients. To meet the 800-milligram iron requirement for pregnancy, during the second and third trimesters of pregnancy a woman must take daily supplements in quantities which will result in her absorbing a minimum of 3 milligrams of iron per day in addition to the amount of iron usually absorbed from food.

Despite exaggerated claims and often misleading advertising, the most commonly prescribed and least expensive supplemental iron preparation remains ferrous sulfate. Since only 10 to 20 percent of dietary iron is absorbed from the intestine, and since ferrous sulfate contains about 20 percent elemental iron, tablets in a dose of 150 milligrams (30 milligrams of elemental iron) per day would allow absorption of the needed quantity of supplemental iron. It is interesting to note that the iron content of several commonly used preparations varies significantly. For example, products containing ferrous gluconate have only 11 percent elemental iron, while preparations with ferrous fumarate contain a high of 30 percent elemental iron. Therefore, to meet the 30 milligram ferrous iron requirement, a woman should consume a daily supplement of either 300 milligrams of ferrous gluconate or 100 milligrams of ferrous fumarate during the second and third trimesters. All iron products should be administered between meals or at bedtime on an empty stomach to facilitate absorption from the intestine. Contrary to popular belief, taking vitamin C with iron supplements will not enhance iron absorption.

Iron therapy is not necessary during the first trimester, when intolerance to this medication is most likely to occur. In fact, iron supplementation in the first eight weeks has been implicated as a possible cause of malformations in the fetus, though this has not been substantiated in any large studies. Most authorities recommend that iron supplements be maintained for two to three months postpartum in order to replenish iron stores which may have been diminished during pregnancy.

Good sources of dietary iron include dried fruits, liver, kidney, prune juice, dried beans, lima beans, dark molasses, fish, egg yolk, raisins, varieties of bread and cereal fortified with iron, and vegetables such as spinach, broccoli, kale, and greens. Certain substances such as carbonates, phosphates, oxalates, fiber-rich foods, and tannates in tea may all be responsible for inhibiting iron absorption from the intestine.

How much calcium do I require?

Calcium is a necessary mineral for proper fetal bone and tooth development. The calcium content of the newborn's skeleton is approximately 30 grams, with most of the accumulation occurring during the last trimester. Even if a woman has an inadequate calcium intake, her fetus is still able to obtain sufficient amounts by extracting it from her bony skeleton. The parasitizing of a mother's bony skeletal by the fetus sounds worse than it really is, since only about 2.5 percent of her total body content of calcium is sacrificed for the sake of the fetus. This small amount will rarely if ever create a negative calcium balance in a well-nourished woman.

Recent laboratory studies and clinical trials suggest that calcium supplementation may be associated with a decreased incidence of hypertension and preeclampsia. It has also been postulated that high doses of calcium cause relaxation of the uterine muscles and inhibition of premature labor. Support for this theory can be found in a 1991 study by doctors at Johns Hopkins Hospital in Baltimore. Women given 2,000 milligrams of calcium a day throughout pregnancy experienced one-third fewer preterm births prior to the thirty-seventh week of pregnancy than an equal number of women receiving a placebo.

The RDA for calcium is 1,200 milligrams for nonpregnant women 11 to 25 years of age, and 800 milligrams for those older than 25. An additional 400 milligrams is recommended during pregnancy and lactation. Milk is unquestionably the best source of calcium, and four glasses daily will satisfy the entire pregnancy RDA. Skim milk has slightly more calcium than either whole milk or low-fat milk. Drinking amounts of milk greater than one quart daily in order to enhance your calcium intake is not beneficial because the high phosphorous content of milk will interfere with its absorption. If you don't enjoy drinking milk, add it in liquid or powdered form to puddings, soups, baked goods, hot cereals, casseroles, and other prepared foods. Other dairy products, such as one cup of yogurt, 1½ ounces of hard unprocessed cheese, such as cheddar and swiss, 1¾ cups of ice cream, or 2 cups of cottage cheese supply an amount of calcium equal to that found in one glass of milk. While there are other natural foods which contain calcium, it is virtually impossible to meet the RDA without the use of dairy products. Fairly good non-dairy sources of calcium include oysters, salmon, sardines, dark green and leafy vegetables, such as broccoli, kale, and mustard greens, and dried figs, dates, apricots, almonds, sesame seeds, and soybeans.

If a pregnant woman is unable to tolerate lactose, the milk sugar, and if dietary solutions cannot be found, a multivitamin containing 250 milligrams of calcium in the form of calcium gluconate, calcium carbonate, or calcium lactate should be taken daily. To promote absorption from the intestine, it is best to take the multivitamin between meals or at bedtime. According to the Institute of Medicine's 1990 recommendations, the daily supplement of calcium should be raised to 600 milligrams for women younger than 25. These higher calcium supplement doses should be taken at mealtime in order to limit interaction with the iron contained in standard prenatal vitamins. Vitamins C and D both aid in calcium absorption from the intestinal tract, so it is a good idea to take your calcium supplement with a dairy product or a citrus fruit or juice.

What can a woman do to relieve leg cramps caused by lower calcium levels?

The characteristic sudden cramps in the back of the calf which some women experience in the last half of pregnancy are believed to be caused by declining serum levels of free calcium obtained from a rise in serum phosphorus. A natural response is to drink more milk. Actually, milk intake should be reduced, because milk contains large amounts of phosphorus as well as calcium, and the phosphorus may impair calcium absorption. Calcium tablets should be taken; but any product containing calcium phosphate should be avoided because it will lower free calcium levels and increase phosphorous concentrations. Another valuable suggestion in relieving leg cramps caused by low calcium levels is to ingest aluminum hydroxide on a daily basis. Trade names of products which contain aluminum hydroxide include Aludrox, Gaviscon, Mylanta, Camalox, Gelusil, Maalox, and Amphojel. Aluminum hydroxide has the effect of lowering phosphate levels by forming inactive aluminum phosphates which are not absorbed into the body from the intestine.

What other minerals are important?

Phosphorous metabolism is intimately related to that of calcium, and the proper balance between these two minerals is necessary for normal bone and tooth development. Phosphorus is also important in energy production and the use of proteins. While both phosphorus and calcium are found in great amounts in milk, there are many foods which lack calcium but supply lots of phosphorus. The RDA for phosphorus is approximately 800 milligrams for the nonpregnant woman, with 1,200 milligrams recommended during pregnancy and lactation. Some representative food servings and their phosphorus contents are: a serving of liver—300 milligrams; a hamburger—165 milligrams; a serving of fish—200 milligrams; and a shredded wheat biscuit—100 milligrams. With these high amounts in many foods, a phosphorus deficiency is never really a nutritional concern for the pregnant woman.

Zinc is an important constituent of enzymes which are vital to the body's metabolism. It aids in protein digestion and in the synthesis of insulin, and plays a role in increasing the blood volume to the brain and other organs of the body. Zinc also speeds the healing of wounds and helps white blood cells fight infection. An adult's RDA for zinc is 15 milligrams, with an additional 5 and 10 milligrams added for pregnancy and lactation, respectively. Most diets which contain adequate amounts of animal protein will easily meet these requirements, and all iron-rich foods are equally abundant in zinc. Fish, oysters, eggs, meat, and milk are the best sources of zinc. Occasional zinc deficiencies have been noted among vegetarians and others who consume large amounts of unprocessed grains, bran, beans, and whole wheat products, since a large amount of phytic acid in these products binds zinc and prevents the body from using it. For such women a multivitamin containing 15 milligrams of supplemental zinc is recommended during pregnancy.

The potential dangers of a zinc deficiency have not been fully elucidated. However, a slight decline in serum zinc concentrations appears to be a normal physiologic adjustment during pregnancy and is not necessarily indicative of inadequate zinc intake. Significant zinc deficiencies, however, have been tentatively linked to a variety of obstetrical complications including inadequate fetal growth, prematurity, respiratory distress, birth defects, preeclampsia, abruptio placenta, and even emotional disorders in children.

Magnesium is an essential nutrient, an important constituent of bone and tissues, and an activator of various proteins and enzyme systems in the body. Articles in popular magazines to the contrary, a magnesium deficiency occurs only under unusual circumstances such as prolonged starvation, chronic malnutrition, alcoholism, diseases causing poor intestinal absorption, and severe diabetes and kidney disease. A nutritional magnesium deficiency has been suspected of predisposing women to premature labor. Magnesium is found in just about all foods; fresh fruits and raw leafy green vegetables supply the greatest amounts. The RDA for magnesium during pregnancy and lactation is 450 milligrams, or 150 milligrams above that recommended for nonpregnant adults. If you eat foods with very high phosphorus content, you may slightly impair your absorption of magnesium.

Iodine is found throughout the body but is concentrated in the thyroid gland. In the past, iodine deficiencies and subsequent goiter formation were noted in a number of states in which inhabitants ingested diets deficient in this mineral. Today, with the use of iodized salt, this is no longer a problem. The RDA for nonpregnant women is 150 micrograms, with an additional 25 micrograms recommended during pregnancy. The nursing woman is advised to ingest 175 to 200 micrograms per day of iodine. However, it is important to remember that too much iodine can suppress thyroid function. For this reason, the recommended daily requirement during pregnancy should not exceed 225 micrograms. Iodine-rich supplements, such as kelp, can bring the pregnant woman dangerously close to this limit.

FLUORIDE

What are the advantages and risks of using fluoride supplements during pregnancy?

It is believed that fluoridation of public water supplies is a safe, effective, and practical way of preventing dental caries and reducing the cost of dental care among children and nonpregnant adults. There is no RDA for fluoride during pregnancy, and it is not contained in any standard prenatal multiple vitamin preparation. While most authorities endorse the use of fluoride supplements during childhood, there is some controversy as to the advantages and safety of these preparations when they are given prenatally. However, the FDA, the AMA, and the American Dental Association have taken a position supporting the safety of fluoride supplementation during pregnancy.

Until more research is available, I would assume that most obstetricians will not be prescribing fluoride supplements for women who have adequate concentrations of fluoride, or approximately 0.7 parts per million, in their drinking water. However, in the absence of adequate fluoride in the drinking water, a daily supplement of 1 to 2.2 milligrams is probably beneficial. The fluoride content of bottled water will practically always have less fluoride than the amounts in public fluoridated water supplies. Only minute amounts of fluoride pass from a woman's bloodstream to her breast milk. Therefore, infants who are completely breast-fed should receive 0.25 milligrams of fluoride supplementation daily, even if the local water source is fluoridated.

Is it safe for a woman to use artificial sweeteners during pregnancy?

There is considerable confusion among women and their obstetricians about the safety of artificial sweeteners such as saccharin and aspartame (trade name NutraSweet) during pregnancy. Most of the negative publicity surrounding the use of saccharin, a nonnutritive sweetener derived from naphthalene, originated from a Canadian study 15 years ago showing an increase in bladder cancer among male rats fed high doses of saccharin. Subsequent biochemical studies on rats, mice, monkeys, and hamsters given high doses of saccharin during their embryonic stage of organ development have not produced cancers or abnormal offspring. When intravenous saccharin was given to rhesus monkeys during the last trimester of pregnancy, researchers noted that it rapidly crossed the placenta and entered the fetal circulation for long periods of time. This effect, however, was not detrimental to the outcome of pregnancy. Unfortunately, there is a paucity of data on the safety of saccharin use during the first three months of pregnancy. As a result, experts on the subject, such as Dr. Robert S. London of Johns Hopkins University School of Medicine, recommend that women not use saccharin immediately before conception or early in pregnancy. In contrast to his concerns about saccharin, Dr. London believes that aspartame may be safely used by the pregnant woman.

The more than 1,500 food products which contain aspartame are appealing to the 100 million Americans who use them because they provide the sweet taste of sugar with only 5 percent of its calorie content. The main fear surrounding aspartame use concerns the safety of the three components resulting from its metabolism: aspartate, methanol, and phenylalanine. Extensive laboratory studies have demonstrated that aspartate does not cross the placenta to any significant degree, and the amount of methanol is too small to cause fetal damage. The chief area of concern regarding aspartame metabolism is its phenylalanine component. Levels of this amino acid are greatly elevated in individuals afflicted with the metabolic disease known as phenylketonuria, or PKU (see Chapter 11). Pregnant asymptomatic carriers of this disease also have higher than normal serum phenylalanine concentrations. If a woman with PKU carefully maintains a phenylalanine-free diet throughout her pregnancy, she is virtually assured of giving birth to a healthy baby; but if she deviates from her diet, her newborn may suffer from severe and permanent mental retardation. Fortunately, scientists have calculated that a pregnant PKU carrier would have to consume almost 200 cans of diet soda daily in order to pose even the slightest threat to her fetus.

Cyclamates are artificial sweeteners which gained great popularity in the past but are now limited in their use. One reason for this was a case report of two infants born with a rare combination of cleft palate, cleft lip, and abnormalities of the hands following maternal use of cyclamates. Subsequent laboratory studies on a variety of animals have failed to reproduce these abnormalities. Studies on laboratory rats have shown an association between cyclamates and bladder tumors, and other research has demonstrated that the drug does cross the placenta and enter the fetal circulation. For these reasons, cyclamates are best avoided during pregnancy.

Sunette is the trade name for acesulfame-K, a noncaloric product which is 200 times as sweet as table sugar. Since it is not metabolized and passes through the intestine unchanged, it should be safe during pregnancy, although proof of its safety is lacking at the present time. Other low calorie sweeteners awaiting FDA approval include alitame and sucralose.

 # *PLANNING MEALS*

What does an ample basic food plan for a pregnant woman contain?

Although many complex nutritional formulas and charts have been devised, a simple and basic food approach is to plan meals according to the four major food groups:

GROUP 1: *PROTEIN*
Two or more servings are recommended daily during the first half of pregnancy, and three or more servings are recommended in the last half of pregnancy and during lactation. This group can include lean meats, chicken, fish, dried beans, and nuts. Cheaper grades of meat are just as nutritious as more expensive ones; a serving is defined as 2 to 3 ounces of lean cooked meat, fish, or poultry without bones. The following servings of food contain equivalent amounts of protein:

- ¼ pound cooked hamburger
- 1 medium fish or meat patty
- 2 frankfurters
- 2 slices of liver
- 2 slices of meat loaf
- 2 medium chicken drumsticks
- 1 chicken leg, including thigh
- 1 medium fish steak
- 1 slice roast meat or poultry 2½ inches ¼ inch

Substitutes for the above are:

- ½ cup cottage cheese
- 3 ounces cheddar, Monterey jack, Swiss, munster, brick, or longhorn cheese
- 1 cup cooked dried beans, peas, or lentils
- ½ cup shelled peanuts
- 4 tablespoons peanut butter
- 3 eggs

GROUP 2: *MILK and MILK PRODUCTS*

Four or more cups of milk are recommended each day. Whole milk, skim milk, buttermilk, reconstituted dried milk, yogurt, and custard are of equal value. The following amounts of cheese equal one cup of milk:

- 1-inch cube cheese
- 1⅓ cups cottage cheese
- 1½ slices (equals 1½ ounces) cheese

GROUP 3: *FRUITS and VEGETABLES*

Four or more daily servings are recommended, and one serving is equal to any of the following:

- ½ to ¾ cup of apple, orange, potato, grapefruit, or cantaloupe
- 1 apple, 1 orange, 1 potato, ½ grapefruit, or ½ cantaloupe
- ½ cup cooked green or yellow vegetables, 1 cup raw vegetables (salad)

GROUP 4: *BREAD and CEREAL*

At least two to three servings during the first half of pregnancy and four to five servings during the second half are recommended. A serving of whole-grain and enriched bread consists of one of the following:

- 1 slice enriched or whole-grain bread
- ½ to ¾ cup cooked whole-grain cereal, such as cracked wheat, oatmeal, brown rice, or rolled wheat
- ½ to ¾ cup cooked enriched cereal, such as grits or cornmeal
- ½ to ¾ cup enriched noodles, macaroni, or spaghetti
- ¾ cup enriched ready-to-eat cereal
- ½ to ¾ cup rice, enriched or converted
- 1 large enriched flour tortilla
- 2 small corn tortillas

To ensure an adequate daily food intake, plan to eat one serving of each of the four groups at breakfast, lunch, and dinner. This allows you an additional serving as a snack each day from Groups 2, 3, and 4 throughout pregnancy, and an additional serving from Group 1 during the last five months. While eating three small meals and three snacks daily may seem excessive, food is more easily digested when served in this manner. It is not healthy for you or your baby to go without food for 8 or more hours. In addition to these recommendations, it is important that you not restrict salt intake and that you use only iodized salt.

You do not have to follow this meal outline fanatically. Some women need additional calories from extra servings or from fat such as butter, margarine, mayonnaise, or salad oil. Discuss your food intake and weight gain with your obstetrician during your prenatal visits.

Liquids are also important, and the drinking of four to six cups of water, broth, tea (one cup maximum daily), or coffee (one cup maximum daily) each day should be encouraged. When shopping for snacks, buy nutritious foods, such as raisins, raw vegetables, nuts, and fruits, and avoid high-calorie, low-nutrition foods, such as candy, cookies, pies, and soft drinks. Processed and refined carbohydrates, such as foods with large amounts of table sugar, provide more "empty calories" than natural carbohydrates. Try not to cook all fruits and vegetables because it will only reduce their vitamin C content.

How important is dietary fiber for the pregnant woman?

Constipation is one of the most frequent discomforts plaguing the pregnant woman. Often the result of diminished intestinal peristalsis which accompanies pregnancy, it is accentuated by the use of iron-containing multivitamins and supplements. Constipation in turn worsens the discomfort caused by enlarging hemorrhoids. Diets rich in fiber help to relieve constipation and prevent conditions associated with fiber-poor diets, such as diverticulitis, hiatus hernia, hemorrhoids, varicosities, and possibly even bowel cancer, heart disease, and diabetes.

There is no RDA for dietary fiber, but adequate amounts can be obtained by a pregnant woman if she eats several servings from a variety of fiber-rich foods such as whole-grain breads and cereals, fruits, vegetables, legumes, and nuts. Fiber is not absorbed by the small intestine but passes through the digestive tract unaltered. Since it is bulky and devoid of energy, it tends to produce satiety without providing excess calories. This benefit is especially significant for overweight women concerned about excessive weight gain during pregnancy.

Can a vegetarian receive adequate nutrition during pregnancy?

There is evidence which suggests that vegetarian diets may prove critical in the prevention of diseases, such as heart disease, cancer, obesity, and osteoporosis, or loss of bone density. In my private obstetrical practice, I have been impressed by the excellent health, knowledge of nutrition, and pregnancy outcome of the vegetarians under my care. My observations are supported by a 1987 report published in the *Southern Medical Journal* in which doctors compared the pregnancy outcome of 775 vegetarians and a control group of women consuming a regular diet. Surprisingly, the two groups were identical in terms of maternal weight gain, length of pregnancy, average newborn birth weight, and Apgar scores (see Chapter 11). One fascinating finding was that only 1 of the 775 vegetarian mothers developed preeclampsia (pregnancy-induced hypertension), an incidence significantly lower than that in the general population.

The main concern is that the vegetarian receive adequate amounts of good-quality protein. The quality of a protein is determined by the amount that is available to the body for use and the number of eight smaller units, called amino acids, which it contains. Protein foods of animal origin are called high-quality proteins because they contain these eight amino acids in optimum amounts which are easily available to the body. Cereal grain proteins favored by vegetarians are considered to be "low-quality" because they lack one of the eight important amino acids, lysine. Fortunately, legumes such as dried beans and peas contain large amounts of lysine, but they are also low-quality proteins because they are deficient in an amino acid named methionine. If cereal and legume proteins are eaten together, the vegetarian will be ingesting a protein of better quality than if either product is eaten alone. If this mixing of proteins is carried out throughout pregnancy, the nutritional value obtained will approach that of the high-quality animal protein eaten by the nonvegetarian. The more liberal vegetarian diet can provide adequate protein with two daily servings of eggs and dairy products. Two daily servings of high-protein nuts and peanut butter are recommended for the stricter vegetarian.

In addition to eating vegetables and grains, the total vegetarian can obtain more daily protein by eating one of the following:

- 1 cup soybeans plus 12 ounces soy milk or soy yogurt
- ½ pound tofu and 1 pint soy milk or soy yogurt
- 1 quart soy milk or soy yogurt and ½ cup soybeans
- 1 cup hydrated TVP (texturized vegetable protein) and 1 cup soy milk or soy yogurt

Additional protein for the lacto-vegetarian is more easily obtained by daily amounts of the following:

- 2 cups cottage cheese
- 1 quart skim milk, low-fat yogurt, or buttermilk

The diet of a total vegetarian may be deficient in calcium, iron, riboflavin, vitamin B_{12}, vitamin D, and zinc. While it is important to try to meet the pregnancy demands for these vitamins with substitute foods, the amounts obtained from available food sources are often inadequate. For this reason, it is important that all vegetarians, and total vegetarians in particular, take supplements containing the important vitamins and minerals.

The greatest risk to a vegetarian comes from dependence on the limited nutritional benefits of a single food source. Macrobiotic enthusiasts, whose diets consist mainly of grain and vegetables, are at great risk of protein, iron, and calcium deficiencies. It is especially important that such individuals take vitamin and mineral supplements throughout pregnancy.

▪ ▪ ▪ *9* ▪ ▪ ▪

MEDICATIONS

*A*lmost all chemical substances can cross the placenta and become concentrated in the fetus. Whether or not a drug causes harm depends on many factors, including the genetic makeup of mother and fetus, the specific chemical structure of the drug, the month of pregnancy in which the drug is used, and the total dose. There are a host of medications that damage the fetus only during early pregnancy, when organ and limb formation take place. Others cause harm only during the last three months, while a third group appears to be most dangerous when administered immediately before delivery.

Effects of medications on the baby do not end at childbirth, since many harmful substances can be rapidly transmitted from mother to nursing infant via the breast milk. Concentrations in the milk vary, depending on the blood supply to the breast, the quantity of milk produced, and the drug's chemical structure, dose, and frequency of administration. While some medications appear only in trace amounts, others are highly concentrated and potentially harmful to the infant, particularly during the baby's first month, when certain enzyme systems which normally metabolize and detoxify drugs are not fully developed.

The list of potentially harmful drugs is expanding daily, and, while a cause-and-effect relationship has not been clearly defined in all instances, the prudent woman should avoid all medication during pregnancy and nursing unless absolutely necessary. On the other hand, many medications have been proven to be safe for use during pregnancy and the postpartum period. Prescription drugs are a cause of less than 1 percent of congenital anomalies, yet many women assign unrealistically high risk to medications known to be harmless. To refuse treatment even when it is medically indicated and necessary is as dangerous as using drugs indiscriminately. When a woman unexpectedly conceives while taking one or more prescription drugs, she should immediately consult her physician regarding potential fetal hazards. Often questions about medications are complex and require an extensive review of the medical literature by a genetics counselor rather than your obstetrician.

This important chapter provides an up-to-date reference for the concerned woman who wants to be sure that any medication she takes is safe for her and her baby.

How does an obstetrician determine if it is safe for a woman to use a particular drug during pregnancy?

The United States Food and Drug Administration (FDA) has established five categories for drugs and medications with regard to possible adverse fetal effects. These are listed in Table 16.

While there are many flaws in this system, it remains more popular than any others that have been introduced to date. Unfortunately, only 40 percent of the drugs and medications listed in the popular *Physician's Desk Reference* (PDR) have been assigned to an FDA category. As a result, obstetricians and their patients are forced to rely on vague laboratory results or limited clinical studies when selecting most medications. Another pitfall of the FDA classification is that manufacturers are not legally bound to adhere to it and often assign their own more generous pregnancy-risk-factor classification to a particular product. One perfect example of this is trimethadione (trade name Tridione), a petit mal drug known to cause abortion and fetal anomalies. While experts agree that Tridione should have an X rating for use in pregnancy, the manufacturer has maintained a D pregnancy-risk-factor classification in its information pamphlets. Of those drugs which are FDA-classified, very few, such as prenatal vitamins, fall into category A. A larger number of drugs fall into category B, and most physicians will not hesitate to prescribe them during pregnancy. From a doctor's point of view, category C is the most difficult to utilize in everyday practice. Unfortunately, the majority of medications commonly needed during pregnancy fall into this category. Although a layperson might be appalled to learn that category D drugs are commonly prescribed during pregnancy, there are often no acceptable alternatives, and the risk encountered in not using them is often far greater. An example of such a drug is phenytoin (trade name Dilantin). Although phenytoin is associated with a risk of fetal abnormalities, grand mal seizures resulting from not using it pose a far greater risk to both the woman and her fetus.

TABLE 16

DEVELOPMENTAL TOXICITY OF DRUGS: DEFINITIONS FROM THE FDA

FDA Category	Definition
A	Controlled studies in women fail to demonstrate a risk to the fetus in the first trimester; there is no evidence of risk in later trimesters; and the possibility of fetal harm appears remote.
B	Either animal reproduction studies have not demonstrated a fetal risk, but there are no controlled studies in pregnant women, or animal reproduction studies have shown an adverse effect (other than decreased fertility) that was not confirmed in controlled studies in women in the first trimester and there is no evidence of a risk in later trimesters.
C	Either studies in animals have revealed adverse effects on the fetus (teratogenic, embryocidal, or other) and there are no controlled studies in women, or studies in women and animals are not available. The drug should be given only if the potential benefit justifies the potential risk to the fetus.
D	There is positive evidence of human fetal risk, but the benefits from use in pregnant women may be acceptable despite the risk—for example, if the drug is needed in a life-threatening situation or for a serious disease for which safer drugs cannot be used or are ineffective.
X	Studies in animals or human beings have demonstrated fetal abnormalities or there is evidence of fetal risk based on human experience or both, and the risk of the use of the drug in pregnant women clearly outweighs any of the benefits. The drug is contraindicated in women who are or may become pregnant.

ANTIBIOTICS

How safe are antibiotics for pregnant and nursing women?

After analgesics (see next section), antibiotics are the drugs most frequently used by pregnant women. Of all antibiotics prescribed, **penicillin** is one of the safest for use during pregnancy. In addition, there are the **synthetic penicillins,** such as ampicillin and amoxicillin, sold under a variety of trade names. Unlike penicillin, these drugs are effective against a broad spectrum of bacteria, such as those commonly associated with urinary and respiratory tract infections. Both penicillin and its synthetic derivatives are classified in category B for use during pregnancy, since both laboratory studies and clinical experience have failed to demonstrate any harmful fetal or maternal effects.

Penicillin, ampicillin, and amoxicillin are rapidly transferred to the breast milk. Babies born with a genetic susceptibility to develop a serious penicillin allergy at a later time may become initially sensitized to these medications while nursing. There are reports in the medical literature of babies who have developed skin rashes, itching, and diarrhea problems following breast-feeding when their mothers have been taking these drugs. For this reason, it is imperative that nursing infants whose mothers are being treated with these antibiotics be carefully and continuously observed for early signs of a drug reaction.

Other **penicillin derivatives** such as methicillin (trade name Staphcillin), oxacillin (trade name Prostaphlin), nafcillin (trade names Nafcil and Unipen), and cloxacillin (trade name Tegopen) are usually reserved for serious or resistant staphylococcus bacterial infections that threaten the life and health of the pregnant woman. The newest semisynthetic penicillin derivatives, known as acylaminopenicillins, have a broad spectrum of activity against many bacterial organisms. Members of this group include mezlocillin (trade name Mez-

lin), piperacillin sodium (trade name Pipracil), azlocillin (trade name Azlin), ticarcillin disodium (trade names Ticar and Timentin), and carbenicillin disodium (trade names Geopen and Pyopen). The safety of all of these penicillin derivatives for use during pregnancy has not been documented, but they do appear to be safe for the developing fetus and nursing infant.

Cephalosporins (trade names Keflex, Duricef, and Ceclor) are a group of antibiotics which have been used extensively by physicians in recent years. Studies show that in the usual therapeutic doses they cross the placenta and produce significant blood levels in the fetus. To date, however, no toxic effects have been reported. Although far less data are available about the safety of cephalosporins when compared to penicillin, most experts believe that they are equally safe for use by pregnant women; they are also placed in category B of the FDA classification. All the cephalosporins are excreted in the breast milk during lactation. To date, laboratory animal studies and human experience have not demonstrated adverse effects on the nursing infant.

Bacterial resistance to penicillins, cephalosporins, and related antibiotics have increased in recent years because many organisms have developed beta-lactamase enzymes that can inactivate these drugs. To counteract this, chemists have developed a new class of antibiotics named **beta-lactamase inhibitors** which, when combined with broad-spectrum antibiotics, block the bacterial enzyme and allow the antibiotic to destroy the bacteria. Clavulanate and sulbactam are the two beta-lactamase inhibitors currently in commercial use. Timentin is the trade name for the combination of clavulanate potassium and the semisynthetic penicillin named ticarcillin. Augmentin combines clavulanate potassium and amoxicillin. Unasyn contains ampicillin and sulbactam. Although there are no well-controlled studies regarding the safety of beta-lactamase inhibitors during pregnancy or lactation, reproductive studies on mice, rats, and rabbits given up to ten times the human dose have not caused impaired fertility or harm to the fetus or nursing infant. All these drugs are listed in category B for use in pregnancy.

Erythromycin is an old and popular antibiotic which is often prescribed for individuals who are allergic to penicillin. Like penicillin, erythromycin has a category B rating for safety in pregnancy. It crosses the placenta in far lower concentrations than does penicillin, and to date there have been no reports of fetal abnormalities or illness resulting from its use during pregnancy. While erythromycin is generally a very safe antibiotic, it may cause impaired though reversible liver dysfunction and a condition called cholestatic hepatitis. Of the erythromycin compounds, erythromycin estolate (trade name Ilosone) is most often associated with this complication. The symptoms—jaundice, severe generalized itching of the skin, weakness, nausea, vomiting, abdominal cramps, and fever—subside when the antibiotic is stopped.

The hormonal changes of pregnancy can cause changes in the liver similar to those produced with Ilosone, and some susceptible women suffer from what is termed recurrent cholestasis during each pregnancy, with symptoms ranging from mild discomfort to severe itching and marked jaundice. Erythromycins in general, and Ilosone in particular, are best avoided by these women and by any women with a history of liver disease. For the pregnant woman who does not have a history of liver disease, erythromycin preparations other than Ilosone can be safely used.

Sulfonamides such as sulfisoxazole, more commonly known by its trade name Gantrisin, are very effective in treating urinary tract infections. Sulfonamides readily cross the placenta to the fetus during all stages of pregnancy, and significant levels may persist in a newborn for several days after birth when the drug is given in the days prior to delivery. Toxicity in the newborn, manifested as jaundice and hemolytic anemia, can be severe;

and for this reason sulfonamides should not be used during the last month of pregnancy. Premature infants are especially susceptible to this complication, so if a woman is at risk of premature labor or has a history of premature labor, it is probably best that she avoid sulfonamides during the last trimester. Aside from this precaution, sulfonamide use at all other times during pregnancy can be considered safe. Based on this information, the sulfonamide risk classification changes from a B for the first 8 months of pregnancy to a D during the last month. Sulfonamides are excreted into breast milk in low concentrations and do not pose a risk to the healthy full-term newborn. However, they are best avoided in breast-feeding women who give birth to premature or ill infants or those who experience jaundice during the first days of life.

Some of the sulfonamide preparations are combined in a single tablet with another drug named **trimethoprim.** The trade names of this popular combination are Septra and Bactrim. Trimpex and Proloprim, which contain only trimethoprim, are also effective antibacterial agents. These, and all drugs which contain trimethoprim, are assigned a pregnancy-risk-factor classification of C for use in pregnancy. Although trimethoprim crosses the placenta and produces similar drug levels in fetal and maternal serum and the amniotic fluid, it has not been associated with congenital malformations. Nevertheless, it is best avoided during pregnancy, especially in the first trimester, because it is a folic acid antagonist. Other drugs in this category have the theoretical potential to cause developmental anomalies. Trimethoprim is excreted in breast milk in low concentrations, and the American Academy of Pediatrics considers it to be compatible with breast-feeding.

Pyridium and **Urised** are the trade names of two urinary anesthetics which are used to relieve symptoms of painful urinary tract infections. Pyridium is available combined with sulfonamides in medications with such trade names as Azo Gantanol and Azo Gantrisin. Pyridium and Urised can safely be taken during pregnancy or breast-feeding.

Tetracyclines are popularly used to treat infections in nonpregnant individuals. However, they are among the most dangerous drugs when prescribed during pregnancy. Deaths from liver failure have been reported in pregnant women given large doses of intravenous tetracyclines as treatment for severe kidney infections.

There are several types of tetracyclines, including familiar products such as Achromycin, Aureomycin, Declomycin, Minocin, Sumycin, Terramycin, and Vibramycin. All are equally dangerous.

Tetracyclines rapidly cross the placenta and, when prescribed during the last half of pregnancy, may be incorporated into fetal bones and teeth during the process of calcification. This may cause a yellow-green discoloration of the deciduous (baby) teeth, underdevelopment of tooth enamel, and a decrease in the growth of the long bones of the fetus. Deciduous teeth will not become stained if a pregnant woman stops using tetracycline after the first trimester. Furthermore, since calcification of the permanent teeth does not begin until after delivery, they can't be stained by tetracyclines taken at any time during pregnancy. While the dental staining caused by in utero exposure to tetracyclines appears to be only of cosmetic significance, of far greater concern is the demonstration of a significant and sometimes irreversible depression of bone growth. Based on these findings, tetracyclines have received a D pregnancy-risk-factor classification from the FDA.

Tetracyclines are excreted in breast milk in very low concentrations. Theoretically, dental staining and inhibition of bone growth could occur in breast-fed infants whose mothers are consuming tetracyclines. However, this theoretical possibility seems remote, and the American Academy of Pediatrics considers tetracyclines to be compatible with breast-feeding.

Chloramphenicol (trade name Chloromycetin) is a potent broad-spectrum antibiotic which is rarely used today because it can cause an unusual but potentially fatal suppression of blood cell formation in the bone marrow. It is metabolized well by the mother but poorly handled by the infant. A high concentration of chloramphenicol in a newborn, especially a premature infant, may result in the "gray baby syndrome," also known as the "gray syndrome," in which 40 percent of affected infants die within a few hours after the onset of symptoms. When the fetus is in utero, the maternal liver enzyme system is able to detoxify the drug, and "gray baby syndrome" does not occur. Chloramphenicol has an FDA pregnancy-risk-factor classification of C. However, there are far safer alternative medications for use during pregnancy, and chloramphenicol is best avoided. Chloramphenicol is excreted in breast milk, and, although its effects on the nursing infant are unknown, it should not be given to a breast-feeding woman.

Nitrofurantoin (trade names Macrodantin and Furadantin) is a drug that has been commonly used for treating urinary tract infections for the past 35 years. Several reports, including the manufacturer's extensive records of more than 1,700 women treated with nitrofurantoin at various stages of pregnancy, have failed to show any evidence of congenital defects or fetal toxicity. As a result, nitrofurantoin has received an FDA pregnancy-risk-factor classification of B. Nitrofurantoin excretion in breast milk is negligible, and the American Academy of Pediatrics considers it to be compatible with breast-feeding.

Nalidixic acid is another popular urinary antibiotic which is more commonly known by its trade name NegGram. As with nitrofurantoin, extensive laboratory and clinical experience with nalidixic acid over many years has produced no harmful fetal effects, and it too has a B pregnancy-risk-factor classification. Nalidixic acid is excreted in breast milk in low concentrations, and maternal ingestion is compatible with breast-feeding.

Nalidixic acid is classified chemically as a fluoroquinolone, or quinolone. Although its efficacy is limited to bacteria causing urinary tract infections, other recently introduced **fluoroquinolones**, such as norfloxacin (trade name Noroxin), ciprofloxacin (trade names Cipro and Perfloxacin), and ofloxacin (trade name Floxin), are potent broad-spectrum antibiotics capable of curing a variety of serious bacterial infections throughout the body. Since little is known about the safety of using the newer quinolones during pregnancy and nursing, it is better to use an older, more established drug whenever possible. Quinolones have been given a pregnancy-risk-factor classification of C, but limited research concerning their safety is somewhat disturbing. For example, immature dogs, rats, and other animal species treated with quinolones experienced degenerative changes in the cartilage of their weight-bearing joints and permanent lameness. Quinolones are believed to be excreted in breast milk in very low concentrations. Nevertheless, they should be avoided in the nursing woman until more is known about their safety.

Clindamycin hydrochloride (trade name Cleocin HCl) is an antibiotic which is unique in its ability to destroy a variety of anaerobic bacteria, which live and reproduce within necrotic tissue and abscesses containing no oxygen. (The most infamous anaerobic bacterium, named *Bacteroides fragilis*, is the culprit in many life-threatening infections.) Experience with clindamycin among pregnant women is limited, but there are no reports linking the antibiotic to congenital defects or fetal complications. It does cross the placenta, and umbilical cord levels in the baby reach approximately half that in the maternal serum. Clindamycin has been given a B pregnancy-risk-factor classification for use in pregnancy. Although clindamycin is excreted in breast milk, the American Academy of Pediatrics considers its use to be compatible with breast-feeding.

The **aminoglycosides** are a group of potent antibiotics which are frequently used to treat serious bacterial infections. They are administered intramuscularly and intravenously and are therefore practically always limited to use within the hospital or a closely supervised outpatient regimen. Streptomycin is the oldest in the group; while still used in the treatment of tuberculosis, it has been replaced in most other instances of infection by newer aminoglycosides such as amikacin sulfate (trade name Amikin), gentamicin sulfate (trade name Garamycin), kanamycin sulfate (trade name Kantrex), and tobramycin sulfate (trade names Nebcin and Tobrex). One great fear associated with aminoglycoside use is that they have the capacity to damage the eighth cranial nerve in the brain. This nerve, named the auditory nerve, is responsible for hearing and balance. Another concern is that prolonged use of aminoglycosides may cause nephrotoxicity, or kidney damage.

All aminoglycosides readily cross the placenta and have the capacity to damage the infant's auditory nerve. To date, there have been more than 30 cases of hearing deficit and auditory nerve damage in infants exposed to streptomycin in utero. Similar effects have been noted for kanamycin. In one report of 391 women who received kanamycin during pregnancy, 9 children, or 2.3 percent, were found to have hearing loss. Interestingly, gentamicin, tobramycin, and amikacin have not been reported to produce auditory nerve damage. This difference may reflect less frequent use, lack of adequate studies, or both. Streptomycin has been implicated in causing spinal cord and bone abnormalities in experimental animals and human beings. The other aminoglycosides have not been similarly indicted. Of all the aminoglycosides, gentamicin has become the most valuable to the obstetrician for treating amnionitis and severe kidney infections during pregnancy, and for prophylactic treatment of mitral valve prolapse and other conditions in which the heart valves are in danger of becoming infected. Studies have demonstrated that gentamicin rapidly crosses the placenta and enters the fetal circulation and amniotic fluid, although no harmful fetal effects have been reported to date. For this reason, gentamicin has been classified by the FDA in category C, while all the other aminoglycosides have been assigned a more restrictive D category.

The longer the fetus is exposed to aminoglycosides, the more likely is the risk of auditory nerve damage. If these antibiotics must be used—and often there is no adequate substitute—they should be administered at the lowest possible effective dose for as short a time as possible. In addition, blood levels of the aminoglycoside should be measured and kidney function evaluated frequently. Since aminoglycosides can be transferred to an infant in maternal breast milk, I advise against nursing if these drugs must be used.

Vancomycin is a potent antibiotic which is often necessary for prophylactically treating penicillin-allergic individuals with mitral valve prolapse and other cardiac conditions in order to prevent damage to the valves of the heart. In a 1989 study published in the *American Journal of Obstetrics and Gynecology*, doctors administered vancomycin to ten pregnant women during the second and third trimesters and found no evidence of impaired hearing or kidney damage in the exposed infants. Vancomycin has a category C pregnancy-risk-factor classification. It is excreted in breast milk, but since its effects on the nursing infant are unknown, it is best avoided.

Newer classes of potent broad-spectrum antibiotics continue to be introduced each year. Often too little is known about them to endorse their use during pregnancy or lactation. One such drug is Primaxin, a combination of the antibiotic imipenem and cilastatin sodium. Imipenem is the first of a class of **carbapenem** antibiotics. Others are bound to be introduced in the near future. Although Primaxin has an FDA pregnancy-risk-factor classification of C and does not cause birth defects when given to laboratory animals in high doses, there are no human studies to support its safety. Another broad-spectrum intravenous antibiotic is aztreonam (trade name Azactam), a member of a new antibiotic group classified as **monobactams.** While aztreonam has also been given an FDA pregnancy-risk-factor classification of C, the manufacturer is quick to point out that it does not know if aztreonam can harm the fetus or nursing infant. The manufacturer suggests that it not be taken by a woman who is nursing.

Table 17 summarizes the safety and risks with the antibiotics discussed above.

Are there any commonly prescribed anti-infective agents which adversely affect either pregnancy or nursing?

Metronidazole (trade names Flagyl and Protostat) has been mentioned as a valuable drug in the treatment of trichomoniasis, nonspecific vaginitis (see Chapter 6), parasitic diseases, and a variety of serious bacterial infections. The use of metronidazole in pregnancy is controversial. While the majority of case reports and reviews have concluded that it is safe, a small number of studies have linked its use to a higher incidence of spontaneous abortions and birth defects. Metronidazole has also been found to be carcinogenic in rodents; although no such association has been found in humans, that is reason enough to avoid its use if at all possible. Many obstetricians, the Centers for Disease Control, and even the manufacturers of metronidazole believe that its pregnancy-risk-factor classification of B is far too generous. In fact, it should never be used to treat trichomoniasis or nonspecific vaginitis during the first trimester, and it is probably best avoided during the second and third trimesters as well. When administered to pregnant women, metronidazole is excreted in the breast milk. The subsequent effects on the infant are unknown. When a single therapeutic dose is taken by a nursing woman, it reaches maximum concentrations in her breast milk 2 to 4 hours later. Studies suggest that metronidazole can probably be taken if nursing is delayed for 12 to 24 hours, when the levels in the milk are minimal.

Antituberculosis drugs may also pose problems. Isoniazid (trade name INH) is an integral part of the plan for treating individuals who contract tuberculosis or whose skin test converts from negative to positive. Duration of treatment is usually 6 to 12 months. One study found twice the expected rate of malformations in a small series of women treated with isoniazid during the first trimester. Other larger studies, including one in which 4,900 women received isoniazid during pregnancy, showed no evidence of fetal anomalies or adverse

TABLE 17

SAFETY OF ANTIBIOTICS DURING PREGNANCY AND NURSING

Drug Class	Generic and Trade Names of Drugs	Suggestions for Pregnancy and Risk Category	Suggestions for Nursing
Aminoglycosides	amikacin (Amikin) gentamicin (Garamycin) kanamycin (Kantrex) streptomycin, tobramycin (Nebein, Tobrex)	All aminoglycosides readily cross the placenta and may cause damage to the auditory nerve of the fetus. Garamycin, category C, possibly safest; all others category D; use only if absolutely necessary for shortest period of time.	Aminoglycosides found in breast milk; best not to nurse if they are used.
Carbapenems	Primoxin (imipenem and cilastatin)	Category C; too little known about it to endorse its use.	Breast milk levels 1% those found in maternal serum.
Cephalosporins	cefazolin (Ancef, Keflex) cefalexin (Keflex) cefadroxil (Duricef) cefaclor (Ceclor) cefotetan (Cefotan) cefamandole (Mandol) cefuroxime axetil (Ceftin) cefoperazone (Cefobid) cefotaxime (Claforan) ceftriaxone (Rocephin) moxabactam (Moxam) ceftizoxime (Cefizox) cephradine (Velosef, Anspor)	Category B; considered safe for use.	Safe for use.
Chloramphenicol	chloramphenicol (Chloromycetin)	Category C; "gray baby syndrome" may occur in newborns; should not be taken in pregnancy.	Found in concentrations in breast milk; not to be taken if nursing.
Clindamycin hydrochloride	clindamycin (Cleocin HCl)	Category B: safe for use.	Excreted in breast milk.

Erythromycin	erythromycin (Ilotycin, Pediamycin, Pediazole, Robimycin, E-Mycin) erythromycin estolate (Ilosone) erythromycin ethylsuccinate (E.E.S., E-Mycine, WyamycinE) erythromycin stearate (Erythrocin, Bristamycin; Ethril, SK-Erythromycin, Pfizer-E Film Coated Tablets)	Category B: safe for use except for erythromycin estolate, may cause liver disorders and cholestatic hepatitis.	Safe for use except if woman has history of liver disease.
Fluoroquinolones	Norfloxacin (Noroxin) ciprofloxacin (Cipro) ofloxacin (Floxin)	Category C; causes artliopathy in immature laboratory animals; avoid if safer options available.	Found in low concentrations in breast milk; avoid if possible.
Monobactams	aztreonam (Azactam)	Category C; too little known about it to endorse its use.	Found in concentrations 1% of maternal serum; too little known to endorse use.
Nalidixic Acid	nalidixic acid (NegGram)	Category B; though clinically similar to fluoroquinolones, extensive use in pregnancy with no adverse fetal effects; safe for use.	Excreted in breast milk in low concentrations; 1 reported case of hemolytic anemia in nursing infant with GGPD deficiency; considered safe.
Nitrofurantoins	nitrofurantoin (Furadantin, Macrodantin)	Category B; safe for use despite theoretical risk of hemolytic anemia in babies with GGPD deficiency or low glutathione levels.	Negligible amounts in breast milk; safe for use.
Penicillins	penicillin G (Bicillin, Wycillin) penicillin V (Betapen-VK, Pen VeeK, Veetids, Ledercillin)	Category B; safe for use.	Safe for use.

TABLE 17 (continued)

SAFETY OF ANTIBIOTICS DURING PREGNANCY AND NURSING

Drug Class	Generic and Trade Names of Drugs	Suggestions for Pregnancy and Risk Category	Suggestions for Nursing
Synthetic penicillins	amoxicillin (Amoxil, Wynox, Polymox) ampicillin (Polycillin, Omnipen, Principen) methicillin (Staphcillin) cloxacillin (Tegopen) nafcillin (Nafcil, Unipen) piperacillin (Pipracil) azlocillin (Azlin) mezlocillin (Mezlin) ticarcillin (Ticar) carbenicillin (Geopen, Pyopen)	Category B; safe for use.	Safe for use but nursing mothers may develop rash, itching, or diarrhea on rare occasions.
Synthetic penicillins and beta-lactamase inhibitors	ticarcillin and clavulanate (Timentin) amoxicillin and sulbactam (Augmentin) ampicillin and sulbactim (Unasyn)	Category B; safe for use.	Same precautions as above.
Sulfonamides	sulfadiazine (Microsulfon) sulfamethizole (Thiosulfil, Urobiotic) sulfamethoxazole (Gantanol, AzoGantanol) sulfasalazine (Azulfidine) sulfisoxazole (Gantrisin, AzoGantrisin)	Category B for first 8 months, but avoid in last month because of neonatal jaundice risk.	Usually safe but avoid if baby premature, ill, or jaundiced.
Sulfonamide combinations	sulfamethoxozole and trimethoprim (Septra, Bactrim)	Category C; see sulfonamide information above; trimethoprim best avoided in first trimester.	Excreted in breast milk in low concentrations; trimethoprim safe for nursing but exercise above precautions with sulfonamides.

Tetracyclines	doxycycline (Doryx, Vibramycin, Vibra-Tabs) tetracycline (Achromycin, Sumycin) minocycline (Minocin) oxytetracycline (Terramycin)	Category D; avoid throughout pregnancy but especially the last 5 months; causes discoloration of baby teeth, underdevelopment of tooth enamel and decrease in growth of long bones.	Very low concentrations in breast milk; risk to nursing infants teeth and bones more theoretical than real; probably safe.
Trimethoprim	trimethoprim (Trimpex, Proloprim)	As above.	As above.
Vancomycin	vancomycin (Vancocin, Vancor)	Category C; use only for those who need prophylaxis for potential heart valve infection and are allergic to penicillin.	Excreted in breast milk; effects on infant unknown, therefore best avoided.

pregnancy outcomes. An association between isoniazid and hemorrhagic disease of the newborn has also been suspected in two infants. Although other reports of this potentially serious reaction have not been found, prophylactic vitamin K is recommended for exposed babies at birth. Isoniazid has a pregnancy-risk-factor classification of C, and much remains to be learned about its effects on the fetus. Untreated tuberculosis, however, remains a far greater threat to a pregnant women and her fetus than does treatment of the disease. Although the use of isoniazid is not restricted if a woman is breast-feeding, babies should be carefully observed for adverse effects which include vomiting, hepatitis, and neurological abnormalities. The American Academy of Pediatrics considers isoniazid to be compatible with breast-feeding.

Rifampin (trade names Rifadin, Rifamate, and Rimactane) is often combined with isoniazid in the treatment of tuberculosis. It, too, has a pregnancy-risk-factor classification of C. Rifampin crosses the placenta to the fetus in significant amounts, but experience with hundreds of women treated during pregnancy has shown no evidence of congenital anomalies. Since only a very small percentage of rifampin given to a women enters her breast milk, it is considered safe for nursing mothers.

If its pregnancy-risk-factor classification of B is any indication of its safety, **ethambutol** (trade name Myambutol) should be safer than isoniazid and rifampin for treating tuberculosis during pregnancy. Clinical experience with hundreds of women have confirmed that this is true. Ethambutol is excreted in breast milk, but the American Academy of Pediatrics considers it to be compatible with breast-feeding.

Ethionamide (trade name Trecator-SC) is used in the treatment of active tuberculosis when the usual medications fail to adequately eradicate the disease. If at all possible, it should be avoided during pregnancy. In one human study, 7 of 23 infants born of mothers treated with ethionamide had anomalies, most commonly of the brain and spinal cord.

Para-aminosalicylic acid (PAS) is no longer as frequently used to treat tuberculosis. Despite one report showing congenital defects in 5 of 43 infants exposed to PAS in pregnancy, most experts agree that it is not harmful to the pregnant woman or her fetus. **Pyrazinamide** is a new and increasingly popular antituberculous agent. Unfortunately, there are no reports of its safety during pregnancy or nursing.

How safe is acyclovir during pregnancy?

Acyclovir (trade name Zovirax) is the only agent capable of effectively treating herpes infections. Whether the drug is administered orally or intravenously, it readily crosses the placenta to the fetus. Acyclovir has been used during all stages of pregnancy, and no adverse fetal effects have been attributed to it. Laboratory research on rats, mice, and hamsters have also failed to produce birth defects or chromosomal damage. Despite this, it has an FDA pregnancy-risk-factor classification of C and should be used only for severe, disseminated life-threatening infections and not outbreaks confined to the genitals during pregnancy.

In 1988, scientists at the University of Utah School of Medicine and Research Triangle Park in North Carolina confirmed the findings of previous studies showing that the concentration of acyclovir in a woman's breast milk is actually more than three times greater than that in her serum. Despite this, no harmful effects have been noted, and a woman receiving acyclovir for a herpes infection can continue to breast-feed her baby.

 ANALGESICS

Analgesics, medications used to relieve pain, are the most commonly prescribed class of drugs during pregnancy, labor and delivery, and the postpartum period.

How safe is aspirin during pregnancy?

Aspirin, or acetylsalicylic acid, is a member of a class of drugs known as salicylates. Until recently, aspirin and salicylate-containing products were consumed by approximately 80 percent of women at some time during pregnancy. While doctors now caution their patients to strictly avoid salicylates, many women fail to heed this advice. Aspirin is an ingredient in a great number of analgesics, including Anacin, Arthritis Pain Formula, Ascriptin, Empirin, Bufferin, Darvon, Alka-Seltzer, Ecotrin, Equagesic, Fiorinal, Percodan, Excedrin, 4-Way Cold Tablets, Norgesic, Soma Compound, Synalgos-DC, Talwin Compound, Vanquish Analgesic Caplets, and Robaxisal. Pepto-Bismol, a popular product for relief of heartburn, indigestion, and traveler's diarrhea, contains bismuth subsalicylate, which is closely related to other salicylates and should not be used during pregnancy.

Laboratory studies on rats and mice given extremely high doses of aspirin early in pregnancy have demonstrated a greater incidence of malformations, although evidence of human malformations is lacking. Reported abnormalities associated with first-trimester aspirin use in animals have included cleft palate and cleft lip, skeletal and facial defects, anencephaly, intestinal abnormalities, and congenital heart disease. Although the data from epidemiologic studies are contradictory, the largest report ever conducted in the United States, involving more than 50,000 pregnant women, found no relationship between first-trimester aspirin use and congenital malformations. In another report published in the *New England Journal of Medicine* in 1989, doctors at Boston University School of Medicine found no link between aspirin use during the first trimester and congenital heart disease.

Use of aspirin during the third trimester is far more hazardous to a woman and her baby than it is during the first six months, as reflected in the change of its pregnancy-risk-factor classification from C to D for the final three months. Aspirin readily crosses the placenta, and significant salicylate concentrations can be found in the cord blood and the newborn's bloodstream. The most serious complication associated with aspirin use late in pregnancy is an alteration in blood platelet adhesiveness, resulting in a higher incidence of maternal anemia and bleeding both before and after delivery, as well as a greater risk of intracranial hemorrhage and death in the newborn infant. Other reported newborn bleeding complications include minute hemorrhages on the skin, blood in the urine, a collection of blood under the scalp, hemorrhage below the conjunctiva of the eye, and hemorrhage from circumcision sites. These complications are especially likely to occur when aspirin is used chronically in significant amounts of more than ten tablets per day, but research has shown that maternal ingestion of as little as 325 milligrams (one adult aspirin) within five days of delivery may cause abnormal platelet changes which could last four to seven days. Premature infants are especially susceptible to intracranial hemorrhage if their mothers take aspirin prior to delivery. For this reason it should not be used during the second half of pregnancy in any woman with a history of premature labor or a likelihood of delivering early.

While a host of obstetrical complications have been attributed to use of daily doses of aspirin greater than one adult tablet or 300 milligrams, researchers have found that amounts of aspirin in the range of 60 to 150 milligrams may help to prevent premature labor, intrauterine growth retardation (IUGR), and preeclampsia. To date, these benefits have been attained without any of the negative effects associated with salicylate use during pregnancy. Though these preliminary reports are encouraging, experts are not yet ready to endorse the use of aspirin as a means of preventing these obstetrical complications.

Prostaglandins are chemical substances produced by the body which have the capacity to stimulate strong uterine contractions. Aspirin is one of several drugs which are classified as prostaglandin synthetase inhibitors. This means that it inactivates the enzymes needed to convert other chemicals to prostaglandins. As a result, when aspirin is taken late in pregnancy, it may actually delay the onset of labor, diminish the strength and frequency of uterine contractions, and increase the length of labor. Prostaglandin synthetase inhibitors, including aspirin, have also been implicated in causing the premature closure or narrowing of a fetal blood vessel near the heart named the ductus arteriosus, which can lead to a serious heart and lung disease in the newborn called pulmonary hypertension. In addition to aspirin, other prostaglandin synthetase inhibitors, medically classified as nonsteroidal anti-inflammatory agents, should also be avoided during pregnancy. These include ibuprofen (trade names Motrin, Advil, Motrin IB, and Nuprin), mefenamic acid (trade name Ponstel), naproxen (trade names Anaprox and Naprosyn), indomethacin (trade name Indocin), diflunisal (trade name Dolobid), sulindac (trade name Clinoril), tolmetin (trade name Tolectin), meclofenamate (trade name Meclomen), piroxicam (trade name Feldene), and flurbiprofen (trade name Ansaid).

Although aspirin is excreted in breast milk, in normal therapeutic doses the effects on a nursing infant would appear to be minimal. However, high maternal doses of more than 15 aspirins per day may cause a baby to develop a generalized body rash and respiratory distress. Research has demonstrated that aspirin and other salicylates reach peak levels in the breast milk two hours after peak levels are attained in the maternal bloodstream. In addition, salicylates are eliminated from the breast milk at a much slower rate. Trace amounts of aspirin can be detected in a woman's breast milk as late as 24 hours after she ingests as little as one aspirin. Despite this, there has never been a case report of a nursing infant suffering from platelet dysfunction or bleeding secondary to maternal aspirin use. The American Academy of Pediatrics recommends that aspirin be used cautiously by a woman during lactation because of potential, but highly unlikely, adverse effects to the nursing infant. If you nurse and use aspirin, you can minimize the risk to your baby by taking it just after nursing, since most of the drug will be metabolized by the next feeding several hours later.

What safe alternatives are there to aspirin for pain relief during pregnancy?

Acetaminophen (trade names Tylenol, Datril, and Phenaphen) does not produce the adverse reactions associated with aspirin use. A safe nonprescription analgesic for short-term use during all trimesters of pregnancy, acetaminophen has a category B pregnancy-risk-factor classification. However, continuous high daily doses may be associated with severe maternal anemia and fatal kidney disease in the newborn. The American Academy of Pediatrics considers acetaminophen to be compatible with breast-feeding.

Phenacetin is an analgesic found in combination with other medications such as aspirin and caffeine. It is metabolized mainly to acetaminophen. It, too, has a pregnancy-risk-factor classification of B. Phenacetin is also considered safe for the breast-feeding woman.

Propoxyphene is the scientific name for one of the most commonly used and abused analgesics prescribed in the United States. Medications which contain propoxyphene include all compounds containing the name Darvon and Darvocet. Wygesic, another frequently used pain medication, contains propoxyphene and acetaminophen. Since the safety of propoxyphene during the first two trimesters of pregnancy has not been established, it has been assigned a pregnancy-risk-factor classification of C. However, there are case reports in the medical literature in which chronic use by pregnant women has resulted in withdrawal symptoms in their newborns. Most researchers conclude that this will not occur if the drug is taken in normal therapeutic doses. Three case reports have linked the use of propoxyphene during pregnancy to congenital abnormalities, but an extensive study of more than 3,000 women exposed to the drug during pregnancy found no such relationship. Propoxyphene use is considered to be compatible with breast-feeding.

Pentazocine (trade names Talwin and Talacen) is a nonnarcotic analgesic which relieves moderate to severe pain. Although pentazocine is often used as a substitute for patients who are addicted, sensitive, or allergic to narcotics, drug dependence may develop following prolonged use. While the safety of pentazocine during pregnancy has not been fully established, there are no reports linking its use with congenital defects. The drug does cross the placenta, and umbilical cord blood levels usually reach a concentration of 40 to 70 percent of those found in the maternal circulation. Chronic maternal use toward the end of pregnancy has resulted in the birth of addicted newborns. For this reason, pentazocine's risk factor when used for prolonged periods in high doses just prior to the onset of labor is a D, compared to a B classification when used in moderate amounts earlier in pregnancy. Women given pentazocine only during labor have experienced no adverse effects. Similarly, their newborns have fared well. Despite this, the manufacturer suggests that the drug be used with caution in women delivering premature infants who are less able to metabolize and inactivate it. Pentazocine is not excreted in the breast milk, so it is an ideal analgesic for the nursing woman who is experiencing moderate to severe pain.

What are ergot alkaloids, and how can they affect the outcome of pregnancy and lactation?

Ergot alkaloids are a group of drugs commonly used for the relief of vascular and migraine headaches. Popular trade names are Cafergot (ergotamine tartrate and caffeine), Sansert (methysergide maleate), Wigraine (ergotamine tartrate and caffeine), and Ergostat (ergotamine tartrate). They should not be taken during pregnancy because they can cause severe uterine contractions, lack of fetal oxygen, and miscarriage. Bellergal-S is the trade name for tablets containing ergotamine tartrate, phenobarbital, and alkaloids of belladona. Although it is effective in the management of disorders characterized by nervous tension, it too should be avoided by the pregnant woman.

Ergot preparations have been reported to enter the breast milk in high concentrations and produce ergotism, or ergot poisoning, in nursing infants. Symptoms of ergotism include weakness, vomiting, diarrhea, weak pulse, and an unstable blood pressure. These drugs also significantly decrease the amount of breast milk.

How safe are the narcotic analgesics during pregnancy and labor?

Although the hazards of narcotic abuse on the outcome of pregnancy have been discussed (see Chapter 5), several of these drugs have been used with great success in the treatment of moderate to severe pain during pregnancy, labor, and the postpartum period.

Codeine is probably the most commonly prescribed narcotic during the first eight months of pregnancy. An even greater degree of pain relief may be safely obtained during pregnancy when codeine is combined with acetaminophen in a single pill. Empracet with Codeine, Phenaphen with Codeine, and Tylenol with Codeine are examples of this effective analgesic combination. Many cough medicines contain codeine as one of their constituents.

Codeine use during the first trimester has been linked to cleft palate and cleft lip in two separate studies. Other reports have found a questionable association with neonatal inguinal hernias, cardiac and circulatory system abnormalities, dislocated hip, and other musculoskeletal defects. One study found a relationship between second-trimester codeine use and gastrointestinal anomalies in the newborn. However, several other large studies involving thousands of pregnant women have failed to show a relationship between codeine and birth defects. As a result of these contradictory findings, codeine has a pregnancy-risk-factor classification of C; however, it changes to D when codeine is used for prolonged periods or in high doses toward the end of pregnancy because there are a few case reports documenting that codeine use in labor can cause neonatal respiratory depression and symptoms of codeine withdrawal.

Codeine passes through the breast milk in very small amounts that are probably insignificant. Consequently, when it is taken in normal therapeutic doses it will not depress the reflexes or respirations of the nursing infant.

Oxycodone is described in the pharmaceutical literature as a semisynthetic narcotic. It is the main ingredient of a pill named Percodan, one of the most abused drugs in the United States. There are no studies which demonstrate either the safety or potential harm of oxycodone on the developing fetus or nursing infant. However, the aspirin in Percodan should discourage a nursing woman from using this medication. The same may be said for Percodan-Demi, even though the dose of oxycodone is one-half that found in Percodan. Percocet is probably a safer alternative during pregnancy, since it contains oxycodone and acetaminophen rather than aspirin. To thoroughly confuse the consumer, there is a nonprescription product named Percogesic Analgesic Tablets for relief of mild to moderate pain. It contains acetaminophen and phenyltoloxamine citrate, but not oxycodone, as one might expect, so it is safe to use during all trimesters of pregnancy as well as the postpartum period. Oxycodone has a pregnancy-risk-factor classification of B, but, as with all other narcotics, this changes to D if it is used for prolonged periods or in high doses at the end of pregnancy.

Oxycodone is excreted into breast milk and reaches peak levels in 1.5 to 2 hours after it is ingested. For this reason, it is best to take an oxycodone-containing product immediately after nursing.

Hydrocodone is another synthetic narcotic analgesic which is combined with acetaminophen in a popular new product named Vicodin ES. Since hydrocodone is relatively new, practically nothing is known about its safety during pregnancy or lactation.

All narcotics pass rapidly from the maternal to the fetal circulation and brain tissues via the placenta. Unfortunately, the fetus metabolizes these drugs and transfers them back to the maternal circulation at a far slower rate than they are received. Narcotics used inappropriately during labor have caused respiratory depression, poor muscle tone, slowing of the heartbeat, and lowered body temperature in the newborn infant.

When a sedative or tranquilizer is used in combination with a narcotic to enhance the narcotic's action, the depressive effects on the baby may be greater. The most popular method for achieving pain relief and sedation during labor is to combine the narcotic meperidine (trade name Demerol) and the antihistamine promethazine (trade name Phenergan) either as an intravenous or intramuscular injection. In addition to providing sedation, promethazine is helpful in combating the nausea and vomiting often induced by meperidine. To minimize the risk of neonatal respiratory depression, the usual dose of each drug should be reduced. The use of narcotics during labor should be restricted in women with specific pregnancy problems such as prematurity and fetal growth retardation since their infants are known to be more sensitive to these drugs.

Meperidine (trade name Demerol), the most popular analgesic used during labor, is excreted into breast milk. In one study of a group of mothers who had received meperidine during labor, the breast-fed infants had higher saliva levels of the drug for up to 48 hours after birth than a similar group that was bottle-fed. When a nursing mother is given an intramuscular dose of meperidine, peak milk levels are reached 2 hours later. Though no adverse effects have been reported in a nursing infant following administration of meperidine to its mother, it is still wise to time the dose

in order to avoid the highest breast milk levels.

Sinusoidal fetal heart rate patterns, often indicative of distress, have been noted with some narcotics. In a 1986 report from Bowman Gray School of Medicine, doctors found a 10 percent incidence with meperidine, and an alarming 75 percent rate with butorphanol tartrate (trade name Stadol). Nalbuphine hydrochloride (trade name Nubain) is a relatively new narcotic analgesic that has also been linked to a sinusoidal heart rate abnormality in the fetus, although the exact incidence is presently unknown.

Most obstetricians have abandoned the use of intravenous and intramuscular **morphine** during labor because it is more likely than other narcotics to produce maternal nausea and infant respiratory depression. Morphine is occasionally helpful in inducing sleep and distinguishing between false labor and early latent phase contractions. However, most of the renewed interest in this narcotic has been the result of its use in epidural anesthetics (see Chapter 12).

Nalbuphine hydrochloride (trade name Nubain) is a relatively new analgesic. Its safety for use during pregnancy has not been confirmed, but animal reproductive studies and human experience have not uncovered any harmful fetal effects. While this drug has been used with success in the relief of pain during labor, it does cross the placenta and may be responsible for causing respiratory depression in the newborn. The safety of nalbuphine hydrochloride for the nursing infant remains unknown at the present time.

Fentanyl (trade name Sublimaze) is a relatively new short-acting narcotic analgesic which can be given as an intravenous or intramuscular injection as well as an epidural or spinal anesthetic. In one study comparing women in labor who received fentanyl every hour as needed to those not requiring analgesia, no statistical differences were found in newborn outcome in terms of the incidence of depressed respirations or Apgar scores. No data are available on the safety of fentanyl on the breast-fed infant, so it is best avoided.

ANTINAUSEANTS AND ANTIEMETICS

What can I do about morning sickness?

Almost 60 percent of all pregnant women experience some degree of nausea and vomiting in early pregnancy. For women pregnant for the first time, the incidence may be as high as 75 percent. While most cases of morning sickness respond to a variety of conservative approaches, home remedies, and helpful hints (see Chapter 2), these measures often prove inadequate for a significant number of women. While I share the concern of pregnant women that medication be taken only when absolutely necessary, it is also true that persistent vomiting can result in consequences far more detrimental to a woman and her fetus than those caused by careful use of drugs to relieve the symptoms.

The safest antinauseant is Emetrol, a pleasant-tasting, mint-flavored liquid available without prescription at any pharmacy. One or two tablespoons, taken at 15-minute intervals until nausea is relieved, is an extremely effective and absolutely safe course of action.

Bendectin was the name of the most popular product ever used for treating nausea and vomiting in pregnancy. It was voluntarily removed from the market in 1983 by its manufacturer as a result of hundreds of lawsuits claiming that Bendectin was responsible for a variety of birth defects. Although several impartial scientific studies and legal decisions have repeatedly absolved Bendectin as a cause of birth defects, the publicity surrounding these cases has permanently undermined patient confidence in its safety. Bendectin contained two innocuous ingredients: pyridoxine (vitamin B_6), which has antinauseant properties and an antihistamine named doxylamine succinate. Although Bendectin is no longer available, its two ingredients may be purchased separately and used either alone or in combination to relieve morning sickness. Vitamin B_6 is sold without prescription as tablets containing 10, 25, 50, 100, and 500 milligrams. Though there are no randomized and controlled studies confirming its efficacy, it has been endorsed by many obstetricians as an antinauseant and antiemetic when taken in an oral dose of 100 milligrams twice daily. If vomiting prevents ingestion of oral pyridoxine, it can be given as an intramuscular injection. The antihistamine doxylamine is sold without prescription under the trade name Unisom Nighttime Sleep Aid. The 25-milligram dose, taken before bedtime, has been used with some success in the treatment of morning sickness. Some women obtain relief of symptoms by breaking the pill in half and taking 12.5 milligrams. The evidence confirming the safety of doxylamine use in pregnancy is impressive. A number of large studies involving thousands of women have detected no adverse fetal or maternal effects. As a result, its B pregnancy-risk-factor classification for pregnancy is well deserved.

Other over-the-counter antihistamines have been used with variable success in combating nausea and vomiting during pregnancy. One of the most popular is dimenhydrinate, more commonly known by its trade name Dramamine. This antiemetic has a pregnancy-risk-factor classification of B. It has been studied intensively and found to be safe for use during pregnancy (see Chapter 7). Benadryl is the trade name for a popular antihistamine and antiemetic named diphenhydramine. It is available as a tablet, liquid, suppository, and intramuscular or intravenous injection. Reproductive studies on rats and rabbits in doses five times the human dose have found no evidence of impaired fertility or harm to the fetus. One study of women who took diphenhydramine during the first trimester found a higher incidence of cleft palate among exposed infants. Other reports, however, have noted no such relationship. Diphenhydramine has a pregnancy-risk-factor classification of C.

Meclizine (trade names Bonine and Antevert), cyclizine (trade name Marezine), buclizine (trade name Bucladin-S), hydroxyzine (trade names Atarax and Vistaril), and perphenazine (trade name Trilafon), which are similar in chemical structure, are classified as piperazine phenothiazines. These drugs are effective antihistamines and antiemetics. While meclizine and cyclizine cause birth defects in animals, several studies involving large numbers of women have concluded that neither drug causes birth defects in humans. Nevertheless, I would be less than enthusiastic about using meclizine or cyclizine unless safer alternatives have first been tried. Both drugs have surprisingly optimistic B pregnancy-risk-factor classifications. Hydroxyzine and buclizine both have category C ratings and pose greater hazards to the fetus than either meclizine or cyclizine. Both have been shown to cause fetal anomalies when administered to pregnant laboratory animals during the first trimester. In one large survey of women using hydroxyzine early in pregnancy, a possible association with birth defects was uncovered. As a result, the manufacturer of hydroxyzine cautions against use of the drug in early pregnancy. Experience with buclizine use during pregnancy was limited to one report of 62 exposed fetuses followed by the birth of 3 malformed children. Based on this information, the manufacturer urges that this drug not be used during the first trimester. While little is known about the effects of perphenazine on the fetus, it has a C pregnancy-risk-factor classification and should be used only if absolutely necessary.

When severe nausea and vomiting of early pregnancy cannot be controlled with any of the above-mentioned medications, use of more potent phenothiazines is usually necessary to prevent the harmful fetal and maternal effects associated with weight loss, electrolyte imbalance, and acidosis. Exposure of more than 2,000 pregnant women to phenothiazines as a group, and especially prochlorperazine (trade name Compazine), did not result in a higher incidence of congenital malformations, perinatal mortality, reduced birth weights, or lower IQ scores of infants tested at one and five years of age. However, in another study, doctors observed 11 malformed children born to 315 women who had taken phenothiazines during the first three months of pregnancy; the anomaly rate of 3.5 percent was significantly higher than the 1.6 percent incidence among mothers not taking phenothiazines. Other reports have been contradictory, but the majority of evidence indicates that phenothiazines are safe for both mother and fetus if used occasionally and in low doses. In addition to prochlorperazine, other popular phenothiazines used to combat morning sickness include chlorpromazine (Thorazine), promethazine (Phenergan), triethylperazine (Torecan), and trimethobenzamide (Tigan). All have a pregnancy-risk-factor classification of C.

Metoclopromide (trade name Reglan) is a relatively new and unique medication which prevents and relieves nausea and vomiting by stimulating the intestinal tract to increase its rhythmic muscular movement or peristalsis. The result is accelerated emptying of food from the stomach and upper intestine. Metoclopromide has a B pregnancy-risk-factor classification. Reproductive studies performed on rats, mice, and rabbits using doses between 12 and 250 times the human dose have shown no fetal harm. Use of metoclopromide during pregnancy is limited, and there are no controlled studies in humans. However, the few instances in which it has been used in pregnancy have demonstrated no adverse fetal consequences.

ANTACIDS AND ANTISPASMODICS

Should I use antacids during pregnancy?

Well-known antacids such as Maalox, Amphojel, Mylicon, Milk of Magnesia, Gelusil, Titralac, Camalox, Di-Gel, Aludrox, Gaviscon, Tums, Rolaids, and Riopan may all be safely used during pregnancy for the relief of heartburn and hyperacidity. Many of these compounds contain, or are combined with, antiflatulents for the relief of excessive gas.

Alka-Seltzer is not recommended during pregnancy since each tablet contains 325 milligrams of aspirin, the amount contained in one adult aspirin tablet. However, Alka-Mints and Alka-Seltzer Advanced Formula are acceptable since they do not contain aspirin.

Tagamet is the trade name for cimetidine, Pepsid is the trade name for famotidine, and Zantac is the trade name for ranitidine, three relatively new and popular drugs for treating duodenal ulcers and other conditions characterized by hyperacidity. Unlike other drugs, cimetidine, ramitidine, and famotidine act by blocking the effects of histamine, the body chemical responsible for the release of acid from the stomach lining. There has been little experience to date with the use of these drugs by pregnant women, but experts believe that they are safe, and all three have been given a favorable B pregnancy-risk-factor classification. Since cimetidine has been available for a longer period of time than the others, more is known about its safety. It rapidly crosses the placenta to the fetus, but there are no reports linking cimetidine use to congenital defects. The American Academy of Pediatrics considers cimetidine to be compatible with breast-feeding. However, too little is known about ramitidine and famotidine to recommend their use while breast-feeding.

What other medications are there for relief of gastrointestinal distress during pregnancy?

Some very popular medications which are prescribed for intestinal disorders are best avoided during pregnancy. One such example is Donnatal, a drug which contains a mixture of ingredients designed to decrease intestinal secretions, spasm, and motility. Unfortunately, each Donnatal capsule, tablet, and liquid teaspoonful contains 16 milligrams of phenobarbital, while a Donnatal Extentab has 48.6 milligrams. Phenobarbital is a barbiturate which may be associated with an increase in fetal abnormalities when taken during the first trimester of pregnancy. When taken late in pregnancy, phenobarbital may be responsible for hemorrhagic disease of the newborn as well as drowsiness, respiratory depression, and withdrawal reactions. As a result of these potential complications, phenobarbital has a D pregnancy-risk-factor classification. The drug accumulates in breast milk and is slowly eliminated. As a result, blood levels in a nursing infant may exceed those of its mother. To date, phenobarbital-induced reactions have been observed in three nursing infants of mothers treated with the drug. Other nonrecommended products which contain phenobarbital are Donnazyme Tablets, Bellergal, Bellergal-S, Kinesed Tablets, Belladenal Tablets, and Belladenal-S Tablets.

Carafate is the trade name for sucralfate, a relatively new medication used to treat duodenal ulcers. Since sucralfate is only minimally absorbed from the stomach and intestinal tract, it is believed to be extremely safe for use during pregnancy and has a pregnancy-risk-factor classification of B. It is not known whether sucralfate is excreted in breast milk, and therefore its use for the nursing woman can not be endorsed.

Atropine and belladona are important active ingredients of several products designed to decrease intestinal irritability and spasm, and reduce excessive intestinal secretions. Each has a pregnancy-risk-factor classification of C, although large studies involving thousands of fetal exposures have failed to find an association between use of either drug and fetal malformations. Atropine is commonly used to reduce a woman's gastric secretions prior to cesarean section anesthesia, a practice that has not been found to cause adverse neonatal effects. To date, it has not been adequately demonstrated if atropine or belladona is excreted in breast milk. Despite this, the American Academy of Pediatrics considers these drugs to be compatible with breast-feeding.

Bentyl is the trade name for a popular antispasmodic named dicyclomine hydrochloride. Both extensive animal research and human experience have confirmed its safety during pregnancy and its B pregnancy-risk-factor classification. Little is known, however, about dicyclomine hydrochloride's concentration in the breast milk or its potential problems for the breast-fed infant.

Isopropamide iodide (trade name Darbid) is a category-C antispasmodic which is best avoided during pregnancy since the iodide it contains may cross the placenta and theoretically could inhibit fetal thyroid function after the twelfth week of pregnancy. In one review, isopropamide iodide use prior to the twelfth week among 180 women produced no fetal abnormalities. Isopropamide also has the capacity to diminish lactation in nursing women.

Pro-Banthine is the trade name for another category-C drug named probantheline bromide. It has the dual capability of slowing excessive gastrointestinal motility and spasm while reducing stomach acid secretions. Experience among pregnant women treated with probantheline bromide over many years has not revealed evidence of fetal toxicity or abnormalities. Limited studies on nursing women suggest that there is no significant excretion of the drug in breast milk. As with other antispasmodics, however, probantheline bromide may inhibit lactation.

Since many gastrointestinal disorders such as spastic colon, colitis, and peptic ulcer are often associated with significant degrees of anxiety and tension, manufacturers have combined the antispasmodic medications with the so-called minor tranquilizers in a single pill. These preparations are mentioned only to be condemned. Fortunately, with the exception of Librax (chlordiazepoxide [trade name Librium] and clidinium bromide), these products have been taken off the market. Librax is best avoided during pregnancy, especially during the first trimester. I also urge nursing women to avoid using minor tranquilizers or medications which contain tranquilizers.

How should I treat constipation during my pregnancy?

For most women, constipation is an annoying problem throughout pregnancy. It occurs because there is a relaxation of the smooth muscles of the intestinal tract, which interferes with the forward wavelike movement called peristalsis. Vitamin preparations which contain iron only serve to worsen this problem. Fortunately, none of the commonly used laxatives and stool softeners have ever been reported to cause harm to the developing fetus.

The woman who is breast-feeding, however, should select a laxative with care, since some may cause increased bowel activity and diarrhea in the nursing infant. Preparations which contain cascara sagrada, such as Peri-Colace, Nature's Remedy Natural Vegetable Laxative, and Milk of Magnesia-Cascara Suspension Concentrated, are most likely to do this and are best avoided. Similarly, laxatives which contain senna, such as Senokot, Senokot XTRA, and X-Prep Liquid, have also been reported to cause diarrhea in a small number of infants whose mothers took greater-than-normal amounts. However, if normal therapeutic doses are maintained, this problem is unlikely to occur, and the American Academy of Pediatrics considers senna use to be compatible with breast-feeding. Phenolphthalein is the chemical found in many nonprescription and prescription products such as ExLax, Argoral, Modane, Phillips' Lax Caps, Feen-A-Mint pills and gum, Doxidan, Correctol Laxative Tablets, and Unilax Stool Softener. While reports concerning the effects of these products on the nursing infant's bowel habits are contradictory, the general conclusion is that they are safe to use if taken in normal therapeutic doses.

What advice do you have for treating diarrhea during pregnancy?

Kaopectate is the trade name for attapulgite, an extremely safe but relatively ineffective antidiarrheal agent. Loperamide hydrochloride (trade name Imodium A-D) is a more potent antidiarrheal drug which has a B pregnancy-risk-factor classification and is considered safe for use during pregnancy. Data relating to the excretion of loperamide hydrochloride into breast milk are lacking.

Most narcotics and narcotic derivatives are potent antidiarrheal agents which act by inhibiting intestinal peristalsis. One of the most popular is Lomotil, the trade name for the combination of diphenoxylate hydrochloride and atropine sulfate. Diphenoxylate hydrochloride is related chemically to meperidine (trade name Demerol) and has a C pregnancy-risk-factor classification. Paregoric is another narcotic antidiarrheal agent which is a mixture of opium powder, anise oil, benzoic acid, camphor, glycerin, and ethanol. It has a B pregnancy-risk-factor classification, and information available to date has convincingly demonstrated that its use is not associated with either major or minor fetal defects.

 # NASAL DECONGESTANTS, ALLERGY AND ASTHMA DRUGS #

Are symptoms of nasal congestion, allergies, and asthma better or worse during pregnancy?

Decongestants and antihistamines are prescribed with far greater frequency during pregnancy, since many women with no previous allergic history will suffer from a condition called "vasomotor rhinitis and sinusitis." This harmless though annoying problem is characterized by nasal stuffiness, mucous congestion, and postnasal secretions. Symptoms may appear at any time during pregnancy, only to mysteriously disappear within one or two days following delivery. Although the cause of vasomotor rhinitis and sinusitis during pregnancy is unknown, doctors believe that it is related to the many hormonal changes which affect women at this time. Women who suffer from hay fever and seasonal allergies characterized by sneezing, runny nose, itching, and excessive tearing of the eyes will often note an intensification of symptoms if rhinitis and sinusitis of pregnancy is also present.

Asthma complicates 1 percent of all pregnancies and is the most common respiratory disease affecting the pregnant woman. While some studies have suggested that symptoms of asthma improve during pregnancy, other reports have found that the frequency and severity of attacks worsen. All experts agree, however, that if asthma is not well controlled immediately prior to conception, the chances of a relapse during pregnancy will be greatly enhanced. Fortunately, most medications for treating asthma in the nonpregnant woman can be used with apparent safety during pregnancy.

What precautions should be taken in treating nasal congestion during pregnancy?

A wide variety of tablets, drops, and sprays are available for the relief of nasal congestion and allergic symptoms. The active ingredient of most nasal decongestants is a class of drugs known as sympathomimetic amines. These compounds achieve their desired decongesting effect by contracting the smaller blood vessels of the nasal passages. Unfortunately, they also have the potential to be absorbed into the maternal circulation and cause the uterine arteries to constrict, thereby reducing uterine blood flow and fetal oxygenation. Oxymetazoline is the longest acting and one of the popular sympathomimetic amines, providing relief from nasal congestion for up to 12 hours. Popular brands containing oxymetazoline include all Afrin products, Coricidin Decongestant Nasal Mist, Dristan Long Lasting Nasal Spray, Duration 12 Hour Nasal Spray, 4-Way Long Lasting Nasal Spray, Neo-Synephrine 12 Hour Nasal Spray, and Vicks Sinex Long-Acting Decongestant. Though oxymetazoline is generally considered safe during pregnancy if used in recommended doses at 12-hour intervals, fetal distress may occur if one does not adhere to these instructions.

Other long-lasting sympathomimetic amine decongestants are naphazoline (Privine Nasal Solution, Privine Nasal Spray, and 4-Way Fast Acting Nasal Spray) and xylometazoline (Otrivin Nasal Spray and Otrivin Nasal Drops). Similar precautions apply to these products as well. Sympathomimetic amines as a class cause birth defects in some animal species, but a clear association between their use and abnormalities in humans has not been established. As a result, all have a category C pregnancy-risk-factor classification. One problem with evaluating their potential to cause fetal harm is that they are often administered in combination with other medications such as antihistamines and antibiotics for treatment of nasal congestion, cough, and upper respiratory infections. Thus, it is often difficult to pinpoint the medication responsible for a particular adverse effect. Certainly, sympathomimetic amines should be used with caution throughout pregnancy, especially during the first trimester.

Phenylpropanolamine, pseudoephedrine, and phenylephrine are examples of shorter-acting sympathomimetic agents which effectively relieve nasal congestion. Phenylpropanolamine is a component of some of the most popularly used over-the-counter cold medicines, antihistamines, and decongestants including Alka-Seltzer Plus Cold Medicine, Allerest Allergy Tablets and Sinus Pain Formula, A.R.M. Allergy Relief Medicine Caplets, Contac, Coricidin, Demazin, Dimetapp, Naldecon, Robitussin-CF, Sinarest Tablets, Sine-Off Snaplets, and Triaminic. A large number of prescription medications also contain phenylpropanolamine. Popular examples include Tavist-D, Ornade Spansule Capsules, and Tuss-Ornade. Like other drugs in its class, phenylpropanolamine has the potential to constrict uterine blood vessels and reduce oxygen flow to the fetus. In one survey of more than 700 women using phenylpropanolamine-containing medications during the first trimester, researchers found a possible association with defects such as hypospadias, eye and ear defects, polydactyly (extra digits), cataracts, and pectus excavatum (abnormal indentation of the sternum or breast bone). The overall malformation rate was 1.4 times greater in infants exposed to phenylpropanolamine when compared to a control group.

Pseudoephedrine is another sympathomimetic agent used to relieve symptoms of nasal congestion, allergic disorders, and upper respiratory infections. It too is a common component of medications containing antihistamines and other ingredients and has a pregnancy-risk-factor classification of C. Some of the more popular products which contain pseudoephedrine include Actifed, Sudafed, Allerest No Drowsiness Tablets, Benadryl Decongestant Tablets and Elixir, Benadryl Plus, Chlor-Trimeton Decongestant Tablets, Contac Nighttime Cold Medicine, Maximum Strength Dristan, Drixoral Plus Extended Relief Tablets and Sustained-Action Tablets, Sinus Excedrin Analgesic, Novahistime DMX, Ornex Caplets, Sinarest No Drowsiness Tablets, Sine-Aid Maximum Strength Sinus Headache Caplets and Tablets, Sinutab Allergy Formula Sustained, Sinutab Maximum Strength Tablets and Caplets, Tylenol Cold Medicine, Tylenol Allergy Sinus Medication, Vicks Formula 44D Decongestant, and Vicks NyQuil Nighttime Cold Medicine.

Since the greatest fear associated with use of products containing pseudoephedrine and other sympathomimetics is narrowing of the arteries carrying oxygen to the fetus, it is encouraging to review the recent findings from the University of Nebraska College of Medicine. In this study, published in *Obstetrics and Gynecology* in 1990, doctors administered a standard 60-milligram dose of pseudoephedrine to 12 healthy women between their twenty-sixth and fortieth week of pregnancy. Blood flow velocities and pulse rate in both the maternal and fetal circulations remained unaltered, leaving the authors to conclude that a normal dose of pseudoephredrine given to a healthy woman in the third trimester was probably safe for her and her infant. Though the American Academy of Pediatrics considers pseudoephedrine to be compatible with breast-feeding, it is advisable to time the dose so as to avoid peak concentrations.

Phenylephrine is a constituent of many products including Dimetane Decongestant Caplets and Elixir, Dristan Decongestant and Nasal Spray, 4-Way Fast Acting Nasal Spray, Neo-Synephrine Nasal Sprays and Nose Drops, Novahistine Elixir, Robitussin Night Relief, and Vicks Sinex Decongestant Nasal Spray. The same warnings that apply to other sympathomimetics in this group also apply to phenylephrine. In one study of more than 1,200 women who used phenylephrine during the first trimester, researchers found a higher incidence of eye and ear defects, syndactyly (webbing of the fingers and toes), skin tags near the ear, and club foot. Although further studies are needed to confirm or refute the significance of these findings, the report would certainly serve as a warning not to use phenylephrine-containing decongestants indiscriminately during pregnancy. Nothing is known about the excretion of phenylephrine in the breast milk or its possible effects on the nursing infant.

How safe are antihistamines during pregnancy?

Antihistamines are useful in the treatment of hives, adverse reactions to medications, sinusitis, and allergic rhinitis or inflammation of the membranes of the nose due to hay fever and specific agents such as dust or molds. Some antihistamines, such as doxylamine, dimenhydrinate, and diphenhydramine, have been successfully used in treating both morning and motion sickness. In a 1977 epidemiologic study of thousands of women treated with antihistamines during the first five months of pregnancy, researchers concluded that brompheniramine, the chemical found in Dimetane, Dimetapp, and Drixoral Antihistamine Nasal Decongestant Syrup, was statistically more likely than other agents to be associated with abnormalities in the newborn. Antihistamines containing diphenhydramine (trade names Benadryl, Sominex, Benylin Decongestant and Cough Syrup, Nytol Tablets, Sleep-Eze 3 Tablets, Unisom Dual Relief Nighttime Sleep Aid/Analgesic), tripelennamine (PBZ Tablets and Elixir), pheniramine (trade names Dristan Nasal Spray, Triaminic Expectorant DH and TR Tablets, Tussirex Syrup, and Poly-Histine Elixir and Polyhistine-D), and chlorpheniramine (trade names Allerest Allergy Tablets and Sinus Pain Formula, Chlor-Trimeton Decongestant Tablets, Contac, Coricidin, Dristan Decongestant/Antihistamine/Analgesic, Novahistine Elixir, Deconamine, Sinarest, Sine-Off Maximum Strength, Sudafed Plus, Triaminic Cold Tablets, Allergy Tablets, Syrup, and Nite Light, Tylenol Cold Medication and Allergy Sinus Medication, and Vicks Formula 44 Cough Medicine) were found to be safe when used judiciously during pregnancy, although the authors were quick to point out the many variables and tenuous conclusions of their studies.

Until recently, one of the main drawbacks of antihistamine use has been the side effect of drowsiness. Newer products such as terfenadine (trade name Seldane) and astemizole (trade name Hismanal) have overcome this problem to a great extent. Unfortunately, too little is known about the safety of these new drugs to endorse their use either during pregnancy or while nursing. In Table 18, I have summarized the safety and risks associated with some of the more commonly prescribed antihistamines during pregnancy.

How safe is the treatment of asthma during pregnancy and nursing?

A wide variety of medications, known as bronchodilators, have been effectively used to dilate, or open, the respiratory passages and relieve the symptoms of wheezing and shortness of breath associated with an acute attack of bronchial asthma. Theophylline (trade names Elixophyllin, Slo-Phyllin, and Theo-Dur), probably the most popular bronchodilator, is considered by many to be the first drug of choice for treating an acute attack of asthma in the pregnant woman. Theophylline is often combined with other medications in pills and liquids (Bronkaid Tablets, Marax, Primatene Tablets, Quibron Liquid and Capsules). Aminophylline is a salt of theophylline which, when given intravenously, is invaluable in aborting an acute asthmatic attack. Both drugs are chemically classified as methylxanthines.

Although theophylline has a pregnancy-risk-factor classification of C, it is generally considered to be safe. Despite extensive use, there are no reports linking theophylline with congenital defects. However, there are occasional problems which may be associated with its use during pregnancy. Doctors from the University of Florida, in their 1986 study, advised that doctors lower the dosage of theophylline during the third trimester in order to reduce the risk of both fetal and maternal toxicity. Another concern about theophylline therapy is based on a 1979 report which found that asthmatic women receiving theophylline had a longer average duration of labor than did untreated women. In another article published in 1979, doctors found that two newborns and their mothers had comparable theophylline blood levels at the time of birth. Transient mild jitteriness and a rapid heart rate have been observed among some newborns whose mothers were found to have high levels of theophylline in their blood.

Theophylline is excreted into breast milk in concentrations 70 percent of those found in maternal serum, and it is cleared slowly from the newborn's circulation. For this reason, experts recommend sustained-release products such as Theo-Dur. Theophylline and aminophylline are chemically similar to caffeine. Therefore, women using these medications and nursing their infants should keep caffeine intake to a minimum. The American Academy of Pediatrics considers aminophylline and theophylline use compatible with breast-feeding.

Instead of theophylline, some specialists prefer to use medications known as sympathomimetics as their first line of treatment for asthma during pregnancy. Others use these agents only if theophylline is unable to abort an acute attack. Unlike the previously mentioned sympathomimetics which are used as decongestants (see page 278), most of the drugs used to treat acute asthma have the capacity to selectively relax the smooth muscles of the respiratory tract without causing undesirable reactions elsewhere, such as constriction of the uterine arteries carrying oxygen to the fetus. Metaproterenol (trade names Alupent and Metaprel), terbutaline (trade names Brethine, Brethaire, and Bricanyl), and albuterol (trade names Proventil and Ventolin) are the most popular and most effect sympathomimetics. Although metaproterenol has a pregnancy-risk-factor classification of C, there are no reports linking its use to birth defects. In addition to its muscle-relaxing effect on the respiratory tract, metaproterenol has been known to relax the uterine muscles, thereby either inhibiting or prolonging labor.

Far more is known about the safety of terbutaline since it is more frequently used by obstetricians to prevent and treat premature labor than to treat asthma. Terbutaline has a pregnancy-risk-factor classification of B, and appears to be a safe

TABLE 18

SAFETY OF COMMONLY USED ANTIHISTAMINES DURING PREGNANCY AND NURSING

Generic and Trade Names of Drugs	Route of Administration	Suggestions for Pregnancy	Suggestions for Nursing
astemizole (Hismanal)	Tablets	Pregnancy category C. No teratogenic effects in animals given 200 times the human dose. No adequate and well controlled studies in pregnant women.	Not known if drug is excreted in breast milk, therefore, use with caution.
brompheniramine (Dimetane, Dimetapp, Drixoral, others)	Tablets, liquid, capsules	Associated with possible increase in birth defects if taken during first five months. Pregnancy category C.	Controversial; one manufacturer considers the drug to be contraindicated for nursing mothers, but the American Academy of Pediatrics considers it safe.
clemastine (Tavist)	Tablets, liquid	No data on human pregnancy available, though manufacturer lists it as pregnancy category B. Laboratory experiments on pregnant rats and rabbits given 500 to 1,000 times the human dose show no fetal abnormalities.	Excreted in breast milk. One case of drowsiness, stiff neck, poor feeding in nursing infant. Use with caution.
chlorpheniramine (Allerest Allergy Tablets, Chlor-Trimeton, Contac, Tylenol Cold Medication, Sinarest, others)	Tablets, liquid, capsules	Probably safe during pregnancy, category B.	No data are available.
dimenhydrinate (Dramamine)	Tablets, liquid, suppositories, intramuscular and intravenous injection	Probably safe during pregnancy, Category B. Should not be used in labor because it can stimulate strong contractions and fetal distress.	Small amounts are excreted in breast milk; effect on nursing infant is unknown.

TABLE 18 (*continued*)

SAFETY OF COMMONLY USED ANTIHISTAMINES DURING PREGNANCY AND NURSING

Generic and Trade Names of Drugs	Route of Administration	Suggestions for Pregnancy	Suggestions for Nursing
diphenhydramine (Benadryl, Sominex, Nytol, Benylin Decongestant, others)	Tablets, capsules, liquid, intramuscular and intravenous injection	Pregnancy category C. Reproductive studies on rats and rabbits in amounts 5 times the human dose found no adverse fetal effects. One study of women using drug in first trimester found an increased incidence of cleft palate. When used with narcotics during labor drug enhances effect of narcotic and can depress newborn.	Excreted in breast milk. No adverse effects reported, but manufacturer considers the drug contraindicated in nursing infants.
doxylamine (Unisom Nighttime Sleep Aid, Contac Nighttime Cold Medicine)	Tablets, liquid	Safe during pregnancy, category B.	No data are available.
pheniramine (Dristan Nasal Spray, Triaminic Expectorant DH, Poly-Histine Elixir, others)	Tablets, capsules, liquid, nasal spray	Pregnancy category C. Possible relationship between first trimester use and respiratory malformations, eye, and ear defects in one study.	No data are available.
terfenadine (Seldane)	Tablets	Pregnancy category C. No evidence of animal teratogenicity, but rats given 63 times and 125 times the human daily dose throughout pregnancy and lactation had poor infant weight gain and lower survival rates. No adequate or well controlled studies in pregnant women.	Manufacturer recommends that it not be used.
tripelennamine (PBZ)	Tablets and liquid	Pregnancy category B. Probably safe. In one study of 100 women using the drug in the first trimester, no adverse fetal effects were noted.	Excreted in breast milk. Manufacturer recommends that it not be used.

triprolidine (Actifed, Alber Act, Actidil) — Tablets, capsules, liquid — Pregnancy category C, but probably safer than most drugs in this category. There are no reports linking the use of triprolidine with congenital defects following experiments with thousands of women over more than 20 years. Animal studies also negative. — Excreted in breast milk. American Academy of Pediatrics considers it safe.

drug for treating asthma at any time during pregnancy. Terbutaline may cause the same maternal and fetal side effects as metaproterenol, but it is more likely to raise the maternal systolic blood pressure. As a result, the American Academy of Pediatrics considers the drug to be compatible with breast-feeding.

Despite its C pregnancy-risk-factor classification, there are no reports linking albuterol use to congenital anomalies. Unlike terbutaline and metaproterenol, albuterol use has been associated with major decreases in maternal systolic and diastolic blood pressure, significant enough to cause fetal distress. No data are available concerning the safety of albuterol use while nursing.

Epinephrine products (trade names Adrenaline, Bronchaid Mist, EpiPen, Primatine Mist, Sus-Phrine, and Medihaler Epi), isoproterenol (trade names Duo-Medihaler, Isuprel, and Medihaler-Iso), and isoetharine (trade names Bronkometer and Bronkosol) are all sympathomimetics which have a limited but often important role in treating asthma. Epinephrine, when given either intravenously or subcutaneously, is invaluable in relieving respiratory distress and bronchospasm caused by an acute and severe asthmatic attack. It is also effective in relieving a wide variety of allergic reactions, nasal congestion, shock, and glaucoma, and it is a lifesaving drug when injected directly into the heart for resuscitation in cardiac arrest. Doctors and dentists frequently use epinephrine in combination with local anesthetics to prolong the action of the anesthetic and reduce bleeding by constricting blood vessels.

In desperate emergencies, epinephrine is the medication of choice, regardless of whether or not a woman is pregnant. However, it is not innocuous, and in the absence of such an emergency safe substitutes should be used. For example, when undergoing routine dental work, a pregnant woman should insist that epinephrine not be combined with local anesthetics. Epinephrine is a potent vasoconstrictor capable of decreasing uterine artery, umbilical cord, and placental blood flow which, if prolonged, can cause a reduction in oxygen reaching the fetus. Epinephrine causes birth defects in some animal species and has a pregnancy-risk-factor classification of C. In one large study of almost 200 women exposed to epinephrine during the first trimester, researchers found a higher incidence of both minor and major malformations. No data are available on the use of epinephrine for women who are breast-feeding.

Isoproterenol is a potent sympathomimetic which is usually administered by inhalation in a solution of water or saline. It is effective in relieving symptoms of asthma, but it may also be responsible for a very rapid fetal and maternal heart rate. Isoproterenol has a C pregnancy-risk-factor classification, and while it has been found to cause congenital defects in some animal species, there are no reports of a similar problem in infants of women using the drug during pregnancy. When a woman uses isoproterenol at the end of her pregnancy it can inhibit the strength and frequency of her uterine contractions and lengthen labor.

Isoetharine is less potent than isoproterenol, but it too has a C pregnancy-risk-factor classification. Little is known about its safety during pregnancy or its effects on the fetus. There are no data available on the safety of either isoproterenol or isoetharine for the breast-fed infant.

Cromolyn (trade name Intal) is a medication which, when used regularly, prevents flare-ups of severe bronchial asthma. It is especially beneficial for individuals in whom the frequency and intensity of asthmatic attacks are totally unpredictable. It is not a bronchodilator or antihistamine and is of no benefit in treating an acute attack of asthma. It is inhaled into the nasal passages through the use of a special inhalator. Animal studies have demonstrated no adverse fetal effects of cromolyn at normal therapeutic levels. Most experts consider cromolyn to be a safe drug for use during pregnancy; it has a B pregnancy-risk-factor classification.

Whereas many medications are dangerous to the fetus when administered during the first trimester, those which contain iodides pose the greatest risk when taken after the twelfth week of pregnancy. The reason is that the fetal thyroid gland begins to function and take up iodides after this time. As a result, iodides given to a mother may cross the placenta and induce congenital goiter formation and hypothyroidism in her newborn. In some instances, the enlarged goiter can actually block the infant's airway and cause respiratory distress. Iodine is frequently found in expectorants and occasionally in bronchodilators. In addition to avoiding the usual saturated solution of potassium iodide, more commonly known as SSKI, pregnant women are advised not to use Elixophyllin-KI Elixir, Mudrane Tablets, Mudrane-2 Tablets, Quadrinal Tablets and Suspension, Tussi-Organidin Liquid, and Theo-Organidin Elixir. Iodides are excreted into breast milk in small quantities. Even though a nursing infant would receive only a small dose, it might be enough to inhibit thyroid function and produce hypothyroidism and goiter.

How safe is cortisone in the treatment of asthma during pregnancy and nursing?

Cortisone is just one of several structurally related chemicals called corticosteroids. In pill, aerosol inhalation, and injectable form they are invaluable in the treatment of severe attacks of bronchial asthma which are resistant to other forms of therapy. In addition, corticosteroids have been used successfully in treating allergic conditions and such serious diseases as adrenal gland insufficiency; the so-called collagen diseases, rheumatoid arthritis and lupus erythematosis; certain kidney diseases; chronic ulcerative colitis; dermatological and eye disorders; shock; and specific types of leukemia and cancer.

Corticosteroids should be administered at any stage of pregnancy if it is determined that they are needed to successfully treat a serious disorder. However, these agents can create some undesirable side effects: fluid and chemical imbalance, abnormal glucose tolerance and diabetes, susceptibility to infections, peptic ulcers which may bleed or perforate, osteoporosis or loss of minerals from the bones, elevation of the blood pressure, generalized muscle weakness, and psychiatric disturbances. High doses of corticosteroids used for long periods of time are responsible for a person's developing a characteristic "moon face," obesity of the body but not the arms and legs, the so-called "buffalo hump" protrusion over the top of the back, striae or purple stretch marks of the skin, acne, and an overabundance of facial and body hair. These serious and distressing side effects are more apt to occur when corticosteroids are administered orally, intramuscularly, or intravenously in high doses for prolonged periods of time. Although there is little clinical information on the safety of corticosteroid nasal sprays and inhalators, most experts believe that they are less likely to cause these unpleasant complications. Therefore, it is best to first try corticosteroid sprays and aerosols for asthma before resorting to more potent treatments. Corticosteroid creams and gels are rarely responsible for any of these serious side effects.

When corticosteroids are administered in the form of nasal and inhalation aerosol sprays, they are rapidly absorbed into the bloodstream and are highly effective in relieving asthmatic symptoms. Beclomethasone (trade names Beclovent, Beconase, Vancenase, and Vanceril), triamcinolone (trade name Azmacort), and flunisolide (trade names Nasalide and AeroBid) are examples of steroids used in this fashion. If these medications do not thwart an acute asthmatic attack, treatment with oral synthetic corticosteroids, such as prednisone or prednisolone, is usually successful. Both are preferable to cortisone during pregnancy because they cause less sodium retention. When an acute attack of asthma occurs during labor, or when all other treatment methods have failed, intravenous hydrocortisone or methylprednisolone should be given.

Once high doses of corticosteroids are taken for more than two or three days, use should taper off gradually to avoid a withdrawal reaction caused by acute adrenal gland insufficiency. Early symptoms of this potentially dangerous condition are fever, muscle weakness, and joint pain. When treating asthma during pregnancy it is important that doctors not use long-acting corticosteroids, such as betamethasone or dexamethasone, which may cause prolonged adrenal gland suppression. Corticosteroids cross the placenta and enter the fetal circulation, and on rare occasions a newborn may also experience temporary adrenal gland malfunction. An obstetrician must alert the pediatrician and newborn nursery to monitor all infants whose mothers take corticosteroids during pregnancy.

Most reports in the medical literature attest to the safety of even high doses of corticosteroids during pregnancy. However, there are some notable exceptions. These medications may pose definite

risks to both a mother and her fetus, and should be prescribed only when absolutely necessary and for as short a period of time as possible. In addition to a corticosteroid user's diminished capacity to respond to the stress of labor, anesthesia, or surgery, she may encounter other problems related to altered blood sugar, sodium retention, and elevated blood pressure.

Laboratory studies on rodents suggest that the use of corticosteroids may be associated with a higher incidence of a variety of fetal complications. However, this has not been substantiated in humans. In the eyes of embryologists, not all corticosteroids are created equal. Prednisone and prednisolone have been judged to be the safest, both having a B pregnancy-risk-factor classification. Only trace amounts of both drugs have been found in breast milk, and the American Academy of Pediatrics considers them to be compatible with breast-feeding, although a woman taking high doses of prednisone or prednisolone is advised not to nurse her infant until at least four hours after her last medication dose.

In contrast to prednisone and prednisolone, cortisone has a pregnancy-risk-factor classification of D. However, this is not necessarily indicative that it is significantly more dangerous to the fetus. Instead, it may simply be a reflection of the fact that it has been used extensively for many more years, resulting in an accumulation of reports associating it with an assortment of congenital anomalies, among them cataracts, cardiovascular defects, cleft lip, clubfoot, and hydrocephaly. While none of these associations has ever been proven conclusively, prednisone and prednisolone are preferable to cortisone during pregnancy.

Despite their C pregnancy-risk-factor classification, beclomethasone and flunisolide aerosol sprays are considered to be safe for use in treating asthma during pregnancy. In one limited experience of 40 women using beclomethasone, researchers noted no increased risk of pregnancy loss or adverse fetal outcome. It is not known if either of these two corticosteroids is excreted in breast milk. Triamcinolone has been assigned a more hazardous D pregnancy-risk-factor classification based on the fact that it causes birth defects in laboratory animals in doses comparable to the highest dose recommended for human use. These toxic fetal effects were noted following aerosol inhalation as well as other routes of administration. Based on this limited information, it is probably best to choose corticosteroid aerosols other than Azmacort during pregnancy.

The safety of various medications used to treat asthma are summarized in Table 19.

How safe is allergy immunotherapy during pregnancy?

Immunotherapy is the process by which a doctor periodically administers small skin injections of allergens, substances to which a person is allergic, to slowly build immunity or resistance to the offending agent. Most allergists believe that it is unwise to initiate immunotherapy during pregnancy, since the severity of a person's response to a particular allergen is occasionally unpredictable. If a pregnant woman is already receiving immunotherapy, it should be continued but administered cautiously to avoid severe reactions. This is especially true during the first trimester, when the smallest amount of allergen should be given. Children born of allergic mothers are 50 percent more likely than other children to develop allergies. For this reason, some doctors are of the opinion that if a mother continues taking allergy shots during pregnancy, her baby may be less sensitive to allergies later in life.

Allergy skin testing is the initial step taken by an allergist to determine the allergens to which a person is most susceptible. As with immunotherapy, caution should be exercised during allergy skin testing. Ideally, allergy and asthma management should begin well in advance of a contemplated pregnancy so that the disorder can be controlled with a minimal amount of medication or immunotherapy.

      # SLEEPING PILLS

Are there over-the-counter sleeping pills which a woman can safely take during pregnancy?

Several popular nonprescription products described as "sleep aids" contain the antihistamines diphenhydramine or doxylamine as their active ingredient. Diphenhydramine-containing products include Excedrin P.M. Analgesic/Sleeping Aid Tablets and Caplets, Nytol, Sominex, Sleepinal Night-time Sleep Aid Capsules, Sleep-Eze 3 Tablets, while doxylamine is found in Unisom Nighttime Sleep Aid. Although they are sold over the counter, products containing diphenhydramine are not innocuous, as evidenced by its C pregnancy-risk-factor classification. Doxylamine, with its B classification, would appear to be the safer choice.

Are there any prescription sleeping pills which may be safely taken by a pregnant woman?

Prescription medications which we commonly refer to as sleeping pills are actually a class of drugs called sedative-hypnotics. There are several categories, and I advise my patients to avoid them all during pregnancy.

Barbiturates are the most commonly prescribed sedative-hypnotics. They are available under a variety of trade names such as Seconal (secobarbital), Nembutal (pentobarbital), Butisol Sodium (sodi-

TABLE 19

SAFETY OF MEDICATIONS USED TO TREAT ASTHMA DURING PREGNANCY AND NURSING

Generic and Trade Names	*Route of Administration*	*Suggestions for Pregnancy*	*Suggestions for Nursing*
Bronchodilators			
Aminophyllin and theophylline (Aminophylline, Elixophylline, Slo-Phyllin, Theo-Dur)	Tablets, capsules, liquid, intravenous, suppositories	Category C risk factor but considered safe for use during pregnancy. Decrease 1 dose often to avoid accumulation in body's bloodstream and possibly longer labor.	American Academy of Pediatrics considers it safe for breastfeeding. May accumulate in breast milk, therefore, observe baby for jitteriness.
Corticosteroids			
beclomethasone (Beclovent, Beconase, Vancenase, Vanceril)	Nasal spray and aerosol inhalation	Category C risk factor. Limited experience with women using beclomethasone shows no fetal problems.	Not known if it is excreted in breast milk.
cortisone (Cortone)	Tablets, intramuscular injection	Category D and associated with sodium retention. Best to use safer alternatives.	No data available.
flunisolide (AeroBid, Nasalide)	Nasal spray and aerosol inhalation	Category C risk factor, but probably considered safe for use in pregnancy.	Not known if it is excreted in breast milk.
hydrocortisone (Hydrocortone)	Tablets, intravenous, intramuscular, and subcutaneous injection	Category C risk factor. Adequate reproductive studies not available.	Excreted in breast milk, but effect on nursing infant is unknown.
methylprednisolone (Medrol, Depo-Medrol, Solu-Medrol)	Tablets, intravenous, intramuscular injection	Category C. Adequate human reproduction studies have not been performed.	Excreted in breast milk, but effect on nursing infant is unknown.
prednisone and prednisolone (Prelone, Predate 50, Hydeltrasol, Deltasone)	Tablets, liquid	Category B risk factor and considered safe for use during pregnancy.	Excreted in breast milk. American Academy of Pediatrics considers it safe for nursing.
triamcinolone (Azmacort)	Aerosol inhalation	Category D risk factor. Best avoided during pregnancy.	Not known if it is excreted in breast milk.
cromolyn (Intal)	Capsules and inhaler	Category B risk factor and considered safe for use during pregnancy.	No data are available.

TABLE 19 (continued)

SAFETY OF MEDICATIONS USED TO TREAT ASTHMA DURING PREGNANCY AND NURSING

Generic and Trade Names	Route of Administration	Suggestions for Pregnancy	Suggestions for Nursing
Iodides			
SSKI, Elixophyllin-KI Elixir, Mudrane Tablets, Mudrane-2 Tablets, Quadrinal Tablets and Suspension, Tussi-Organidin Liquid, Theo-Organides Elixir	Liquid, tablets	Category X, contraindicated.	Excreted in breast milk, therefore, best not to take while nursing.
Sympathomimetics			
albuterol (Proventil, Ventolin)	Aerosol inhaler, liquid, tablets	Category C risk factor, though there are no reports linking it to congenital defects. May cause drop in maternal blood pressure, elevated blood sugar. Decreases uterine contractions and has been used to treat premature labor.	No data are available.
epinephrine (Adrenalin, Bronkaid Mist, EpiPen, Primatene Mist, Medihaler Epi, Sus-Phrine)	Intravenous and subcutaneous injection, aerosol inhaler	Category C. A potent vasoconstrictor which can reduce O_2 flow to the fetus. Use only for emergencies.	No data are available.
isoetharine (Bronkometer, Bronkosol)	Aerosol inhaler	Category C risk factor, though there are no reports linking it to congenital defects.	No data are available.
isoproterenol (Duo-Medihaler, Isuprel, Medihaler-Iso)	Aerosol inhaler, intramuscular, intravenous, and subcutaneous injection	Category C risk factor, though there are no reports linking it to congenital defects. May inhibit uterine contractions.	No data are available.

metaproterenol (Alupent, Metaprel)	Aerosol inhalant, tablets, liquid	Category C risk factor but no reports linking it to birth defects. Fetus may have rapid heart rate and newborn may have low blood sugar. Drug relaxes uterine muscles and may delay or prolong labor.	No data are available.
terbutaline (Brethine, Brethaire, Bricanyl)	Aerosol inhalant, liquid, subcutaneous injection	Category B risk factor. Considered safe during pregnancy and commonly used to prevent labor. May cause rapid maternal and fetal pulse and raise maternal systolic blood pressure.	Excreted in breast milk in low concentrations. American Academy of Pediatrics considers it safe for breast-feeding.

um barbital), Phenobarbital (phenobarbital), and Amytal (amobarbital).

All barbiturates have a pregnancy-risk-factor classification of D, and each has the ability to rapidly cross the placenta and reach high concentrations in the fetal liver and brain. The evidence linking barbiturates to congenital defects varies among the different drugs in this group. For example, despite several hundred first-trimester exposures of pregnant women and their fetuses to both pentobarbital and secobarbital, neither one has been found to cause malformations or chromosomal abnormalities. In contrast, amobarbital seems most deserving of its D pregnancy-risk-factor rating. In one survey of 273 women who received amobarbital during the first trimester, an alarming 95 of the exposed infants were born with major or minor malformations. Infant outcome associated with phenobarbital use during pregnancy has been difficult to confirm despite the fact that this drug has been used since 1912. The reason is that phenobarbital is more often used in combination with other potent drugs to treat epilepsy rather than alone as a sleeping pill. However, one large survey of more than 1,400 infants exposed to phenobarbital in utero has demonstrated no link to either major or minor birth defects. Phenobarbital has

the capacity to cause a condition named hemorrhagic disease of the newborn if it is taken in the hours before delivery.

The American Academy of Pediatrics cautions that nursing infants of mothers who require phenobarbital daily be carefully observed for sedation. It has also been suggested that these infants undergo periodic monitoring of their phenobarbital blood levels. A far saner approach would be not to breast-feed if you take phenobarbital. The shorter-acting barbiturates are far less likely to cause similar problems. In fact, the American Academy of Pediatrics lists secobarbital as a drug which is compatible with breast-feeding.

Halcion, Dalmane, Doral, and Pro Som are popular trade names for sleeping pills with the scientific names of triazolam, flurazepam, quazepam, and estazolam, respectively. All are chemically classified as benzodiazepines, the same family of drugs as some of the more popular minor tranquilizers (see page 290). Benzodiazepines have a pregnancy-risk-factor classification of X and should not be used during pregnancy. Several studies, including the most recent from Gottenburg University in Sweden, have linked first-trimester benzodiazepine use to birth defects. The benzodiazepines are excreted in breast milk. Since little is known about their effects on a nursing infant, the manufactures of Halcion, Dalmane, and Doral recommend that they not be given to nursing women. Recent reports linking Halcion use to adverse psychiatric reactions and hallucinations have severely limited its use in the United States.

Chloral hydrate (trade name Chloral Hydrate Capsules), an effective sedative popularly used as a rectal suppository in years past to allay apprehension during the early stages of labor, is no longer recommended for this purpose. Despite its C pregnancy-risk-factor classification, there is no known association between its use and fetal anomalies. For this reason, chloral hydrate would be preferred over the barbiturates if sedation was necessary during pregnancy. While chloral hydrate is excreted in breast milk, the amount is not sufficient to depress an infant if used in the normal recommended doses, and the American Academy of Pediatrics considers the drug to be compatible with breast-feeding.

Glutethimide (trade name Doriden) has not been studied adequately to recommend its use during pregnancy or nursing. However, withdrawal symptoms have been exhibited by infants born to mothers dependent on this drug, and reports suggest that it may have prolonged adverse neonatal

effects. It has a pregnancy-risk-factor classification of C.

Ethchlorvynol (trade name Placidyl) is an excellent drug for the treatment of insomnia. However, pregnant rats given ethchlorvynol have shown a higher percentage of stillbirths and a lower survival rate beyond the neonatal period. For this reason, heed the manufacturer's suggestion that this category-C drug not be used during the first and second trimesters. During the third trimester, ethchlorvynol has been associated with central nervous system depression and withdrawal symptoms in the newborn. It is not known if ethchlorvynol is excreted in breast milk, and there are not enough data available to endorse its use by a nursing mother.

Methyprylon (trade name Noludar) is a sedative-hypnotic which has been given a B pregnancy-risk-factor classification by its manufacturer. Reproduction studies performed on rats and rabbits given up to nine times the maximum recommended human dose have revealed no evidence of fetal abnormalities. There are, however, no adequate or well-controlled studies in humans to endorse its use. It is not known whether methyprylon is excreted in breast milk.

TRANQUILIZERS AND DRUGS USED IN PSYCHIATRY

What are minor tranquilizers?

The minor tranquilizers are a group of drugs that are used medically for the relief of acute anxiety and nervous tension. Unfortunately, they are indiscriminately abused by too many people who are either unaware or unconcerned that these medications may be habit-forming and a cause of emotional and physical dependence. Valium is classified as a benzodiazepine. Other popular mi-

nor tranquilizers in this group include chlordiazepoxide hydrochloride (trade names Librium and Libritabs), chlorazepate dipotassium (trade name Tranxene), prazepam (trade name Centrax), alprazolam (trade name Xanax), lorazepam (trade name Ativan), and most recently oxazepam (trade name Serax). All are mentioned only to be scorned and strictly avoided. While these benzodiazepines are classified as minor tranquilizers, all have the capacity to cause major problems for the fetus and newborn, and should not be used by a pregnant or nursing woman. Benzodiazepines have a category D pregnancy-risk-factor classification.

In recent years, buspirone (trade name Buspar) has gained great popularity as an antianxiety drug. It is less likely than other tranquilizers to cause drowsiness and other unpleasant side effects. Its greatest advantage, however, is that it does not cause physical or psychological dependence. Unlike other minor tranquilizers, buspirone has a relatively safe pregnancy-risk-factor classification of B. Extensive studies performed on various laboratory animals given many times the maximum human dose have found no evidence of impaired fertility, chromosomal abnormalities, or fetal damage. However, buspirone's manufacturer is quick to point out that there are no adequate or well-controlled studies to prove its safety in human pregnancy and that animal studies do not always translate to a successful outcome in a human's pregnancy. There are no data available as to whether or not buspirone is excreted in breast milk.

Meprobamate (trade names Equanil and Miltown), although a different chemical class of minor tranquilizer than the benzodizepines, also has a D pregnancy-risk-factor classification. While several researchers have found no relationship between its use and adverse fetal effects, others have noted just the opposite. One report of women who used meprobamate during the first six weeks of pregnancy found a rate of 12 abnormalities per 100 live births, compared to only 2.6 per 100 among women who used no medications. The most frequently found abnormalities involved the heart; joint and skull defects were also reported. Other studies have linked first-trimester meprobamate use with a significant rise in the incidence of cleft lip and cleft palate, deafness, and defects of the diaphragm, abdominal wall, eyes, and central nervous system. Meprobamate is excreted in breast milk. Although the effect on the nursing infant is not known, a breast-feeding woman should be aware that the concentration of meprobamate is two to four times greater in her breast milk than in her bloodstream. As a result, it is best avoided.

What are the dangers associated with the use of antidepressants during pregnancy?

Many drugs are employed in the treatment of depression, but none has received as much media attention and popularity as fluoxetine hydrochloride, better known by its trade name Prozac. Following its introduction in 1987, it has rapidly become the most frequently prescribed antidepressant in the United States and has been hailed by some as a miraculous wonder drug. Although Prozac has FDA approval only for the treatment of depression, enthusiastic medical practitioners have claimed success in treating anxiety, addictions, bulimia, panic attacks, and obsessive-compulsive disorders. Unlike other antidepressants, Prozac decreases one's appetite, and some doctors have even attempted to use it as a part of a weight reduction program. This side effect would appear to be a significant reason for not using Prozac during pregnancy. As clinical experience with this drug has increased, psychiatrists have come to learn that as many as 15 percent of their patients experience worrisome side effects associated with its use. Included among these has been intense agitation, tremors, manic behavior, and preoccupation with suicide. Some critics have sarcastically labeled it "the suicide pill" rather than a wonder drug.

The manufacturer of Prozac has given it a surprisingly generous B pregnancy-risk-factor classification based on the fact that studies on rats and rabbits given doses 9 to 11 times the maximum daily human dose experienced no fetal complications. Unfortunately, there are no adequate and well-controlled studies in pregnant women to support this B rating, and the drug should be used only when absolutely necessary. Nursing women should be equally cautious, since one study found breast milk concentrations equal to one-fourth the levels in the maternal bloodstream.

In the years prior to the introduction of Prozac, antidepressants came in two basic varieties: tricyclics and monoamine oxidase inhibitors, or MAOIs. Though still widely used today, sales of these drugs have been clearly eclipsed by Prozac. Tricyclic products include amitriptyline (trade names Elavil and Endep), nortriptyline (trade names Aventyl and Pamelor), amoxapine (trade name Asendin), protriptyline (trade name Vivactil), desipramine (trade names Norpramin and Pertofrane), doxepin (trade names Adapin and Sinequan), and imipramine (trade names Tofranil and Imavate). Examples of MAOIs include tranylcypromine (trade name Parnate), phenelzine (trade name Nardil), and isocarboxazid (trade name Marplan).

The tricyclic antidepressants have not been subjected to adequate clinical investigation to endorse their use during pregnancy. Amitriptyline, nortriptyline, and imipramine have been assigned D pregnancy-risk-factor classifications, while all the others in this group are in category C. Isolated case reports have linked imipramine, amitriptyline, and nortriptyline to limb deformities in exposed fetuses, although subsequent larger studies have demonstrated no such relationship. Withdrawal symptoms in newborns have been reported in a few instances during the first 30 days of life when women have taken tricyclic antidepressants late in pregnancy. Although there are no animal studies firmly linking the tricyclics to congenital anomalies, researchers have demonstrated that animals exposed to tricyclics in utero can suffer behavioral and neurochemical disturbances lasting well past termination of drug exposure and occasionally into adulthood.

Most studies have found that only minimal amounts of tricyclics are excreted in the breast milk, and their effect on the nursing infant remains unknown. There is one case report in the medical literature of a nursing infant who became pale, limp, and almost stopped breathing after its mother was treated with high doses of doxepin for depression. While this is only one isolated case, it should make obstetricians and their patients conscious of the potential dangers of taking tricyclics while nursing.

Dangerous maternal elevations of blood pressure may occur when MAOI antidepressants are combined with certain medications or a variety of foods such as cheese, sour cream, yogurt, wine, beer, liqueurs, caviar, pickled herring, raisins, chocolate, bananas, and meats prepared with tenderizers. Although very little is known about the fetal effects of MAOIs, the limited information available is somewhat worrisome. Despite their C pregnancy-risk-factor classification, all have been linked to a higher incidence of anomalies among infants exposed to MAOIs during the first trimester. No data are available about the safety of these drugs for the breast-fed infant.

Bupropion hydrochloride (trade name Wellbutrin) is a new antidepressant which is chemically unrelated to all other antidepressants. Reproduction studies on rabbits and rats at doses up to 15 to 45 times the human daily dose have revealed no evidence of impaired fertility, miscarriage, or fetal compromise. In rabbits, however, there was a slightly higher incidence of fetal anomalies in two reports, but no specific defects could be isolated. Considering these findings and the fact that there are no adequate well-controlled studies of this drug for nursing women, the manufacturer's B pregnancy-risk-factor classification would appear to be overly generous, misleading, and potentially dangerous.

Trazodone hydrochloride (trade name Desyrel) is another new and chemically different antidepressant about which too little is known. It has a C pregnancy-risk-factor classification. Although there have been no adequate or well-controlled studies on trazodone's effect on human pregnancy, animals given 15 to 50 times the human dose experienced higher miscarriage and congenital anomaly rates. Therefore, it should be used only when absolutely imperative. Trazodone is excreted in breast milk, but its effect on the nursing infant is unknown.

What drugs are used to treat the more severe psychiatric disorders, and how can they affect the outcome of pregnancy?

Unfortunately, half the medications used to treat severe emotional disorders and various forms of psychotic and deranged behavior are prescribed by nonpsychiatrists who often fail to recognize their potentially harmful effects on the pregnant woman.

Manic-depressive psychosis is a fairly common and very serious psychiatric disorder characterized by unpredictable and dangerous mood swings. It is treated most often with lithium carbonate. Lithium, however, has a D pregnancy-risk-factor classification and has been reported to cause severe abnormalities, and its use should be avoided by pregnant women and women likely to conceive. Following maternal ingestion, lithium levels in the amniotic fluid actually exceed those in the maternal bloodstream. Studies of infants exposed to lithium carbonate during the first trimester of pregnancy have revealed a 9 percent incidence of severe anomalies of the heart and its great vessels. Defects of the central nervous system and the external ears have also been noted. The most vulnerable period for the fetus is between the eleventh and ninetieth day following conception. As a result of the severity of these abnormalities, a registry of lithium-exposed babies has been established in order to determine more precisely the types of anomalies that may be associated with the use of this drug.

In contrast to the many reports linking maternal lithium use to severe fetal complications, a 1992 multicenter study of 138 women found no such relationship. The reasons for the discrepancy between this study and others remains unknown at the present time.

Women receiving lithium therapy during the last two trimesters of pregnancy should not restrict their sodium or salt intake and should never take diuretics. When sodium intake is restricted, lithium excretion is reduced and lithium intoxication may result. Two separate case studies from Copenhagen and Texas, published in *Obstetrics and Gynecology* in 1990, found that maternal lithium use could cause polyhydramnios, the abnormal accumulation of excess amounts of amniotic fluid. This occurs because lithium stimulates the fetus to urinate in greater amounts, and urine is the major source of amniotic fluid. If at all possible, avoid lithium in the last month of pregnancy, since it may cause neonatal toxicity at birth. Lithium is excreted in breast milk at one-quarter to one-half the concentrations of maternal serum levels; therefore, mothers receiving lithium therapy should not breast-feed.

Haloperidol (trade name Haldol) is frequently used to treat psychotic disorders. There have been two cases of severe limb malformations following maternal use of haloperidol early in the first trimester. Other investigators, however, have not found these defects. In one study of 98 women who received haloperidol during the first trimester, doctors uncovered no abnormalities or adverse fetal effects. During labor, the drug has been administered without causing neonatal depression. Haloperidol is excreted in breast milk in concentrations of approximately 60 to 70 percent of those found in the maternal plasma. While no adverse effects have been reported in nursing infants, the American Academy of Pediatrics classified haloperidol as an agent whose effect on the nursing infant is unknown but may be of concern.

Many antipsychotic agents are derived from a basic chemical class called phenothiazines, the same drug category of some of the previously mentioned antihistamines. Examples of some of the popular phenothiazines used in psychiatry include chlorpromazine (trade name Thorazine), promazine (trade name Sparine), trifluoperazine (trade name Stelazine), trioridazine (trade name Mellaril), fluphenazine (trade name Prolixin), and perphenazine (trade name Estrafon). Chlorpromazine has been available for the longest period of time, and more pregnant women have used it than any other phenothiazine. The overwhelming majority of studies have found it to be safe for both mother and fetus if used occasionally in low doses. In one survey of 142 fetuses exposed to chlorpromazine during the first trimester, United States researchers found no evidence of malformations, reduced birth weight, or impaired IQ when the children were evaluated at four years of age. Opposite results were found in one French study of 57 exposed infants, 4 of whom experienced a variety of defects including microcephaly, clubfoot, syndactyly (fusion of the digits), and cardiac defects. Chlorpromazine has been used in labor to promote analgesia and amnesia. However, as many as 20 percent of the women treated experienced a marked and unpredictable fall in blood pressure. Use of chlorpromazine in high doses during the last ten days of pregnancy may cause jaundice, depressed reflexes, lethargy, and poor muscle tone in the newborn; symptoms may persist for as long

as three weeks. While chlorpromazine is excreted in breast milk in very low concentrations, women who take it and breast-feed should carefully observe their babies for the earliest signs of drowsiness and lethargy.

Chlorpromazine and the other phenothiazines used in psychiatry all have a pregnancy-risk-factor classification of C. Although some reports have attempted to link first-trimester use of trifluoperazine to limb and cardiac defects, these findings have been refuted in larger and more extensive studies. Very little information is available about the safety of other phenothiazines in this group, but all are believed to be reasonably safe when used in low doses for limited periods of time. Virtually nothing is known about their excretion in breast milk or their potential to harm the nursing infant.

 ANTICONVULSANTS

What problems may be encountered during pregnancy by a woman who is treated for seizure disorders?

Two million Americans, including 800,000 women of childbearing age, have epilepsy. Obstetricians and neurologists caring for the pregnant epileptic often face difficult decisions. Anticonvulsant medications, invaluable in the control of seizures, may involve a significant risk of fetal damage, while discontinuing the medication may precipitate seizures which could cause even greater harm to the pregnant woman and her fetus. Studies suggest that seizure frequency is increased in 30 to 45 percent, unaltered in 50 percent, and decreased in anywhere from 5 to 20 percent of pregnant women. Women who carry a male fetus are twice as likely to deteriorate as those carrying a female, and there are curious case reports in the

medical literature of women who have had seizures when carrying a male child and none when carrying a female. The reasons for this phenomenon are presently unknown.

Dilantin is the trade name of the most commonly prescribed anticonvulsant. It is generically named phenytoin and belongs to a class of drugs called hydantoins. Mephenytoin (trade name Mesantoin) is another popular hydantoin. In 1964, a relationship between hydantoin use and congenital malformations was first noted. Since then, numerous reports have confirmed these findings. A review of the literature indicates that an epileptic pregnant woman taking phenytoin, either alone or in combination with other anticonvulsants, has a two to three times greater risk for delivering a child with congenital defects over the general population. Some authors have also described a group of abnormalities termed the "fetal hydantoin syndrome" (FHS). This occurs in 11 percent of infants exposed to hydantoins in utero and consists of a variety of abnormalities of the face, skull, and limbs. Impaired prenatal and postpartum growth and mental retardation are often observed in conjunction with FHS. However, more often than not, symptoms may be subtle and difficult to diagnose.

Fatal hemorrhage in newborns has been reported following maternal anticonvulsant therapy with hydantoins. Studies show that newborns suffering from this form of hemorrhage lack vitamin K, which is associated with clotting of blood. Bleeding usually occurs within 24 hours of birth and may involve the brain, lungs, and abdominal organs of the infant.

As if these potential problems weren't bad enough, 11 separate case reports have suggested that exposure to hydantoins in utero may be responsible for causing a variety of unusual childhood tumors and cancers. For this reason, hydantoin-exposed infants should be closely observed for several years, since tumor development may take that long to express itself. Based on all these potential complications, is it any wonder that phenytoin has a D pregnancy-risk-factor classification?

Phenytoin is excreted in breast milk in low concentrations, and researchers believe that it poses little risk to the nursing infant if maternal doses are kept within the normal therapeutic range. The American Academy of Pediatrics considers phenytoin compatible with breast-feeding.

Phenobarbital, a barbiturate, is often prescribed in the treatment of epilepsy. Use of phenobarbital is associated with a slightly increased rate of birth defects, especially cleft palate, cleft lip, and congenital heart disease. However, specific malformations are difficult to confirm because other anticonvulsants are usually taken in combination with it. As with phenytoin, phenobarbital has a pregnancy-risk-factor classification of D and is also capable of suppressing vitamin K-dependent clotting factors, leading to hemorrhagic disease of the newborn. However, the incidence of major malformations associated with phenobarbital use is believed to be significantly lower than it is with phenytoin. Fetal barbiturate addiction and neonatal withdrawal have been observed in infants exposed to phenobarbital in utero. Since phenobarbital-induced sedation has been observed in a small number of nursing infants, women using this drug while breast-feeding should be instructed to carefully observe their infants for sedation. It is probably far more logical for the phenobarbital-dependent epileptic woman not to nurse her baby.

Primidone (trade name Mysoline) is an anticonvulsant which is almost identical in chemical structure to phenobarbital. Although little is known about its side effects or potential to cause fetal damage, the same precautions should be used when prescribing it during pregnancy and nursing. Primidone has a D pregnancy-risk-factor classification.

Trimethadione (trade name Tridione) is used to control the mild seizures called petit mal. The relationship between fetal exposure and malformations is more firmly established with this drug than with any other anticonvulsant, and it should never be used during pregnancy. Equally dangerous is paramethadione (trade name Paradione), which is also used in the treatment of petit mal; in one study, doctors reported 13 prenatal deaths among 53 women using trimethadione or paramethadione during pregnancy. Both have D pregnancy-risk-factor classifications, but most experts believe that an X classification would be more suitable. The safety of trimethadione for use during lactation is unknown at the present time.

Carbamazepine (trade name Tegretol) is a popular drug with a C pregnancy-risk-factor classification. It has been used successfully in the treatment of all forms of epilepsy. However, it rapidly crosses the placenta and attains fetal blood levels ranging between 50 and 80 percent of those found in the maternal circulation. Until recently, neurologists often recommended that carbamazepine be used as the anticonvulsant of choice during pregnancy since it was believed to be safer for the fetus than other medications. However, a 1989 study published in the *New England Journal of Medicine* throws doubt on this conclusion. Dr. Kenneth Lyons Jones and his associates at the University of California in San Diego detected a pattern of fetal malformations associated with carbamazepine. Although the abnormalities were classified as "minor" by Dr. Lyons and his colleagues, they are nevertheless worrisome and of great concern to pregnant epileptics receiving carbamazepine and doctors contemplating prescribing it. Recent reports have also linked carbamazepine exposure during pregnancy with a higher incidence of spina bifida. Carbamazepine is excreted in breast milk in concentrations 20 to 60 percent of those in maternal serum, but levels detected in the nursing infant's bloodstream are extremely low. The American Academy of Pediatrics considers carbamazepine to be compatible with breast-feeding.

Depakene is the trade name for valproic acid, a medication used to treat brief and usually mild petit mal seizures as well as other convulsive disorders. Like other anticonvulsants, it has the capacity to cross the placenta, enter the fetal circulation in high concentrations, and cause serious consequences. Complications associated with valproic acid use during pregnancy have included major and minor congenital abnormalities, intrauterine growth retardation, jaundice and potentially fatal liver toxicity, clotting defects, and fetal distress. Although it is listed as a D pregnancy-risk-factor classification drug by some, most experts believe it should be in category X and never used in pregnancy. In one recent study from the Netherlands, doctors reported neural tube defects in three babies out of 120 exposed to the drug between the seventeenth and thirtieth day after conception. Other predominant major defects have involved the heart, face, skull, and limbs.

Levels of valproic acid in breast milk are only about 3 percent of those in maternal serum, and no adverse effects in the nursing infant from this exposure have been reported. The American Academy of Pediatrics considers valproic acid to be compatible with breast-feeding.

The so-called "succinimide anticonvulsants" used in the treatment of petit mal epilepsy include ethosuximide (trade name Zarontin), methsuximide (trade name Celontin), and phensuximide (trade name Milontin). Ethosuximide is a C pregnancy-risk-factor classification drug and the agent of choice for treating petit mal epilepsy during pregnancy. Although there are sporadic and poorly documented case reports of fetal abnormalities associated with ethosuximide use, most authorities believe that its potential for causing birth defects is far less than that of other drugs used to treat petit mal in pregnancy. While ethosuximide freely enters the breast milk in concentrations similar to those in maternal serum, no adverse effects on the nursing infant have been reported, and the American Academy of Pediatrics considers it to be compatible with breast-feeding. There is practically no information available on the effects of methsuximide or phensuximide on the fetus or nursing infant, but for reasons which are incomprehensible the former has a C, while the latter has a D pregnancy-risk-factor classification.

Clonazepam (trade name Klonopin, formerly Clonopin) is an anticonvulsant that is chemically and structurally similar to the benzodiazepine tranquilizer named diazepam (trade name Valium). Benzodiazepines in general, and clonazepam in particular, have been reported to cause lethargy, poor muscle tone, respiratory arrest, and low blood oxygen levels in babies when the drug is taken by a woman at the end of pregnancy. While no congenital defects have been linked to clonazepam use early in pregnancy, experience with this drug is limited to only a small number of cases. Clonazepam is excreted in breast milk at levels one-third those found in maternal plasma. There is one case in the medical literature of a nursing infant who experienced respiratory distress believed to be secondary to its mother's use of clonazapam. Based on this report, experts recommend that infants exposed to clonazapam through breast-feeding be closely monitored for lethargy and respiratory depression.

What advice do you have for the pregnant woman with a convulsive disorder?

Ideally, you should have a full evaluation by a neurologist before you try to conceive. It is sometimes discovered that a particular medication you are taking is unnecessary, especially if you have been free of seizures for several years and your brain wave pattern is normal. Sometimes the medication you are taking can be changed to another that is less likely to cause abnormalities. If you are taking trimethadione or paramethadione, it should be discontinued before a contemplated pregnancy and replaced with a safer alternative. Even if a woman cannot forego anticonvulsants entirely, changing from a combination of drugs to a single agent reduces the likelihood of a major fetal malformation, microcephaly, or growth retardation by more than 30 percent. It is also safer to administer drug therapy in small increments up to four or five times a day to sustain uniform drug levels, since wide fluctuations can interfere with normal fetal growth. You should be aware that even if you take no medication and experience no seizures during pregnancy, your chances of giving birth to an infant with anomalies are still two to three times that of the general population.

If you require hydantoins, be assured that you have nearly a 90 percent chance of giving birth to a normal child. If you are taking phenobarbital, your risk of giving birth to a deformed infant is probably significantly less than the 11 percent figure quoted for hydantoins. If your doctor decides that these medications must be taken during pregnancy, you should heed that advice, since the risk of maternal and fetal damage may be greater if severe and uncontrolled convulsions occur. It is important to monitor maternal serum levels to detect decreasing concentrations and to adjust the dosage accordingly.

Pregnancies complicated by epilepsy require fetal monitoring with periodic diagnostic ultrasound examinations beginning in the first trimester and nonstress testing during the last trimester (see Chapter 11). Maternal serum alpha fetoprotein testing should be performed between the fifteenth and eighteenth week to detect neural tube defects, especially if a woman has used valproic acid during the first trimester.

Be sure that your baby receives an intramuscular injection of vitamin K (trade name AquaMEPHYTON, generic name phytonadione) in the delivery room if you have been treated with hydantoins, trimethadione, primidone, or phenobarbital before delivery. This will prevent a bleeding disorder caused by a depletion of coagulation factors by the anticonvulsant.

Treatment with anticonvulsants may result in lowered serum folic acid levels, so pregnant women with epilepsy should receive a daily supplement of 1 milligram. Experts now suggest that folic acid supplementation be started before conception (see Chapter 8). Women taking hydantoin anticonvulsants over a period of time are at greater risk of a vitamin D deficiency in themselves and in their fetuses. This can be corrected with the vitamin D found in all prenatal vitamins.

After delivery, your baby should be carefully examined for congenital malformations and the nursery alerted to perform clotting factor and platelet counts every 2 to 4 hours during the first 24 hours of life. Infants exposed to phenobarbital should be observed for drowsiness and barbiturate withdrawal symptoms. Withdrawal is characterized by hyperexcitability, tremor, restlessness, difficulty in sleeping, poor sucking, and possibly seizures.

ANTICOAGULANTS

What are anticoagulants, and how may they cause problems during pregnancy?

Anticoagulants are lifesaving medications which prevent clotting of blood. A thrombus is defined as a clot attached to the wall of an artery or vein. When in a vein (phleb), it is often accompanied by inflammation (itis). Thrombophlebitis is most common in the veins of the legs and pelvis and may be either superficial or deep. The superficial variety is located just beneath the surface of the skin in the varicose veins which may develop with childbirth. Few women have serious complications from superficial thrombophlebitis, but thrombophlebitis of the veins deep in the legs and pelvis presents a real threat to a woman's life. Unfortunately, deep thrombophlebitis may occur without any warning symptoms. When one of these deep clots becomes dislodged from the wall of the vein, it travels through the circulation and is called an embolus. If this embolus reaches the lung, it is then called a pulmonary embolus. There it may block the opening of a large oxygen-carrying blood vessel, causing instant death. Anticoagulants are invaluable in preventing the formation and spread of thrombophlebitis and pulmonary emboli. They are also essential in the prevention and treatment of certain types of stroke and heart disease. During pregnancy, anticoagulants are effectively used as prophylaxis against clot formation in women with a previous history of deep vein thrombophlebitis and pulmonary emboli. This is a worthwhile precaution in view of the fact that a woman who has experienced a thromboembolism during pregnancy faces a 12 percent risk of a recurrence in a subsequent pregnancy. Previous placement of a heart valve prosthesis also warrants anticoagulant use during pregnancy.

Anticoagulants are either oral or injectable. Examples of oral preparations are warfarin (trade names Coumadin and Panwarfin) and bishydrox-coumarin (trade name Dicumarol). The injectable anticoagulant is heparin sodium. Heparin can be administered intravenously or subcutaneously, but it should not be given intramuscularly because it may produce a blood clot at the injection site. During the first trimester, especially between the sixth and ninth week, oral anticoagulants may cause what is called the fetal warfarin embryopathy syndrome. This syndrome, which occurs in 15 to 25 percent of exposed infants, is characterized by underdevelopment of the cartilage of the nose, stippled cartilage on x-ray examination of the vertebral column and long bones, small fingers and hands, atrophy of the nerves of the eye, cataracts leading to blindness, retarded physical and mental development, and microcephaly. The incidence of spontaneous abortion is greater among infants exposed to oral anticoagulants during each of the three trimesters. If oral anticoagulants are taken by a mother in the second trimester, fetal hemorrhage may occur along with developmental defects such as microcephaly, blindness, and mental retardation. Fetal and placental hemorrhage have been reported following maternal use of oral anticoagulants during the last trimester, while stillbirth and neonatal death rates are also significantly higher. Coumadin derivatives have been assigned a D pregnancy-risk-factor classification, but many authorities believe that an X rating is more appropriate. However, there are important medical conditions, such as prevention of clot formation on an artificial heart valve, where these agents are more effective than heparin. Under these circumstances, doctors have prescribed heparin for the first 12 weeks and the last month of pregnancy, to reduce the risks of anomalies and newborn hemorrhage, respectively, while switching to coumadin derivatives for the reminder of the pregnancy.

If anticoagulant therapy is necessary during pregnancy, heparin is preferred, but it may not be totally innocuous. On a positive note, despite extensive use of heparin by thousands of women over a period of many years, there are no reports linking it to congenital defects. Despite this, in one study, maternal use of this drug was associated with a 12 percent incidence of stillbirths and a 30 percent rate of prematurity. However, this poor pregnancy outcome might not have resulted from the use of heparin but from the underlying disease conditions which demanded its use. The most recent study, published in 1989 by doctors at McMaster University in Ontario, Canada, found that pregnant women who received prophylactic heparin were at no greater risk than other women of experiencing premature births, spontaneous abortions, stillbirths, neonatal deaths, or congenital anomalies. Heparin has a C pregnancy-risk-factor classification.

Osteoporosis is an abnormal loss of minerals from the bones which may be aggravated with prolonged use of heparin. When osteoporosis is severe, it can cause fractures of the bones of the vertebral column. Studies from England suggest that pregnant women may be more prone to this complication than nonpregnant women. Prolonged heparin use may also be associated with a reduction in the number of platelets needed for blood coagulation. In the days immediately following delivery, heparin use may be associated with a 50 percent risk of postpartum hemorrhage.

Most medical textbooks advise against the use of oral anticoagulants while breast-feeding for fear that they will anticoagulate the baby. However, recent studies have clearly demonstrated that warfarin does not enter the breast milk and cannot possibly cause harm to the nursing infant. Bishydroxycoumarin is equally safe, and the American Academy of Pediatrics has classified both of these anticoagulants as compatible with breast-feeding. However, other less-popular coumadin derivatives such as ethyl biscoumacetate and phenindione (not used in the United States) do enter the breast milk in concentrations sufficient to cause hemorrhage in the nursing infant and must never be used.

How safe are the medications used to dissolve blood clots once they have formed?

Thrombolytics are enzymes which dissolve blood clots once they have formed. Examples include urokinase (trade name Abbokinase), alteplase (trade name Activase), and streptokinase (trade names Streptase and Kabikinase). These agents often play a lifesaving role in breaking down pulmonary emboli, coronary artery thrombosis, and arterial thrombosis in the extremities. Because of the significant risk of hemorrhage associated with their use, thrombolytics should be used only in acute emergencies during pregnancy and the postpartum period.

Its manufacturer has assigned urokinase a B pregnancy-risk-factor classification, but this is far too generous in view of the fact that only one case report of its use in human pregnancy has been located. Animal studies in rats and mice with urokinase have revealed no harmful fetal consequences. More experience has been gained with use of streptokinase during pregnancy, and although it has a C pregnancy-risk-factor classification, there are no reports linking its use to congenital defects. The minimal amounts that cross the placenta are not sufficient to cause excessive fibrinolysis or bleeding problems in the fetus. One researcher has treated 24 women with streptokinase in the second and third trimesters without fetal complications. There are no data available on the excretion of thrombolytics in breast milk or their safety for the nursing infant.

ANTIHYPERTENSIVES

Which medications should be avoided and which may be safely used in the treatment of hypertension during pregnancy?

Hypertension is an abnormal elevation of the blood pressure which occurs in approximately 5 to 10 percent of the adult population. The cause of the high blood pressure is unknown 90 percent of the time. There is a form of hypertension which occurs specifically after the twentieth week of pregnancy, known as preeclampsia, eclampsia, and toxemia. Pregnancy-induced hypertension completely subsides following childbirth.

A wide variety of antihypertensive agents have been advocated for use during pregnancy. Of these, some are less than ideal and others are unquestionably a poor choice.

Reserpine is the perfect example of a popular antihypertensive medication that has a pregnancy-risk-factor classification of D and should not be used during pregnancy. In addition to causing too sudden a drop in the blood pressure during exercise or change in position, it may also be responsible for an increase in stomach acid secretion, peptic ulcer, and frequency of bowel movements. Of even greater concern is a study of 48 fetuses exposed to reserpine in the first trimester. Eight percent experienced developmental defects, including microcephaly, abnormal dilatation of the kidneys and ureters, and inguinal hernia. Unpleasant fetal effects include lethargy, severe nasal congestion, poor appetite, and bradycardia, or an abnormally slow heart rate. Reserpine is excreted in significant quantities in breast milk, but no clinical reports of adverse effects in the nursing infant have been located. Popular antihypertensive brands that contain reserpine are Regroton, Diupres, Diutensen-R, Renase-R, Salutensin, Serpasil, Ser-Ap-Es, Hydropres, and Hydromox R.

Inderal is the trade name for propranolol, a drug used in the treatment of hypertension as well as a variety of disorders such as angina, hyperthyroidism, and abnormalities of the heart rate and rhythm. Propranolol and other drugs of similar chemical structure are classified as beta-blockers. Examples of some of the newer and more popular beta-blockers include labetalol (trade names Trandate and Normodyne), nadolol (trade name Corgard), pindolol (trade name Visken), timolol (trade names Timolide and Blocadren), acebutolol (trade name Sectral), atenolol (trade name Tenormin), metoprolol (trade name Lopressor), betaxolol (trade name Kerlone), and penbutolol (trade name Levatol).

While pindolol and acebutolol have been assigned pregnancy-risk-classifications of B by their manufacturers, all the other beta-blockers have a less favorable C rating. The most clinical experience has been gained with propranolol and labetalol, but virtually nothing is known about most of the other products.

American physicians have been reluctant to prescribe beta-blockers during pregnancy because of isolated case reports of fetal growth retardation, a higher stillbirth rate, prolonged labor, and, following delivery, respiratory distress, jaundice, low blood pressure, abnormally low blood sugar (hypoglycemia), and an abnormally slow heart rate (bradycardia) for as long as three days. Two separate studies have demonstrated an abnormal fetal nonstress test and a poor heart rate response to sound stimulation following maternal treatment with propranolol. More recent reports and a 1988 review of the use of propranolol and other beta-blockers have been more favorable than earlier studies. For example, despite extensive investigation there are no reports linking beta-blocker use to birth defects. In addition, labetalol has been found to increase uteroplacental blood flow, and it may also play a role in reducing the incidence of respiratory distress syndrome in premature infants by increasing the baby's production of pulmonary surfactant (see Chapter 11). When a group of pregnant women with severe hypertension were treated with pindolol, they gave birth to babies with an average birth weight of 3,285 grams, or almost 700 grams (1½ pounds) more than babies born of mothers treated with atenolol. Despite these positive findings, beta-blockers must be used with caution during pregnancy, especially in the days just prior to delivery. Newborn infants of women taking a beta-blocker should be closely observed for 72 hours after birth for respiratory depression, hypoglycemia, low blood pressure, and bradycardia.

Beta-blockers are excreted into breast milk at levels which appear to be too low to cause adverse reactions. The breast milk concentration for propranolol is believed to be less than 40 percent of its concentration in the maternal bloodstream, with peak concentrations occurring between two and three hours after a dose. Peak levels of labetalol parallel those of propranolol. One researcher calculated that a nursing infant would absorb only 1/100th of a normal pediatric dose of propranolol, and that this amount was safe. To eliminate even the slightest risk to a nursing infant, experts suggest that a woman postpone feeding for three to four hours after ingesting a beta-blocker. The American Academy of Pediatrics considers propranolol, labetalol, nadolol, timolol, and metoprolol to be compatible with breast-feeding. Too little is known about the other beta-blockers to endorse their use during nursing.

In addition to beta-blockers, there is a category of antihypertensives known as alpha-blockers. Terazosin (trade name Hytrin) and prazosin (trade name Minipress) are two examples. Both have a pregnancy-risk-factor classification of C, although experience with the drugs is too limited to endorse their use during pregnancy or nursing.

Diazoxide (trade name Hyperstat) is a potent antihypertensive agent which is given intravenously in combating severe hypertensive emergencies. Its manufacturer has given it a pregnancy-risk-factor classification of C. Unpleasant maternal side effects, such as severe hypotension (low blood pressure), salt and water retention, and elevation of the blood sugar, limit its usefulness. Studies in pregnant monkeys and sheep demonstrate that diazoxide readily crosses the placenta, with fetal concentrations of the drug equaling maternal levels one to two hours after injection. Prolonged hyperglycemia, or abnormal elevations in the blood sugar, have been noted and are believed to be caused by the drug's capacity to destroy the insulin-producing cells in the fetal pancreas. Diazoxide is also a potent uterine muscle relaxant capable of inhibiting uterine contractions during labor. As a result, oxytocin is often needed during labor if a woman has been given diazoxide. At the present time, the effects of diazoxide on the nursing infant are unknown.

ACE is an acronym for Angiotension Converting Enzyme Inhibitors, a new class of antihypertensive drugs. Members of this group include captopril (trade name Capoten), enalapril (trade name Vasotec), and lisinopril (trade names Zestril and Prinivil). Although ACE inhibitors are effective in lowering blood pressure, preliminary studies suggest that they are best avoided by pregnant hypertensive women. All three ACE inhibitors have been given pregnancy-risk-factor classifications of C by their manufacturers, but scientists believe that this classification is unwarranted in view of the fact that these drugs may compromise fetal kidney function to the point of causing in utero renal failure. A 1991 published report on this subject from the Netherlands found that kidney dysfunction was more likely to occur with enalapril than with captopril. The authors of this study correctly concluded, "There are strong reasons for not using angiotensin converting enzyme inhibitors in pregnancy unless the likely benefit is considered great enough to outweigh the substantial negative consequences of their use." As a result of a growing number of studies indicating ACE inhibitors as a cause of hypotension and kidney failure in exposed fetuses, the FDA ordered that manufacturers change their package inserts to reflect these dangers. As of May 1992, the new labeling must warn of the fetal risks of using ACE inhibitors during the second and third trimesters and the need to find safer alternatives.

If an ACE inhibitor must be used during pregnancy, experts recommend that it be given at the lowest possible dose, and that periodic ultrasound examinations be performed in order to evaluate fetal kidney function and amniotic fluid volume. In addition to kidney failure, severe hypotension has been observed in newborns exposed in utero to both captopril and enalapril. In animal species, captopril use has been associated with a higher incidence of spontaneous abortions and stillbirths.

Captopril is excreted in breast milk in very low concentrations, and the American Academy of Pediatrics considers it to be compatible with breast-feeding. No data are available on the safety of nursing for women being treated with enalapril and with lisinopril.

Calcium channel blockers are a new class of antihypertensive medication which have a category C pregnancy-risk-factor classification. Examples include verapamil (trade names Calan and Isoptin), nifedipine (trade names Procardia and Adalat), nicardipine (trade name Cardene), and diltiazem (trade name Cardizem). The contractile process of heart muscles, smooth muscles lining blood vessels, and the myometrium, or muscle of the uterus, are all dependent upon the movement of calcium ions into their cells through specific channels or openings. Calcium channel blockers prevent this from happening without changing serum calcium concentrations. Obstetrical researchers in Europe have described several instances in which calcium channel blockers successfully reversed a congenitally abnormal and rapid fetal heart rate. Calcium channel blockers have also been used as tocolytics, uterine muscle relaxants which stop premature labor.

Although there are no reports linking calcium channel blockers to congenital defects, the use of these drugs during pregnancy remains controversial. Several studies performed on pregnant sheep,

rabbits, and monkeys in 1987 and 1988 demonstrated that calcium channel blockers can drop the maternal blood pressure to perilously low levels; this can cause reduced uterine blood flow and low oxygen levels in the fetus. Limited studies in human pregnancy have been more favorable. For example, a 1990 report from Finland measured fetal blood flow patterns with a Doppler ultrasound device following use of nifedipine by ten women at the end of pregnancy and noted no significant changes in blood flow pattern in the umbilical arteries. Decreased resistance to blood flow was noted in the uterine arteries, allowing more oxygen to reach the fetus.

All calcium channel blockers are excreted in the breast milk, and the few studies to date have found no problems associated with nursing. In one report, investigators calculated that a nursing baby would ingest less than 5 percent of the maternal nifedipine dose and this would present no dangers to its health. Of the calcium channel blockers, only verapamil has been officially sanctioned by the American Academy of Pediatrics as being compatible with breast-feeding. To minimize the amount of a calcium channel blocker ingested by a nursing infant, a woman should delay feeding her baby for 3 to 4 hours after taking the drug.

Clonidine (trade names Catapres and Combipres) is another potent antihypertensive with a pregnancy-risk-factor classification of C. Clonidine easily crosses the placenta, and its concentrations are equal in maternal serum and umbilical cord blood at birth. Reproduction studies on animals have not shown that clonidine produces malformations, but they did find a higher incidence of fetal loss. There are no reports linking the use of clonidine to congenital defects in humans, but experience is limited. When used by the pregnant woman in the last trimester, clonidine has not been known to cause hypotension in the newborn. Maternal problems encountered with clonidine—such as sodium and fluid retention, bowel disturbances, drowsiness, and abnormal lowering of the blood pressure—may discourage pregnant women from using this drug. Clonidine is excreted into breast milk in concentrations two times those of maternal serum, and it has been detected in the bloodstream of nursing infants. The significance of this finding is unknown as is the safety of using clonidine while breast-feeding.

Sodium nitroprusside (trade names Nipride and Nitropress) has proven to be a lifesaving medication for rapidly lowering severe elevations of blood pressure during pregnancy. Although there are no reports linking sodium nitroprusside to birth defects, animal studies have shown that this drug rapidly crosses the placenta and is metabolized to the poisonous chemicals cyanide and thiocyanate. However, fetal cyanide poisoning will not occur if the drug is used in the recommended therapeutic doses for short periods of time. Occasionally, sodium nitroprusside can cause a precipitous drop in blood pressure, which may decrease blood and oxygen flow to the fetus. Sodium nitroprusside has a pregnancy-risk-factor classification of C, and virtually nothing is known about its excretion in breast milk or its safety for the nursing infant.

The two safest and most effective antihypertensive agents for use during pregnancy are methyldopa (trade name Aldomet) and hydralazine (trade name Apresoline). Despite its pregnancy-risk-factor classification of C, methyldopa has been endorsed by most medical authorities as an ideal antihypertensive for long-term use during pregnancy because it does not impair the flow of blood and oxygen to the fetus. Methyldopa's safety to the fetus has been documented in several clinical trials involving thousands of pregnancies over the past two decades. Compared to hypertensive patients who are untreated, those receiving methyldopa have lower spontaneous abortion rates, increased birth weights of their babies, fewer premature deliveries, and decreased neonatal mortality. Methyldopa is not without maternal side effects such as

drowsiness, depression, salt retention, and constipation.

In addition to its low concentrations in breast milk, methyldopa has been found to stimulate the secretion of prolactin hormone from the pituitary gland; this may have the positive effect of increasing the quantity of breast milk. While the safety of methyldopa in lactating women has not been documented in any large clinical studies, the American Academy of Pediatrics considers it to be compatible with breast-feeding.

Reported side effects of hydralazine in adults have included sodium and water retention, weight gain, flushing, nasal congestion, headaches, dizziness, and palpitations, but most patients tolerate the drug extremely well. One rare but bizarre complication of hydralazine use is the presence of symptoms closely resembling those of a serious collagen disease named lupus erythematosis. Fortunately this condition is reversible once the drug is discontinued. Hydralazine has a pregnancy-risk-factor classification of C. There are conflicting reports in the medical literature on the effects of hydralazine on the blood flow to the uterus and placenta. This is an important determination because the amount of oxygen received by the fetus is directly related to the amount of blood reaching the uterus and placenta. The majority of research conducted on pregnant sheep seems to indicate that hydralzine increases the uterine blood flow. Animal studies on mice and rabbits indicate that hydralazine may produce cleft palate and malformations of the facial and skull bones. Extensive clinical experience in human pregnancy, however, has not revealed any such abnormalities. Bleeding and a low platelet count have been reported in three newborns whose mothers used hydralazine daily throughout the third trimester.

Hydralazine is excreted into breast milk. Although there is little information available to document either its safety or hazards, the American Academy of Pediatrics considers it to be compatible with breast-feeding.

DIURETICS

How safe are diuretics ("water pills") during pregnancy?

Diuretics are agents which increase the amount of urine excreted. Better known as "water pills," diuretics are medically valuable in the treatment of hypertension, heart failure, and a variety of disorders characterized by edema, the swelling of tissues with fluid. Premenstrual edema is often successfully relieved with diuretics.

In the past, diuretics were frequently used to relieve the normal physiological edema which accompanies pregnancy. Some doctors even proposed that they be used prophylactically to prevent the development of toxemia. However, convincing research has demonstrated that the routine use of diuretics during normal pregnancy exposes a mother and her fetus to unnecessary hazards while in fact doing nothing to prevent toxemia. By inhibiting the normal physiologic expansion of the plasma volume during pregnancy, diuretics may actually predispose to IUGR, preterm labor, and preeclampsia (pregnancy-induced hypertension). Unfortunately, diuretics are still prescribed too often for pregnant women in this country.

Edema during pregnancy is rarely a cause for concern. The so-called dependent edema of pregnancy is characterized by swelling of the ankles and results from restriction of blood flow through the veins of the legs and pelvis by the enlarged uterus. The vena cava is a huge vein which carries blood to the heart from the lower part of the body. It runs behind and to the right of the enlarged pregnant uterus. Often the only treatment necessary to relieve edema during pregnancy is to lie on your left side in bed for several hours at a time. This will prevent the floppy uterus from falling against the vena cava, thereby increasing the amount of blood that is carried from the lower extremities. Other helpful measures in reducing edema are elevating the legs and wearing support stockings. When these simple measures fail, and edema is severe enough to cause great discomfort in the legs or numbness or pain in the hands, a short course of diuretic therapy is occasionally appropriate.

Of all diuretics, the thiazide group of drugs is the most commonly prescribed during pregnancy. Popular thiazides are chlorothiazide (trade name Diuril), hydrochlorothiazide (trade names HydroDIURIL and Esidrix), trichloromethiazide (trade name Naqua), bendroflumethiazide (trade name Naturetin), methclothiazide (trade name Enduron), benzthiazide (trade name Exna), methyclothiazide (trade name Aquatensen), and polythiazide (trade name Renese). Aldactazide, Capozide, Diutensen, Enduronyl, Apresazide, Inderide, Lopressor HCT, Maxzide, Zestoretic, and Vaseretic are trade names of compounds which contain thiazides in combination with other drugs.

Although often casually prescribed, thiazide diuretics have a dangerous pregnancy-risk-factor classification of D and should rarely if ever be prescribed during pregnancy. Maternal complications associated with thiazide use include a chemical imbalance caused by excessive loss of sodium and potassium, inflammation of the pancreas, hyperglycemia (abnormal elevation of the blood sugar), and hyperuricemia (abnormal elevation of the blood uric acid level). While most studies have found no link between thiazide use and congenital abnormalities, one large survey of 233 infants exposed during the first trimester did note a slight increase. A far greater number of fetal and neonatal problems have been associated with maternal thiazide use during the last trimester.

Although thiazides are excreted in breast milk in low concentrations, they may be responsible for decreasing the quantity of breast milk. Despite this, the American Academy of Pediatrics considers the following thiazides to be compatible with breast-feeding: chlorothiazide, hydrochlorothiazide, chlorthalidone, and bendroflumethiazide.

Furosemide (trade name Lasix) is a very potent diuretic with a pregnancy-risk-factor classification of C. It readily crosses the placenta and fetal concentrations of furosemide equal maternal levels 8 hours after a dose is taken. To date, no abnormalities have been reported among infants of mothers treated with furosemide during pregnancy. Probably the only two valid reasons for using this potent diuretic during pregnancy are severe congestive heart failure and kidney disease requiring immediate and massive excretion of urine. Furosemide, like other diuretics, will decrease the quantity of breast milk. Its concentration in breast milk and its effects on the nursing infant have not been adequately studied.

Ethacrynic acid (trade name Edecrin) and bumetanide (trade name Bumex) are potent "loop diuretics," meaning that they exert their effect on an anatomic site in the kidney known as Henle's loop. Limited experience with ethacrynic acid use in pregnancy has not shown an increased incidence of malformations or adverse fetal effects. Nevertheless, the drug has a category D pregnancy-risk-factor classification because of concerns that its exaggerated diuretic effects may decrease placental blood flow and fetal oxygenation. No data are available on the safety or concentrations of ethacrynic acid in breast milk, but its manufacturer advises against its use if a woman is breast-feeding. Far less is known about the safety of bumetanide. It has a pregnancy-risk-factor classification of C based on its safety in pregnant laboratory animals and a limited number of pregnant women. It is not known if bumetanide is excreted in breast milk, but the manufacturer suggests that nursing not be undertaken when a woman is using this drug.

Spironolactone (trade name Aldactone) is not as potent a diuretic as ethacrynic acid. It has been found to cross the placenta, but its effects, if any, on the fetus have not been determined. It has a pregnancy-risk-factor classification of D based on

animal research showing feminization of male fetuses exposed to spironolactone. While its effects on the nursing infant are unknown, the American Academy of Pediatrics considers spironolactone to be compatible with breast-feeding.

Indapamide (trade name Lozol) is a new class of diuretic and hypertensive agent known as an indoline. Its manufacturer has bestowed upon it a very generous category B pregnancy-risk-factor classification based on studies demonstrating its safety in pregnant rats, mice, and rabbits given more than 6,000 times the therapeutic human dose. However, there are no reports in humans that confirm the manufacturer's optimistic evaluation. Nothing is known about indapamide's excretion in breast milk.

Can cholesterol-lowering drugs cause harm if used during pregnancy?

There are a host of new medications on the market which are known as cholesterol reducers, or hypolipidemics. Some lower the levels of triglycerides, lipoproteins, and the so-called "bad" or low-density lipoprotein-cholesterol (LDL-C), while others are less selective in their effects and also reduce the concentration of the "good," or high-density lipoprotein-cholesterol (HDL-C). Practically nothing is known about the effects of these agents on the fetus and nursing infant.

Of the hypolipidemics, only lovastatin (trade name Mevacor) has a pregnancy-risk-factor classification of X, based on research showing that rat fetuses exposed to 500 times the maximum recommended human dose experienced bone malformations. Its manufacturer also cautions against using the drug if a woman intends to nurse her baby. Cholestyramine (trade names Questran and Colybar) and colestipol (trade name Colestid) are probably the two safest hypolipidemics for the pregnant women because they are not absorbed from the intestinal tract. However, the manufacturer cautions that they may interfere with the absorption of fat-soluble vitamins into the bloodstream. The manufacturer of gemfibrozil (trade name Lopid) has assigned it a relatively safe pregnancy-risk-factor classification of B despite the fact that there are no studies proving its safety for pregnant women. Although experimental pregnant animals given several times the normal adult dose of gemfibrozil have not experienced adverse fetal effects, concerns have been expressed that it may cause liver nodules and liver cancer. Dextrothyroxine sodium (trade name Choloxin) and probucol (trade name Lorelco) also have a pregnancy-risk-factor classification of B, and pregnant rats, rabbits, and

mice given between 50 and 100 times the maximum human dose have experienced no complications. There are, however, no adequate or well-controlled studies in pregnant and nursing women to document their safety. Clofibrate (trade name Atromid-S) is one of the most popular hypolipidemics. Although there are no animal or human studies to confirm its safety, it has a pregnancy-risk-factor classification of C; its manufacturer states that it should not be used if a woman is breast-feeding.

 CARDIAC DRUGS

How can drugs which are used to treat abnormal heart rhythms alter the outcome of pregnancy?

Digitalis and its derivatives are frequently prescribed in the treatment of heart failure and other cardiac conditions characterized by abnormal heart rate and rhythm. The most popular drugs in this group are digoxin (trade name Lanoxin) and digitoxin (trade name Crystodigin). Since digitalis preparations are so essential to the health of the person being treated, it is a relief to know that they have been given to a large number of pregnant women for varying periods of time without any reports of fetal ill effects or anomalies. All digitalis preparations readily pass from the maternal to the fetal circulation in increasing concentrations as pregnancy progresses, and theoretically they could cause abnormal slowing of the fetal heart rate. However, with the exception of one fetal death in the medical literature resulting from a maternal digitoxin overdose, this does not appear to be a problem. In the unlikely event that digitalis intoxication of the fetus is to occur, it is most likely to happen during the eighth month of pregnancy. Digitalis and its derivatives have a pregnancy-risk-

factor classification of C. Digitalis derivatives are excreted into breast milk in low concentrations, and no adverse effects in the nursing infant have been reported. The American Academy of Pediatrics considers digoxin to be compatible with breast-feeding.

Quinidine is another commonly prescribed drug used in the treatment of abnormalities of the cardiac rate and rhythm. Some popular trade names of quinidine preparations are Duraquin, Quinaglute, Cardioquin, Quinidex, and Quinora. Quinidine has been assigned a pregnancy-risk-factor classification of C. It has been used to treat cardiac arrhythmias in pregnant women for approximately 70 years, and to date there are no reports linking its use to congenital defects. Most doctors conclude that if a woman requires the drug, she can be reasonably certain that it will not adversely alter the outcome of her pregnancy. While quinidine has been shown to freely pass into the breast milk in a concentration similar to that found in the mother's bloodstream, the American Academy of Pediatrics considers it to be compatible with breast-feeding.

Disopyramide (trade name Norpace), a popular

drug for treating cardiac arrhythmias, has a pregnancy-risk-factor classification of C. While experience is limited, animal studies and human pregnancies in which disopyramide has been used have not been associated with congenital defects or fetal growth retardation. Even though one study found that it caused premature uterine contractions, most reviews consider disopyramide to be safe for use during pregnancy. Disopyramide is excreted into breast milk in relatively high concentrations, but the American Academy of Pediatrics considers it to be compatible with breast-feeding.

Lidocaine (trade name Xylocaine) is widely used as a local anesthetic but may also be administered intravenously in treating life-threatening cardiac arrhythmias. It has a pregnancy-risk-factor classification of C but appears to present minimal fetal risk when administered in the usual therapeutic doses. In one study, researchers found that offspring of mothers receiving lidocaine had significantly lower scores on tests of muscle strength and tone than did infants that were not exposed. There are no data available on the safety of lidocaine for infants who are breast-fed.

Procainamide (trade names Pronestyl and ProcanSR) is another antiarrhythmic medication with a pregnancy-risk-factor classification of C. It does not appear to have adverse fetal effects and is approved for nursing infants by the American Academy of Pediatrics.

Mexiletine (trade name Mexitil) is one of the newest medications used for treating cardiac arrthmias. Although it has a pregnancy-risk-factor classification of C, practically nothing is known about the safety of its use during pregnancy. Laboratory tests on rats, mice, and rabbits at four times the maximum human dose have produced no abnormalities. A 1987 study from the University of North Carolina found that concentrations of mexiletine are higher in breast milk than in maternal plasma, which the investigators cautioned could potentially cause problems for the nursing infant.

 # THYROID MEDICATIONS

What problems may be encountered when using medications to treat thyroid disease during pregnancy and nursing?

Since uncontrolled thyroid gland disease will worsen a woman's chances for a successful pregnancy outcome, it is imperative that the diagnosis be made and treatment begun as early as possible, ideally before pregnancy. Normal pregnancy induces a number of changes in thyroid function studies, some of which may confuse the unenlightened physician interpreting these laboratory tests. As a result, medications are too often prescribed when they are not really needed.

The chances of a pregnancy in a woman with an underactive thyroid gland (hypothyroidism) ending in spontaneous abortion are greatly increased. The obvious treatment for a poorly functioning thyroid gland is thyroid hormone replacement therapy. Thyroid extracts containing the two natural hormones of the thyroid gland, thyroxine and triiodothyronine, are the most popular. In spite of widespread use of thyroid hormone, there have been only a few isolated case reports of children born with congenital malformations following maternal use of these preparations, and most authorities consider thyroxine and triiodothyronine to be extremely safe.

If a hypothyroid newborn is not promptly treated with adequate amounts of thyroid hormone, permanent mental retardation and cretinism may develop. Thyroxine and triiodothyronine, when ingested by nursing women, have actually helped prevent permanent damage to infants born with severe hypothyroidism. In one study, 12 of 15 nursing infants born with hypothyroidism had average intelligence compared to only 12 of 32 formula-fed infants. Thyroxine and triiodothyronine are excreted in breast milk in small amounts, and a woman using these medications can safely nurse her infant.

The treatment of maternal hyperthyroidism, or excessive thyroid activity, is far more complex and unpredictable than that of hypothyroidism. Although the details of the various treatment regimens endorsed by different specialists are beyond the scope of this discussion, the most popular method involves suppression of excessive maternal thyroid function with either propylthiouracil or methimazole (trade name Tapazole). Unfortunately, both drugs readily cross the placenta and have the capacity to induce severe hypothyroidism, goiter, and even cretinism in the developing fetus. Therefore, these drugs should be used at the lowest dose capable of maintaining thyroid function at its upper limits of normal. Under ideal conditions, the drug can be stopped completely two to three weeks prior to delivery in order to minimize the risks to the fetus.

Despite a pregnancy-risk-factor classification of D, propylthiouracil is considered the drug of choice for the treatment of hyperthyroidism during pregnancy. Its use has not been associated with fetal anomalies, but methimazole has been linked to a specific ulcerlike scalp defect among exposed infants. Propylthiouracil is not concentrated in breast milk to any significant degree, and women taking this drug can safely breast-feed their babies. Since the remote potential for neonatal hypothyroidism exists, experts recommend that the nursing infant's thyroid function be tested every two to four weeks. The American Academy of Pediatrics considers propylthiouracil compatible with breast-feeding.

Methimazole also has a pregnancy-risk-factor classification of D, but doctors consider it to be far less desirable than propylthiouracil for treating hyperthyroidism in the pregnant and nursing woman. In addition to the previously mentioned scalp defects, isolated reports of umbilical abnormalities, cataracts, and other anomalies have been reported in association with methimazole use during pregnancy. However, the majority of studies have found it to be a drug free of fetal complications. Although methimazole is excreted into breast milk in greater concentrations than propylthiouracil, it will not pose a risk to a nursing infant provided that the mother is treated with the lowest effective dose and the baby's thyroid function is monitored at frequent intervals.

Iodides have also been used to suppress thyroid activity. Ingestion of iodides after the twelfth week of pregnancy is not recommended, since they may cause hypothyroidism and goiter in the fetus. Use of radioactive iodine as a diagnostic test of thyroid function or in the treatment of thyroid disease is absolutely not recommended during pregnancy. Iodides are also excreted in breast milk, but in much lower concentrations. However, since milk ingestion by the baby could theoretically depress the functioning of its thyroid gland, women who use iodides should not nurse.

Propranolol (trade name Inderal) is an antihypertensive medication which is gaining popularity in the treatment of hypothyroidism. The safety of its use during pregnancy and nursing has been previously discussed (see page 300).

ANTIDIABETIC MEDICATIONS

How safe are the medications used for treating diabetes during pregnancy?

To ensure a successful pregnancy outcome for diabetic women and those who develop pregnancy-related or gestational diabetes, it is vital that blood sugars be carefully controlled and monitored throughout pregnancy. There are two classes of medications used to control diabetes: oral hypoglycemics and injections of insulin.

Oral hypoglycemics act by stimulating the synthesis and release of insulin from the pancreas. They should not be used during pregnancy because they are unable to lower blood sugar levels as precisely as insulin and they may be associated with adverse fetal effects. Given to a mother at the end of pregnancy, oral hypoglycemics pass into the fetal circulation and stimulate the fetal pancreas to secrete excessive amounts of insulin, which may cause a dangerous lowering of the newborn's blood sugar.

Tolbutamide (trade name Orinase) is the oldest and most popular oral hypoglycemic. It has been assigned a pregnancy-risk-factor classification of D by the FDA and a more generous C rating by its manufacturer. Although tolbutamide has been associated with an increased incidence of congenital defects in animals, such a relationship has not been clearly demonstrated in pregnant women. Neonatal thrombocytopenia, or an abnormally low platelet count, persisting for as long as two weeks, has been associated with maternal use of tolbutamide toward the end of pregnancy. Although tolbutamide is excreted into breast milk, it is the only oral hypoglycemic deemed compatible with breastfeeding by the American Academy of Pediatrics.

Glyburide (trade names Micronase and Dia-Beta) and glipizide (trade name Glucotrol) are the two newest oral hypoglycemics. They are preferred by some endocrinologists because of their greater potency and the fewer side effects associated with their use. While nothing is known about the effects of glyburide on the fetus or nursing infant, its manufacturer has given it a totally unrealistic pregnancy-risk-factor classification of B based on limited studies with rats and rabbits showing no harmful fetal effects. Glipizide's manufacturer has bestowed an even more bizarre C pregnancy-risk-factor rating on it even though there have been no studies conducted in humans and laboratory research has found it to be "mildly feto-toxic" in rats exposed during pregnancy.

There is no evidence to show that insulin produces abnormalities in humans, and it is unquestionably the drug of choice for treating diabetes during pregnancy. It has a pregnancy-risk-factor classification of B, and the fact that it is a naturally occurring constituent of the blood attests to its safety. If taken by a diabetic mother, insulin will not enter her breast milk and therefore will pose no hazards for the nursing infant.

 # ACNE MEDICATIONS

What are the hazards associated with the use of acne medications during pregnancy?

Isotretinoin (trade name Acutane) is a synthetic derivative of vitamin A which has proven to be unmatched in treating severe and recalcitrant acne. Unfortunately, it is also one of the more deadly and disfiguring fetal toxins. Isotretinoin was first marketed in 1982, but it was not until the end of 1983 that reports linking it to a higher spontaneous abortion rate and characteristic fetal defects, known as the "isotretinoin teratogenic syndrome," first appeared. Among fetuses exposed to isotretinoin between 1982 and 1986, researchers have found a 25 percent incidence of anomalies involving the central nervous system, skull, face, heart and great vessels, and thymus, in addition to a spontaneous abortion rate of at least 20 percent and a significantly higher incidence of stillbirths and neonatal deaths. In addition, more subtle mental deficiencies have been noted in seemingly unaffected children as they have grown older. Equally tragic consequences have been associated with the use of etretinate (trade name Tegison), a drug similar in chemical structure to isotretinoin which is used in the treatment of psoriasis. The critical period of exposure in human pregnancy occurs between the second and fifth weeks following conception, although less obvious defects may occur before and after this time.

Concern has been expressed that birth defects may occur even if a woman stops using isotretinoin prior to conception. This fear has been allayed to a great degree by a report published in the *Archives of Dermatology* in 1989, in which doctors studied the pregnancies of 88 women who conceived between 2 and 60 days following their last isotretin-

oin dose. There were 8 spontaneous abortions (9 percent), 75 normal births (85 percent), and 4 (4.5 percent) infants with congenital malformations. The malformations, however, were not characteristic of those associated with in utero exposure to isotretinoin. This study concluded that if a woman stops using isotretinoin just prior to conception, she need not fear that her fetus will suffer from its toxic effects.

Unlike isotretinoin and etretinate, which both have pregnancy-risk-factor classifications of X, retinoic acid or tretinoin (trade name Retin-A) appears to be safe, as evidenced by its pregnancy-risk-factor classification of B. Retinoic acid is approved for the treatment of acne, but some researchers have used it experimentally for treating wrinkles, brown aging spots, and even skin cancer. Studies have convincingly demonstrated that the amount of retinoic acid absorbed into a person's body is minuscule, even when used in the highest concentrations over several body sites.

Antibiotics are frequently prescribed in the treatment of acne, and tetracyclines are the most popular. Unfortunately, their use is contraindicated during pregnancy (see page 261). Safer alternatives include penicillin and its derivatives, cephalosporins, erythromycin, and clindamycin.

⋅⋅⋅ *10* ⋅⋅⋅

ENVIRONMENTAL
and OCCUPATIONAL HAZARDS
of PREGNANCY

*M*any pregnant women encounter serious problems related to a wide variety of toxins in their home and work environments. Scientists have proven that ubiquitous pollutants, such as dioxin and PCPs, can cause medical illnesses as well as reproductive failure. Insulating a house or painting and preparing a room for a baby brings with it questions about the effects of these chemicals on the developing fetus. Misconceptions about the dangers of video display terminals, radon, and radiation released by microwave ovens and television sets often add to the pregnant woman's anxiety, as do fears that she must find a new home for a beloved pet cat, bird, or turtle to be sure that the potentially serious diseases which are caused by these animals will not harm her fetus.

Exposure to fumes, noxious chemicals, asbestos, noise pollution, and radiation pose definite hazards to a pregnant woman. Knowledge of these hazards and the methods of preventing or at least minimizing their effects is invaluable to the outcome of a successful pregnancy. A woman's concerns about exposure to toxins and pollutants do not necessarily end at the moment of birth, since concentrations of certain contaminants in breast milk often exceed those found in the bloodstream.

Your medical history is not complete unless your obstetrician asks where you and your partner presently work and where you have worked during the past five years. Hobbies and outside activities must also be investigated to find out if you are exposed to possible pollutants. In the future, obstetricians can expect to play an increasingly important role in determining pregnancy disability for exposure to toxic substances and in protecting women from workplace and environmental hazards. This chapter deals with the many questions and concerns about the home and occupational environments of the pregnant woman.

EMOTIONAL STRESS

Do stress and anxiety affect pregnancy?

Although there is little scientific data available on this subject, several clinical investigations have concluded that anxiety-prone women are more likely to experience spontaneous abortion and still-birth and to produce babies of diminished birth weight. This information is especially relevant today because growing numbers of women are experiencing job-related anxieties. In a recent survey of 40,000 working women, 95 percent considered their jobs to be either "somewhat stressful" or "very stressful."

Based on animal research and clinical experience, scientists have concluded that some anxious pregnant women release an abundance of epinephrine and norepinephrine. These body chemicals, classified as catecholamines, enter the circulation of susceptible women and narrow the uterine arteries which carry oxygen to the fetus. They also increase the uterine muscle tone, further reducing the amount of oxygen transmitted to the fetus. It should be noted, however, that an equal number of studies have shown no relationship between mental stress and adverse pregnancy outcome.

Pregnant or not, we all experience mental stress and anxiety in our daily lives, and there is incontrovertible proof that emotional factors can cause physical changes such as increased muscle tension, faster breathing, a more rapid heartbeat, and elevated blood pressure. Chronic stress can lead to physical and emotional problems ranging from fatigue and insomnia, ulcers, and heart disease. Job strain has been defined as a situation in which the psychological demands at work were high but the individual's latitude in decision making and ability to control the pace of work was limited. Certainly, many pregnant and nonpregnant women are employed in jobs which fit this description, and the medical consequences of such stress demand further study.

In a 1990 study by researchers at the University of North Carolina, 786 working women were evaluated for the effects of job stress on the outcome of their pregnancies. This report, published in the *American Journal of Public Health*, concluded that preterm birth and low-birth-weight infants were not associated with job stress in the total sample of women studied. However, a small subgroup of 70 women, opposed to working outside of their home and employed in jobs with low control and high levels of psychological stress, gave birth to infants who weighed 500 grams (about 1 pound) less than those born to women who worked in less stressful positions. In another study published in 1970, doctors evaluated the "anxiety-proneness" of 150 women tested on the Taylor Manifest Anxiety Scale; the more anxiety-prone women gave birth to smaller babies. Similar results were reported in a 1986 report from the University of New South Wales in which women with the highest levels of anxiety were more likely to experience pregnancy complications such as hypertension, preeclampsia, and premature births. In addition, their infants were slower to nurse than infants born to less anxious women.

While childbirth education classes, the support of family and friends, an understanding doctor and hospital nursing staff, and a homelike environment in the labor room all help to allay fears brought on by pregnancy, there still remains a small group of women who are simply unable to rid themselves of these fears, and the fear of labor in particular. For some women, the stress of labor triggers excessive catecholamine release and jeopardizes fetal well-being. Sometimes anesthesia techniques, such as epidural, can eliminate the perception of pain during labor and delivery and provide a more favorable environment for the infants of anxiety-prone individuals. One very important study from Yale University compared the relationship between a woman's psychological characteristics, as tested during the last trimester of her first pregnancy, and the amount of pain medication and sedation which she received during labor. Among the 64 women studied, it was found that the amount of medication which was administered by an obstetrician during labor was based more on the woman's psychological state during pregnancy than her actual requirements during labor; those demonstrating high anxiety during pregnancy tended to receive the largest amounts of analgesics and sedatives during labor even though they did not necessarily require medication. If, as is believed, an anxiety-ridden woman is more apt to give birth to a compromised infant, the added insult of unneeded medication can only worsen the chances of survival.

 # PHYSICAL STRESS

Can jobs which require physically demanding work adversely alter the outcome of pregnancy?

While many women now work until the onset of labor, some evidence in the medical literature suggests that this trend may be ill advised. Several studies support the view that lack of rest during the last two to four weeks of pregnancy may have an unfavorable effect on the fetus. When European working women of poor socioeconomic levels were allowed rest in maternity homes for several days prior to delivery, a significant decrease in perinatal mortality was observed among those resting for longer than one week.

In a 1982 study from the Pennsylvania State University College of Medicine, researchers analyzed the work activity of 7,722 women during pregnancy. They found that those who worked past their twenty-eighth week gave birth to infants weighing 150 to 400 grams (5.3 to 14 ounces) less than women who did not work. They also noted a higher incidence of placental infarcts among some working women. A placental infarct is an area of dead tissue in the placenta caused by impairment of its blood supply from the uterus; extensive infarcts can be responsible for growth retardation and even fetal death. The investigators found that large infarcts, having a diameter of 3 centimeters or more, occurred with a very high frequency of 250 per 1,000 births among women who did "stand-up work" after their thirty-seventh week. Included in this group were retail sales workers, private household workers, and laborers. Women who quit this type of work before their thirty-third week had only 47 infarcts per 1,000 births, while the incidence for those who quit between the thirty-third and thirty-seventh weeks was 96 per 1,000 births. Women who did "sitting work" throughout pregnancy, such as clerical workers and students, experienced large infarcts at a rate of 51 per 1,000, compared with 53 per 1,000 for women who remained at home. Several articles published since 1982 have confirmed and expanded upon the findings of the Pennsylvania State University researchers. Despite these findings, the researchers found no evidence to prove that working women were more likely to give birth to babies with long-term mental or physical impairment. However, such reports do suggest that if you have a "stand-up" job, it might be advisable to curtail this activity during the last two months of your pregnancy.

NOISE POLLUTION

Can excessive environmental noise affect the outcome of pregnancy?

There is increasing scientific evidence that exposure to noise, especially unexpected and uncontrollable noise, is associated with hearing loss, high blood pressure, heart disease, insomnia, and nervous disorders. As with other forms of stress, "noise pollution" may also increase maternal catecholamine release and decrease fetal oxygenation. Studies conducted as early as 1941 noted that maternal emotional agitation induced by harsh sound profoundly decreased the fetal heart rate. It is known that fetuses hear some of the sounds to which their mothers are exposed; however, the protective uterine and amniotic fluid environment screens out most of the noise. In 1991, Finnish researchers exposed a group of 27 pregnant volunteers to measured amounts of noise transmitted through headphones, thereby eliminating any direct fetal stimulation. All of the women were in their third trimester. Maternal catecholamine levels and fetal and uterine blood circulation remained unaltered throughout the period of testing. This is a reassuring sign for pregnant women who enjoy listening to loud music on personal stereos.

In studies on the effects of noise on the outcome of pregnancy conducted on pregnant women living near busy airports, it was found that babies born of women living in close proximity to Los Angeles International Airport had a higher incidence of birth defects such as anencephaly, spina bifida, abdominal hernia, cleft lip, and cleft palate; the stillbirth rate was higher among women living closest to London's Heathrow Airport; and expectant mothers living near Osaka International Airport had lower levels of human placental lactogen and gave birth to babies with lower birth weights than pregnant women living in quieter areas of Japan. In 1988, researchers from Montreal, Canada studied the effects of occupational factors in more than 100,000 pregnancies and found that women exposed to excessive amounts of noise at work were more likely than other women to give birth to a low-birth-weight infant.

In a rather disturbing study published in the *American Journal of Industrial Medicine*, doctors conducted hearing tests on 131 children whose mothers were exposed to excessive levels of industrial noise for a minimum of one month during pregnancy. They found hearing deficits in as many as 40 percent of infants whose mothers were exposed to the highest noise levels over the greatest number of pregnancy days. Smaller amounts of environmental noise over shorter periods of time also produced hearing deficits, but to a lesser degree.

 ## *CARBON MONOXIDE*

Aside from cigarette smoke, how can the pregnant woman inhale noxious carbon monoxide fumes?

Whether you smoke or are exposed to the "sidestream" or "secondhand" smoke of others, cigarette smoking in the home or work environment will put you and your fetus in jeopardy (see Chapter 5). Carbon monoxide is one of the most dangerous pollutants found in cigarette smoke, but it is also produced by cars, trucks, furnaces, and industrial machinery. Carbon monoxide concentrations are heaviest in the air around big cities. In one survey, it was found that in the South Pole the carbon monoxide concentration was 0.02 parts per million, compared to 13 parts per million in midtown Manhattan. On occasion, levels in high traffic areas in New York City have been reported to be as high as 40 parts per million. In some sections of Los Angeles, carbon monoxide levels have reached an amazingly high 100 parts per million.

Even low levels of carbon monoxide, absorbed repeatedly, could deprive the fetus of some of the oxygen needed to develop normally. For this reason, pregnant women should not work around cars and trucks, near furnaces, or in any confined space where there is heavy smoke or fumes.

The rising costs of home heating fuel have resulted in the widespread use of energy-efficient kerosene heaters. However, a report published in the October 1982 issue of *Consumer Reports* has concluded that these devices are responsible for the release of dangerous amounts of toxic chemicals such as carbon monoxide, carbon dioxide, nitrogen dioxide, and sulfur dioxide. With respect to the carbon monoxide levels, the *Consumer Reports* medical consultants determined that several hours' exposure to a kerosene heater was especially hazardous to people with heart disease, pregnant women and their fetuses, newborns, and those with respiratory disease.

 # *HAIR DYES*

What are the dangers involved if a woman works with or uses hair dyes during pregnancy?

Although much has been written about the potential for chemicals used in permanents and hair dying to cause cancer and birth defects, there has never been a published scientific study which supports this assertion. Laboratory research, however, has found that many hair dye ingredients are chemicals which are closely related to known carcinogens. Of the chemicals contained in the hundreds of hair dyes on the market, laboratory studies suggest that phenylenediamine, toluenediamine compounds, and resorcinol are the chemicals most likely to be associated with birth defects.

There are several studies in which pregnant rodents exposed to hair dye formulations equivalent to 100 times the usual human dose failed to uncover fetal abnormalities or adverse pregnancy outcomes. Human experience with hair dyes, although incomplete, is somewhat disconcerting. In a 1978 published report from England, there was a statistically significant excess of chromosomal damage and breaks among women who dyed their

hair. If it is substantiated that chromosomal damage is more likely among men and women with dyed hair, the potential exists for transmitting these abnormalities to the fetus.

It should come as no surprise that studies sponsored by the hair color industry have failed to note an association between hair dye use and cancer or complications of pregnancy. Based on these conflicting reports it is difficult for a woman to decide whether or not to use hair dyes during pregnancy or before a planned pregnancy. Many potential harmful carcinogens and mutation-inducing agents remain in all hair dye formulas. The public should not feel secure until the laws are changed so that the chemicals in cosmetics and hair dyes undergo the same premarket testing and FDA approval policies as those in foods and drugs.

In addition to concerns about the hazards of exposure to hair dyes, hairdressers and beauticians are exposed to a variety of dangerous occupational chemicals including acetone, aerosol propellants, benzyl alcohol, hair spray resins, hallogenated hydrocarbons, and chemicals in nail polish. Moreover, women in this profession often have to stand for prolonged periods of time, and this may be one of several determinants of premature labor (see page 350).

What hair dyes and cosmetics can a pregnant woman use?

Those who use hair dyes usually know little about the contents of the products which they apply to their scalp. Thanks to research by *Consumer Reports*, many of these questions can now be answered.

Coal-tar chemicals are found in permanent, semipermanent, and temporary hair dyes. While none are safe, permanent dyes have the greatest potential for harm. These products are usually advertised as "shampoo-in" dyes and are sold in two-part kits which contain coal-tar chemicals in one bottle and hydrogen peroxide "developer" in the other. The two liquids are mixed together just before use and shampooed into the hair shaft. The color lasts until the hair grows out in about four to six weeks.

Semipermanent hair dyes do not contain peroxide but have chemicals that penetrate the hair shaft. The color generally lasts for three to four weeks. While these products are probably safer than the permanent hair dyes, their coal tars still penetrate the skin and may be absorbed into the bloodstream. Temporary hair dyes, also known as rinses, contain coal-tar dyes that coat rather than penetrate the hair shafts. As a result, there is less of a likelihood for absorption of the dyes into the scalp. These products are usually removed with the next shampooing. This should not lull the consumer into a sense of security, since *Consumer Reports* investigators encountered a great deal of secrecy surrounding the exact ingredients of these products. Chemicals in temporary hair dyes, bearing names such as Direct Brown 1:2, Direct Blue 6, and Acid Black 107, when traced to their laboratory origins, were found to contain several coal-tar derivatives that have long been suspected of causing cancer and chromosomal damage.

Henna is a dye which has the advantage of being a plant substance rather than a coal-tar chemical. Henna products are carefully regulated by the FDA. These products are perfectly safe, but the only color produced is an orange-red. If any henna-containing products boast that they can produce colors other than orange-red, check the label to be sure that coal-tars have not been added.

Metallic dyes, known as "progressive dyes," are applied daily and cause a gradual darkening of the hair. These products contain a metallic salt, such as lead acetate, which reacts with sulfur to produce a pigment that colors the hair. In evaluating the safety of lead acetate, the Food and Drug Administration has concluded that the amount which penetrates the skin and is absorbed into the body is far too little to produce toxic effects. However, it is important that these products not be used if there is a cut or abrasion of the scalp because too much of the chemical may then be absorbed into the body. The effects of lead on the outcome of pregnancy can be quite significant.

Since the safety of hair dyes has been questioned, the best advice is to avoid these products if you are pregnant or are of childbearing age. This is especially true for products which contain coal-tar chemicals, since there is no doubt that they have the potential to damage chromosomes and cause cell changes or mutations. Theoretically, the changes produced in a woman's immature unfertilized ovarian follicles could be transferred to offspring at a later date.

If you insist on using hair dyes, products containing henna would appear to be the safest. Unfortunately, not everyone wants to have orange-red hair. Metallic dyes are probably safe for use during pregnancy. Of the products which contain coal tars, I would surmise that the permanent hair dyes are the most dangerous, followed closely by the semipermanent dyes. If you want to use hair dyes, use a technique that involves minimal contact between the dye and your scalp. Hair dye enters the bloodstream through the scalp, not the hair shaft; the dye has to touch the scalp in order to penetrate the skin and be absorbed. Frosting, tipping, streaking, highlighting, and painting involve less scalp contact than permanent dyes applied in the form of shampoos. Hair painting and highlighting should be applied along the shaft in a direction away from the scalp.

Red dye No. 3 is a food coloring chemical which is also used in cosmetics and externally applied medications, ointments, and salves. Tests in rats have shown that this dye may be responsible for thyroid tumors and other cancers. Although nothing is known about the effects of Red dye No. 3 on humans, the FDA is currently supervising studies directed at determining its safety.

ANESTHETIC GASES

Is it true that pregnancy complications are more common among operating room nurses and other hospital employees who are exposed to anesthetic gases?

Since 1967, reports from Russia, Denmark, Great Britain, and the United States have concluded that women who are continually exposed to trace amounts of anesthetic gases when working in operating rooms are at greater risk of aborting or giving birth to babies with congenital abnormalities. Research at New York University College of Dentistry suggests that dentists, wives of dentists, and dental technicians may also be threatened by the effects of anesthetic gases. However, other investigators have reached different conclusions.

At the present time, no one can say with certainty if continued employment in an area in which general anesthesia is used is detrimental to the outcome of pregnancy. However, since doubt exists, it would be wise for the pregnant operating room nurse or aide to transfer to a different area of the hospital, especially during the first trimester. Women employed as dentists and dental technicians are best advised to stay out of rooms in which nitrous oxide anesthesia is being used. Similarly, if you need extensive and prolonged dental work during pregnancy, you should select a local anesthetic, such as Novocain (procaine) or Xylocaine (lidocaine), rather than nitrous oxide.

The concentration of anesthetic gases in a dental office or an operating room can be easily measured and can be reduced to concentrations of less than 1 percent by use of modern scavenging systems which remove the gas through the ventilation system. If you are a pregnant operating-room employee, it is not unreasonable to insist on knowing the concentration of anesthetic gases in your work area. If the levels are above 1 percent, you should demand that corrective measures be taken to improve the situation.

Can dental personnel experience pregnancy-related problems other than those caused by anesthetic gases?

Aside from exposure to x-rays, which is totally preventable (see page 329), few people are aware of the fact that exposure to mercury vapors is an occupational hazard for dentists and dental assistants. These vapors are produced in the preparation of mercury amalgams used for filling cavities. A dental office is considered to be contaminated if the mercury content in the air is equal to or greater than 0.05 milligrams per cubic meter. Based on a 1987 review of this subject, it is estimated that 10 percent of dental offices in the United States have unacceptably high levels of mercury in the air. In actual practice, there are less than a handful of documented cases of mercury poisoning among dentists and their technicians, but it is well documented that mercury easily passes through the placenta to the fetus, and that the fetus is far more sensitive to its toxic effects than is its mother (see page 320). Although this problem is extremely rare, if you work in a dental office, you can ask to have the air analyzed for mercury vapors. It should be emphasized that dental patients with mercury amalgam fillings are at no risk for mercury toxicity.

What is ethylene oxide, and what effect can it have on pregnant workers?

Ethylene oxide is a commonly used gas which may be encountered by women who work in areas of hospitals and clinics where equipment is steril-ized. In addition to causing severe irritation of the skin and mucous membranes, ethylene oxide is classified by the Occupational Safety and Health Administration (OSHA) as a carcinogen and pos-sible reproductive hazard. One study in Finland noted that nurses exposed to ethylene oxide had a higher incidence of spontaneous abortion than un-exposed nurses. In addition, chromosomal abnor-malities in a person's white blood cells have been found to occur more frequently following ethylene oxide exposure. The OSHA has set the ethylene oxide exposure limit at 1 part per million over an eight-hour work shift for women employed as ster-ilizer operators.

 HEAVY METALS

What heavy metals pose the greatest threat to the pregnant woman and her fetus?

In discussing exposure to heavy metals we are pri-marily concerned with lead, mercury, and cad-mium. Nickel and selenium have not yet been proved to be harmful to the human fetus.

How extensive is the threat of lead toxicity in our society?

Until recently, it was commonly believed that lead poisoning was limited to babies and young chil-dren who ate particles of lead paint peeling from the walls in old buildings. Scientists and environ-mentalists have made us aware that lead is a ubiq-uitous toxin which has become a public health problem for all segments of our society.

Workers employed in industries which use lead are especially susceptible. The industries present-ing the greatest risks for lead poisoning are lead smelting, brass foundries, storage battery man-ufacturing, ship building, paint manufactur-ing, printing, ceramics, ammunition, stained-glass manufacturing, and pottery glazing. Individuals who work in or frequent indoor firing ranges are often exposed to extremely high lead levels. If you or your husband are employed in any of these in-dustries, you are entitled to ask your employer for proof that concentrations of lead in the air have met federal safety standards. If not, use of a respi-rator is required until the standards are met. Other safety precautions mandated by the OSHA include frequent monitoring of lead levels in the air, the wearing of protective clothing, changing clothes and washing hands before eating, and never eating in the work area. Washing thoroughly and chang-ing clothes before leaving work helps to prevent the introduction of lead dust particles into the home. Unfortunately, any level of lead in the blood is too much, and exposures that were considered to be safe in the past are now deemed hazardous by the Environmental Protection Agency.

Water may also be a source of lead contamina-tion where it is acidic or where old lead pipes are still in use. Lead from plumbing can also dissolve into your drinking water, especially if the water stays unused in the pipes for several hours. For this reason, it is a good idea to flush lead out of your plumbing by letting the cold water run for 3 to 5 minutes before taking a drink. Hot water has higher levels of lead than cold water, so it is best not to use hot tap water for instant coffee or soup, cocoa, cereal, and baby formula and other infant food. While public drinking fountains and electric water coolers found in offices, schools, and buildings produce cold water, many also have lead-lined tanks which release lead at levels exceeding the Environmental Protection Agency limits.

Table wines, especially those with foil-wrap covering the outside rim and cork, are a recently discovered source of lead exposure. If you drink an occasional glass of wine during pregnancy, avoid products that are foil-wrapped. If your bottle does contain foil, you can reduce your lead exposure by removing the foil and the cork and wiping the rim with a wet cloth or one moistened with vinegar or lemon juice before pouring the wine.

Lead-soldered food cans are another source of lead. Fortunately, as of 1990 only 35 percent of domestically manufactured food cans contain lead, compared to 90 percent ten years ago. However, the number of imported cans with lead solder is believed to be significant. Defective ceramic ware can also release toxic levels of lead when food is served or stored in them. This problem is worsened by the acidity of food and beverages like tomato sauce and orange juice. Approximately 60 percent of the dinnerware sold in the United States is imported from a number of countries, with products from Mexico City, Italy, Spain, Portugal, and Hong Kong most often found to be leaking excessive amounts of lead. In contrast, ceramic ware from Japan is the safest because it must meet rigid safety standards before it is exported. Since it is often difficult if not impossible to tell if a food can contains soldered lead or if a ceramic plate is likely to leak lead into your food, you can determine this by purchasing a lead-detection kit from Frandon Enterprises, 511 North 48th Street, Seattle, Washington 98103, telephone (800) 332-7723 or Lead-check Swabs, HybriVet Systems, P.O. Box 1210, Framingham, Massachusetts 01701, telephone

(800)262-5323. Both kits cost less than $30.00. Another excellent source of information about lead toxicity is the Environmental Protection Agency Public Inquiries Center (PM-215), 401 M Street, S.W., Washington, D.C.

It has become fashionable to buy and renovate old homes, many of which have lead-base paints. Removing and handling these paints can increase the pregnant woman's risk of lead exposure. Cosmetics such as surma and kohl or folk remedies pose a significant risk to a woman and her fetus. Finally, dolomite or bone meal should not be used by the pregnant or lactating woman to meet calcium requirements because of the relatively high concentration of lead in many commercial preparations.

What are the effects of lead on pregnancy outcome?

Lead crosses the placenta and is present in umbilical cord blood at nearly the same concentrations as in maternal blood. Even when a pregnant woman is exposed to significant amounts of lead in her environment, she will practically always be asymptomatic, though several studies have confirmed that she will be more likely to experience an elevation of blood pressure during labor. The fetus is far more susceptible to lead's toxic effects. At least 25 percent of infants born in urban areas have significant levels of lead in their umbilical cord blood, a finding that has been linked to high infant mortality rates, preterm delivery, low birth weights, possible chromosomal aberrations, structural malformations, and lower intellectual and cognitive skills in childhood. Several researchers support the belief that even low levels of in utero exposure to lead result in lower IQ scores, poorer memory, and inferior academic achievement in childhood, and probably throughout one's lifetime.

Fortunately, there is a simple blood test which can detect early signs of lead poisoning. Women who fear they may have been exposed to high levels of lead can have this test performed at a cost of about $20.00 at most commercial laboratories.

What are the hazards associated with mercury poisoning during pregnancy?

Mercury has been responsible for several tragedies in the past, when pregnant women ate food contaminated with mercury from polluted waters or pesticides sprayed on farm produce. Mercury vapors may be inhaled in the work environment of dentists, dental hygienists, dental technicians (see page 317), and laboratory technicians and workers. Individuals employed in the production of electrical products, catalysts, thermometers, paints, amalgams, pesticides, and wood chemical processing agents are all subject to the dangers of mercury poisoning. Today, however, the principle source of contamination is rain containing traces of mercury from coal-burning power plants, municipal incinerators, and smelters. Other contamination comes from lake and ocean sediments previously polluted with mercury. In a 1979 study reported in the *Archives of Environmental Health*, scientists studied the chromosomes of workers in a chemical plant who were exposed to mercury vapors. Although these individuals appeared to be in good health, they were found to have a relatively high incidence of chromosomal breaks and gaps. Some of these abnormalities persisted long after the high concentrations of mercury in their bloodstream returned to normal. As recently as 1991, French researchers noted a significant increase in the rate of spontaneous abortion among wives of men occupationally exposed to mercury.

Despite its known toxicity, mercury has been widely used in many household products, such as latex paint, to preserve their shelf life. Fortunately, it was banned by the FDA as a paint additive in 1990. However, products manufactured before this date may still be sold.

High levels of mercury may on rare occasions cause severe neurologic and kidney diseases in an adult, but most individuals do not experience symptoms. The fetus, however, is extremely sensitive, and mercury readily passes into its bloodstream and brain to cause damage. Some reports show that the average mercury level in the baby's umbilical cord blood is 20 to 30 percent greater than the corresponding mercury concentration in maternal blood. Cerebral palsy, severe mental retardation, tremors, seizures, and kidney and liver disease have been noted among many infants whose mothers showed no symptoms of illness. In some instances, infantile poisoning worsened following the ingestion of mercury-contaminated breast milk. The diagnosis of elevated mercury levels can be determined by a blood or urine test on a scalp hair sample. Concentrations of mercury dust and vapors in the working environment can also be measured with special instruments.

Research has proven that fish caught in most United States waters are unlikely to be contaminated with mercury, except those taken in new man-made reservoirs, lakes heavily affected by acid rain, and lakes in the Everglades. However, a daily diet of fish with high concentrations of mercury, such as shark, swordfish, tuna, or red snapper among the salt water fishes and northern pike or walleye among the fresh water fishes, may be potentially dangerous for pregnant women.

What effect does cadmium have on pregnancy outcome?

Cadmium is often discharged into sewage systems by the electroplating industry and into the air by deterioration of rubber tires, and is a constituent of tobacco smoke. Cadmium may cause severe toxicity in the form of liver, kidney, heart, and lung disease. Abnormalities in the body's blood cells are also frequently observed. Chronic cadmium exposure may increase a woman's risk of cancer, reduce fertility, and lead to anomalies in her offspring. All this is easily avoided if air standards for cadmium levels in fumes and dust are met. If you work in a factory where cadmium is used, you can have the concentrations of the metal in your urine checked to be sure that your working environment is safe.

PHENOLIC GERMICIDES

What is hexachlorophene, and how can it cause pregnancy complications among medical and dental personnel?

Hexachlorophene, better known by the popular trade name of pHisoHex, is a potent antibacterial disinfectant first introduced in the United States in 1941. It rapidly gained popularity throughout the world and was soon added to soaps, face lotions, hair tonics, acne medications, antiperspirants, and toothpaste. A University of Washington study which found that brain damage occurred more frequently among newborn infants who were routinely washed with hexachlorophene solutions led the FDA to restrict the marketing of hexachlorophene to physician and hospital use. Several studies have confirmed hexachlorophene's unusual ability to rapidly penetrate the broken skin, enter the bloodstream, and migrate quickly into the cells of the brain, liver, and other organs. In a report from France, infants accidentally exposed to high concentra-tions of hexachlorophene in talcum powder suffered severe brain damage.

During pregnancy, hexachlorophene easily passes from mother to fetus via the placenta. In 1978, Swedish doctors reported that severe congenital malformations occurred 50 times more frequently in newborn infants born of hospital workers who washed their hands with a 1 to 3 percent concentration of hexachlorophene soap from 10 to 70 times daily during the first three months of pregnancy. Subsequent research on laboratory animals in the United States has confirmed the relationship between hexachlorophene use and birth defects. Burdeo is the trade name of a lotion which also contains hexachlorophene and must not be used by the pregnant woman. Newborns should be washed with germicides other than pHisoHex, unless there is a contagious bacterial infection in the nursery which is resistant to all other disinfectants.

Birth defects will result only if exposure to hexachlorophene occurs during pregnancy, and especially in the first three months.

PARASITES FROM PETS

Does a cat present risks to a pregnant woman?

Yes. Of all diseases caused by household pets, none has aroused more attention and concern among pregnant women than toxoplasmosis. This disease, caused by a microscopic protozoan named *Toxoplasma gondii*, is commonly transmitted by contact with infected cat feces or by the handling or eating of infected undercooked or raw meat, particularly pork, lamb, and goat. Infectious *Toxoplasma gondii* cysts persist in as many as 10 percent of mutton, 25 percent of pork, and 10 percent of beef samples. Adults who contract the disease usually have no symptoms and never know they have acquired it. When symptoms are present, they consist of a mild illness characterized by a low-grade fever, cough, headache, lethargy, and lymph node enlargement. According to a 1988 study from the National Institute of Neurological and Communicative Disorders and Stroke, maternal toxoplasmosis may increase a woman's risk of thrombophlebitis and asthma during pregnancy. Unfortunately, during pregnancy the organism crosses the placenta in 45 percent of all cases and severely damages or kills the fetus. Although many people consider toxoplasmosis to be a rare disease, the alarming truth is that it is the most common worldwide human parasitic infection, and one-third of all pregnant women have antibodies in their blood suggestive of previous exposure to *Toxoplasma gondii*. Epidemiologists have determined that a woman's chances of contracting toxoplasmosis for the first time during pregnancy are approximately 1 in 1,000. More than 3,000 infants are born with toxoplasmosis each year.

Toxoplasmosis is one of a group of diseases which cause similar defects in the developing fetus. They are called the TORCH complex, with the TO standing for toxoplasmosis. The other members of the infamous group are rubella (R), cytomegalovirus (C), and herpesvirus (H). If a woman contracts toxoplasmosis during the first trimester of pregnancy, it is estimated that her fetus will have a 17 percent risk of becoming infected. Of this 17 percent, 80 percent will be stillborn or show severe manifestations of the disease such as microcephaly (abnormally small head), hydrocephaly (abnormally large head), cerebral calcifications, blindness due to destruction of the retina, and convulsions. Blood platelet deficiencies and abnormal enlargement of the liver and spleen are also frequently seen. Although the likelihood of transmission of the disease to the fetus increases as pregnancy progresses, the severity of congenital manifestations becomes milder. For women infected during the second trimester, 25 percent of their infants will be infected, and 30 percent of this group will have severe defects. Among women infected during the third trimester, 65 percent of the fetuses will become infected, but few will show obvious problems at birth although problems may develop later.

Toxoplasma gondii undergoes a complex life cycle. The adult form of the organism invades body cells, multiplies, and then forms cysts within body tissues. If these cysts rupture, protozoa are released and the life cycle is repeated. Scientists have discovered that the cat intestine is unique among all animal species because it is here that little sacs, called oocysts, are formed when a cat contracts the disease. These oocysts are filled with *Toxoplasma gondii* organisms, and once formed they are passed daily in a cat's feces. This potential for disease dissemination may persist throughout the lifetime of the cat. If its feces are disturbed, the oocysts may become airborne and inhaled into the mouth or nose of a susceptible person. Cockroaches and flies are also capable of transmitting oocysts from cat feces to exposed foods.

A woman who has been exposed to toxoplasmosis before pregnancy or during a previous pregnancy will develop antibodies and immunity against reinfection and will rarely, if ever, transmit the disease to the fetus of her present pregnancy. The diagnosis of previous exposure to toxoplasmosis can be ascertained by an antibody blood test. More often than not, a woman's initial antibody testing is performed during the first trimester. The presence of IgG antibodies at this time makes it impossible for a doctor to know for certain if the toxoplasmosis exposure is old or recent. This problem can be resolved, however, by repeating the IgG titres over a period of three to four weeks; a fourfold rise during this time suggests acute infection.

A more reliable method for confirming a recent exposure to toxoplasmosis is to perform IgM antibody tests on all women with IgG antibodies. These antibodies appear soon after a primary toxoplasmosis attack, reach their peak a few weeks later, and usually disappear within eight to ten months. With few exceptions, the presence of IgM antibodies in a pregnant woman's bloodstream is a virtual confirmation of a recently acquired infection and the risk of fetal infection.

What steps should I take to avoid contracting toxoplasmosis?

There is no need to throw out the family cat as soon as the diagnosis of pregnancy is confirmed. However, extreme caution should be taken to avoid infection. While it is best that other family members empty the litter box, you can do this provided that it is done at least once each day. The reason for this is that the oocysts in the cat feces are not infectious for the first 24 hours. Oocysts have the capacity to survive in soil and water for as long as 18 months and, if the litter box is not completely and carefully emptied, infection after the first 24 hours is possible. Periodically disinfect metallic litter boxes for five minutes with nearly boiling water to help to kill oocysts, but assign this job to another family member. Wear gloves when handling litter boxes or other materials that may be contaminated with cat feces. This is especially important when gardening in an area where cat feces may have been deposited. Whenever you touch your cat, wash your hands thoroughly. Handwashing should also be thorough before each meal, since oocysts can be transmitted from the hands to the mouth. Keep house cats indoors, away from possible sources of infection such as infected mice and other animals. In addition, do not feed cats raw meat. Since outdoor cats have a higher risk of acquiring toxoplasmosis, it is best that they be kept outdoors and away from the immediate environment of the pregnant woman. Pregnancy is not the time to introduce a stray cat into the household.

Most cases of toxoplasmosis are acquired by eating raw or poorly cooked meat. Smoking or curing meats in brine are effective measures against *Toxoplasma gondii* oocysts. It is a good idea to wear gloves when handling raw meat; if you don't, be sure to avoid touching the mucous membranes of your mouth and eyes at these times. Always wash your hands and all kitchen surfaces after they come in contact with raw meat.

A woman with a high toxoplasmosis antibody titre prior to pregnancy need not take these precautions, because her fetus will not be in jeopardy.

How is toxoplasmosis treated during pregnancy?

In an impressive study of 746 documented cases of maternal toxoplasmosis, published in the *New England Journal of Medicine* in 1988, French physicians clearly proved that early and vigorous antibiotic treatment of an infected pregnant women will reduce the incidence of congenital disease and the spread of infection to her fetus. Unfortunately, one never knows until after the baby is born if treatment was initiated early enough. For this reason, most women opt for therapeutic abortion when the disease is diagnosed with certainty during the first 24 weeks of pregnancy.

If a woman elects to be treated, the drug of choice is spiramycin. It has been used extensively in Europe and there are no reports linking it to maternal or fetal complications. Spiramycin is available in the United States only by special request from the FDA. The combination of sulfonamides and pyrimethamine has also proven effective against *Toxoplasma gondii*. Pyrimethamine, however, has been linked to congenital defects when used during the first trimester and is best avoided at that time. Sulfonamides may cause neonatal jaundice if a woman uses them in the last month but have proven to be safe during the remainder of pregnancy (see page 260).

Is there anything else that pregnant women need to know about cats?

Cat-scratch disease is usually a mild, self-limited illness caused by a cat infected with a rod-shaped bacterial organism. Although the disease results mostly from cat scratches, it can also be introduced through a bite or lick. Within three to five days after exposure to an infected cat, a person will usually note a small pimple near the contact site. Within two weeks, enlarged and tender lymph nodes will appear, often accompanied by fever, loss of appetite, and headache. Approximately 12 percent of infected people experience severe illness in the form of an infected rash, liver disease, bone damage, and encephalitis. While the effects of cat-scratch disease on the fetus are unknown, the fever and debilitation associated with more severe cases can only be harmful. Until 1990, it was believed that antibiotics were incapable of curing cat-scratch disease. However, research by doctors at

Vanderbilt University School of Medicine has demonstrated that gentamicin, a potent antibiotic, has shown promising results.

What problems may be encountered by the pregnant dog owner?

Assuming that your dog is not rabid, you should be able to safely enjoy the company of your canine friend during pregnancy. However, an increasing number of recent medical reports have dealt with the growing problem of parasitic diseases that may be passed to humans from woman's best friend.

One such disease, named toxocariasis, is caused by the roundworm *Toxocara canis*. (In the cat, this organism is equally infectious and is named *Toxocara cati*.) Although this disease is relatively unknown, public health officials estimate that it may be one of the more common parasitic infections in the United States. *Toxocara canis* eggs contain infective-stage larvae which are passed with the dog's feces and may be found in streets, soil, sandboxes, lawns, and gardens. While all age groups are at risk, the disease is most prevalent among children 1 to 14 years of age. Although previously considered a mild disease, there is growing concern that severe damage to the eyes, brain, lungs, liver, and other organs may occur. Nothing is known about its effect on the outcome of pregnancy. However, one must assume that a mother's debilitation resulting from this disease can only mean trouble for her baby.

Heartworm, another dog infection, can also be transmitted to humans. This disease, named dirofilariasis, is caused by a parasite named *Dirofilaria immitis*. Transmission to humans takes place when one of several types of mosquitoes, infected with the microscopic larvae while feeding on the blood of infected dogs, bites the human skin surface. Pregnant women are advised to have their pet dogs examined for parasites at regular intervals by a veterinarian. Dogs that run loose are more likely to contract a parasitic disease, and therefore more careful supervision is necessary during pregnancy. Pregnancy is not the time to adopt a stray.

What are the health hazards associated with owning other pets?

Pet turtles are known to be a frequent source of salmonella bacterial infections in humans. Salmonella is the same organism which causes food poisoning. It has been estimated that almost 15 percent of the nearly 300,000 cases of salmonella-associated infections reported in the United States each year result from contact with contaminated turtles or the water in which they live. Most cases occur in children who handle the turtles and then touch their hands to their mouths. However, salmonellosis in adults may also be contracted in this manner. If you own a pet turtle or plan to buy one, make sure to do it through a reputable dealer who is willing to certify that the animal is free of salmonella. If you have young children, discourage them from touching the turtles or the water in which they swim. When you are pregnant, it is probably best to wear gloves when cleaning the tank, changing the water, or handling the turtles.

Psittacosis, or ornithosis, commonly known as parrot fever, is an infectious disease of birds caused by a microscopic parasite named *Chlamydia psittaci*. Transmission of the infection to humans often occurs following contact with infected pets, such as parrots and parakeets, although all birds, including pigeons, ducks, turkeys, and chickens, may also infect humans. Psittacosis is almost always transmitted to humans by inhalation of the organism into the respiratory tract. On rare occasions it may be acquired from the bite of a pet bird; there are no cases of infection acquired through eating poultry products. In the lungs, *Chlamydia psittaci* causes inflammation or pneumonitis, fever, and a generalized weakness. From this site it may spread to the liver and spleen and also enter the bloodstream.

One can contract the disease by spending only a few minutes in an environment previously occupied by an infected bird. As with other infectious diseases of this type, the best advice is to avoid contact with infectious birds. The treatment of choice for this disease is tetracycline antibiotics. However, their use is not recommended during pregnancy, and less predictable antibiotic alternatives must be employed.

 # FIFTH DISEASE

What is fifth disease, and what are its effects?

Fifth disease is usually considered a mild viral illness that primarily affects children but which can spread easily to adults. Very little is known about how it is transmitted, but the respiratory tract appears to be the most likely portal of entry and excretion. The official name of fifth disease is erythema infectiosum, and the causative organism is one of the smallest DNA viruses, known as the human parvovirus B19. The word erythema means red, an appropriate name in view of the fact that the chief symptom of the disease in children is a scarlet red or "slapped cheek" rash covered with a raised fiery flush resembling the effects of a hand-slap. The rash also covers the bridge of the nose, but not the mouth area, and is usually followed after a day or two by a secondary rash on the cheeks, upper arms, chest, and thighs lasting one to two weeks. The rash is variable: at first blotchy and then assuming a paler, dull-red pattern resembling lace or net. Adults who contract fifth disease are more likely to escape the rash but experience joint pain and a flu-like illness. By the time a person with fifth disease develops a rash or joint pain they are no longer contagious. Twenty percent of adults with fifth disease are totally asymptomatic but can spread the disease from their respiratory tract during the first two to three weeks after exposure.

Fifth disease follows the seasonal pattern of most epidemic viral infections with outbreaks occurring in the late winter or early spring. It is less infectious than chicken pox or measles. Fear of the disease is based on several recent reports linking maternal parvovirus infections to adverse pregnancy outcomes. Pregnant teachers, day-care workers, pediatricians, pediatric nurses, and others in close contact with children are most susceptible. Women in households where children introduce fifth disease face a 50 percent chance of contracting it. While much remains to be learned about the effects of a parvovirus infection on the fetus, it is known that maternal infection during the first trimester may result in a 20 percent risk of spontaneous abortion. The disease, however, is not associated with an increased incidence of congenital abnormalities. After the first trimester, the virus has the capacity to cross the placenta and destroy red blood cells in the fetal circulation and bone marrow. This in turn may cause pronounced anemia, hydrops, or heart failure, characterized by massive edema and enlargement of the liver and spleen, and even stillbirth. Prematurity is common among affected fetuses. If a stillbirth is going to occur, it is likely to happen within four to six weeks following the maternal illness. The risk of such a complication is far less likely after the twentieth week. One reason for optimism is that 50 percent of all pregnant women already have IgG antibodies to fifth disease, indicative of previous exposure and immunity. As a result, their pregnancies are not at risk even if they are exposed to children with the disease. In addition, once a woman has had fifth disease during a pregnancy, she will never get it again in a subsequent pregnancy.

While recent publicity surrounding fifth disease has understandably stimulated requests for routine parvovirus B19 screening for all pregnant women and women contemplating pregnancy, the Centers for Disease Control and the American College of Obstetricians and Gynecologists both strongly advise against it, characterizing such screening as an unnecessary and expensive precautionary measure.

However, if a woman is exposed to a parvovirus B19 epidemic during pregnancy, she should be removed from the infectious environment and tested. If testing shows the absence of antibodies, indicative of no previous exposure and susceptibility to fifth disease, a work transfer or temporary leave of absence is advised until the epidemic subsides. Return to the environment should be avoided until 21 days after the onset of illness of the last reported case. A susceptible pregnant woman who has had direct contact with a person with fifth disease should be retested in three weeks if her initial antibody test is negative, since she may convert from negative to positive during this time. The presence of antibodies named IgM is diagnostic of a recent infection. Any pregnant woman who has recently worked in a place that is known to be epidemic for fifth disease and who develops a rash, joint pain, or a flu-like illness should also be tested.

If antibody testing indicates a recent infection, careful serial ultrasound monitoring should be employed to detect the earliest evidence of fetal hydrops. Umbilical cord blood sampling obtained during pregnancy or at birth enables a doctor to detect the presence of anemia and IgM antibodies in an infant's circulation. If anemia and hydrops develop in utero and the baby is too immature to be delivered, recent studies have shown that in utero blood transfusions directly into the blood vessels of the umbilical cord can successfully reverse the disease process.

Occasionally, an abnormally elevated maternal serum alphafetoprotein (AFP) determination can offer a clue to the presence of an infection in the fetus. This occurs because the virus attacks fetal liver cells, causing them to release excessive amounts of AFP into the amniotic fluid and maternal serum. Though AFP testing between the fifteenth and eighteenth week of pregnancy is performed primarily as a screening test for the presence of neural tube defects, the presence of an elevated AFP and a normal spine and skull should alert a physician to explore the possibility of fifth disease in a fetus. Some researchers have found that the highest levels of maternal AFP are often directly related to an unfavorable fetal prognosis.

ULTRASOUND

What are the potential dangers of ultrasound?

The images produced with diagnostic ultrasound result from the reflection of high-frequency sound waves from tissues with different densities and acoustic properties. When diagnostic ultrasound is used medically, the wave frequency is very high, but the intensity of the sound wave is extremely low. As a result, the ultrasound energy is incapable of causing ionization in tissues, alterations in the genetic make-up of cells, mutations, cancer, or birth defects. Despite the exposure of millions of women and their fetuses to both diagnostic ultrasound and ultrasonic monitoring of the fetal heart rate over a period of at least 20 years, there is no evidence to show that these procedures are harmful. Follow-up studies of children exposed to diagnostic ultrasound in utero have detected no physical or developmental difficulties when compared to a control group, and more studies are being conducted. If anything, it would appear that ultrasound should be used more frequently in place of x-ray procedures, which are far more hazardous (see page 329).

Higher intensities of ultrasound are also used medically as a form of heat therapy for sore muscles of the shoulder, neck, hip, and back. Although heat is produced over the area being treated, it does not raise a person's body temperature and can be safely used during pregnancy, provided it is not applied to the abdomen over the area of the pregnant uterus.

 # *NONIONIZING RADIATION*

How dangerous is the radiation emitted by household appliances such as microwave ovens, radios, and television sets?

Radiowaves and microwaves are forms of invisible penetrating electromagnetic waves of energy known as nonionizing radiation. Both are used extensively for communication, in industry, for medical purposes, and in the home. In addition to the microwave oven and communication microwaves, other sources of nonionizing radiation include word processors, video display terminals (VDTs), radios and frequency modulation (FM) radiowaves, televisions, long-distance telephone and telegraph transmissions, citizens band (CB) radios, radar, taxi dispatch lines, high-voltage power lines, satellite communications towers, cathode ray tubes, diathermy, visible, ultraviolet, and infrared light, certain burglar alarms, "electronic" garage door openers, electric toys, electric blankets, and heated water beds.

Unlike the ionizing radiation produced by x-ray machines, nuclear weapons, and nuclear power plants, nonionizing radiation does not generally have enough energy to cause serious mutations or genetic damage. This is not to imply, however, that scientists are unconcerned about the safety of this increasingly popular form of energy. Research conducted to date has been inconclusive and controversial. It has been suggested, but not proven, that high levels of nonionizing radiation in humans may be associated with a greater incidence of cancer, nervous disorders, cataracts, sterility, genetic damage, spontaneous abortion, birth defects, heart disease, and even death.

The FDA has the authority to regulate the levels of nonionizing radiation emitted from consumer products. Microwave ovens manufactured after 1976 have had to meet rigid requirements so that they release amounts of radiation well within the limits of safety. Microwave ovens manufactured before 1976 sometimes develop gaps between the door and the frame which allow higher emissions of radiation. If doorframes of these older models are not kept clean during use, radiation can leak out. However, be assured that even if your oven has a significant leak, microwave intensity, like all electromagnetic radiation, dissipates so rapidly with each centimeter from its source that maternal or fetal injury is practically impossible. Even if you were to use your leaking microwave oven ten times daily, standing at a distance of 2 inches from the door, you would still not come close to reaching your total daily limit for nonionizing radiation. Likewise, it is highly unlikely that a woman's TV could emit enough radiation to cause problems during pregnancy. Although FM radiowaves are far more penetrating than those emitted by television sets, they will not alter the outcome of pregnancy.

Is there a limit recommended for exposure to nonionizing radiation?

Yes. The United States Occupational Safety and Health Administration (OSHA) has recommended that exposure to nonionizing radiation for workers be limited to 10 milliwatts per square centimeter, or $10mW/cm^2$. Sadly, this standard is not mandated by law, and many workers are exposed to amounts significantly higher. In one study, levels as high as $21mW/cm^2$ were found in the upper floors of office buildings located close to radio and TV transmitters. The highest exposure level found was 1,000mW/cm². Amounts of nonionizing radiation in this range would, in the opinion of most scientists, pose significant hazards to maternal and fetal health.

The amount of scientific evidence linking nonionizing radiation in the work environment to an adverse pregnancy outcome is minimal at best. Several investigations of workers employed in high voltage stations have met with mixed results. Some have noted an increased incidence of congenital malformations in offspring and an increased risk of cancer, particularly leukemia. Other reports have found no such relationship.

If you are pregnant and work with radio-frequency equipment, satellite communications, or other significant electromagnetic sources, it is not unreasonable to ask your employer or union representatives to verify that the suggested standard of 10mW/cm² is being met. The same advice applies to women working in the upper floors of office buildings which are in close proximity to radio and TV transmitters.

What are the reproductive risks associated with use of video display terminals, or VDTs?

The adverse publicity and fear associated with use of VDTs by pregnant women had its origins in the early 1980s with reports of spontaneous abortions and birth defects among several groups or clusters of VDT operators in the United States and Canada. Further worldwide investigations since then have clearly shown that the birth defects described were nonspecific and not the type caused by radiation. Authorities also point out that the clusters of miscarriages were undoubtedly random occurrences. Since millions of American women use VDTs and at least 15 percent of all pregnancies end in spontaneous abortion, it is not difficult to envision several women at the same workplace experiencing similar pregnancy complications.

Further fanning the flames of VDT anxiety and panic was a highly publicized but flawed 1988 study by doctors at the Northern California Kaiser-Permanente Medical Care Program in Oakland, California. They surveyed 1,600 working women two and one-half years after their pregnancies and found that those who operated VDTs for more than 20 hours per week in early pregnancy were twice as likely to miscarry as workers not using VDTs. Unfortunately, what failed to receive headlines was the finding that the high miscarriage rates only occurred among low-level clerical workers and not in supervisors or other professionals using VDTs with equal frequency. This neglected bit of important information would appear to place the blame for higher pregnancy failures on factors other than the VDT.

A far more meticulous and convincing study was published in 1991 by Dr. Teresa M. Schnorr and her associates at the National Institute of Occupational Safety and Health (NIOSH) and the American Cancer Society. This report, published in the *New England Journal of Medicine*, found that spontaneous abortion and stillbirth rates among telephone operators who used VDTs throughout their eight-hour workday were equal to operators not using VDTs.

The vast majority of VDTs emit the same or smaller amounts of radiation than most television sets. The radiation emitted is usually so weak that extremely sensitive instruments must be used to detect any output at all. VDTs also emit harmless levels of ultraviolet, infrared, microwave, very low frequency (VLF), and extremely low frequency (ELF) electromagnetic radiation. Although it is possible that all of these forms of radiation may be released from any VDT, extensive measurements in the United States and Europe have determined that the levels, even under the worst of conditions, are still well below acceptable limits for exposure.

Based on all available information, official government agencies, including the NIOSH, the FDA, and OSHA, as well as several reputable research organizations all agree that there is no association between VDT use and reproductive problems.

How much radiation is released at indoor suntanning centers?

Under names such as Plan-A-Tan, Tantrific Sun, and Sum Tan, indoor suntanning centers give customers courses of treatment with ultraviolet light cabinets that surround the user with high-intensity sunlamps. Although ultraviolet radiation may burn a pregnant woman's skin and may be associated with precancerous and cancerous diseases of the skin, premature wrinkling, sun plaques, skin atrophy, pigment abnormalities, and corneal and retinal injuries, it will not cause the chromosomal damage or congenital defects associated with ionizing radiation.

 IONIZING RADIATION

How can ionizing radiation in the form of diagnostic x-rays affect the developing fetus?

Unless it is absolutely essential, all diagnostic x-rays should be avoided during pregnancy, especially during the first trimester, when the rapidly dividing and differentiating fetal tissues are most susceptible to radiation damage. Despite innumerable warnings and prominently placed signs in radiology offices and hospital x-ray departments, too many fetuses continue to be inadvertently radiated before the diagnosis of pregnancy is confirmed. In my own personal experience, I have cared for two women over the past five years who underwent upper gastrointestinal series, involving multiple x-rays of the stomach, esophagus, and duodenum, for what was belatedly diagnosed as severe cases of morning sickness. The period of major fetal organ development occurs between the second to eighth week following conception, that is, from the fourth to tenth week after the last menstrual period. Excessive amounts of radiation administered during this time may be associated with abnormalities of the central nervous system, especially microcephaly or an abnormally small head. Mental retardation and eye defects such as cataracts, retinal degeneration, and optic atrophy are also likely to occur. Similar doses of radiation given during the first two weeks of pregnancy are unlikely to cause fetal anomalies but may be more apt to result in a spontaneous abortion.

High doses of diagnostic radiation after the eighth postconception week and during the last two trimesters, although less likely to cause malformations, are certainly not innocuous. The central nervous system, gonadal system, and tooth buds continue to grow and develop until the moment of birth, and too many x-rays may lead to a significant degree of permanent growth retardation. Mental retardation and more subtle intellectual deficiencies are most likely to occur following x-ray exposure between the eighth and fifteenth postconception week, but exposures throughout pregnancy may result in permanent, though less obvious, intellectual impairment as well. Fortunately the risk of producing fetal abnormalities is slight when diagnostic x-ray procedures are used judiciously and conservatively during pregnancy.

A rad is defined as a measurement of radiant energy absorbed in body tissues. While it is theoretically possible for any dose of radiation to cause anomalies if administered at a critical time during the first trimester, a higher incidence of malformations is only likely when doses greater than 20 rads are absorbed by the fetus. To receive this dangerous amount, a woman would have to undergo several diagnostic x-ray procedures directed at her lower abdomen (see Table 20). In their most recent 1990 report, the National Research Council estimated that a threshold for intellectual deficiency, but not necessarily gross mental retardation, may exist at 20 to 40 rads for fetuses exposed

TABLE 20

ESTIMATED RADIATION DOSES TO THE FETUS FROM COMMONLY USED X-RAY PROCEDURES

Examination	Reported Range (in millirads)
A. Low-dose group	
1. Dental	.03 to 0.1
2. Upper spine	8 to 55
3. Chest	0.2 to 53
4. Shoulder	0.5 to 3
5. Neck	Less than 50
6. Head	Less than 50
7. Mammography	Less than 50
B. Moderate-dose group	
1. Upper G.I. series	5 to 1230
2. Gallbladder study	14 to 1600
3. Lower thigh	1 to 50
4. CAT scan of head	Less than 100
5. CAT scan of chest	Less than 1000
6. CAT scan pelvimetry	Less than 230
C. High-dose group	
1. Lumbar spine (mid back)	20 to 2900
2. Lumbosacral (lower back)	73 to 3870
3. Pelvis	40 to 1600
4. Hip and upper thigh	73 to 1370
5. Intravenous pyelogram (IVP)	70 to 5400
6. Lower GI series (barium enema)	28 to 12,600
7. Abdomen	18 to 1400
8. X-ray pelvimetry	200 to 5400
9. Radionuclides except iodide	7 to 3800
10. Iodide radionuclide	100 to 3000 to fetal body; 15,000 to 6,000,000 to thyroid

between the critical eighth and fifteenth weeks.

Unfortunately, the damage caused by radiation cannot always be measured by the presence of an obvious abnormality. Even if a baby appears perfectly normal at birth, radiation can cause mutations or changes in the structure of the genes and chromosomes within its body cells. No statistics are available which accurately show the probability of inducing a mutation in humans at specific radiation doses, and chromosome and gene changes have been found in human embryos after only minimal radiation exposure. Therefore, it is best to assume that there is probably no safe dose with respect to mutation induction, and even the lowest levels of radiation have the potential to cause fetal genetic change. This is especially relevant because mutations induced in the immature germ cells of a fetal ovary and testes may be passed to succeeding generations where they may appear as obvious defects and abnormalities.

Several epidemiological studies of large numbers of pregnancies suggest that radiation exposure in utero significantly increases the risk of childhood malignancy. While all types of cancers have been reported, leukemia is by far the most common, and even fetal doses as low as 0.2 to 0.5 rads have been implicated. It should be noted that some studies, including one of almost 40,000 pregnant women, have shown no association between diagnostic radiation during pregnancy and later childhood cancer.

Most authorities, including the National Council on Radiation Protection and Measurements, maintain that 5 rads or less present such a low risk to the fetus that pregnancy termination is unwarranted. This dose does not appreciably increase an infant's risk of congenital defects or mental and physical retardation. Following a fetal exposure of 5 to 10 rads, therapeutic abortion is strongly recommended. This level is more difficult to reach than is commonly realized. For example, if you were to receive dental x-rays, a chest x-ray, and an upper gastrointestinal series, the total dose to your fetus would still be less than 2 rads.

Table 20 lists the amount of radiation in millirads (1/1,000 rad) which is absorbed by the fetus during various x-ray procedures.

There is a wide range of radiation doses for each procedure. Rather than refuse all x-rays during pregnancy, be sure that the radiologist uses the most modern equipment and the most meticulous technique, in which the fewest number of x-rays are taken. Also listed in Table 20 are estimates of radiation doses for computerized axial tomography (CAT) scan, a relatively new technique used in diagnosing a variety of medical, surgical, and gynecological conditions.

Radionuclides are radioactive substances used in nuclear medicine. The fetal effects of a particular radionuclide will depend upon the type and energy of its emission, the disposition of the substance in the body, the dose, the placental permeability, and fetal accumulation, which can vary widely depending on the radionuclide. Doses to the fetus from standard procedures are low, but it is usually recommended that pregnant women not undergo nuclear medicine procedures. Of all radionuclide materials, radioactive iodide delivers the most dangerous amount of radiation to the fetal body and thyroid gland. After the twelfth week of pregnancy, the fetal thyroid gland has an affinity for iodine which is 20 to 50 times that of the maternal thyroid gland. Consequently, if a pregnant woman is given therapeutic radioactive iodine, it may cause destruction of the fetal thyroid gland and hypothyroidism.

Can x-rays taken before pregnancy affect subsequent births?

A 1980 study from the University of Hawaii and earlier studies show that x-ray exposure before conception more than doubled the chances of subsequent offspring for developing cancer. Although these have been less extensively studied, it has been noted that benign tumors of childhood such as polyps, papillomas, lipomas, or fatty tumors, fibromas, adenomas of the kidney, hemangiomas, neurofibromas, and dermoid cysts on the ovary occur more often among children born of women who had been irradiated before pregnancy. There is some evidence to suggest that preconceptual irradiation of a man also increases the risk of benign and malignant tumors in his offspring.

The researchers from the University of Hawaii theorize that diagnostic x-rays induce damage and changes in the immature sperm and egg cells prior to fertilization. These defects are then passed on to the susceptible fetus at the time of fertilization.

What is x-ray pelvimetry, and why is there so much controversy surrounding its use?

Simply stated, pelvimetry is a measurement of the maternal pelvis. While a doctor may obtain a general idea of the size of a woman's pelvis by careful physical examination and palpation of the pelvic bones, the use of anteroposterior (front to back) and lateral (side) x-ray is a more accurate method of achieving this. Computerized tomography, or CT, pelvimetry, is a new technique which is as accurate as x-ray pelvimetry but exposes the fetus to no more than 230 millirads, compared to a range of 160 to 4,000 millirads with x-ray pelvimetry. Ultrasonic techniques have replaced x-ray procedures for the diagnosis of a wide variety of pregnancy complications, but they are of no value in accurately assessing the diameter of the maternal birth canal.

In the past, x-ray pelvimetry was often used by obstetricians before and during labor to determine the relative size and shape of a woman's pelvis in relation to the size of the baby. These measurements were often considered crucial to determining whether or not a cesarean section was necessary. Today most obstetricians have completely abandoned pelvimetry because of the amount of radiation to which the fetus is subjected. If one possibly valid indication for pelvimetry still remains, it is when a doctor is contemplating the vaginal, rather than cesarean, delivery of a baby in a frank breech position (see Chapter 12), although many authorities would vociferously reject this reason as well. In addition to the obstetrical hazards associated with a breech delivery, pelvimetry performed on a baby in this position exposes its gonads to greater amounts of radiation than when the head of the baby is in the pelvis.

In addition to concerns about the radiation risks of pelvimetry, some doctors have questioned the clinical value of the information acquired. Several reviews of the subject have concluded that pelvimetry is of little prognostic value in determining which women require cesarean section.

In my own practice, I no longer order pelvimetry examinations. If a woman's contractions are of adequate quality but her labor is not progressing, a cesarean section is indicated even if the x-ray tells me that the dimensions of her pelvis are adequate for a vaginal delivery. And if a 9-pound baby is in a breech position during a woman's first labor, there is no need to routinely order pelvimetry because a cesarean section is a certainty.

If your doctor determines that you need x-ray pelvimetry, it is not unreasonable to discuss your concerns and to voice your objections. Remember, the overwhelming majority of these examinations will not influence the outcome of your labor but will create a slight though significant cancer risk to your baby.

What other sources of ionizing radiation may the pregnant woman be exposed to?

Until 1987, low levels of background radiation and fallout were believed to account for an average of approximately 170 millirems per year of radiation exposure for every United States resident. (A rem measures the amount of tissue damage produced by one rad of x-rays.) Since then this estimate has been raised to 360 millirems because radon, which has always been present in our environment, had not been previously figured into these calculations. Radon, radioactive rocks, soil, minerals in the body, particles from space, and other forms of cosmic radiation account for more

than 80 percent of a person's yearly radiation exposure (see Figure 43), with amounts varying according to where one lives and works. For example, background radiation doses at sea level may be as low as 70 millirems per year, versus 1,000 millirems in some mountainous regions of the United States. The federal standard for maximum annual permissible total-body radiation in the general public is 500 millirems per year, while that for radiation workers is ten times this limit.

No subject in recent years has generated as much publicity and fear as that of radon, a colorless, tasteless, odorless gas produced naturally by the breakdown of uranium in soil, rocks, some building materials, water used in the home, and utility natural gas. Radon's breakdown products, in turn, include isotopes that emit high-energy alpha particles which, when inhaled over a period of months and years, may induce 5,000 to 20,000 lung cancers annually. While the EPA has described radon as the nation's most damaging cancer-causing pollutant and second-leading cause of lung cancer, all studies to date have failed to document an epidemic of disease or death traceable to radon. Many experts deplore the government's "radon hysteria" and claim that the perils of radon have been greatly exaggerated. At the present time, there are no studies linking radon exposure in the home to adverse fetal or maternal complications.

Radon, thorium, and other naturally occurring radioactive materials are common in the earth's crust. The potential danger occurs after these elements have been brought to the surface and spread through the environment by such basic industries as oil and gas production, mining, fertilizer manufacturing, and burning coal for electricity. Naturally occurring radiation from industries other than the nuclear industry is the largest source of available radiation exposure in the United States.

Damage to humans caused by environmental accidents such as the Three Mile Island nuclear power plant leak in 1979 and the Chernobyl nuclear accident in 1986 is difficult to assess. While

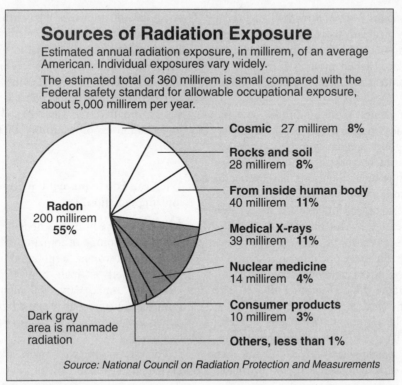

Sources of Radiation Exposure

Estimated annual radiation exposure, in millirem, of an average American. Individual exposures vary widely.

The estimated total of 360 millirem is small compared with the Federal safety standard for allowable occupational exposure, about 5,000 millirem per year.

Radon 200 millirem **55%**

Dark gray area is manmade radiation

Cosmic 27 millirem **8%**

Rocks and soil 28 millirem **8%**

From inside human body 40 millirem **11%**

Medical X-rays 39 millirem **11%**

Nuclear medicine 14 millirem **4%**

Consumer products 10 millirem **3%**

Others, less than 1%

Source: National Council on Radiation Protection and Measurements

Figure 43

The New York Times/Nov. 20, 1987

initial evaluation of women who were pregnant and living within a 10-mile radius of the Three Mile Island has detected no increase in infant mortality rates, long-term studies of up to 25 years are needed before definite conclusions can be reached. In a 1988 study published in the *American Journal of Obstetrics and Gynecology*, doctors from the University of Bologna in Italy found high levels of radioactivity in the breast milk and placentas of 15 women in the year following the Chernobyl accident. Fortunately, Finnish investigators in their 1989 report noted no significant differences in the incidence of malformations or perinatal deaths among children born in the area of Chernobyl fallout between August 1986 and December 1987. Less highly publicized but equally dangerous radiation leaks have occurred throughout the United States in recent years: at the nuclear-weapon fuels plant Savannah River, Aiken, South Carolina; at a

nuclear weapons plant in Rocky Flats, Colorado, only 16 miles from the center of Denver; and at other United States nuclear sites, including the Feed Materials Production Center, in Fernald, Ohio, and the Hanford Reservation in the state of Washington. The effects of this radiation exposure on the thousands of plant workers and residents of nearby towns may not be known for decades.

Many women are exposed to ionizing radiation through jobs such as medical and dental x-ray technicians, radiologists, and nurses. Those employed in industries that manufacture radioisotopes for medicine, science, and industry are also vulnerable. Other unrecognized sources of radiation include work with luminous-dial paints for watches and clocks and baggage x-ray security machines at airports. Laboratory technicians working with electron microscopes receive low levels of ionizing radiation, as do thousands of female physicists and research technicians who work with high-voltage x-ray machines on a daily basis. In contrast to rigid hospital regulations, the monitoring of dentists, dental technicians, dental hygienists, radiologists, and x-ray technicians in private offices is almost nonexistent.

Radiation is greatest at high altitudes, and frequent fliers and women who work as flight attendants throughout pregnancy receive greater exposure than women working on the ground or those taking infrequent flights. It has been estimated that cosmic radiation given off by the stars, the sun, and sunspots at 30,000 feet is about seven times that at sea level. This translates to an extra 160 millirems per year for the average flight attendant. Travelers on the Concorde are exposed to even greater amounts of radiation because it attains altitudes well above those of most jet aircraft. The earth's magnetic fields tend to concentrate radiation at both polar regions, so that flights following these routes will expose passengers and crew members to higher radiation levels. More planes than ever before are now flying between North America and Asia or Europe over the North Pole, a route in which radiation levels are four times greater than flights passing over the equator. On some routes, the annual radiation doses for crews are higher than the average for workers in a nuclear power plant or industrial setting where x-rays or radiation sources are used (see Table 21). (For more details on radiation exposure during air travel, see page 200.)

What can I do to prevent unnecessary exposure to ionizing radiation?

Diagnostic medical and dental x-rays are easily the greatest source of ionizing radiation to which the pregnant woman is subjected. Government radiation experts estimate that 30 percent of such x-rays are unnecessary, and many that are performed during pregnancy could be omitted or postponed without adversely altering the outcome of treatment.

There is nothing wrong with asking your doctor or dentist to explain why an x-ray is necessary be-

TABLE 21

NUMBER OF WORKERS IN VARIOUS OCCUPATIONS EXPOSED TO RADIATION AND ESTIMATED ANNUAL DOSE RATE

Source	Number of Workers Exposed	Percent Women	Average Dose Rate (mrems/year)
Medical x-rays	195,000	80	300–350
Dental x-rays	171,000	85	50–125
Radiopharmaceuticals	100,000	20	260–350
Commercial nuclear power plants	67,000	5	400
Fuel processing and fabrication	11,250	10	160
Particle accelerators	10,000	—	Unknown
X-ray diffraction units	10,000– 20,000	—	Unknown
Electron microscopes	4,400	60	50–200
Airline crew and flight attendants	40,000	90	160

fore submitting to it. And, of course, inform your doctor that you are pregnant when you are. If necessary, request the opinion of another doctor or dentist. In the case of x-ray pelvimetry, you're in a difficult bargaining position during labor, and it is much easier to resolve this question during your initial prenatal visits.

While it is often more convenient to be x-rayed with the archaic equipment used by most family physicians, the machines found in modern radiology offices and teaching hospitals can give more accurate information with considerably less exposure to ionizing radiation.

If you agree with your doctor that an x-ray procedure is clearly necessary, insist on consulting with a radiologist before having the films taken. Techniques can be modified so that the maximum amount of information may be achieved with the lowest number of exposures. To protect your fetus

and your ovaries from scattering of rays, be sure to request a lead shield or apron over your abdomen when your x-ray examination involves parts of the body other than the lower abdomen and pelvis. A lead shield over your thyroid gland is also a wise precaution.

Women exposed to ionizing radiation in medical and industrial settings should wear film badges for monitoring. These badges, read at three-month intervals, determine the amount of radiation accumulated during the preceding three months. A woman working in such a setting and planning a pregnancy should request a monthly badge reading to ensure that her dose has remained within safe limits. A far better idea is to transfer to a safer job before conception and throughout pregnancy. As previously stated, any dose of ionizing radiation is too much for the fetus, and efforts should be directed toward lowering these levels to zero.

HALOGENATED HYDROCARBONS

What are halogenated hydrocarbons, and how can they affect the outcome of pregnancy?

Halogenated hydrocarbons are a group of agricultural and industrial chemicals which are known to be toxic to the liver and kidneys. Members of this group include the infamous polychlorinated and polybrominated biphenyls (PCBs and PBBs), vinyl chloride, trichloroethlene, perchloroethylene (also known as tetrachlorethylene), vinylidine chloride, oxychlordane, heptachlor epoxide, and many other compounds of similar chemical structure. Geneticists are concerned because the percentage of children born with congenital defects has doubled in the past 30 years; they believe that this is from PCBs and more than 2,000 other mutation-causing agents currently in our environment. As a result of a woman's increased metabolic rate during pregnancy, it is believed that she may be more

susceptible to absorption of these agents at this time. Halogenated hydrocarbons readily enter the breast milk and may increase the nursing infant's risk of chemical toxicity and cancer.

PCBs are used as plasticizers, heat-exchange fluids, and insulation material in transformers and other electrical devices such as capacitors. Other common products which utilize these compounds include lubricants, pesticides, cutting oils, adhesives, wax extenders, inks, sealants, caulking compounds, and paper coating. Although the production of PCBs was officially terminated by the Environmental Protection Agency in 1979, federal regulations do not prohibit the use of existing supplies. Industrial and electrical plants have discharged their PCBs into nearby sewers and streams, thus contaminating them. While some manufacturers have worked with the Environmental Protection Agency in locating and cleaning up hazardous waste sites, many more have allowed illegally dumped PCBs to remain hidden and leak into our water supplies.

PCBs may enter the body by ingestion, inhalation, or through the pores of the skin. Excessive amounts of PCBs in the body cause a characteristic "cola-colored" complexion. One study of ten affected newborns found that their mothers had used a specific brand of cooking oil during pregnancy; the source of contamination was in the manufacture of the oil, from the erosion of pipes containing PCBs used for heat transfer. Although the "cola-colored" complexion faded, these children were smaller in size and shown to be more likely to have eye defects and other abnormalities when compared to children who were not exposed to PCBs. More recent animal experimentation and human experience has shown a clear relationship between maternal PCB intake and fetal intrauterine growth retardation (IUGR). In one study of women who ate significant amounts of PCB-contaminated fish from Lake Michigan and the St. Lawrence Seaway before and during pregnancy, newborns were 160 to 190 grams (5.6 to 6.7 ounces) lighter and had smaller head sizes than nonexposed infants. Exposure to PCBs need not be in the form of ingested food in order to affect the outcome of pregnancy. In a 1989 report published in the *American Journal of Epidemiology*, doctors studied 200 pregnant women exposed to PCBs in the manufacture of capacitors and found that they were more likely than nonexposed individuals to have elevated PCB blood levels and give birth to infants of lower birth weights. In addition to these problems, PCBs have been suspected of causing liver cancer, reproductive failure, allergic skin diseases and acne-like eruptions, nausea, dizziness, eye and nasal irritation, and asthmatic bronchitis. The transfer of PCBs via breast milk is quite significant, and nursing infants may appear lethargic and lacking in muscle tone.

Some species of fish absorb higher amounts of PCBs than others. Eels, for example, have been found with PCB levels as high as 700 parts per million because, as bottom-feeders, they ingest the silt where PCBs are in greatest concentrations. Freshwater fish, such as bass, carp, whitefish, trout, pike, and catfish, and some saltwater fish, such as flounder, sardines, sole, and herring, are most frequently contaminated. East Coast salmon, swordfish, and shark are known to have high PCB levels as well. A 1991 *Consumer Reports* survey of supermarket fish found that 43 percent of the salmon and 25 percent of the swordfish tested contained PCBs. Shellfish that are filter feeders can also accumulate large amounts of PCBs. Offshore ocean fish such as cod, red snapper, pollock halibut, yellowfin tuna, and haddock are usually free of PCBs. A diet that limits potentially contaminated varieties of fish can prevent accumulation of PCBs during pregnancy, and health experts advise that women who expect to become pregnant avoid fish known to have high PCB levels in the months prior to conception. The highest PCB breast milk concentrations in North America were observed in Eskimo women in northern Quebec in 1987. Their diets for centuries have included large amounts of fish taken from rivers and coastal waters contaminated with industrial wastes.

PBBs are similar in chemical structure to PCBs. They were manufactured as a fire-retardant by the Michigan Chemical Corporation and sold under the name of Firemaster PB-6. This product is no longer being produced. While some researchers have theorized that persons who ingested PBBs in breast milk as infants may be more susceptible to cancer as adults, there are no data at the present time to support this supposition.

Vinyl chloride is probably one of the most widely used chemicals in the United States. This halogenated hydrocarbon has its greatest use in the manufacture of plastic plumbing pipes and conduits. It is also used for wire cables in electrical systems but may be found in such diverse products as flooring, garden hoses, and clothing. Significantly, almost 5 million workers are exposed to vinyl chloride gas in factories throughout the United States.

Vinyl chloride can induce brain, liver, lung,

and lymph node cancers among workers exposed to its vapors. Exposure during pregnancy to vinyl chloride and chloroprene, a chemically similar compound used in the synthetic rubber industry, may be associated with higher rates of birth defects. In some studies, chromosomal aberrations have been found, and increased fetal mortality was noted among wives of vinyl chloride workers. Men exposed to vinyl chloride may have low sperm counts and abnormal sperm. Studies also show that these men are more likely to father children with tumors and cancer.

Trichloroethylene and vinylidine chloride are two halogenated hydrocarbons which are suspected of being cancer-inducing agents. The former is occasionally used in inhalers for the relief of pain during labor. It also serves as a degreasing agent for metals and as an extractant in foodstuffs. Recently, trichloroethylene has been found in contaminated household water supplies via its release into the soil. Studies by the Environmental Protection Agency suggest that long, steamy, hot showers may be the greatest source of this chemical pollutant. Vinylidine chloride is widely employed in the manufacture of plastics.

Pregnant women working in dry cleaning may be exposed to tetrachlorethylene, also known as perchloroethylene. Vapors from this solvent can be detected in a home for a week or more after clothes are brought back from the cleaners. During the postpartum period, occupational exposure to tetrachlorethylene has been associated with liver disease in breast-fed infants.

What advice would you give to the nursing woman who is concerned about contamination of her breast milk with PCBs?

While animal studies and human experience have demonstrated that high doses of PCBs in a woman's body are hazardous to her nursing infant, there is no proof that trace amounts of these chemicals are detrimental. PCBs are everywhere in our environment. Of the 1,038 samples of breast milk studied by the Environmental Protection Agency, only 9 were totally free of PCBs.

I would concur with La Leche League's recommendation that nursing mothers avoid exposure to PCBs if at all possible. General precautions suggested for nursing mothers are that they avoid eating freshwater fish, or at least limit such meals to one per week, and that they not work at jobs involving possible exposure to PCBs. Nursing women are also advised not to lose great amounts of weight over a short period of time. PCBs are stored in body fat, and rapid weight loss through a crash diet might release large amounts from the body fat to the breast milk. In general, women have higher PCB concentrations at first lactation; levels decline with time spent breast-feeding.

Some scientists have recommended that all women planning to nurse their infants first have the PCB level measured in their milk. Women whose milk contains more than 1 part per million are advised not to nurse. Unfortunately, such analyses are not widely available at this time and are often too expensive to order routinely.

DIOXIN

What is dioxin, and how can it affect the outcome of pregnancy?

Dioxin is a chlorinated manufacturing impurity that contaminates many industrial products, in-cluding wood preservatives, sealants, pesticides, and bleached paper products such as coffee filters, milk cartons, uncoated paper plates, paper towels, tampons, and disposable diapers. There are actually as many as 75 dioxins, but the chemical agent known as 2, 3, 7, 8, tetrachlorodibenzo-p-dioxin (TCDD) is the most hazardous and the one most often used synonymously with dioxin. TCDD has gained a reputation as one of the most toxic chemicals ever synthesized, and its lethal effects have been observed in laboratory studies on rats and mice. Cancer, birth defects, adrenal hemorrhage, hair loss, weight loss, impaired immunity, liver and peripheral nerve dysfunction, and blood disorders have all been observed in animals exposed to dioxin. Chloracne, a severe form of acne which has been described in humans exposed to high levels of dioxin, may appear from two days to several weeks following exposure and is remarkably resistant to the usual acne treatment regimens. The relationship between dioxin exposure and cancer in humans has been debated heatedly by scientists and epidemiologists. In the most recent report, published in the *New England Journal of Medicine* in 1991, doctors from the Centers for Disease Control noted a significantly higher death rate from all cancers, but especially those of the respiratory system as well as two rare malignancies named soft-tissue sarcoma and non-Hodgkin's lymphoma, among more than 5,000 dioxin-exposed workers. Many of the cancers followed exposure periods of at least 1 year and often did not appear until 20 or more years later.

Although dioxin has been linked to birth defects in experimental laboratory animals, proof of similar problems in humans is lacking. In 1976, an industrial accident near Seveso, Italy, dispersed TCDD over a wide area and exposed thousands of women to this chemical. While early reports suggested that this accident resulted in higher rates of spontaneous abortions and fetal malformations, subsequent research has clearly refuted this claim. The overwhelming number of studies to date have failed to note an association between TCDD exposure and impaired fertility or birth defects.

Dioxins are readily transmitted to a woman's breast milk, but their effects on the nursing infant remain unknown at the present time.

 ## *PESTICIDES*

How can exposure to pesticides alter the outcome of pregnancy and nursing?

The word "pesticide" encompasses approximately 600 chemical ingredients found in more than 50,000 insecticides, herbicides, and fungicides sold in the United States each year. It is estimated that one-fourth of these products have the potential to cause toxicity, sterility, and chromosomal changes among individuals who are exposed to relatively high concentrations. While it has been claimed that infants exposed in utero to these toxins will suffer from a higher incidence of birth defects, this has never been scientifically proven in any large-scale studies. Similarly, the effects of exposure to low concentrations of pesticides are unknown at the present time. One disconcerting report published in the *American Journal of Public Health* in 1988 noted that women living in agricultural communities, in which pesticide use is extensive, were at an increased risk of bearing children with congenital limb defects. Of equal concern is the finding that many of these chemicals, especially the chlorinated hydrocarbons, such as benzene hexachloride, are readily transmitted to a nursing infant in the breast milk.

Pesticides that have been associated with a variety of serious adverse effects are listed in Table 22.

To protect yourself and your babies from the effects of pesticides on foods, avoid use or exposure to pesticides in a home or garden, lawn, or greenhouse. If you must use one of these agents, scientists

TABLE 22

SOME COMMONLY USED PESTICIDES

Pesticides	Crops Affected	Comments
Mancozeb (fungicide)	Apples, onions, potatoes, tomatoes, grains	Laboratory studies suggest increased risk of cancer and birth defects.
Captan (fungicide)	Various fruits and vegetables including apples, cherries, lettuce, tomatoes, blueberries, apricots, grapes, plums	Laboratory studies suggest increased risk of cancer and birth defects. Banned on brussels sprouts, carrots, grapefruits, oranges, peas, sweet corn, tangerines, soy beans, squash, cauliflower, cucumbers, potatoes, pumpkins, tomatoes.
Folpet (fungicide)	Grapes, apples, melons	Cancer in laboratory animals.
Parathion (insecticide)	Various fruits and vegetables	Cancer and nervous system damage in laboratory animals.
Malathion (insecticide)	Fruits, vegetables, and ornamental plants	Low risk of toxicity, but metabolized slower by newborns than adults. Crosses placenta, but no increased rate of birth defects following fetal exposure.
Chlorthalonil (fungicide)	Various fruits, vegetables, peanuts	Potential for cancer, reproductive failure, and kidney problems.
Diazinon (insecticide)	Sod farms, grasses	Responsible for deaths of ducks and Canada geese.
Alachlor (herbicide)	Various forms of vegetation	Potential risk for cancer in humans appears very low.
Cyhexatin (miticide)	Apples, citrus fruits, and nuts	May pose a risk of birth defects in fetus.
EBDC (fungicide)	Tomatoes, potatoes, sugar beets, wheat, sweet corn, grapes, cranberries, almonds, asparagus, figs, onions, peanuts	Banned by EPA on 50 food crops including apples, melons, carrots. A metabolite named ethylenethiourea may cause cancer of thyroid, liver, and pituitary gland.
Dinoseb (herbicide)	Used to kill weeds in crops of lentils, peas, chickpeas in the Northwestern states and raspberry and other berry crops that grow on canes	May cause birth defects and sterility in males, extremely toxic.
Organochlorines (Chlordane, Heptachlor, Aldrin) (insecticides)	All three banned in 1975 except for killing termites	One study in rats showed an increased risk of cataracts with heptachlor. However, entire milk supply of Oahu, Hawaii, contaminated with heptachlor in the past with no subsequent birth defects. Impaired cellular immunity in mice exposed to chlordane.

recommend that you wear gloves and a disposable face mask. A pregnant or nursing woman should try to avoid foods that are suspected of containing pesticide residues. Fruits and vegetables should be peeled or thoroughly washed. However, not all pesticide residues can be removed in this fashion. For example, apples, tomatoes, and cucumbers are often coated with a fungicide mixed with wax, thereby making it impossible to rinse off. Pesticides known as systemics become an integral part of the plant's chemistry and can't be removed.

How should household pesticides be used during pregnancy?

There are no known studies linking normal use of household pesticides with an increased incidence of birth defects. However, to be on the safe side, it is best to wait until after the first trimester to spray pests such as roaches, fleas, spiders, flies, and ants within your home. In addition to delegating the job of spraying to someone else, be sure to completely cover all food and do not allow spraying of your clothing. Stay out of your house for at least 24 hours in order to allow the pesticides to settle. Ideally, someone other than yourself should come in and scrub down all the eating surfaces in your home and air out the house before you go back in.

 ASBESTOS

What are the dangers associated with asbestos exposure during pregnancy?

Until its hazards were publicized in the 1970s, asbestos was widely used for insulation in thousands of American homes, public buildings, and schools. Asbestos fibers released into the air when these structures are renovated or demolished can be inhaled into the respiratory tract and lungs over a period of time and cause characteristic debilitating scarring known as asbestosis, lung cancer, a

tumor of the lining of the lung and abdominal cavity known as mesothelioma, and other malignancies.

Pregnant women need not fear that acute asbestos exposure will adversely affect the outcome of pregnancy. Inhaled particles lodge in the respiratory tract and are too large to enter a person's bloodstream or cross the placenta. Despite this reassurance, I do not believe that pregnancy is the optimum time to undertake any asbestos-removal or sealing project in the home.

 FORMALDEHYDE

What problems may be encountered from formaldehyde exposure during pregnancy?

Formaldehyde is one of the most common organic chemicals, appearing as both a natural component of food and a metabolite of the human body. It is used extensively in industry as a binding

resin and preservative, and it plays an important role in the manufacture of textiles, wrinkle-resistant clothing, wood products, plumbing, automobiles, insulation, plastics, disinfectants, embalming fluid, leather, dyes, inks, paper, electrical equipment, cosmetics, glues, photographic film, and even some medications. An estimated 2 million people are exposed to formaldehyde in the workplace, with 10 percent of these individuals receiving a significant concentration of 0.5 part per million parts of air during an eight-hour work shift. More than half of exposed individuals work in the apparel industry.

The common symptoms of formaldehyde toxicity are tearing and itching of the eyes, headache, sneezing, frequent colds, flu-like symptoms, nasal infections, cough, shortness of breath, eczema-like skin rash, a general feeling of fatigue, sore throat, insomnia, and loss of appetite. The severity of reported symptoms have ranged from mild to incapacitating.

The EPA and the OSHA have recently stated that they regard formaldehyde as a probable human carcinogen, but scientific proof for this conclusion is minimal at best. While some epidemiologic studies have found higher rates of cancer among workers in the textile industry, other reports have found no such relationship. One reassuring article, published in the *Journal of the American Medical Association* in 1988, studied the health consequences of chronic formaldehyde inhalation among 109 workers and found no evidence of permanent respiratory impairment after an average exposure period of ten years. This report refutes earlier studies linking formaldehyde exposure to chronic and permanent lung damage.

Although earlier animal research and human studies suggested that maternal exposure to formaldehyde could cause chromosomal damage, mutations, and birth defects, these assertions have been totally refuted by all recent experience. Formaldehyde is simply not the reproductive villain it was previously believed to be. Both the OSHA and the EPA have concluded that there is no evidence linking maternal formaldehyde exposure to fetal toxicity, chromosomal abnormalities, birth defects, or an adverse pregnancy outcome.

HOUSE PAINTING

What precautions should I take while preparing and painting my baby's room?

There is no danger associated with painting during pregnancy, provided that the room you're working in is well ventilated to dispel any fumes. It is safer to leave a window open and feel uncomfortably cold than to inhale noncirculating air. In addition to paints, work with floor and furniture polishes is also associated with noxious fumes, and the same precautions must be followed. Avoid using all these agents in confined and windowless spaces.

Lead-based paints are dangerous and must never be used to paint a baby's room. If you are renovating a house that was built before World War II, there is a good chance that the paint in the walls contains lead. In tearing down walls or scraping paint, a do-it-yourselfer may expose herself and her family to dangerously high concentrations of lead dust. Until it was banned by the FDA in 1990, mercury was widely used as an additive to indoor latex paints in order to preserve their shelf life. Unfortunately, products manufactured before this date may still be sold. Recent studies have demonstrated that vapors from mercury-laced latex paint can be absorbed into a person's bloodstream and reach dangerously high levels (see page 320).

Polyurethane paints and coatings are often preferred on floors because of their luster and the fact that they resist weathering. Polyurethane paints contain chemicals known as diisocyanates, and until recently the most popular products contained toluene diisocyanate (TDI). Unfortunately, manufacturers are now limiting TDI use because of studies confirming that it may induce asthma, severe lung infections, and respiratory distress. These symptoms often persist even after exposure to TDI ceases. Other diisocyanate compounds, such as hexamethylene diisocyanate, would appear to be a safer choice, though this has not been scientifically proven. Pregnant women should avoid all contact with polyurethane spray paints, and workers using them should wear appropriate respiratory protective gear.

Extensive exposure to spray paint which contains M-butyl ketone (MBK) may be associated with severe neurological abnormalities. Pregnant women should avoid working with this chemical.

Use of turpentine and other liquid paint-stripping agents should also be considered hazardous during pregnancy. The main ingredient in most paint removers is methylene chloride, which rapidly metabolizes to carbon monoxide, a colorless, odorless, deadly gas. Exposure to methylene chloride for two or three hours can reduce oxygen levels in maternal and fetal blood to dangerously low levels. Pregnant women with heart disease are extremely susceptible to even a slight decrease in oxygen concentrations. Such individuals should be advised not to use paint removers and varnishes that contain methylene chloride during pregnancy.

 ## TOXIC CRAFTS MATERIALS

What hazards may be encountered if I work with arts and crafts materials during pregnancy?

There is a growing concern among artists, photographers, hobbyists, and craftswomen about the hazards of the materials with which they work. Sixty percent of the 90 million people engaged in arts and crafts in this country are women. Statistical analysis of artists' obituaries reveal an unusually high incidence of urinary bladder cancer. Male artists appear to be particularly prone to kidney and brain tumors, while females are more likely to die of rectal, lung, and breast cancers. Blood disorders and severe damage to the lungs, kidneys, liver, and brain have also been reported following chronic exposure to toxic art materials. Solvents used by painters may be responsible for irritation of the eyes and nose, chronic cough, sleep disturbances, headaches, drowsiness, and disorientation.

Although there are no large-scale studies, scientists believe that most fumes, dust, sprays, and chemicals found in art materials have the capacity to enter the body through the skin, nose, mouth, and respiratory tract and then pass into the mater-

nal bloodstream and across the placental barrier. In addition, the amount necessary to damage the fetus is much smaller than that which can injure an adult. The most sensitive time for these chemicals to alter normal development is from the eighteenth to sixtieth day after conception.

Art chemicals, especially heavy metals and solvents, can be found in a woman's breast milk several hours after exposure. Animal studies show that nursing increases lead absorption from the intestine, leading ultimately to higher levels of lead in the breast milk. In one study, methylene chloride, a popular solvent found in paint strippers and other art materials, was shown to be present in women's milk up to 17 hours after exposure had ended.

What precautions can pregnant artists and hobbyists take to reduce their exposure to toxic art materials?

If you are an artist, or are involved in crafts as a hobby, you must inform your obstetrician of all the materials that you use in your work. Manufacturers are required to provide you with Material Safety Data Sheets, detailing the ingredients, possible hazards, and precautions to take when using a particular product. During pregnancy, try to substitute less hazardous materials whenever possible and store materials safely. Table 23 lists some non-toxic substitutes for commonly used art supplies as recommended by the Center for Safety in the Arts.

It is important that you not eat or drink in or near your work area, and be sure to wash your face

TABLE 23

SAFER ART MATERIAL SUBSTITUTES

Type Hazardous Products	Substitutes
Dusts and powders	
1. Clay in dry form.	Talc-free, premixed clay.
2. Ceramic glazes or copper enamels.	Water-based paints, acrylic-based waterproofing products.
3. Cold-water or other commercial dyes.	Vegetable and plant dyes (onion skins, tea, flowers, etc.) or food dyes.
4. Instant papier-mâchés	Papier-mâchés made from black and white newsprint and white paste.
5. Powdered tempera colors.	Liquid paints or premixed paints.
6. Dusty pastels, chalks, or dry markers.	Wax crayons, oil pastels, dustless chalk.
Solvents	
1. Turpentine, shellac, toluene, rubber cement thinner; solvent-based inks, alkyd paints, rubber cement, etc.	Water-based products.
2. Solvent-based inks.	Water-based inks with safe pigments.
3. Aerosol spray paints.	Water-based paints.
4. Epoxy, instant glue, airplane glue, etc.	White glue, library paste, wheat paste.
5. Permanent felt-tip markers.	Water-based markers.
Toxic metals	
1. Lead used in stained glass projects.	Colored cellophane or black paper.
2. Pigments, metal filings, metal enamels, ceramic glazes, metal casting products, etc., that may contain arsenic, cadmium, chrome, mercury, lead, manganese, etc.	Approved materials that are free of toxic metals.
Miscellaneous	
1. Photographic chemicals.	Blueprint paper of Polaroid cameras.
2. Acid for etching, etc.	Print-making techniques not based on dangerous chemicals, such as soap prints, potato prints, woodcuts, etc.
3. Scented felt-tip markers.	Water-based markers.
4. Casting plaster for hand prints, etc.	Avoid body-part casting in products that produce heat as they dry; alternative can be medical plaster.

and hands before eating. Use only soap and water, never solvents, to clean your skin. Wear protective clothing, and remove it when leaving the work area. Safety goggles should be worn when grinding, sanding, welding, or working with chemicals that could splatter. It is vital that you wear a mask over the nose and mouth when working with powders, dusts, and fumes. Surgical gloves or gloves made of nitrile or neoprene can often be used to prevent chemicals from entering through the skin. Always cover powdered materials and store liquid solvents and paints in sealed containers. It is important that you not soak brushes in open containers of solvent. The safest way to get rid of solvents is to allow them to evaporate outside or under an exhaust hood. Clean up all spills immediately, avoiding contact with your skin. Clean your work area often, using a vacuum cleaner, wet mop, or moist rag. Do not sweep the floor or brush dust off shelves.

Most important, be sure you have proper ventilation in your working environment, not just an open window. In general, there are two basic types of ventilation: general or dilute ventilation and local exhaust ventilation. Local exhaust ventilation is better because it traps the toxic agents at their source and exhausts them before the air in the room becomes contaminated.

Two excellent sources of information regarding the safety of art materials are the Center for Safety in the Arts Incorporated, 5 Beekman Street, Suite 1030, New York, New York 10038, and Arts, Crafts, and Theater Safety, 181 Thompson Street, No. 23, New York, New York 10012, telephone (212) 777-0062.

 ## OTHER ENVIRONMENTAL POLLUTANTS

What other environmental pollutants should I try to avoid?

The colorless liquid solvent **benzene** is used to manufacture a wide array of products including plastics, textiles, polyurethane foam, pharmaceuticals, and pesticides. Emissions of benzene are also present in automobile exhausts and cigarette smoke. Dry cleaning establishments also use abundant amounts of benzene. It is estimated that more than 1 million American workers receive some exposure to benzene, and this has been proven to increase a person's risk of leukemia and chromosomal breaks. Exposure to benzene and other organic solvents may increase a woman's risk of bearing children with central nervous system defects.

Toluene, carbon disulfide, trichlorethylene, n-hexane, and methyl-n-butyl are widely acknowledged to be the most toxic solvents. **Carbon disulfide,** a colorless, volatile, and extremely flammable liquid which generates toxic vapors that can inadvertently be inhaled, is used in the production of viscose rayon and cellophane and the manufacture of carbon tetrachloride, as well as in vulcanizing rubber, fumigating grain, chemical analysis, degreasing, dry cleaning, and oil extraction. Animal experimentation and human experience suggest that carbon disulfide is toxic to the male and female reproductive systems as well as to the fetus. Women exposed to high doses of this solvent have reported a higher incidence of spontaneous abortion and premature births. While carbon disulfide does not appear to produce congenital malformations, impaired behavioral and sensory development has been reported in infants whose mothers were exposed to toxic fumes during pregnancy.

Trichlorethylene is a solvent used in many industries, including aircraft painting. At least six animal studies have shown a relationship between trichlorethylene use and lymphoma, liver, lung, and kidney cancer. In one study of 92 children less than ten years of age with brain tumors, doctors found a strong association with maternal and paternal exposure to trichlorethylene and other chemicals used in the aircraft industry.

Occupationally induced liver damage has been reported to occur with exposure to **dimethylform-amide** (DMF), a solvent widely used for manufacturing acrylic fibers and polyurethanes. In a 1987 study of 45 workers exposed to DMF, 30 had abnormal liver enzyme studies as a result of DMF's absorption through the skin and respiratory tract. Other chemicals capable of producing liver damage are carbon tetrachloride, kepone (chlordecone), and monovinyl chloride.

A host of other industrial chemicals are suspected of causing birth defects. Included among these are styrene, acetone, denatured alcohol, alkylphenol, dichloromethane, methanol, xylene, methylethylketone, petrol, butanol, and ethylene oxide. Of this group, **ethylene oxide** arouses the most suspicion. It is used in the production of hospital supplies and antifreeze, and as a fumigant for dried fruit and cereals. Ethylene oxide exposure has also been linked to a higher incidence of bone marrow cancer.

Diethylene glycol dimethyl ether and ethylene glycol monethyl ether acetate are two chemicals used in manufacturing semiconductor chips for computers. Researchers at Johns Hopkins University recently found that ten of thirty workers exposed to these chemicals experienced miscarriages. The extent of this problem may include the aerospace and printing industries since they use chemicals as well.

Spray adhesives have a wide variety of uses in the home. In 1973, the Consumer Product Safety Commission suddenly banned all spray adhesives because of a report which claimed they caused chromosomal and genetic damage among men and women using them, but at the present time there is no proof that chromosomal damage results from their use.

Nitrosamines are widely distributed carcinogens and mutation-inducing chemicals which may enter the body by inhalation, ingestion, or absorption through the skin. They are formed when chemicals called nitrites combine with substances known as amines. Various nitrosamines have been found in foods, cosmetics, alcoholic beverages, cigarette smoke, and many industrial processes, including leather-tanning, rocket fuel, and rubber and tire manufacture. Vegetarian diets also contribute to the level of nitrosamine exposure. Naturally high amounts are found in beets, spinach, celery, lettuce, and turnip greens, although the concentration in these foods varies according to the soil, fertilization, and harvesting conditions. Although there is no direct evidence that nitrosamines cause cancer in humans, a number of epidemiologic studies of the tire industry have reported a high incidence of cancer when the nitrosamine levels are most likely to be high.

A study sponsored by the National Science Foundation reported the presence of a nitrosamine named N-nitrosodimethylamine (NDMA) in 6 of 7 scotch whiskies and in 18 brands of beer. Since the concentration of NDMA is higher in beer than in scotch, beer probably constitutes a hazard to the pregnant woman. A woman will often drink beer during pregnancy rather than "hard liquor" because of its lower alcoholic content. While such women may diminish their chances of giving birth to a baby with the fetal alcohol syndrome, they may be exposing their unborn infants to a different risk. For this reason, if you must have an alcoholic beverage during pregnancy, a glass of wine is probably your best bet.

From their extensive study of environmental and occupational health hazards, scientists have come to realize that toxins produce specific organ system manifestations and symptoms. Knowledge of these relationships will often help in the early diagnosis and rapid initiation of treatment. The Health Systems Agency of New York City has provided a valuable table for early identification of some of these environmentally related symptoms.

TABLE 24

ENVIRONMENTAL AND OCCUPATIONAL HEALTH HAZARDS AND MANIFESTATIONS

Organ System (Primarily Affected)	Manifestations Acute and Chronic	Environments and Practices Conveying an Increased Risk of Developing Disease	Chemical and Physical Agents
Skin	Dermatitis Skin cancer	Electroplating; photoengraving; metal cleaning; wood preserving; food preserving; contact with foods and cosmetics; use of household chemicals and soaps	Hydrocarbon solvents; beryllium; arsenic, zinc oxide, PCB, nickel, dioxane, soap, pentachlorophenol, bismuth, alcohol, drugs
Respiratory System	Acute pulmonary edema and pneumonitis Asthma Chronic lung disease Lung cancer	Construction and insulation; textile manufacturing; painting; arc-welding; meat wrapping; animal handling; in-flight airline services; radiological work; exposure to traffic exhausts, dust, and industrial air pollution; improper ventilation and heating	Arsenic, asbestos, chromium, iron oxide, ionizing radiation, beryllium, ozone, nitrogen oxides, textile dusts, nickel, carbonyl, aerosolized plastics (e.g., vinyl chloride, teflon), dusts, fumes, vapors, TMA
Cardiovascular System	Arrhythmias Angina Intermittent circulatory disease of the legs Arteriosclerosis	Exposure to traffic exhaust; diesel engine operation; sewage treatment; cellophane and plastic manufacturing; motor vehicle repairing; extreme hot/cold; contact with synthetic film and hazardous agents in art and hobby supplies; pest extermination	Carbon monoxide, hydrogen sulfide, barium, organophosphates, freon, glues and solvents, heat and cold

TABLE 24

ENVIRONMENTAL AND OCCUPATIONAL HEALTH HAZARDS AND MANIFESTATIONS (Continued)

Organ System (Primarily Affected)	Manifestations Acute and Chronic	Environments and Practices Conveying an Increased Risk of Developing Disease	Chemical and Physical Agents
Gastrointestinal System	Abdominal pain, nausea Vomiting, diarrhea, bloody stools Hepatic necrosis Hepatic cancer Hepatic fibrosis	Jewelry making; dry cleaning; refrigerant manufacturing; food processing; chemical handling; printing; contact with lead-based paints and components of batteries and electrical equipment; consumption of improperly handled food.	Heavy metals (e.g., lead, cadmium), carbon tetrachloride, chlorinated hydrocarbons, phosphorus, beryllium, arsenic, nitrosamines, vinyl chloride, aflatoxin, bacterial toxin
Genitourinary System	Amino acid (protein) in the urine Chronic renal disease Bladder cancer	Plumbing; soldering; exterminating; textile manufacturing; contact with components of batteries	Cadmium, lead, mercury, organic dyes, halogenated hydrocarbons
Nervous System	Headache/convulsions/ coma Extrapyramidal disorders Peripheral neuropathy	Wood working; painting; exposure to traffic exhausts; fireproofing; plumbing; soldering; manufacturing of textiles and petrochemicals; contact with pesticides and battery components; consumption of improperly prepared food	Mercury, manganese, lead, carbon monoxide, boron, fluoride, organophosphates, hexane, organic solvents, wood preservatives (pentachlorophenol)
Auditory System	Hearing loss (and stress reactions)	Subway operations; metal working; construction; activities involving loud music	Loud noise, high frequency noise

TABLE 24

ENVIRONMENTAL AND OCCUPATIONAL HEALTH HAZARDS AND
MANIFESTATIONS (Continued)

Organ System (Primarily Affected)	Manifestations Acute and Chronic	Environments and Practices Conveying an Increased Risk of Developing Disease	Chemical and Physical Agents
Ophthalmic System	Eye irritation Cataracts	Petroleum refining; chemical handling; paper production; laundering; contact with photographic films; glass blowing	Nitrogen oxides, acetic acid, formaldehyde, radiation
Reproductive System	Spontaneous abortions Birth defects Infertility	Operating room procedures; contact with pesticides and contact with battery components	Anesthetic gases, ionizing and nonionizing radiation, lead, chemicals (dioxane) pesticides (DBCP)
Hematological System	Dangerous decrease in the number of blood cells, leukemia, lymph node enlargement, and anemia	Dye manufacturing; dry cleaning; chemical handling; contact with hazardous agents in art and hobby supplies; contact with rodent excreta, rodent bites	Benzene, arsenic, organic dyes, arsine, nitrates, drugs, lead
Nasal Cavity and Sinuses	Inflammation Cancer	Welding; photoengraving; manufacturing of glass, pottery, linoleum, textile, wood and leather products; contact with battery components	Arsenic, selenium, chromium, nickelcarbonyl, wood

WHEN TO STOP WORKING AND RIGHTS OF PREGNANT WORKERS

How long should I continue to work and what limitations, if any, should I continue to observe?

In the past, if a woman was discovered to be pregnant, she was quickly discharged from her job or refused employment. Many misunderstandings and taboos about work during pregnancy still exist, but, in general, normal pregnancy is no longer treated as an illness. Obstetricians have come to learn that their patients are often capable of working at a variety of jobs until late in pregnancy. However, there are many differences between individuals and pregnancies, and two healthy women working at identical jobs often show different capacities for activity and productivity at this time. For this reason, women and their obstetricians must work together to make intelligent decisions about working and stopping work during pregnancy. Remarkably few guidelines have emerged from the medical literature to help physicians determine how long, how strenuously, and under what conditions pregnant women may safely continue to work. Often, decisions made about employment are extremely difficult and challenging, and involve economic, physiologic, and social factors as well as obstetrical considerations.

Obviously, jobs that are dangerous or cause physical or mental exhaustion should be given up, if possible, and a temporary transfer to an easier job arranged to enable the pregnant woman to prolong her working career during pregnancy. The American College of Obstetricians and Gynecologists, in cooperation with the National Institute for Occupational Safety and Health, published "Guidelines on Pregnancy and Work" in 1977. In general, the College recommends that physical exertion at work be somewhat reduced because the greater blood volume of pregnancy increases oxygen consumption and places greater demands on the circulatory system. In addition, loss of balance and coordination, combined with relaxation of joints and musculature, increases the likelihood of experiencing muscle sprains and injuries if the pregnant woman's job requires heavy lifting or excessive physical exertion.

The American Medical Association has established general guidelines for determining how long women should work during pregnancy, based on their type of employment. These are outlined in Table 25. There are many exceptions to these guidelines. If you prefer to work or must work until late in pregnancy, you should be allowed to do so provided that you are examined and evaluated by your doctor at weekly intervals during the last six weeks of pregnancy. Regardless of the type of job you hold, try to take frequent breaks and elevate your legs periodically. If you are sedentary most of the day, stretch your legs or take a short walk for a few seconds every hour. Women employed in more physically demanding jobs should limit heavy lifting and straining, excessive stair climbing, and prolonged standing. Take a short break whenever you experience shortness of breath. During the last trimester, it is a good idea to spend your lunch hour resting on your left side.

Following an uncomplicated vaginal birth, most women are physically able to return to work after six weeks. Full recovery following a cesarean section usually takes an additional two weeks, provided you are returning to a sedentary job. Strenuous work requiring heavy lifting and physical exertion should not be resumed until ten weeks after surgery.

Are there certain women who should definitely not work during pregnancy?

Yes. Most knowledgeable obstetricians would agree that certain women should not be allowed to

TABLE 25

GENERAL GUIDELINES FOR WORK DURING PREGNANCY

Job function	Week of gestation		
	First trimester 1 2 3 4 5 6 7 8 9 10 11 12	Second trimester 13 14 15 16 17 18 19 20 21 22 23 24 25	Third trimester 26 27 28 29 30 31 32 33 34 35 36 37 38 39 40
Secretarial, light clerical, professional, managerial			40
Seated; light tasks (prolonged or intermittent)			40
Standing			
Prolonged (>4 hrs)		24	
Intermittent (>30 mins/hr)			32
(<30 mins/hr)			40
Stooping and bending below knee level			
Repetitive (>10 times/hr)		20	
Intermittent (<10 >2 times/hr)			28
(2 times/hr)			40
Climbing Vertical ladders and poles			
Repetitive (>4 times/8-hr shift)		20	
Intermittent (<4 times/8-hr shift)			28
Stairs			
Repetitive (>4 times/8-hr shift)			28
Intermittent (<4 times/8-hr shift)			40
Lifting			
Repetitive			
>50 lbs		20	
<50 >25 lbs		24	
<25 lbs			40
Intermittent			
>50 lbs			30
<50 >25 lbs			40
>25 lbs			40

SOURCE: *American Medical Association, Council on Scientific Affairs: Effects of pregnancy on work performance. Printed before House of Delegates at annual meeting, June 19–23, 1983.*

work during pregnancy, including those in the following categories:

- Those who have delivered two previous premature infants weighing less than 5 pounds.
- Those who have a history of an incompetent cervix, have had surgery for an incompetent cervix, or have had more than one spontaneous midtrimester abortion.
- Those with uterine malformations, such as a septum (wall) in the uterus or a double uterus, who have lost a fetus in the past.
- Those with heart disease who experience shortness of breath when doing less than a normal amount of activity.
- Those with diseases classified as hemoglobinopathies, such as sickle cell disease and thalassemia, and those with severe anemia regardless of its cause.
- Those with significantly elevated blood pressure before or during pregnancy.
- Those with moderately severe lung and kidney disease.
- Those with third-trimester bleeding, premature rupture of the amniotic membranes, placenta previa, or abruptio placenta.
- Those who are expecting a multiple birth.
- Those with long-standing and severe forms of diabetes characterized by narrowing of the blood vessels carrying oxygen to the uterus. (Most diabetics, however, do not have this problem and are usually able to work until early in the third trimester.)

What should pregnant women know about their legal rights and medical benefits during pregnancy?

The most important legislation ever passed for the pregnant working woman was the 1978 amendment to Title VII of the 1964 Civil Rights Act. Simply stated, the Federal Pregnancy Discrimination Act prohibited job discrimination based on pregnancy, childbirth, or related medical conditions. While most employers are usually sympathetic and supportive of the pregnant worker, many others become unresponsive and even hostile to the point of demanding an immediate resignation. Remember, you cannot be penalized, demoted, denied a promotion, or forced to resign simply because you are pregnant.

The most important factor to consider is your ability to do your job. If you can function as you did before pregnancy, the fact that you are pregnant should in no way determine how you are treated. Furthermore, even if you are partially disabled by pregnancy, you need not necessarily resign. If your employer regularly assigns light work to other partially disabled employees, he or she is obliged to do the same for you. If you are temporarily unable to work, your employer should give you the same rights as other employees who are temporarily disabled by accidents or illnesses, including the same medical insurance benefits provided to other workers. Finally, you should be permitted to return to your job or one equivalent in pay and status without loss of seniority, just as are other employees who have temporary disability conditions.

While we continue to await a Federal policy on parental leave, a growing number of states have taken the initiative of passing their own parental leave and job protection laws. Each states' regulations are different, and it is important that you familiarize yourself with those of your particular state. If you live in a state that does not address the issue of maternity leave, it is entirely up to your company to determine your benefits. Maternal and financial benefits vary significantly from one company to another. Ask about the exact coverage provided by your corporate and private health insurance plans. Many women assume that because their employer's group health insurance plan provides some maternity benefits every pregnancy-related bill will be covered. Unfortunately, this is often not the case. Be sure to determine if your policy includes items such as special tests, additional hospital stay, hospital nursery costs, and medications. Some policies also require that you pay the bills and then await reimbursement.

Disability payments cover the period of time from when you stop working to have your baby until you return to your job following delivery. Most employers treat pregnancy as any other temporary medical disability and continue your salary and benefits while you are away from the office. They will compensate you only while you are unable to function on the job for physical reasons. More often than not, there will be no provisions for spending time at home with your baby after you give birth. However, if you are forced to stop working because of a pregnancy-related complication, your employer must treat your condition like any other medical disability and provide the same medical benefits, disability insurance, and leave that your company offers to employees with other medical conditions or disabilities. Some companies allow you additional sick leave as part of your maternity leave. Others offer partial disability while continuing other benefits. Be sure that your employer is not among those miserly few who offer no disability payments.

From a financial point of view, it is better that you continue working for as long as you can rather than to quit on a specific predetermined date prior to your due date. Delivery dates are usually unpredictable, and if you or your doctor have miscalculated and you are late, you could use up several weeks of maternity leave before your baby is born. In addition, by leaving voluntarily before it is medically necessary, you might disqualify yourself from your company's health insurance, disability, and sick pay provisions.

If your employer does not have a temporary disability plan, you may qualify for full or partial unemployment or temporary disability benefits from your state. To find out about the benefits for which you may be entitled, check with your local state employment office.

If I am being treated unfairly at work because I am pregnant, what are my options?

If you believe that you are being unfairly treated because you are pregnant, object to your personnel director or union shop steward. To determine exactly what your rights are and the legality of your claim, contact your state's human rights commissioner. Many cities have a human rights commission that handles sex discrimination cases. Check the government pages of your local telephone book.

An excellent source of help is the 9 to 5 Office Survival Hotline, run by the National Association of Working Women. The hotline operates between 10 A.M. and 4 P.M. (Eastern Time) each weekday and can help you with legal questions about hiring, promotions, and firings. The calls are free if you dial 1-(800) 245-9865. The Women's Legal Defense Fund, (202) 887-0364, can furnish you with invaluable and accurate information about the legality of your claim. The local branch of the American Civil Liberties Union, the National Organization for Women, or the Equal Employment Opportunity Commission can also furnish you with this information. A short but comprehensive booklet entitled *Sex Discrimination in the Workplace: A Legal Handbook* is an excellent reference book available for $7.95 from the Women's Legal Defense Fund, 2000 P Street, N.W., Suite 400, Washington, D.C. 20036.

What can I do if my request for transfer to a safer job during pregnancy is denied?

If you believe that you are being exposed to potentially harmful substances or hazardous work conditions, you should bring it to the attention of your local union representative. Your employer is bound by Occupational Safety and Health Administration regulations to furnish you with detailed information on the names and amounts of all substances in your work environment. Often, a letter from your physician explaining why you should be transferred to a safer job will bring instant results. If these measures fail, call the Office of Public Information of the National Institute of Occupational Safety and Health at (800) 356-4674.

11

The NEW OBSTETRICAL TECHNOLOGY

Pregnant women today are far more knowledgeable than their predecessors about their own bodies and about childbirth. Terms such as amniocentesis, chromosomal analysis, and fetal monitoring are not foreign to them. But many women and men have reacted to this new technology with skepticism and antagonism. In the eyes of many expectant parents, the new medical technology has only helped to further depersonalize the birth experience and intensify the rift between parents and what they see as uncaring, scientifically oriented obstetricians. The recent surge in midwifery and home births in the United States is a direct result of widespread dissatisfaction with technically competent, but emotionally deficient obstetricians and the hospitals in which they work.

Despite the significant drawbacks of our new technology, even the most skeptical person would have to agree that modern obstetrical discoveries have been an invaluable comfort to women. Just ask any 40-year-old who has recently carried a pregnancy to term, secure in the knowledge that her baby would not be born with a chromosomal abnormality. Similarly, many babies are alive today because laboratory studies determined the ideal time for delivery to occur without fear of respiratory complications.

Some doctors enjoy impressing their patients with their medical double-talk and the complicated names of various tests. In fact, there is no test so complex that its indications and interpretations cannot be accurately explained to the layperson. This chapter evaluates some of the newer obstetrical tests and procedures. It is not my purpose to convert all pregnant women to board-certified obstetricians, but rather to help you understand these procedures and decide if you need them.

AMNIOCENTESIS

What is amniocentesis and how is it performed?

Amniocentesis is the sampling of the amniotic fluid from the pregnancy sac, or bag of waters, which surrounds the fetus in order to evaluate the well-being of the fetus. Through analysis of the amniotic fluid, it is now possible for doctors to detect the sex of the fetus, chromosomal abnormalities, alpha-fetoprotein (AFP) levels suggestive of neural tube defects, a wide variety of heredity diseases, the severity of Rh disease, the presence of infection, and the maturity of a baby's lungs during the third trimester. To obtain amniotic fluid, a needle is passed through the skin of the abdominal wall and the uterine muscle into the amniotic sac. Amniocentesis is only mildly uncomfortable and does not require anesthesia or analgesia.

Despite the introduction of chorionic villus sampling (CVS; see page 359), amniocentesis remains the primary diagnostic technique for detecting genetic disorders. It is most often performed between the fifteenth and eighteenth week of pregnancy, a time frame in which an adequate quantity of amniotic fluid is present, thereby minimizing the risk of fetal or placental injury.

Amniocentesis is a very simple procedure which may be easily performed in a hospital's outpatient department or an obstetrician's office. Wearing sterile gloves, the doctor cleans the skin over the needle site with an antiseptic solution. The ultrasound probe, encased in a sterile cover, locates the safest insertion site and the depth of penetration needed for the needle to reach the amniotic sac. As the needle is inserted, its path is followed by continuous ultrasound viewing so that corrections can be made for needle depth and for avoiding the fetus and umbilical cord in the event of a sudden fetal movement or change of position. The discomfort experienced during the procedure is minimized if the needle is inserted rapidly. Correct placement is confirmed by a free flow of clear amniotic fluid through the tip of the needle. After

amniocentesis is completed, the needle is rapidly withdrawn and the baby is observed under ultrasound to be certain that all is well. The entire procedure usually takes no more than 5 minutes, but the information obtained lasts a lifetime.

Waiting until the fifteenth to eighteenth week of pregnancy to undergo amniocentesis for genetic analysis is often an unnerving experience. This delay is extended because it usually takes an additional 7 to 14 days to obtain the results of the amniotic fluid culture. The strong emotional bond that a mother develops toward her baby when the pregnancy is this far advanced makes the decision to terminate the pregnancy, in the event of an abnormality, an extremely painful one. In addition, midtrimester abortions are more difficult to perform and have significantly higher complication rates. For these reasons, many women opt for CVS, a procedure performed between the ninth and eleventh gestational week (see page 359). Another option employed by a growing number of obstetricians has been early amniocentesis prior to the fifteenth week of pregnancy, and in some cases as early as the tenth week. This technique, however, is probably best left in the hands of a select group of experts rather than your local obstetrician.

What are the risks of amniocentesis?

When the fetal position, umbilical cord site, and placental location are determined by ultrasound immediately before and during amniocentesis, the incidence of complications will be extremely low. However, even in the best of hands, it is not a totally innocuous procedure. Trauma to the fetus, placental and umbilical cord hemorrhage, injury to maternal structures, inadvertent rupture of the amniotic membranes, uterine and amniotic fluid infections, premature labor, and spontaneous abortion have all been reported.

The passage of fetal red blood cells into the maternal circulation following a midtrimester amniocentesis may be far more common than is currently believed; it was 8.4 percent in one study. This is especially significant for Rh-negative women who may become sensitized by Rh-positive fetal cells in approximately 1 percent of all procedures. To prevent this complication, all nonsensitized Rh-negative women should receive a prophylactic injection of Rh-immune globulin or D immunoglobulin (trade names RhoGAM, Gamulin Rh, HypRho-D, and Rho-D Immune Globulin) at the time of the amniocentesis. The one exception to this rule is when a woman and her spouse are both Rh-negative, thereby eliminating the risk of sensitization (see page 397).

Fortunately, severe complications are infrequent, and several large studies have confirmed that fetal loss following amniocentesis between the fifteenth and eighteenth week occurs in 1 out of 200 pregnancies, for an incidence of 0.5 percent. Some studies suggest that there is an increased risk of pregnancy loss following amniocentesis prior to the fifteenth pregnancy week.

Inadvertent fetal injuries caused by the amniocentesis needle are rare, and those identified after delivery usually appear as faint, 2 to 5 millimeter dimple-like marks on the skin. Minor maternal complications, such as transient vaginal clotting, uterine cramps, and minimal amniotic fluid leakage occur approximately 1 percent of the time and almost always subside spontaneously. Long-term follow-up studies on infants born after amniocentesis have failed to reveal gross neurologic or developmental problems that can be attributed to the procedure.

Who should undergo amniocentesis for genetic indications?

The current practice in the United States is to advise genetic amniocentesis for women who are or will be 35 years old or more at the time of delivery. However, there is no reason to arbitrarily adhere to this age as an absolute cutoff. In my practice, many women between the ages of 30 and 34 have availed themselves of amniocentesis since the risk of Down syndrome and several other chromosomal abnormalities rises progressively after 30 (see page 402 and Table 28). Some geneticists recommend the procedure for women married to men older than 55, based on minimal evidence that chromosomal abnormalities in sperm increase in frequency after this age; other studies show no such relationship. In addition, any woman, regardless of her age, who has given birth to a child with a chromosomal abnormality should be encouraged to undergo a diagnostic amniocentesis since she faces a 1 percent risk of delivering a child with the same or a different chromosomal defect. A family in which one parent is a known carrier of a genetic disease is at especially high risk of conceiving an abnormal infant. Asymptomatic chromosomal breaks, inversions, and translocations in a parent can lead to full expression of these abnormalities in the fetus. Similarly, pregnancies among women who are known carriers of serious X-linked diseases, meaning that they are carried by healthy females but appear in 50 percent of all males, must have the fetal sex verified with amniocentesis and appropriate measures taken if it is male (see page 398). When both parents are discovered to be carriers of one of the increasing number of autosomal recessive diseases which may be diagnosed in utero, amniocentesis is mandatory. The same is true for autosomal dominant conditions (see page 404).

Amniocentesis is occasionally indicated when a woman's prenatal alpha-fetoprotein (AFP) blood test is abnormally elevated, suggesting that she is at risk for giving birth to an infant with a neural tube defect such as anencephaly or spina bifida. However, the new sophisticated ultrasound machines have the capability of viewing the anatomical details of the skull and vertebral column with such clarity that fewer amniocenteses need to be performed for elevated AFP levels. This, however, has been offset by a greater number of abnormally low AFP levels, a finding which is predictive of Down syndrome and other chromosomal abnormalities 40 percent of the time. An even newer blood test, known as a triple screen or AFP_3, measures a woman's levels of AFP, hCG (human chorionic gonadotropin), and UE_3 (unconjugated estriol) and can predict Down syndrome and other chromosomal abnormalities 65 percent of the time. As this test becomes more popular, an even greater number of women under 35 will be undergoing amniocentesis in order to diagnose these chromosomal disorders.

As mentioned in Chapter 2, spontaneously aborted fetuses are significantly more likely to be chromosomally abnormal. It is believed that if a woman has experienced three or more spontaneous abortions prior to her present conception, she will be at a significantly greater risk of giving birth to an infant with a genetic defect. Similarly, if her husband's previous wife experienced several miscarriages, the odds are slightly greater that he may be contributing chromosomally abnormal sperm to the present union. Some geneticists believe that couples with this type of history should be offered diagnostic amniocentesis.

 # AMNIOCENTESIS AND RESPIRATORY DISTRESS SYNDROME (RDS)

How is amniocentesis used in the last few weeks of pregnancy to determine the respiratory status of the fetus?

The leading cause of death among newborn infants, particularly premature infants, is respiratory distress syndrome (RDS). Infants suffering from RDS, formerly known as hyaline membrane disease, lack a substance named surfactant, which is produced by the cells lining the small air spaces (alveoli) within the lungs. Surfactant prevents the baby's lungs from collapsing with each expiration by reducing the surface tension in the lining of the alveoli. As a result, newborns with sufficient amounts of surfactant rarely succumb to RDS. When adequate concentrations of surfactant are present in the fetal lung, some is transported into the amniotic fluid. Its concentration in the amniotic fluid can then be measured if the sample is obtained via amniocentesis.

The components of surfactant are chemicals called phospholipids, with lecithin (L), sphingomyelin (S), and phosphatidylglycerol (PG) being the most important. The relationship between the concentrations of lecithin and sphingomyelin in the amniotic fluid, termed the L/S ratio, is the basis for one of the most important laboratory tests available to obstetricians. When the concentration of lecithin is at least twice that of sphingomyelin, meaning that the L/S ration is 2/1 or greater, there is a 97 percent likelihood that the newborn will not develop RDS. PG appears in the amniotic fluid at about the 36th week of pregnancy and increases in amount from that point on. The presence of even a small amount of PG in the amniotic fluid is a virtual certainty of fetal lung maturity.

There is no longer any excuse for a newborn to develop RDS just because a doctor decides to induce labor for his or her convenience or for the convenience of a patient. Similarly, a prescheduled, nonemergency cesarean section should hardly ever result in the birth of a baby who develops RDS. Judicious use of ultrasound and amniocentesis, when indicated, before induction of labor or a scheduled nonemergency cesarean section, in which a woman's due date is not absolutely certain, should prevent this physician-induced complication from occurring.

What else does the study of amniotic fluid reveal about the maturity of the fetus?

Prior to the discovery of surfactant, doctors used a variety of other amniotic fluid tests to determine a baby's overall body maturity and health. While none of these nonsurfactant tests of fetal maturity give an accurate prediction of fetal lung maturity, they are still performed today in many laboratories as confirmation and in situations where the fetal lung profile is questionable, contradictory, or borderline.

One fascinating test involves examination of a sample of amniotic fluid after it is stained with Nile blue sulfate dye. The presence of unusual-looking orange cells which clump together and do not have a nucleus is often indicative of fetal maturity. A related skin test for fetal maturity is the quantitative assessment of squalene levels in the amniotic fluid. Squalene is a major component of vernix caseosa, a white, sebaceous deposit which totally covers the fetal skin at 34 to 37 weeks but is then reduced in amount and only found in the skin folds of the full-term fetus. As squalene totally disappears from the skin of the postmature fetus, its concentrations in the amniotic fluid increase.

Creatinine is a chemical which is easily measured in the serum and urine in order to determine a person's kidney function. The concentration of creatinine in the amniotic fluid increases significantly during the last four weeks of pregnancy, providing an indication of fetal maturity in 85 percent of all cases.

The breakdown, or hemolysis, of circulating red blood cells yields a yellow pigment named bilirubin. Exact measurements of bilirubin concentrations in the amniotic fluid are accomplished with a special light meter called a spectrophotometer. Bilirubin is first found in the amniotic fluid as early as the twelfth week of normal pregnancies. It decreases in amounts during the second half of pregnancy and eventually disappears during the last four weeks. Its absence from the amniotic fluid provides some assurance that a baby is mature, but

it is not specific enough to be used as a sole test for determining if a jeopardized infant should be delivered early.

What are the shake and tap tests, and how accurately do they determine fetal lung maturity?

The shake and tap tests are two rapid and inexpensive methods of determining if amniotic fluid surfactant is present in concentrations sufficient to prevent RDS in the newborn. The shake test, also known in its more sophisticated version as the foam stability index (FSI), provides an estimate of fetal lung maturity in 20 to 30 minutes and requires no complicated technology. The shake test is performed by mixing amniotic fluid with various dilutions of alcohol and water in a test tube and then vigorously shaking the mixture for 15 seconds. If surfactant is present in sufficient concentrations, a ring of bubbles and foam will form. If the ring of foam persists for at least 15 minutes after the mixture is shaken, the risk of respiratory distress will be very low.

The great advantage of the FSI is that it takes such a short time to interpret the results. This is vital in situations where decisions must be made within minutes. Most problems with this test and all other surfactant determinations have arisen with false-negative results, in which the quantity of surfactant is adequate but the ring of foam does not persist for 15 minutes. In fact, 75 percent of babies with FSIs consistent with lung immaturity do not develop RDS. For this reason, shake test and FSI results that are negative for lung maturity should always be confirmed by a more precise test.

The tap test is another rapid and inexpensive test for fetal lung maturity. It derives its name from the fact that a test tube containing amniotic fluid, hydrochloric acid, and diethyl ether is briskly tapped with the index finger of the person performing the test. Tapping creates an estimated 200 to 300 bubbles in the ether or top layer. In amniotic fluid from a mature fetus the bubbles quickly rise to the surface and break down, while bubbles from an immature fetus remain or break down slowly. If no more than 5 bubbles persist in the ether layer after 10 minutes, the baby's lungs are considered to be mature.

Is there a way to speed up fetal lung maturation if there is a threat of premature labor and RDS in the newborn?

Since the principle defect in infants who develop respiratory distress syndrome (RDS) is the limited amount of surfactant coating their lung tubules, a great deal of research has focused on finding a drug that will hasten lung maturation by increasing surfactant concentrations. The urgency of this quest is prompted by the fact that 50 percent of babies born at a gestational age below 33 weeks develop RDS and 15 percent die of the disease. Survivors often suffer from bronchopulmonary dysplasia, a chronic lung disease of childhood.

As previously mentioned, the principle phospholipid components of surfactant are lecithin (L) and phosphatidylglycerol (PG); when lecithin is abundant and PG is present, RDS will not occur. To date, maternal intramuscular administration of corticosteroids (cortisone-like drugs) have shown the greatest promise in raising fetal surfactant levels. Betamethasone, dexamethasone, hydrocortisone, and methylprednisolone have all been used with varying degrees of success. Usually two injections are given 24 hours apart, with the major biologic effects occurring at 48 hours after initiating therapy.

The long-term effects of corticosteroids on the infants exposed in utero have not been fully established. While preliminary evidence in human beings is encouraging, the results of some animal experiments have been somewhat pessimistic. In a 1979 report, monkeys exposed to betamethasone had smaller head circumferences than those not exposed. Rats similarly treated were noted to have lower body weights and smaller brains, hearts, livers, kidneys, and adrenal glands. Subsequent studies, however, have not supported these findings.

Some doctors oppose the use of betamethasone and other cortisone preparations, such as dexamethasone and hydrocortisone, because of their potential maternal hazards.

What measures can be taken following delivery to prevent premature infants from developing RDS?

In an attempt to both prevent and treat RDS in its earliest stages, scientists have devised various aerosol and liquid surfactant concoctions which can be delivered to a newborn's lungs by a catheter or tube placed into the trachea. When used prophylactically, surfactant is usually reserved for newborns weighing less than 3 pounds (1,350 grams) at birth, and best results are obtained when treatment is initiated almost immediately following the baby's first breath. Therapeutic benefits diminish when treatment is delayed and the disease is well-established. Surfactant preparations are also effective in heavier babies suffering from RDS. Of the many studies evaluating the efficacy of surfactant therapy, most have concluded that treated infants experience significant improvement in respiratory function and have an RDS-associated mortality rate one-half that of untreated babies. Treated infants also require one-third to one-half less time in the neonatal intensive care unit. While some researchers have noted a reduction in other prematurity-associated complications, such as brain hemorrhages, retinopathy (eye disease), and necrotizing enterocolitis, others have reported no such surfactant-related benefits.

As mentioned (see previous question), corticosteroids given to a woman in danger of giving birth prematurely will help to mature her fetus's lungs and prevent RDS. Little is known, however, about the effects of corticosteroids given to a newborn infant.

AMNIOINFUSION

What is amnioinfusion and how is it used to treat obstetrical complications?

Amnioinfusion is the filling of the uterine cavity with normal saline after the membranes have ruptured. This relatively new procedure has captured the enthusiasm of obstetricians who have used it to correct complications of labor such as abnormal fetal heart rate decelerations, the presence of thick meconium, oligohydramnios (decreased amniotic fluid associated with prematurity), intrauterine growth retardation, and postmaturity. Recently amnioinfusion has been used to instill antibiotics directly into the uterine cavity as a method of preventing and treating fetal and maternal infections following premature rupture of the membranes.

The procedure itself is simple. An intrauterine pressure catheter is inserted into the uterus and attached to tubing connected to an intravenous solution of 1,000 milliliters of normal saline. The usual saline infusion rate is approximately 20 milliliters per minute, and no more than 1,000 milliliters should be infused at any one time. It is not unusual for the infused fluid to leak out over a period of time, but the procedure can be repeated later in labor.

The characteristic fetal heart rate abnormality associated with umbilical cord compression is known as a variable deceleration. As this pattern becomes repetitive and more ominous during labor, it can compromise fetal oxygenation and cause fetal distress. Ultrasound studies have demonstrated that amnioinfusion expands the amniotic space and forms a protective cushion of fluid around the umbilical cord, thereby protecting it from compression. The success rate of amnioinfusion in correcting variable decelerations has ranged from a low of 15 percent in some studies to a high of 70 percent in others.

The presence of fetal distress in labor can often be verified retrospectively by studying the pH of the umbilical cord blood vessels immediately at birth. Several studies have confirmed that newborns of women treated with amnioinfusion for variable deceleration have higher, meaning healthier, pH values than untreated newborns.

CVS

What is CVS and why do some doctors prefer it to amniocentesis for genetic analysis?

The chorion is a membrane which helps to form the early fetal portion of the placenta. CVS stands for chorionic villus sampling, a relatively new technique for studying chromosomal abnormalities and genetic defects in the fetus. The cells obtained for analysis come from villi, or hair-like projections of tissue, in the chorion frondosum layer of the first-trimester placenta. As seen in Figure 44, the chorion frondosum is that part of the chorion which attaches directly to the uterine lining. (See also Figure 45.) The most popular method for obtaining CVS specimens is the transcervical technique, in which a catheter is passed through the cervix under ultrasound guidance. Approximately 10 to 25 milligrams of chorionic tissue are then aspirated into a collection syringe and prepared for analysis. Transabdominal CVS, recently popularized in Europe, allows access to chorionic villi through an ultrasound-guided needle inserted into the lower abdomen.

In order to obtain an adequate sample of tissue for analysis and to minimize fetal and maternal complications, CVS is usually performed between

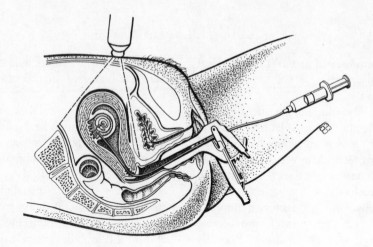

Figure 44 *Transcervical CVS*

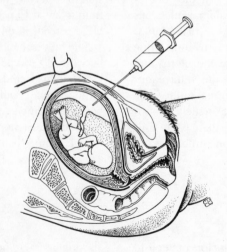

Figure 45 *Transabdominal CVS*

the ninth and eleventh week of pregnancy. The aspirated chorionic tissues contain rapidly dividing cells that can be used for direct chromosomal analysis. As a result, a preliminary report is usually available in 24 to 48 hours, while confirmatory cultures can be obtained in less than seven days. In contrast, amniocentesis is most often performed between the fifteenth and eighteenth week of pregnancy and requires 7 to 14 days to obtain an adequate number of cultured cells.

Are there any disadvantages associated with CVS?

Even the most ardent proponent of CVS will reluctantly admit that it is more hazardous to the fetus than amniocentesis. Statistically, 1 pregnancy out of every 200, or 0.5 percent, will be lost as a result of complications arising from amniocentesis performed between the fifteenth and eighteenth week of pregnancy. A 1989 National Institute of Child Health and Human Development-supported study of seven American hospital centers performing CVS found that the procedure was responsible for a 0.8 percent increase in fetal loss above the 0.5 percent risk quoted for amniocentesis. These results were confirmed in another 1989 study from the University of Toronto which reported an excess CVS risk of 0.6 percent among 2,000 women undergoing the procedure. These statistics are quoted from a handful of medical centers where large numbers of CVS procedures are performed by skilled physicians possessing extensive experience with the technique. Many experts believe that a more realistic fetal loss rate in less-experienced hands ranges from 2 to 4 percent above that quoted for aminocentesis.

Whether one uses the transvaginal or transabdominal CVS method, the skills required are far greater than those needed to perform amniocentesis, a procedure which can be easily accomplished by most obstetricians in an office setting. Accessibility to the small number of hospitals and private clinics with CVS capability is also a problem, since these facilities are overcrowded and overburdened with requests.

The excellent success rates quoted for CVS apply to procedures performed between the ninth and eleventh week of pregnancy. When it is attempted before or after this time period, pregnancy losses rise to an unacceptably high 6 to 7 percent.

Bleeding and cramping are the two most common side effects following CVS, occurring in approximately one-third and one-fifth of all procedures, respectively. Both symptoms, practically nonexistent following amniocentesis, may persist for a few hours to several weeks. Leakage of small amounts of amniotic fluid is an uncommon but worrisome complication which has aroused the concern of several authorities. One expert, Dr. Ronald J. Wapner, of Jefferson Medical College of Philadelphia, has described the "oligohydramnios syndrome," a potentially lethal fetal condition characterized by minimal or absent amniotic fluid during the second trimester and subsequent spontaneous abortion. The leakage of blood and amni-

otic fluid responsible for causing this problem usually has its origin immediately following first-trimester CVS. Dr. Wapner has theorized that the procedure causes either a hematoma (collection of blood) or a low-grade infection in the chorion; this weakens the amniotic membranes, predisposing them to leakage, infection, and abortion. In their 1989 national study, Canadian investigators also expressed concern that six stillbirths occurred after the twenty-eighth week of pregnancy among 1,000 women undergoing first-trimester CVS. In contrast, there was only one stillbirth among an equal number of women undergoing midtrimester amniocentesis.

There are currently five separate reports in the medical literature showing a relationship between CVS and the development of fetal limb malformations, sometimes accompanied by a shortened tongue and an underdeveloped lower jaw. In the latest study published in *Obstetrics and Gynecology* in 1992, doctors at the University of Illinois College of Medicine found limb defects in 4 of 394 fetuses subjected to CVS between the ninth and twelfth week of pregnancy. It is believed that this complication is caused by the formation of clots in the blood vessels at the chorionic villus sampling site, which lead to a reduction in the amount of blood and oxygen flowing to the fetal limbs and jaw. As a result of these findings, the use of CVS has declined precipitously over the past two years.

Maternal or fetal infections following transcervical CVS are far less common than cramping or bleeding, but the severity of such infections is usually far greater. There are several cases in the medical literature of women who have experienced near-fatal septic shock following transcervical CVS. Fortunately, this complication has not been reported following the transabdominal method. Women scheduled for transcervical CVS should be scrupulously examined for any evidence of chlamydia, gonorrhea, or herpes beforehand.

One of the greatest drawbacks of CVS, when compared to amniocentesis, is that the villi cannot be used to measure alpha-fetoprotein (AFP) levels.

As a result, the procedure is unable to detect neural tube defects such as anencephaly and spina bifida. To rule out a neural tube defect, a blood test must be performed during the sixteenth week of pregnancy. If the results are abnormal, amniocentesis may then be necessary. An occasional CVS problem is the contamination of the uncultured cells with maternal rather than fetal chromosomes, a problem rarely seen with amniocentesis.

What is embryoscopy and how successful is it in obtaining villi for CVS?

Embryoscopy is a new technique for visualizing the developing fetus and placenta via a viewing instrument passed through the cervix. A powerful fiberoptic light source attached to the embryoscope allows direct chorionic villus sampling (see Figure 46).

In an article published in the *American Journal of Obstetrics and Gynecology* in 1990, doctors from the Yale University School of Medicine reported their results in performing embryoscopy in 100 women prior to a scheduled first-trimester termination of pregnancy. The embryo was easily visualized in 96 of the 100 procedures. Since embryoscopy is performed without anesthesia or with only local anesthesia to the cervix, it would appear to be a promising technique for visualizing early fetal anomalies and for obtaining chorionic villi for analysis. One serious complication, however, appears to be the risk of inadvertent rupture of the amniotic membranes, leading to fetal and maternal infection and spontaneous abortion. This is least likely to occur if embryoscopy is performed between the seventh and eleventh week of pregnancy. Other potential complications include hemorrhage and fetal eye injuries caused by exposure to the bright fiberoptic light. A great deal more research will be needed on the immediate and long-term risks of embryoscopy before it can be considered to be a safe and reliable diagnostic technique.

Amnioscopy is identical to embryoscopy, but it is performed during the last trimester rather than the first.

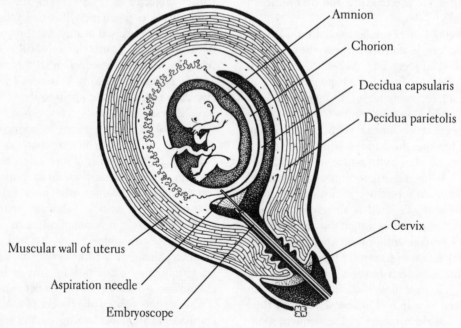

Amnion

Chorion

Decidua capsularis

Decidua parietolis

Cervix

Muscular wall of uterus

Aspiration needle

Embryoscope

Figure 46 *Embryoscopy*

FETOSCOPY

What is fetoscopy and how is it used in obstetrics?

A fetoscope is a viewing instrument which has a diameter that is slightly greater than a large needle. It is placed through the abdominal wall and into the amniotic sac in much the same manner as in amniocentesis (see Figure 47) and is usually performed between the eighteenth and twenty-second week of gestation. The fetoscope contains a high-powered fiberoptic light source which allows a view of the fetal and placental surfaces; but due to the small diameter of the fetoscope, the area observed at any one moment is quite limited. Fetal abnormalities, such as cleft lip and cleft palate, limb defects, and spina bifida, have all been diagnosed through the fetoscope. The instrument is equipped with a biopsy forceps which can be used to obtain a small piece of the baby's skin for chromosomal and biochemical studies. The prenatal diagnosis of a variety of congenital skin diseases is also possible with this technique. By inserting a tiny needle into the placenta and umbilical cord, doctors have been able to obtain samples of fetal blood for analysis. The fetal blood type and the assessment of fetal anemia can be established in this fashion, as can the diagnosis of disorders such as sickle cell anemia, beta-thalassemia, hemophilia, von Willebrand's disease, innumerable metabolic disorders, chromosomal abnormalities, and viral and other infections. Blood transfusions and injection of medications into the umbilical cord have also been reported.

The development of expertise in fetoscopy is very difficult, and at the present time its use is limited to a very few medical centers in the United States. The procedure must be considered a research tool because of the increased risks to the fetus and mother compared to other methods of prenatal screening and diagnosis. Fetal hemorrhage, accidental rupture of the amniotic membranes, premature labor, and second-trimester abortion are all possible complications.

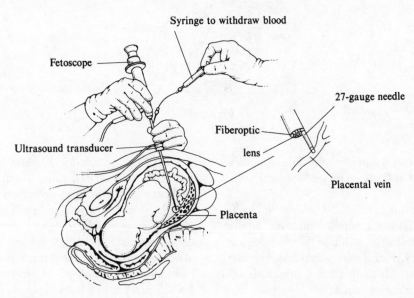

Figure 47 *Fetoscopy*

PUBS

What is PUBS, and when and how is it performed?

PUBS is an acronym for percutaneous umbilical cord blood sampling, a technique for obtaining blood from an umbilical cord vessel via an ultrasound-guided needle passed through the maternal abdomen and uterine wall. (See Figure 48.) Cordocentesis and funicentesis are two names used synonymously with PUBS. The procedure also enables doctors to inject lifesaving transfusions of drugs and blood directly into the fetal umbilical vein. PUBS accomplishes most of the diagnostic and therapeutic goals of fetoscopy with only a fraction of its complication rates, leading many neonatalogists to predict that this procedure will revolutionize the fields of genetics and intrauterine fetal therapy.

PUBS cannot be performed prior to the eighteenth week of pregnancy because the umbilical vein is too narrow until then to allow entry of the 20- to 22-gauge spinal needle needed to obtain an adequate fetal blood sample. Therefore, PUBS is not designed as a technique to replace earlier and safer techniques such as CVS and amniocentesis. Once PUBS is performed, however, it can be repeated periodically or initiated when necessary throughout the second and third trimesters. The procedure causes minimal discomfort and can usually be accomplished under local anesthesia to the maternal abdomen, occasionally combined with mild sedation.

Although PUBS has gained worldwide popularity since its introduction in 1982, the procedure is certainly not innocuous and should only be performed in large medical centers by personnel skilled in both ultrasonography and perinatology.

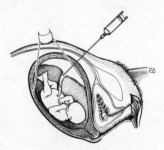

Figure 48
PUBS Procedure

What are some of the present and future medical and obstetrical indications for performing PUBS?

Although amniocentesis and chorionic villus sampling (CVS) are generally employed for the prenatal diagnosis of cytogenetic disorders in early pregnancy, PUBS may occasionally be necessary after the eighteenth week if previously obtained cell cultures are inadequate or if confusing chromosomal findings need clarification. When a woman first appears for prenatal care after the twentieth week and requires immediate genetic evaluation, PUBS will allow direct fetal blood sampling and cytogenetic analysis within 48 hours. These rapidly obtained results are especially important if the findings are abnormal and abortion needs to be performed prior to the legally allowable cutoff of 24 weeks. Between 10 and 15 percent of fetuses experiencing severe intrauterine growth retardation (IUGR) during the second and third trimesters are later found to have serious chromosomal abnormalities. When PUBS is performed late in the second trimester or during the third trimester, it may be too late to perform an abortion, but the information is still helpful in planning for delivery and the postpartum care of the baby. In addition, when fetal chromosomal abnormalities are found to be incompatible with life, an unnecessary emergency cesarean section for fetal distress can be avoided.

Without access to the fetal circulation, doctors are often unable to determine if a maternal infection has been contracted by the fetus. PUBS allows blood samples to be analyzed and cultured for a variety of pathological organisms such as rubella, varicella, cytomegalovirus, toxoplasmosis, and syphilis. An even more significant test of fetal infection is the presence of disease-specific immunoglobulin M or (IgM) antibodies. IgM antibodies are found only in the presence of acute infection and are too large to pass from the maternal to the fetal circulation across the placenta. Therefore, their presence in the PUBS blood sample is a virtual certainty that the fetus is infected. This information is vital since many of these fetuses will demonstrate abnormalities, and the presence or absence of IgM is often a determining factor as to whether or not a woman will undergo a second-trimester abortion.

PUBS-obtained blood samples have been successfully used to evaluate fetal health by measuring the acidity or pH of the blood, combined with carbon dioxide, oxygen, lactic acid, glucose, and lipid levels.

Erythroblastosis fetalis is the presence of severe fetal anemia and heart failure caused by a blood incompatibility between an Rh-negative woman and her Rh-positive fetus. Fortunately, it is infrequently seen today because of the introduction of Rh-immune globulin, or D immunoglobulin. When Rh-incompatibility is suspected, PUBS is invaluable in determining the blood type of the fetus and the degree of anemia that is present. It

also provides a channel through which periodic transfusions of fresh blood cells can be given until the baby is mature enough to be delivered. Several so-called isoimmune conditions can be similarly diagnosed and treated. Fetal heart failure may also result from diseases such as cardiac malformations, congenital heart block, abnormal heart rhythms, hyperthyroidism, and infections. PUBS is often helpful in elucidating the cause of these problems. A baby with thrombocytopenia, or an abnormally low platelet count, may experience a cerebral hemorrhage when subjected to the forces of labor and a vaginal delivery. By obtaining a fetal platelet count via PUBS, obstetricians are now able to determine which women require a cesarean section and which ones can safely attempt a vaginal birth. Inherited fetal blood diseases such as sickle cell anemia, beta-thalassemia, and hemophilia A and B can all be diagnosed with PUBS, but recent advances in molecular biology have enabled doctors to do this with greater safety using CVS or amniocentesis.

What are some of the complications associated with PUBS?

PUBS is a procedure which should be performed only for very specific and limited indications by physicians who are skilled in the technique. Such experts are presently located in a select number of large United States medical centers.

The most frequent complication is bleeding from the umbilical cord, which may occur in 15 to 20 percent of all procedures. Fortunately, such bleeding is most often harmless and stops spontaneously within 2 minutes. Pregnancy loss rates attributed directly to PUBS have been quoted to be as low as 1 in 200, or 0.5 percent, in the most experienced medical facilities; but based on a 1989 sampling of ten centers worldwide, a more realistic rate is approximately 2 percent. Fetal death may result from an umbilical cord blood clot or a laceration of the umbilical vein causing excessive fetal blood loss. Amniotic fluid contamination and subsequent infection may also vary from a low of 2.4 percent in some reports to an unacceptably high 15 percent in others. While PUBS will initiate labor 1 percent of the time, it can usually be stopped with tocolytic, or uterine-muscle-relaxing, drugs.

 ## NEWBORN UMBILICAL CORD BLOOD SAMPLING

What can be learned about the health of a newborn by studying the blood in its umbilical cord?

If a 4- to 8-inch segment of the umbilical cord is doubly clamped immediately after delivery, the blood in the umbilical artery and vein can be analyzed for its acidity, or pH, as well as its oxygen and carbon dioxide concentrations. This has proven to be the most accurate method of immediately assessing the health of a baby at the moment of birth and for determining if hypoxia, or a serious lack of oxygen, is present. Cord blood analysis helps a doctor differentiate between more ominous conditions and harmless incidents of acute asphyxia and respiratory acidosis resulting from a transient interruption of the normal blood flow between the fetus and the placenta that may occur during labor. When the umbilical cord blood analysis confirms the diagnosis of respiratory, rather than metabolic, acidosis, it is a comforting sign for an obstetrician and pediatrician, since these babies respond rapidly to minimal resuscitation and transient ventilation in the delivery room. In contrast, babies with metabolic acidosis often require more vigorous management in the pediatric intensive care unit.

 ## THE APGAR SCORE

How does the Apgar score compare to umbilical cord blood analysis in evaluating the health of a newborn?

Until the introduction of postpartum umbilical cord blood sampling, obstetricians relied solely on the Apgar score for evaluating the health of newborns and for determining whether or not asphyxia was present at birth. The Apgar score is the number which is derived by evaluation of the newborn's color, heart rate, respirations, reflexes, and muscle tone. Each of these five factors is given a value of either 0, 1, or 2, with an Apgar of 10 being awarded to the healthiest babies. Apgar scores are given to newborns at 1, 5, and 10 minutes of life, and low scores at 5 and 10 minutes are more indicative of a serious problem than a low score at 1 minute. Although the Apgar score still serves as an important and universally accepted method of evaluating a newborn's general condition, it does not accurately reflect the degree of asphyxia and metabolic acidosis that a baby may have experienced during pregnancy and labor; and it is almost valueless in predicting if a threat of cerebral palsy exists. Only umbilical cord blood analysis of the pH, oxygen, and carbon dioxide values allows such a precise determination.

Congenital anomalies, prematurity, and maternal drug administration are examples of situations which may result in a low Apgar score, but not necessarily asphyxia or maternal acidosis. Between 56 and 62 percent of depressed newborns, as evidenced by 1- or 5-minute Apgar scores of less than 7, have normal cord pH values, thus ruling out the diagnosis of birth asphyxia. When the Apgar score is the only available method for determining if asphyxia is present, the American Academy of Pediatrics requires that all three of the following criteria be met: an Apgar score of 0 to 3 at 10 minutes, early onset of seizures, and prolonged loss of muscle tone in the newborn. The lack of specificity of the Apgar score as a predictor of birth asphyxia leading to cerebral palsy is attested to by the National Collaborative Perinatal Project data showing that 55 percent of children who later developed cerebral palsy had high 1-minute Apgar scores of 7 to 10, while 73 percent had 7 to 10 Apgars at 5 minutes of life. Conversely, 80 percent of newborns who survive despite dismally low Apgar scores of 0 to 3 at 10 minutes are found to be free of major neurological handicaps when they reach school age.

While no one has suggested that the Apgar score be abandoned as a method of evaluating a newborn's condition, it should be used in conjunction with more precise modalities such as electronic fetal heart rate monitoring, scalp pH determinations during labor, and umbilical cord blood analysis at the moment of birth.

 ## *LAPAROSCOPY AND PELVISCOPY*

What is laparoscopy and how is it used in pregnancy?

A laparoscope is an instrument with a diameter slightly larger than a pencil. It contains a powerful fiberoptic light source which, when inserted through the navel, allows visualization of the upper abdominal and pelvic contents.

The injection of two or more liters of carbon dioxide into the abdomen moves the intestine out of the lower pelvis and makes viewing of the pelvic organs easier. Specially designed instruments can then be passed through the laparoscope, or through tiny accessory incisions in the lower abdomen, to accommodate a variety of procedures. When the laparoscopic procedure is completed, the carbon dioxide is removed from the abdomen, and the tiny incisions in the navel and other sites are closed with absorbable sutures. The sutures are then covered with a Band-Aid, hence the name "Band-Aid surgery." Another synonym for laparoscopy and pelviscopy is "belly-button surgery." The procedure may be performed under general or local anesthesia.

One of the most important uses of laparoscopy is in the diagnosis of an ectopic pregnancy (see page 61), one located outside its normal site in the uterine cavity. If laparoscopy confirms the presence of an ectopic pregnancy, it must be surgically removed through a lower abdominal incision. Removal of a tubal pregnancy through the laparoscope was first described in the medical literature in 1973 by this writer. Since then it has been successfully accomplished by many other doctors.

Diagnostic laparoscopic procedures performed beyond the sixteenth week of pregnancy are potentially dangerous because the large uterus may be injured by the instrument as it passes through the umbilicus.

In the days immediately following childbirth, laparoscopic tubal sterilization may be performed instead of the traditional tubal ligation. This is easily accomplished by coagulation, or burning, of the tubes. Despite impressive statistics from several medical institutions, most doctors have never performed this operation postpartum, and some have even claimed that it is hazardous. My experience with the technique on more than 100 postpartum women at Norwalk Hospital in Connecticut has been excellent. There have been no complications, and all patients have experienced significantly less discomfort and a shorter hospitalization than those undergoing the abdominal procedure. There is also the added benefit of no visible scar. One great advantage of the procedure over the abdominal postpartum operation is that it may be performed on the second or third day following delivery rather than immediately after. This gives a woman more time to decide if she really wants the operation.

 ## AFP TESTS

How is AFP testing used to detect fetuses with neural tube defects?

Once a woman has given birth to a baby with a neural tube defect such as anencephaly and spina bifida, her odds of giving birth to a second affected infant increase to 2 to 5 out of 100. After two such births, the chances of a third are 6 to 10 out of 100.

The failure of the fetal neural tube to close properly occurs during a well-defined period between the seventeenth and thirtieth day after ovulation. While some neural tube defects may be mild, others are severe, and the baby may die after the first few days. When the neural tissue is not covered by the scalp or skin, it is called an open neural tube defect. Anencephaly is the most abnormal open defect. It is characterized by incomplete closure of the fetal skull and retarded development of the brain, and it is invariably fatal. Open spina bifida is caused by an incomplete closure of the lower spine with exposure of nerve tissue of the lower back. It is often associated with paralysis of the legs and blockage of the fluid which surrounds the brain and spinal cord. The result is hydrocephaly, or an abnormally large head, caused by the accumulation of obstructed fluid. In contrast, when the spina bifida defect is closed, or covered with normal skin, an affected individual is most likely to be perfectly healthy and asymptomatic.

Most open neural tube defects can be diagnosed before the twentieth week of pregnancy by the measurement of a protein, named alpha-fetoprotein (AFP), in the amniotic fluid and maternal bloodstream. AFP is produced by all fetuses. Under normal circumstances, its concentrations in the fetal bloodstream and the amniotic fluid increase until the fifteenth week of pregnancy, and then they drop precipitously. Traces of AFP also cross the placenta and enter the maternal circulation. Maternal blood levels, however, follow a different pattern, rising slowly during the second trimester and reaching a plateau during the third trimester. When a pregnancy is complicated by an open neural tube defect, AFP levels in the amniotic fluid and maternal bloodstream are extremely high between the fifteenth and twentieth week.

A blood test should be used as the initial screening for neural tube defects rather than amniocentesis, except when amniocentesis is performed because of other suspected abnormalities or the mother's advanced age. This blood test has its greatest accuracy when performed between the fifteenth and eighteenth week of pregnancy. Then, almost all cases of anencephaly and at least 80 percent of open spina bifida defects can be detected. If this initial maternal serum AFP (MSAFP) test is elevated, many experts suggest that the test be repeated immediately to be sure it is not in error. If it is still high, ultrasound examination is then performed in order to demonstrate these abnormalities or to uncover benign causes for the test result, such as the presence of twins or a pregnancy that is further along than expected. A growing number of experts are of the opinion that a second blood test wastes valuable time and should be bypassed in favor of a so-called Level I, or screening, ultrasound, to find the cause of the abnormally high MSAFP. When this examination fails to solve the mystery of the elevated MSAFP, most authorities recommend that amniocentesis be performed and that the fluid be tested for both AFP and acetylcholinesterase, a nervous system enzyme. If the amniotic fluid levels of these two substances are normal, a woman can be assured that she is not carrying a fetus with a neural tube defect. However, high concentrations of AFP and acetylcholinesterase will confirm the presence of either a neural tube defect or another structural anomaly. More precise identification of the defect can usually be accomplished with a Level II ultrasound, a procedure which employs sophisticated high-resolution equipment and requires a great deal more time than the standard office Level I ultrasound. Level II ultrasound is performed by a select group of skilled ultrasonographers located in major United States medical centers.

When the findings of either the amniocentesis or Level II ultrasound confirm the presence of an anomaly, genetic counseling is mandatory, and a woman should be offered the option of a midtrimester abortion. For parents who elect not to undergo an abortion, Level II ultrasound is invaluable in determining the exact location and extent of the spinal lesion. A couple can then be counseled about what they can reasonably expect regarding the neurological function of their child. Pinpointing the lesion with an early Level II ultrasound allows time to plan for delivery in a medical center staffed with pediatric and surgical teams experienced in dealing with these serious birth defects.

MSAFP testing should be routinely offered to all woman between the sixteenth and eighteenth week of pregnancy. The strongest argument in favor of screening is that 95 percent of women at risk of bearing a child with a neural tube defect have no previously affected child or family history of neural tube abnormalities. The blood tests are painless and easy to perform, and the high yield of 5 to 10 abnormal fetuses per 100 amniocenteses makes these tests extremely worthwhile. Even when ultrasound and amniocentesis reveal no obvious cause for an elevated MSAFP, the test may still serve as an omen of potential complications later in pregnancy. Several reports have indicated that a woman with an unexplained MSAFP elevation faces a 20 to 30 percent risk of complications such as preterm birth, premature rupture of membranes, intrauterine growth retardation, preeclampsia, abruptio placenta, and stillbirths. Therefore, such pregnancies should be classified as high-risk and carefully monitored.

 AFP_3

How does the AFP$_3$ test improve the accuracy of standard AFP testing?

In addition to determining AFP concentrations, the AFP$_3$ blood test, or so-called triple screen, also measures levels of the pregnancy hormone known as human chorionic gonadotropin (hCG) and a type of estrogen named estriol. When this so-called three-marker or triple screen test is characterized by a low MSAFP, a high hCG, and low estriol, the detection rate for Down syndrome in a woman under 35 may be as high as 55 to 65 percent when confirmed by amniocentesis. Despite its improved accuracy over standard AFP testing, AFP$_3$ screening should not be substituted for amniocentesis in women 35 years of age and older, since it will still miss at least 35 percent of Down syndrome and other age-related chromosomal defects.

ULTRASOUND

What is ultrasound and how are the various ultrasound instruments used in obstetrics?

The medical use of high-frequency sound waves, or ultrasound, has revolutionized the practice of obstetrics and gynecology. This painless and safe diagnostic technique has provided significantly more information about the status of a woman's pregnancy than had ever been achieved with the use of potentially harmful x-ray examinations. The intensity of diagnostic high-frequency sound waves is extremely low and well within the upper limits of safety. When ultrasound was first introduced, its use was limited to a select number of major medical centers. Today, however, the development of relatively inexpensive, portable, high-resolution imaging equipment has enabled three out of four practicing obstetricians to have an ultrasound machine in their offices. It is impossible to imagine how a doctor could practice obstetrics today without having immediate access to an ultrasound machine.

An ultrasound machine generates sound waves when a current is applied to its probe or transducer. The transducer is moved gently over the skin of the abdomen during an abdominal ultrasound examination, while a specially designed transducer is inserted for vaginal ultrasound procedures. A pulse of sound waves, moving at a frequency too high for the human ear to hear, passes through the surface tissues and into the abdominal cavity. As the sound waves are bounced back to the transducer from the structures deep within the abdominal cavity, an image, displayed as a picture on a fluorescent screen, is created. Since tissues of different densities reflect sound differently, the trained ultrasonographer is usually able to identify abdominal and pelvic structures and interpret abnormalities which may be present. To diminish the loss of ultrasound waves at the point where the transducer meets the skin or vagina, a large amount of mineral oil or gel is first applied liberally to these surfaces.

Vaginal ultrasound is far superior to abdominal ultrasound in diagnosing and treating pregnancy and its complications during the first trimester. The close proximity of the vaginal transducer to the pregnancy sac and fallopian tubes allows doctors to visualize the early pregnancy sac and detect abnormalities such as a blighted ovum, missed abortion, and ectopic pregnancy. Vaginal ultrasound guidance is also invaluable in performing chorionic villus sampling (CVS) for genetic testing between the ninth and eleventh gestational week (see page 359). An increasing number of fetal abnormalities are being detected when vaginal ultrasound is performed at the end of the first trimester, but the technique is not nearly as accurate for this and most other purposes during the second and third trimesters, when abdominal ultrasound is used almost exclusively.

Doppler ultrasound, named after Christian Johann Doppler, an Austrian physicist who discovered it, measures the velocity of blood flowing through the circulatory system. The small handheld ultrasound devices used by most obstetricians to hear the fetal heartbeat in their offices employ the simplest form of Doppler sound waves, known as continuous-wave Doppler. Similar devices secured to a woman's abdomen are used for external fetal heart rate monitoring during labor and for nonstress and stress testing in the last trimester (see page 384). These machines provide no diagnostic information other than the fetal and maternal heartbeats. Newer and more sophisticated continuous-wave Doppler devices are capable of measuring and graphically recording characteristic velocity waveforms of blood passing through the umbilical artery. Researchers have found that resistance to blood flow, as occurs with placental malfunction, IUGR, and fetal distress, will alter the waveform appearance and help in the early diagnosis of a jeopardized pregnancy.

The pulsed-wave Doppler can do everything that the continuous-wave Doppler can do, but it has the added capability of measuring blood flow within the fetal heart and great vessels, and it clearly delineates the presence and severity of heart disease in the fetus. Pulsed-wave Doppler can also measure and record blood flow velocity in the fetal vena cava, hepatic (liver) veins, renal (kidney) arteries, and intracranial blood vessels. With the newest Doppler advance, known as color-flow imaging, the recorded image is color-coded so that it looks like an arteriogram of blood flow with the velocity superimposed upon a real-time image. This method holds great promise for pinpointing congenital heart defects in utero. The cost of the equipment and the skills needed to perform and interpret pulsed-wave readings limit its use to medical centers.

What information can be gained about fetal anomalies by using ultrasound during the second and third trimesters of pregnancy?

Whether ultrasound is performed as a general screening procedure or for the purpose of diagnosing a specific problem, it must be done in a systematic and thorough manner. A second- and third-trimester ultrasound examination is incomplete and inadequate if it does not include a complete survey of the maternal pelvic organs, an estimation of gestational age, the number of fetuses present and their position, fetal physiology and anatomy, including a view of the four heart chambers, amniotic fluid volume, and the location and condition of the placenta. In addition, estimates of fetal weight should be routinely calculated during the last trimester.

The presence of fetal central nervous system anomalies, such as anencephaly and spina bifida, can be confirmed with ultrasonography during the second trimester. An initial screening or Level I ultrasound should uncover most defects of the fetal spine. Occasionally, however, a more intensive Level II examination with a higher resolution machine is needed to diagnose smaller defects. The diagnosis of hydrocephaly, an abnormally large fluid-filled head, can usually be made during the second trimester before grossly abnormal changes have developed. An unusually small fetal head, or microcephaly, is easily diagnosed by midtrimester ultrasound. Craniofacial malformations such as cleft palate and cleft lip, abnormal facial bones, and underdevelopment of the jaw are also readily detected.

Gastrointestinal obstruction in the fetus may be caused by a variety of conditions such as esophageal and duodenal atresia (narrowing) and tracheoesophageal fistula (abnormal communication between the trachea and esophagus). Other gastrointestinal abnormalities readily diagnosed by ultrasound include omphalocoele (large umbilical hernia) and gastroschisis (herniation of intestinal contents due to absence of abdominal wall musculature), and diaphragmatic hernia. Making the precise diagnosis prior to delivery is vital in planning the timing and method of delivery and for the emergency medical and surgical treatment of these abnormalities.

Fetal urine production usually begins late in the first trimester, and the urinary bladder should be visualized by the second trimester. Under normal circumstances, the fetal kidneys should be easily seen on ultrasound by the eighteenth gestational week. In a healthy fetus, the bladder fills and empties itself of urine every 20 to 45 minutes, and this can usually be seen on ultrasound. The kidneys are one of the most common organs involved in congenital malformations. A marked diminution of amniotic fluid, or oligohydramnios, should lead a doctor to suspect bilateral renal agenesis, an invariably fatal disease characterized by insufficient kidney function. Hydronephrosis, or swelling of the fetal kidneys, is a fairly common condition which usually resolves soon after birth. Cystic diseases of the kidneys can also be detected, as can abnormalities and obstruction of the urinary bladder.

Genital anomalies detected by ultrasound include fetal ovarian cysts and tumors and abnormal male genitals. The scrotum can often be delineated, as can abnormal fluid collections called hydroceles.

Every ultrasound examination performed after the eighteenth week of pregnancy should include a view of the four chambers of the heart. This simple screening procedure will help to identify 60 to 90 percent of fetuses with major forms of heart disease. Women suspected of carrying a fetus with congenital heart disease should be referred for a detailed echocardiogram and Doppler color-flow imaging to assess the size of the cardiac chambers, the thickness of the heart muscle, and the blood flow patterns within the heart and its great vessels. A precise diagnosis of fetal heart disease prior to delivery allows time to prepare for delivery and in some cases to administer in utero fetal therapy (see page 395). Hydrops fetalis, or fetal heart failure, can be seen ultrasonically as a collection of fluid under the fetal scalp, in the lungs, neck, and abdominal cavity. This medical emergency often necessitates immediate delivery. Babies with severe cardiac defects should be delivered in large medical centers where they can be treated by specialized pediatric and surgical teams.

Malformations within the lungs as well as the bones of the thorax and chest cavity can be readily diagnosed with ultrasound. A diaphragmatic hernia is a defect in the diaphragm which allows the stomach and intestine to fill the chest cavity, causing compression and underdevelopment of the lungs and displacement of the heart from its normal position. Antenatal detection of a congenital diaphragmatic hernia allows doctors the time to plan for immediate resuscitation and surgery of these critically ill infants at birth. The normal umbilical cord contains two umbilical arteries and one umbilical vein. These three blood vessels can be seen ultrasonically during the second and third trimesters. Fewer than 1 out of every 100 fetuses have only one umbilical artery, and these infants have a 10 to 24 times higher incidence of major congenital anomalies as well as a greater likelihood of IUGR and preterm delivery. The presence of one umbilical artery should alert an obstetrician of the possibility of these complications.

Abnormalities of the fetal skeletal system, such as bone deformities, abnormally short or long bones, demineralization, and fetal fractures, often help doctors diagnose a wide variety of congenital defects and rare inherited diseases. The various types of dwarfism can be distinguished from one another with ultrasound. Polydactyly (extra digits) are often a clue that other more serious congenital anomalies coexist. Since bone disorders are frequently associated with cardiac anomalies, the diagnostic work-up should also include fetal echocardiography.

How accurate is ultrasound in diagnosing Down syndrome?

While it would be an invaluable asset to identify Down syndrome fetuses with a screening ultrasound examination rather than amniocentesis during the second trimester, this goal is not likely to be realized in the foreseeable future. When ultrasound is performed between the fifteenth and twentieth week of pregnancy, Down syndrome fetuses are more likely than normal fetuses to have a thickened skin fold of the neck, abnormally short femurs or thigh bones, and an abnormal fifth digit of the hands.

In a report published in the *New England Journal of Medicine* in 1987, doctors from Harvard Medical School found that 12 of 28 fetuses with Down syndrome had neck skin folds of 6 millimeters or more, while 19 of 28 were found to have abnormally short femurs. When these two sonographic signs were both present, the detection rate for Down syndrome soared to 82 percent. Unfortunately, several investigative groups have been unable to reproduce the original findings of the Harvard researchers, and many experts now conclude that ultrasound's accuracy in diagnosing Down syndrome leaves much to be desired. The main problem is that there are simply too many chromosomally normal fetuses that happen to have short femurs and thick skin folds of the neck. As a result, the use of ultrasound as a diagnostic screening test for Down syndrome will subject too many healthy fetuses to the risks of amniocentesis. For the present, the only prenatal tests that can identify Down syndrome and other chromosomal defects with absolute certainty are chorionic villus sampling, amniocentesis, and percutaneous umbilical cord blood sampling, or PUBS (see discussions this chapter).

How is ultrasound used in the new technique of pregnancy reduction?

Thousands of women previously unable to have children have been assisted in conceiving with a variety of techniques such as induction of ovulation, in vitro fertilization (IVF), and zygote intrafallopian transfer (ZIFT). A small but significant number of pregnancies achieved with these methods are complicated by three or more fetuses, thereby significantly increasing the risk of spontaneous abortion, premature labor, and a variety of serious maternal and fetal complications. Surviving infants are often born so early that they either die during the neonatal period or are irreversibly damaged because of their extreme prematurity.

Selective multifetal pregnancy reduction or termination is a procedure in which the number of fetuses is reduced to a safer and more manageable number, specifically one or two, with the hope of improving the survival of the remaining fetuses. This is best performed between the tenth and twelfth week of pregnancy by passing a needle into one or more of the fetal gestational sacs under either vaginal or abdominal ultrasound guidance. Abortion is accomplished either by aspirating or suctioning the gestational sac into a syringe or by injecting a small but lethal dose of calcium gluconate or potassium chloride into the targeted sac. While the ethical issues surrounding the use of selective pregnancy reduction for the above-mentioned reasons will continue to evoke heated

discussion in our society, the procedure does offer an option to pregnant women facing extremely difficult obstetrical and emotional decisions.

Medical experience with multifetal pregnancy termination during the first trimester is limited to a handful of medical centers in the United States. The procedure requires great expertise, and even in the best of hands the entire pregnancy will be lost 15 percent of the time.

How accurate is ultrasound in determining fetal sex?

The fetus develops well-formed external genitals at 13 to 14 gestational weeks, but they cannot be seen reliably with ultrasound until approximately 18 weeks. The discovery of fetal gender may be hindered by a variety of factors, including an upward position of the fetal back, crossed legs, breech or buttocks-down position, maternal obesity, diminished amniotic fluid volume, and the presence of loops of umbilical cord passing between the legs.

While the resolution of the newest ultrasound machines has improved the accuracy of predicting fetal gender during the second trimester, it should not be relied upon in critical situations such as the diagnosis of so-called X-linked or sex-linked diseases (see page 398). Under these circumstances, chorionic villus sampling (CVS) or amniocentesis is mandatory.

How can ultrasound be used to accurately determine gestational age and the presence of intrauterine growth retardation (IUGR)?

The accurate assessment of fetal gestational age is essential to the management and successful outcome of pregnancy. This is especially crucial in the timing of delivery in high-risk pregnancies and pregnancies complicated by either prematurity or postmaturity. Basing a woman's due date on her recollection of her last menstrual period often proves inaccurate, especially when periods are irregular. One study showed that the due date of 25 percent of women was changed after they underwent routine ultrasound screening.

The most accurate method of determining gestational age is the so-called crown-rump length (CRL), a measurement of the distance from the top of the fetal head to the base of the spine. Unfortunately, the CRL loses its reliability after the first trimester and is therefore valueless in diagnosing problems of fetal growth later in pregnancy.

The distance between the outside edges of the two parietal bones of the fetal skull is known as the biparietal diameter (BPD). Normal fetuses, regardless of their eventual weight differences at birth, have similar BPDs between the eighteenth and twenty-eighth week of pregnancy. Two biparietal measurements taken at four-week intervals at this stage of pregnancy may be plotted on a graph and should accurately determine the duration of pregnancy within five to eight days.

To accurately assess gestational dates and the presence of IUGR, doctors are using a variety of other measurements in combination with the BPD. One of the most useful is the fetal abdominal circumference. Not only can ultrasound measurements of the head and abdominal size diagnose IUGR in 90 percent of the cases, they can also determine if it is symmetrical (type I) or asymmetrical (type II). This distinction is important because it gives an obstetrician valuable clues as to the cause and severity of the fetal problem. When growth retardation is symmetrical, meaning that the fetal head and body both lag in growth, one can assume that the insult causing this condition most probably originated early in pregnancy. Chromosomal abnormalities and first trimester viral infections, such as rubella, are examples of conditions which cause this type of growth retardation. In contrast, asymmetrical growth retardation results from an insult in the latter part of pregnancy and comprises at least 80 percent of all cases of IUGR. Its cause is more often conditions that lead to a malfunctioning placenta, such as hypertension and preeclampsia, and is characterized by a reduction in blood flow and oxygen transport to the fetus. To compensate for this lack of oxygen and nutrients over a prolonged period of time, the fetal blood flow is diverted to the brain at the expense of the abdominal organs such as the intestines, liver, and kidneys. Asymmetrical, or type II, growth-retarded newborns tend to do well if they survive delivery and will rapidly catch up in weight and development in the weeks following delivery. In contrast, babies born with the more ominous type I, or symmetrical growth retardation, are often permanently impaired.

There are several other ultrasonic measurements, which, when used in conjunction with the fetal biparietal diameter, help to improve the accuracy of gestational dating. One of the most popular and easiest to determine is the length of the fetal femur, or thigh bone. Other fetal bone lengths that have proven helpful in determining gestational age include those of the foot, the orbit or eye sockets, the humerus (upper arm bone), the tibia (bone of the lower leg), and the clavicle (collarbone).

Ossification, or bone-forming, centers are located at the ends, or epiphyses, of the long bones of the body. The timing of the bone growth is specific for each bone, with some ossification centers developing during fetal life and others throughout childhood. The DFE, or distal (furthest away from the body) femoral epiphysis, and PTE, or proximal (closest to the body) tibial epiphysis, usually form during the last three to four weeks of pregnancy. The presence of DFEs and PTEs on an ultrasound examination helps to confirm gestational age. More important, virtually 100 percent of fetuses with DFEs and PTEs will also have pulmonary maturity.

Doctors at Yale University School of Medicine have reported great success in measuring the transverse cerebellar diameter (TCD) within the fetal brain. From the fifteenth to the twenty-fourth week of gestation, the fetal cerebellar measurement in millimeters is equal to the gestational age in weeks. TCD measurements, however, lose their predictability as a measure of gestational dates during the last trimester.

Can any of these ultrasound calculations accurately predict the weight of the fetus?

With the use of modern ultrasound technology, fetal weight can be estimated with reasonable accuracy. These determinations are as important for timing the delivery of a severely growth-retarded infant as they are for deciding if a macrosomic infant, or one larger than 4,000 grams (8 pounds 13 ounces), should be delivered vaginally or by cesarean. The most widely used equation for determining fetal weight is based on measurements which combine the biparietal diameter (BPD) and the abdominal circumference. When the fetal head is deep in the pelvis late in pregnancy or when there is a breech, or buttocks-first, position, it is sometimes difficult to obtain an accurate BPD measurement (see page 374). In such cases, logarithmic charts which plot the femur length and abdominal circumference may be used with almost equal accuracy.

Unfortunately, the ability to predict fetal weight is least accurate in the situations for which it is most needed—the macrosomic infant weighing more than 4,000 grams (8 pounds 13 ounces) and the premature or growth-retarded infant weighing less than 1,500 grams (3.3 pounds). In a 1988 study, doctors from Harvard Medical School estimated more than 1,300 fetal weights within a week prior to delivery. They found that 74 percent of the newborns had birth weights within 10 percent of the ultrasound estimates. However, only 65 percent of macrosomic infants weighing more than 4,000 grams were correctly identified prior to birth. Other investigators have reported similar disappointing results. These findings are somewhat disconcerting in view of the trend in recent years to perform cesarean section prior to the onset of labor in order to avoid the severe maternal and fetal injuries that may result from the vaginal birth of a macrosomic infant. Conversely, false ultrasound predictions of macrosomia have resulted in a greater number of unnecessary cesarean sections. To improve the accuracy of predicting the weight of a macrosomic infant, Dr.

Creigh I. Hirata and his colleagues at the University of Southern California found that the best ultrasound results were achieved by using equations based on fetal abdominal circumference and femur length, rather than those relying on head and other body measurements. However, regardless of which formula is used, our present ultrasound technology does not allow obstetricians to precisely gauge the weight of macrosomic infants or determine the likelihood of a safe vaginal birth.

A higher incidence of ultrasound errors has been reported when estimating weights of severely premature and growth-retarded infants. However, encouraging results have been presented by Dr. Bruce W. Pielet and his associates at Northwestern Medical School, who performed ultrasound examinations on 61 infants weighing less than 1,700 grams (3 pounds 12 ounces) within one week of birth. Formulas incorporating head and abdominal circumferences and femur lengths were associated with an impressive mean percentage weight error of only 11 percent. Of even greater importance was a 7.7 percent mean percentage weight error among infants weighing only 750 grams (1 pound 10 ounces).

How can ultrasound be used to determine the cause of vaginal bleeding during the second and third trimesters?

One of the most important uses of ultrasound is the evaluation of vaginal bleeding during the second and third trimesters of pregnancy. Premature separation of the placenta from the uterine wall (abruptio placenta) occurs when a blood clot forms behind the placenta and actually shears it off from its attachment to the wall. In addition to uterine bleeding, maternal symptoms often include a tense, tender abdomen and shock due to blood loss. This potentially catastrophic situation for both mother and fetus can often be diagnosed in its early stages with ultrasound.

Less serious conditions, such as bleeding from a small sinus at the edge of the placenta, may be readily distinguished from the more severe abruptio placenta. Structural abnormalities of the placenta as well as variations in its size and its maturity may also be diagnosed. An ultrasound scan accurately demonstrates the placental location in relation to the cervix so that preparations for cesarean section may be made when indicated. However, a doctor should not perform a cesarean section based on a second-trimester report of placenta previa (placenta situated over the cervix) since the placenta will almost always migrate to a normal position as pregnancy progresses. This can be confirmed by a repeat ultrasound examination during the third trimester.

How can Doppler ultrasound measurements of the umbilical cord be used to monitor fetal well-being?

Continuous-wave Doppler ultrasound imaging (see page 370) can be used to measure and record the velocity of the blood as it flows through the two fetal umbilical arteries. Under normal circumstances, blood flow increases as pregnancy progresses, but complications such as hypertension, IUGR, diabetes, and placental pathology may impede this process and produce abnormal umbilical artery velocity waveforms.

Systole is that part of the heart-pumping cycle in which the heart muscles contract, while diastole represents the relaxation of the muscles and the filling of the heart with blood. The difference between the fastest systolic velocity (S) and the peak diastolic velocity (D) seen on a Doppler display screen is called the S/D ratio.

In fetuses that are not affected by IUGR, the umbilical artery S/D ratio decreases as the gestational age increases. This is due to the loss of placental vascular resistance and the increase in fetal blood pressure as pregnancy progresses. After 30 weeks gestation, the S/D ratio should be less than 2.8. When there is impairment of the placental vascular system, there is an elevation in the S/D ratio. During the third trimester, a ratio of 3 or greater is considered abnormal. A sign of severe placental impairment is the absence of the diastole peak.

However, the most ominous and urgent finding, indicative of impending fetal death, is the inversion of the diastolic wave, suggestive of a reversal of blood flow caused by almost complete impedance of blood as it passes through the umbilical artery.

Literally hundreds of articles have espoused the value of Doppler umbilical artery waveforms in the early diagnosis of IUGR and for distinguishing the small but healthy fetus from one in distress, although some experts have been less impressed than others with the predictive value of this technique. It has been proposed that Doppler umbilical artery blood flow velocity waveforms be used as an admission test for diagnosing fetal distress among patients in labor. In a 1991 study published in *Obstetrics and Gynecology*, doctors did Doppler studies on 575 laboring women both before, during, and after uterine contractions. Unfortunately, no association was found between abnormal flow velocity waveforms and umbilical cord complications, meconium-stained amniotic fluid, abnormal fetal heart rate tracings, the incidence of cesarean sections for fetal distress, or low Apgar scores. In this study, Doppler compared poorly in accuracy to standard electronic monitoring as a screening method for assessing fetal well-being during labor.

Should ultrasound be routinely performed on all pregnant women?

The overwhelming consensus of patient and physician opinion favors routine ultrasound screening during pregnancy. It is estimated that approximately 80 percent of American women are currently examined with ultrasound at some point in pregnancy. In contrast, ultrasound screening is the norm in most European countries, while women in Germany receive two routine examinations during the course of pregnancy.

The three greatest benefits of routine screening are early diagnosis of multiple births, accurate dating of gestational age, and the early detection of fetal anomalies. Other benefits include the diagnosis of the placental location, amniotic fluid volume, IUGR, and gynecologic diseases such as ovarian cysts and fibroids. Emotional benefits, such as relief of anxiety and early bonding with the fetus, may also accrue.

The best time to perform a single-screening abdominal ultrasound examination is between the eighteenth and twentieth gestational week. At this point, between 55 and 75 percent of previously unsuspected major fetal abnormalities can be diagnosed, depending on the skill of the ultrasonographer. In addition, there is still time for genetic counseling and performance of a midtrimester abortion if requested. If a woman elects to continue with her pregnancy, the precise diagnosis of a fetal defect improves the chances for survival because in utero therapy may be possible and delivery can be planned in a medical center capable of performing immediate postpartum pediatric surgery (see page 396). If it is determined that a woman is carrying a fetus whose anomalies are incompatible with life, an unnecessary cesarean section for an abnormal fetal heart rate pattern, IUGR, or fetal distress can be avoided.

If financial concerns did not enter into this discussion, I would personally perform ultrasound examinations on all of my obstetrical patients during the twelfth, eighteenth, and thirty-fourth weeks. The first would be a high-resolution vaginal ultrasound, so that gestational age could be accurately assessed with a crown-rump measurement. The presence of multiple fetuses could also be determined with a vaginal ultrasound examination at this time. High-resolution vaginal ultrasound has enabled doctors to detect an increasing number of birth defects during the first trimester. Pregnancy termination is an easier and safer procedure, and is emotionally far less devastating for a woman at this point than during the second trimester.

In addition to the previously stated benefits of abdominal ultrasound screening between the eighteenth and twentieth weeks, gestational dating can help to confirm the findings of a first-trimester crown-rump measurement.

A third ultrasound examination, performed at 34 weeks, can detect most cases of IUGR, abnormal fetal positions, placenta previa, and derangements in amniotic fluid volume. Unfortunately, the cost of performing three ultrasound examinations on all women during pregnancy is prohibitive.

What are the potential dangers of ultrasound?

When ultrasound is used for diagnostic purposes, the wave frequency is very high, but the power of the sound wave is extremely low. Despite the exposure of millions of women and their fetuses to diagnostic ultrasound and Doppler ultrasonic monitoring of the fetal heart rate over a period of at least 20 years, there is no evidence to show that these procedures are harmful. Newborns exposed to in utero ultrasound have similar Apgar scores, birth weights, lengths, head circumferences, anomalies, and neonatal infections when compared to newborns who do not receive ultrasound examinations. Follow-up studies of children exposed to ultrasound in utero have detected no physical or developmental difficulties when compared to unexposed control groups. Several of these studies have been extremely sophisticated and detailed in scope.

Pulsed-wave Doppler ultrasound is a sophisticated method of evaluating the blood flow in the fetal heart and circulatory system when cardiovascular problems are suspected (see page 370). This technique requires a higher power output than the continuous-wave Doppler machines which are applied to the maternal abdomen to monitor the fetal heart rate or measure umbilical artery blood flow velocity. The FDA has expressed concern that the power output of some of the pulsed-wave Doppler instruments have the potential to generate heat in the body tissues and create air bubbles within the tissues. While both effects are theoretically possible, they have never been demonstrated in a clinical situation. The fetus is well protected by the mother's abdominal and uterine walls and the amniotic fluid, thereby lessening the power intensity of the beam as it passes deeper to reach the fetus. There is no doubt that the risk of fetal injury secondary to diagnostic ultrasound is far more theoretical than it is real.

FETAL BREATHING MOVEMENTS

What can be learned by studying fetal breathing movements during pregnancy and labor?

A pregnant woman is unable to perceive fetal breathing movements (FBM), but they can be readily detected with the use of a standard real-time ultrasound machine. While research has shown that the assessment of fetal breathing patterns can be of some value when incorporated with other tests of fetal well-being, initial predictions that it would be used as the sole index of fetal health have been unfulfilled.

We eagerly await the newborn infant's first breath at birth; however, the patterns of breathing activity and use of the muscles of respiration actually begin in utero. The entire chest cavity moves when a fetus breathes, but amniotic fluid, rather than air, is inhaled and exhaled. Faint breathing movements may be seen as early as the eleventh week, with a periodic pattern appearing at about 24 weeks of pregnancy. The onset of regular breathing activity first becomes obvious at about the thirty-fourth week, and some investigators have claimed that this observation can be used to assess fetal age.

Data from several studies have demonstrated that healthy human fetuses make breathing movements about 30 to 35 percent of the time during the last ten weeks of pregnancy, compared to 14 percent of the time between the twenty-fourth and twenty-eighth gestational weeks. When fetal breathing does occur at any time after the twenty-fourth week, it is usually a very rapid 40 breaths per minute on average, or approximately three times that of the normal adult respiratory rate.

Apnea is defined as the absence of breathing movements, and it is not unusual to see this in the fetus for varying periods of time throughout pregnancy. While some researchers have claimed that the absence of fetal breathing movements after 30 minutes of ultrasound observation could identify a fetus in distress, Dr. Laurence D. Devoe of the

Medical College of Georgia stated that such a conclusion was overly pessimistic. In 1987 and 1989 studies on fetal breathing rates, he found that 70 percent of the fetuses who did not breathe during this time frame experienced normal pregnancy outcomes. Gasping motions, rather than breathing, are a more ominous indication of fetal distress than no breathing at all.

Dr. Kenneth Boddy and his associates at the University of Edinburgh have made some interesting and important observations of FBMs under a variety of conditions. For example, the second twin has a lower rate of FBMs and a longer period of apnea than the first-born twin, confirming the clinical impression that first-born twins have a higher survival rate. A reduction in breathing movements may also be associated with a mother's disturbed emotional state. Cigarette smoking reduces fetal breathing for as long as 90 minutes, while maternal alcohol consumption exerts a similar effect for up to 1 hour (see Chapter 5). Active labor causes fetal breathing to diminish and usually cease even among healthy fetuses. Even in the absence of infection, premature rupture of the amniotic membranes is associated with a significant reduction of FBMs. Conversely, the claim that the presence of fetal breathing movements is a reassuring sign that infection isn't present is nothing more than a dangerous presumption.

Exercise initially reduces and later increases FBMs. Drugs may affect FBMs as well. When diazepam (Valium) is administered intravenously to women in labor, there is a marked reduction in FBMs during the next 2 hours, followed by a return of normal. Doctors at the University of Western Ontario in Canada who observed FBMs during the last trimester reported a significant increase during the 2 to 3 hours following meals. This pattern appeared to coincide with levels of maternal plasma glucose.

The observation that FBMs normally decline or

cease within 72 hours of the onset of labor has prompted several investigators to study whether or not this information could help differentiate true from false labor among women with premature uterine contractions. In a study published in the *British Journal of Obstetrics and Gynaecology* in 1987, doctors from Edinburgh analyzed the predictive value of absent FBMs in 64 women presenting with threatened premature labor between 26 and 36 weeks gestation. All 17 fetuses without FBMs delivered within 56 hours. In contrast, 42 of 47 patients, or 89 percent, with FBM continued their pregnancies for at least 56 hours, with 70 percent of this group continuing for at least one more week. A second 1987 study from the University of Michigan found almost identical results.

Much remains to be learned about the significance of fetal breathing movements. At the present time, they would appear to have their greatest use when combined with other indications of fetal well-being.

How common are fetal hiccups, and what are their significance?

Fetal hiccups are a harmless and common phenomenon occurring in approximately 2 percent of all pregnant women during the third trimester. Unlike fetal breathing movements, they are easily perceived by a woman as being hiccups, appearing as abrupt, repetitive movements. They have a tendency to occur at the same time of day for each woman and often persist in the newborn following delivery.

Although the reflex of hiccuping is extremely similar to that of gasping, the fetus does not inhale amniotic fluid because the covering over the trachea, or glottis, closes during a hiccup.

 FETAL BODY MOVEMENTS

What is known about in utero fetal body movements, and how can this information be used as a test of fetal well-being?

While most women first experience fluttering movements between the seventeenth and twentieth week of pregnancy, real-time ultrasound enables us actually to observe twitching motion at the seventh to eighth week, independent limb movements by 10 to 12 weeks, and combined movements of the limbs, head, and body by 16 weeks. Real-time ultrasound has also enabled doctors to document the accuracy of a woman's perception of fetal movement during the third trimester. Based on the findings of several studies, it has been determined that a mother will detect between 75 and 85 percent of all movements.

Mothers usually characterize fetal movements as weak, strong, or rolling. In general, weak movements occur most often at 20 weeks, decrease in frequency until 36 weeks, and then increase until delivery. Strong and rolling movements slowly increase in frequency until about 37 weeks and then decrease. The total number of movements, rather than changes in a woman's perception of the type of movements present, is the more important determinant of fetal health in the third trimester.

The type of fetal movements observed on real-time ultrasound often depend upon the health and maturity of the fetus. Those suffering from intrauterine growth retardation (IUGR) exhibit markedly fewer and less clearly defined movements than the healthy fetus. Fetal maturity will also influence the number and type of fetal movements exhibited. Ultrasound studies conducted by researchers at the University of Western Ontario in 1988 found that fetuses of 24 to 28 weeks move more frequently than those older than 30 weeks.

While there is a gradual decrease in the percentage of time spent moving and the total number of movements as a fetus matures, the movements of the older fetus last longer, are more organized, and are characterized by well-defined periods of rest and activity.

Doctors at Hadassah-Hebrew University Hospital in Jerusalem have studied fetal body movements during pregnancy and found that the daily-fetal-movement recording (DFMR) rises from an average of 200 in the twentieth week to approximately 500 in the thirtieth week. From this point, the number of daily movements gradually declines to an average of 282. One important observation was the wide range of normal DFMRs, from a low of 50 to a high of almost 1,000. The actual number, however, is of much less significance than a sudden change from active to inactive, since this may portend fetal distress.

Using continuous real-time ultrasound monitoring for 12 to 24 consecutive hours, researchers found that the fetus moved an average of 90 times every 12 hours at 32 weeks compared to 50 times every 12 hours at 40 weeks. Others have found an average of 31 movements per hour over a 24-hour period during the last ten weeks of pregnancy, with fetuses spending 10 percent of their time moving. In contrast, fetuses between 24 and 28 weeks move approximately 13 percent of the time. Some studies have shown a distinct periodicity to fetal movement, with the greatest number occurring between the hours of 8 P.M. and 11 P.M. In a 1988 report, doctors found an increase in movement between the hours of 11 P.M. and 8 A.M. among 24- to 28-week-old fetuses, with a significant lessening of periodicity among more mature fetuses. Fetal movements have been noted to diminish in number following maternal cigarette smoking and alcohol ingestion and in association with sedative and narcotic use. Studies are controversial, but the overall conclusion is that fetal movements appear to be unrelated to maternal food intake. One study found an increase in movements following maternal administration of intravenous glucose, while a contradictory report found that fetal movements increased after maternal blood glucose concentrations reached abnormally low levels.

It is unknown why fetal movements decrease slightly in number during the last two to three weeks of pregnancy. One theory routinely quoted in most obstetrical textbooks is that the relative decrease in the amount of amniotic fluid and uterine volume restricts fetal movement. If this is so, fetal motion following rupture of the amniotic membranes should be markedly decreased. Dr. William F. Rayburn of Ohio State University has decisively disproved this theory. In his article published in the *American Journal of Obstetrics and Gynecology*, he noted that fetal movements occurred more than twice as frequently following rupture of the amniotic membranes. In addition, maternal perception of fetal motion following membrane rupture was as accurate as when membranes were intact.

Fetal movement may decline slightly at the end of pregnancy, but one must never believe the myth that complete cessation of movement at the end of pregnancy, for several hours at a time, is a healthy sign that labor is imminent. It is more likely to indicate that the baby is in severe distress and that the doctor should be notified immediately. He or she in turn would be well advised to instantly perform a nonstress test (NST) or biophysical profile (see next question). If either of these is abnormal, immediate delivery should be strongly considered. Remember, a " quiet" fetus is more likely to be a sick fetus than one with a placid disposition.

At the present time, there are no universal criteria for determining the number of perceived or recorded fetal movements indicative of fetal distress. The Hadassah-Hebrew University group regards less than three perceived movements per hour as abnormal. When this occurs, patients are asked to chart fetal movements for 6 to 12 hours; those with no fetal movements after 12 hours are delivered immediately. Other experts use three or fewer movements over a 24-hour period as an ominous sign of fetal distress. Doctors at the University of Pennsylvania consider a fetus to be distressed when its mother perceives fewer than 10 movements in 12 hours, while those at Ohio State University define "alarming fetal movement" as less than two movements recorded per hour for two consecutive days. In one study, women were divided into a group reporting 10 or more fetal movements over 12 hours and those noting fewer than 10 movements over this period of time. There were no perinatal deaths in the group with greater fetal activity compared to two deaths among women with decreased activity. Similarly, neonatal complications, such as fetal distress in labor and abnormal heart rate monitoring, were 5 percent and 22 percent, respectively.

The "daily-fetal-movement count" is a system used in many hospitals and is based on daily counts by the pregnant woman for 30-minute periods, three times daily. If the woman notes fewer than three fetal movements during one of these time periods, fetal movements are counted for 12 hours. The "movement alarm signal" of impending fetal death is fewer than four fetal movements in a 12-hour period. Another simple method is known as

the "count to 10" technique. This is performed by having a woman record how long it takes to feel 10 movements in the evening before bedtime. The average time to achieve this goal is 20 minutes, since this time period often coincides with the baby's wake cycle. If it takes more than 2 hours to feel the 10 movements, notify your obstetrician immediately. If you are not a night person, count fetal movements starting at 9 A.M. With this technique, you should feel the tenth movement before 6 P.M. The differences in time needed to achieve the 10 movements are the result of normal circadian variations that all healthy fetuses experience.

Also considered "abnormal" is a drop of 50 percent or more in the number of fetal movements on two consecutive days. For example, a drop from seven movements on one day to three on the next would be a cause for concern. A marked decrease in fetal movement has been found to precede ominous fetal heart rate changes by one to four days. A progressive decline in fetal activity is equally important, even if the total number of movements is still within the normal range.

 # BIOPHYSICAL PROFILE

What is the biophysical profile, and how is it used to identify the distressed fetus?

The biophysical profile (BPP) was first introduced in 1980 and since then has gained worldwide acceptance as an accurate means of assessing fetal health during the last trimester. By measuring five fetal biophysical components—breathing movements, body movements, fetal tone, amniotic fluid volume, and heart rate reactivity on a nonstress test (see page 383)—the BPP has been found to be more reliable than the use of only one or two of these indicators. Each of the five elements of the BPP are assigned a score of two points when nor-

mal and a score of zero if abnormal. (See Table 26.) Thus, the highest score possible for a healthy fetus is 10, while a total of 0 would indicate severe distress. It has been suggested that the nonstress test not be included as part of the BPP, but many physicians continue to rely on it and use it effectively.

A normal biophysical profile score of 8 to 10 is a reassuring sign that the fetus is healthy and will remain so until the test is repeated one week later, provided that the amniotic fluid volume is adequate. While BPP testing is less reliable in women with insulin-dependent diabetes and those with prolonged pregnancies, even under these circum-

TABLE 26

COMPONENTS AND NUMERICAL SCORES OF THE BIOPHYSICAL PROFILE

Biophysical Variable	Normal (BPS = 2)	Abnormal (BPS = 0)
Fetal breathing movements	At least one episode of FBM of at least 30 seconds' duration in 30 minutes' observation	Absent FBM or no episode of ≥ 30 sec in 30 min
Gross body movement	At least three discrete body-limb movements in 30 min (episodes of active, continuous movement considered a single movement)	Two or fewer episodes of body-limb movements in 30 min
Fetal tone	At least one episode of active extension with return to flexion of fetal limb(s) or trunk (opening and closing of hand considered normal tone)	Either slow extension with return to partial flexion or movement of limb in full extension or absent fetal movement
Reactive FHR	At least two episodes of FHR acceleration of ≥ 15 bpm and of at least 15 seconds' duration associated with fetal movement in 40 min	Fewer than two episodes of acceleration of FHR or acceleration of <15 bpm in 40 min
Qualitative AFV	At least one pocket of AF that measures at least 1 cm in two perpendicular planes	Either no AF pockets or one pocket <1 cm in two perpendicular planes

FBM—fetal breathing movement, FHR—fetal heart rate, bpm—beats per minute. AFV—amniotic fluid volume, AF—amniotic fluid

stances it is still a valuable addition to prenatal testing. In a 1987 study involving almost 20,000 BPPs, doctors found an in utero death rate of fewer than 1 per 1,500 pregnancies in the presence of a normal test. At the other end of the scale, BPPs of 0 to 4 are associated with an infant mortality rate of 28 percent. Of the five components of the BPP, fetal breathing and the nonstress test are usually the first to become abnormal. As the fetal condi-

tion worsens, movement and tone become compromised as well. As noted in Table 27, the volume of amniotic fluid and the amniotic fluid assessment of fetal maturity are often pivotal in timing delivery when BPP scores are in the equivocal range of 4 to 6. A composite BPP score of 2 or less is an obstetrical emergency requiring immediate delivery.

TABLE 27

INTERPRETATION AND MANAGEMENT OF BIOPHYSICAL PROFILE SCORES

Score	Interpretation	Recommended Management
10	Normal infant, low risk for chronic asphyxia	No fetal indication for delivery; repeat test weekly except in diabetic patient or postterm pregnancy (twice weekly).
8–10 with normal fluid	Normal infant, low risk for chronic asphyxia	No fetal indication for delivery; repeat test as above.
8–10 with decreased fluid	Suspect chronic fetal asphyxia	Deliver.
6	Possible chronic fetal asphyxia	Deliver if amniotic fluid volume is reduced; if normal fluid at greater than 36 weeks with favorable cervix, induce labor; if less than 36 weeks or L/S ratio <2:1 or cervix unfavorable, repeat test in 4–6 hours; if repeat test <6, deliver; if repeat test >6, observe and repeat per protocol.
4	Suspect chronic fetal asphyxia	Repeat testing within 4–6 hours; if BPP score <6, deliver.
0–2	Almost certain fetal asphyxia	Deliver immediately.

 FETAL MONITORING

What is fetal monitoring and how is it used to assess fetal well-being?

In recent years, electronic monitoring has become the most frequently employed method of assessing fetal health during the last trimester of pregnancy and throughout labor. Great controversy has arisen between consumer groups and obstetricians over the use and possible abuse of this new electronic gadgetry. However, most experts agree that it has been invaluable in the early diagnosis of fetal difficulties and in the management of high-risk pregnancies.

Many obstetricians and delivery-room nurses would like you to believe that the interpretation of fetal monitoring recordings is beyond your limited comprehension. While there are a small percentage of tracings that are complex and confusing, most are easily interpretable and surprisingly simple to understand.

There are two basic methods of electronic fetal monitoring: external (noninvasive) and internal (invasive). With the external technique, a Doppler ultrasonic transducer is strapped to the maternal abdomen over the area where the fetal heartbeat is most easily heard. The heartbeat is recorded on a strip of graph paper which runs through the monitoring machine. A second detector, known as a tocodynamometer, is strapped to the upper abdomen at a point over the top of the uterus. This detector records the frequency and strength of the uterine contractions as well as most fetal movements. Alterations in the fetal heartbeat in relation to both fetal movement and uterine contractions are of great importance in determining if the fetus is in jeopardy.

Internal, or invasive, fetal monitoring involves the placement of monitoring devices into the uterus through the vagina. With this method, the fetal heartbeat is recorded from a tiny spiral electrode attached to the baby's scalp. A specially designed catheter, inserted through the cervix, monitors the uterine contractions from within.

Internal fetal monitoring usually gives a more accurate recording of fetal heart rate and uterine contractions than the external method. However, it can only be used during active labor when the amniotic membranes are ruptured and the cervix is sufficiently dilated to allow insertion of the spiral electrode and the uterine pressure catheter. During labor, a doctor may elect to use only the external equipment, a combination of one external device and one internal method, or two internal monitors.

How is external monitoring used to evaluate fetal status before labor begins?

The normal fetal heart rate usually ranges between 120 and 160 beats per minute, although a rate 20 beats above or below this standard does not necessarily mean fetal distress. Under normal conditions, the fetal heart rate fluctuates from one moment to the next. This fluctuation, called beat-to-beat variability, is a sign of a healthy infant who has a reactive and functioning nervous system. The fetal heartbeat that resembles a straight line on the electronic monitor is an ominous sign of asphyxia, or central nervous system depression.

The nonstress test (NST), or fetal heart rate acceleration determination (FAD), is the most commonly used method of assessing the condition of the fetus during the last trimester. It is extremely simple to perform and to interpret. The Doppler ultrasonic transducer is placed over the maternal abdomen at the point where the fetal heartbeat is

most easily detected, while the tocodynamometer is positioned over the fundus, or top, of the uterus. The heartbeat is recorded on the fetal monitor's paper strip. A nonstress test is considered by most authorities to be normal or reactive when two or more fetal movements over a period of 20 minutes are immediately followed by an increase of the fetal heartbeat by at least 15 beats per minute, for a minimum of at least 15 seconds. Unfortunately, the definition of what constitutes adequate fetal reactivity is not universally agreed upon. Some obstetricians use an observation period of only 10 minutes, while others require a minimum of four fetal heart rate accelerations within the 20-minute time frame. One variation of the NST is to have the pregnant woman press a button, which she holds in her hand, whenever she detects fetal movement. This is recorded as an arrow on the paper monitor strip and allows for a clearer picture of the relationship between fetal movement and heart rate acceleration. Although the tocodynamometer may not record, and the woman may not discern, every fetal movement, it really doesn't matter. Several studies have confirmed that when fetal heart rate accelerations meet the criteria for a reactive NST, it is a virtual certainty that the fetus has moved.

When the criteria for heart rate accelerations are not met, a nonstress test is termed nonreactive. This is a potentially serious sign which requires a contraction stress test (CST) or a biophysical profile (see page 381). Of all NSTs performed, fewer than 10 percent will be nonreactive and necessitate further testing.

Occasionally, the nonstress test will be unsatisfactory because the fetus is in a sleep cycle and does not move during the 20-minute observation period. This is not necessarily worrisome, since many healthy infants experience periods of sleep lasting as long as 75 minutes. This situation can usually be remedied by giving a glucose-rich beverage or by gently shaking the maternal abdomen in order to arouse the fetus. Failure of the fetus to respond within 40 minutes, however, classifies the test as nonreactive and indicates that a problem may exist. A nonstress test may also be falsely nonreactive if a woman is positioned incorrectly during the test. All NSTs should be performed in the so-called Fowler's, or semi-sitting, position or in the left-lateral, or left-sided, position in order to prevent compression of the aorta by the enlarging uterus.

A reactive nonstress test implies that a fetus possesses reactive nervous and cardiovascular systems. While there have been notable exceptions to this rule, a reactive test usually indicates that the fetus is not distressed and is healthy enough to survive for at least one more week in the uterus, and the obstetrician need not plan an immediate delivery. This assumption proves to be incorrect—that is,

the fetus dies within a week of a reactive NST—in fewer than 1 percent of all women tested. Many obstetricians now favor use of NSTs as often as every other day and even daily in particularly complicated pregnancies.

A well-known obstetrical aphorism is that the NST often makes a healthy baby appear unhealthy but rarely makes an unhealthy one appear healthy. In other words, a nonreactive NST readily identifies fetuses at risk, but the test gives a falsely abnormal result 50 to 80 percent of the time. Therefore, if your NST is nonreactive, don't panic. The odds are that the biophysical profile and the contraction stress test (see page 386) will confirm that all is well.

SOUND AND VIBRATORY STIMULATION

How is sound and vibratory stimulation used as a form of nonstress testing?

The main disadvantage of standard nonstress testing is that too many healthy fetuses demonstrate nonreactive heart rate patterns, falsely suggesting fetal distress. Researchers have discovered that fetal heart rate accelerations can be stimulated in as many as 50 percent of these cases simply by applying intermittent bursts of pure-tone sound or vibrations to the maternal abdomen, in the region of the fetal head, for periods ranging from 1 to 10 seconds. Following this so-called vibroacoustic stimulation, most healthy fetuses exhibit at least two heartbeat accelerations of at least 15 beats per minute, lasting at least 15 seconds, over a 10-minute period of time. Vibrations produce more predictable fetal heart rate accelerations than sound, and doctors have reported success with a variety of ingenious vibratory devices, including electric toothbrushes, electronic artificial larynxes,

and a specially designed vibroacoustic stimulating device.

When a healthy fetus is viewed with real-time ultrasound during vibroacoustic stimulation, it will demonstrate an increase in movement, and this accounts for its accelerated heart rate. Also noted are reduced and irregular respiratory movements for up to 1 hour and a greater amount of head turning, mouth opening, tongue protrusion, hand to head movement, and rapid eye movements. These reactions are thought to represent a startle response of the fetus as it is aroused from a state of sleep to one of wakefulness.

Some physicians have expressed concern about the immediate and long-term consequences of in utero vibroacoustic exposure. However, preliminary data appear encouraging, with incidence rates for meconium staining, low Apgar scores, and cesarean section equal among NST and vibroacoustic-exposed infants.

Despite studies with promising results, widespread endorsement of vibroacoustic stimulation as a test of fetal well-being will only be achieved through standardization of testing techniques and long-term follow-up of thousands of exposed infants.

 # CONTRACTION STRESS TEST (CST)

What is a contraction stress test (CST), and when is it used?

While it is usually not performed as the initial screening test for evaluating fetal well-being, the contraction stress test (CST), or oxytocin challenge test (OCT), is invaluable in studying the fetus suspected of being in jeopardy. This is especially true when the nonstress test is either nonreactive or inadequate for proper interpretation.

To perform this test, the fetal heartbeat and uterine contractions are recorded with external monitoring devices in a manner identical to that used for the NST. However, maternal perception of fetal movement is not recorded. The CST is meaningful only if three uterine contractions take place over a period of 10 minutes and each contraction lasts approximately 40 seconds. Some women have these contractions spontaneously during the third trimester without being in labor, but 85 to 90 percent require a dilute solution of intravenous oxytocin (trade name Pitocin) to stimulate the required number of contractions. You need not fear that this procedure will inadvertently induce labor prematurely because only minimal amounts of oxytocin are used at a controlled rate of flow.

Under normal conditions, the fetal heart rate does not decrease following a uterine contraction. However, in the presence of a poorly functioning placenta and a severely distressed infant, the contractions of the uterus cause a decrease in oxygen flow to the baby. This in turn results in a drop in the fetal heart rate beginning as the contraction intensity peaks. The lowest level of the heart rate is usually recorded approximately 30 seconds after the contraction is most intense. When the fetal heart rate shows this characteristic decline in response to more than 50 percent of the uterine contractions, the CST is termed positive. Doctors have given this pattern of fetal heart rate change a variety of names, including late decelerations, late dips, and Type II dips. Regardless of the name, this pattern indicates that fetal distress may be present and immediate delivery should be considered if the fetus is mature. This is especially true when a positive contraction stress test is preceded by a nonreactive NST.

A negative CST means that the fetal heart rate does not decelerate following the peak of the contraction. This is a reassuring indication that there is no fetal distress. A negative contraction stress test implies that a woman possesses sufficient placental function to maintain the fetus safely in utero for at least one more week. This is true even in the presence of a nonreactive nonstress test. The test must be repeated weekly and occasionally biweekly as long as it remains negative.

The NST and CST complement each other as predictors of fetal well-being. When both the CST and the NST are in agreement that the fetus is distressed, there is a very high probability that this is so. However, either test used without the other is associated with an unacceptably high incidence of tests which falsely show a healthy fetus to be distressed. It is generally believed that the CST is a somewhat earlier predictor of fetal compromise than the NST. In one large study comparing the two tests, there were eight times fewer stillbirths when the CST was used as the primary screening test. Depending upon which study one reads, the risk of an intrauterine death within one week of a negative CST ranges between 0.4 and 7 per 1,000 tests performed. The fact that the NST is more commonly used than the CST is based more on logistical considerations, cost, and the time needed to perform each test. On average, a CST takes 2 hours to achieve the three desired contractions in a 10-minute time period.

While a reactive NST in a high-risk pregnancy is very reassuring that the fetus will survive for at least one more week, the one disturbing exception to this rule appears to be the postterm pregnancy. Several studies have demonstrated that the CST may be the more appropriate initial test for detecting a postmature infant in distress. If the NST is to be used to evaluate the postmature fetus, it should be performed at least twice a week.

Are there any women who should not undergo a contraction stress test?

If a woman has a history of premature labor, or if examination reveals that she has an incompetent cervix or that she may start labor before her estimated delivery date, the use of oxytocin is not recommended because it may be just enough of a stimulus to trigger labor in her sensitive uterus. This advice also applies to women with premature rupture of the amniotic membranes, because contractions may induce premature labor or disperse bacteria which are capable of causing a uterine infection. In the presence of placenta previa, abruptio placenta, and undiagnosed uterine bleeding, a CST should not be performed.

Most cesarean sections are performed through an incision in the lower segment of the uterus. However, on rare occasions it is necessary to do the surgery through the muscles in the upper part of the uterus. This is called a classical cesarean section, and its scar is far more likely to weaken and rupture if the uterus is stimulated to contract. For this reason, if a previous classical cesarean section has been performed, a CST is not recommended. Finally, the presence of multiple fetuses and hydramnios (excessive amount of amniotic fluid) may overly distend the uterus and make oxytocin stimulation more hazardous. If the CST is performed under these circumstances, it must be done with great care, using the lowest possible dose of intravenous oxytocin.

Can the CST be performed using nipple stimulation?

To reproduce the results of the CST without the inconvenience of using intravenous oxytocin, doctors have devised the nipple stimulation contraction stress test. It has long been known that nipple stimulation results in the release of oxytocin from the pituitary gland and subsequent uterine contractions. By firmly massaging the nipples manually or with a breast pump, between 60 and 100 percent of pregnant women will note contractions almost immediately. This method has the advantage of taking less time than the CST, an average of 24 minutes versus 2 hours for the CST. It is also less expensive and more acceptable to most women. Nipple stimulation has also been used effectively as a means of ripening the cervix for labor, inducing labor, improving the quality of contractions during labor, reducing postpartum hemorrhage, and for the more rapid expulsion of the placenta following childbirth.

While the contraindications to the nipple stimulation contraction stress test are identical to those for the CST, researchers have expressed concern that the risk of unpredictable uterine hyperstimulation may be far greater. Some studies have reported hyperstimulation rates as high as 30 percent, while others have noted a more optimistic incidence of 2 to 3 percent. Women undergoing a nipple stimulation contraction stress test must be closely monitored for evidence of hyperstimulation.

What is the significance of fetal heart rate changes which occur during labor?

When labor contractions produce late fetal heart rate decelerations, or Type II dips, it is an indication that the baby may be in jeopardy. Late decelerations begin at or after the peak of the uterine contraction and return to the baseline rate only after the contraction has ended. While an occasional late deceleration is no cause for alarm, repetition of the pattern and its presence following more than 50 percent of all contractions is considered to be an ominous sign. Of particular concern is the presence of late decelerations accompanied by a baseline heart rate showing minimal variability. Under these circumstances, 25 percent of babies will be distressed at birth. Late decelerations can sometimes be converted to normal by the pregnant woman's taking simple measures such as turning on her left side, assuming the knee-chest position, and breathing oxygen through a face mask or nasal catheter. If labor is being induced or stimulated, stopping the oxytocin often improves the heart rate within seconds. If all of these measures fail, prompt vaginal or abdominal delivery is often indicated.

Doctors have described two other classic fetal heart rate patterns which may appear frightening but are usually harmless. One is known as an early fetal heart rate deceleration, or Type I dip. This pattern can easily be identified. It begins with the onset of the contraction and returns to normal with or before the end of the contraction.

Early decelerations are believed to be caused by mild compression of the baby's head with each contraction, and they become more pronounced as labor progresses. Another type of deceleration is referred to as nonuniform, or variable. It derives from the fact that it may or may not occur in relation to the contractions and it differs in appearance from those which precede and follow. Variable decelerations may be caused by mild compression of the umbilical cord which can occur if the cord is draped around the baby's neck or body or is knotted. Conditions which cause oligo-

hydramnios, or diminished amniotic fluid volume, such as postmaturity and rupture of the amniotic membranes, are often associated with cord compression and variable decelerations. While most variable decelerations are not a cause for concern, others which reach a level of 70 beats per minute or last at least 60 seconds at a time may indicate fetal distress. In addition, when the return or recovery of the heartbeat to the baseline becomes excessively prolonged, so that the first half of the deceleration has the appearance of a "V" but the second half resembles a "U," this may indicate fetal jeopardy.

A fetal tachycardia, meaning a heart rate greater than the normal limit of 160 beats per minute, may be an indication of fetal distress caused by oxygen deprivation. This is especially true when it persists for prolonged periods of time and is accompanied by other fetal heart rate abnormalities. A moderate tachycardia, defined as a rate of 160 to 180 beats per minute, is not nearly as ominous as rates above 180 beats per minute. Maternal fever is probably one of the more common causes of a rapid fetal heart rate, but other conditions such as hyperthyroidism, certain drugs and medications, prematurity, infection, and fetal heart disease and anemia may also produce this effect.

An abnormally slow fetal heart rate, or bradycardia, may be associated with fetal distress. The lower limit of the normal fetal heart rate is 120 beats per minute, but a range between 100 and 119 beats during labor is usually not a cause for concern. During the second, or pushing, stage of labor, bradycardias ranging between 80 to 100 beats per minute are not uncommon and are not necessarily worrisome. However, severe bradycardias of less than 80 beats per minute which persist for 3 minutes or more are a worrisome sign that fetal distress and acidosis may be present.

Despite all of our modern technology, the diagnosis of fetal distress during labor remains imprecise. Reports by several authors suggest that even the most ominous fetal heart rate patterns are associated with, at most, a 50 to 65 percent incidence of newborn depression, as judged by low Apgar scores. This represents a dismal 35 to 50 percent false prediction of fetal compromise and a major contributing factor to the soaring cesarean section rates in the United States.

 ## FETAL SCALP TESTS

How is fetal scalp blood obtained, and what is the significance of an abnormal test?

The pH measurement is a laboratory test which determines the relative acidity of the blood in the capillaries of the fetal scalp. The blood specimen obtained from the scalp usually reflects the degree of acidity present in the rest of the fetal bloodstream, and an abnormally low pH level, or acidosis, is often associated with a severe lack of oxygen and fetal distress.

The technique of obtaining a fetal scalp blood specimen is painless, safe, and easy to perform. An endoscope, a funnel-shaped viewing device with a light attached to its end, is inserted through the cervix and placed firmly against the fetal scalp. For this to occur, your cervix must be at least two centimeters dilated and the amniotic membranes ruptured. After the scalp is prepared so as to minimize bleeding, one or two superficial scalp incisions are made with a small knife blade placed within the endoscope. The blood which forms is collected in a special tube and immediately analyzed for its pH. Pressure applied to the scalp with a cotton swab will stop the blood flow within seconds. The procedure can be repeated periodically throughout labor, in some cases as often as every 15 to 30 minutes.

The major advantage of fetal scalp blood sampling is that it will often clarify the significance of a confusing or abnormal heart rate pattern noted on the electronic monitor. In one study, only 5 percent of infants with a normal scalp pH required a cesarean section for fetal distress. It is estimated that judicious use of this technique has reduced by at least 50 percent the incidence of unnecessary cesareans for what falsely appears to be fetal distress on the electronic monitor.

Despite the advantages of fetal scalp blood sampling, it remains an underutilized technique which is used in fewer than 5 percent of American obstetrical units. Of late, an increasing number of obstetricians have found fault with the procedure and have cast doubt about its ability to predict fetal distress. One reason quoted for its lack of popularity is that the fetal pH status changes so rapidly during labor that the pH can be in the favorable range one minute and in the acidotic range the next. As a result, the condition of a newborn is often unrelated to the pH obtained during labor. In fact, it has been reported that 10 percent or more of infants with a fetal scalp blood determination below the critical level of 7.20 will have Apgar scores above 7. Conversely, an equal number of babies with low Apgar scores are born following reassuringly high pH levels. Another disadvantage of fetal scalp pH sampling is the patient discomfort and inconvenience associated with performing and repeating the procedure at frequent intervals throughout labor. Technical difficulties in obtaining the blood samples are often frustrating for some obstetricians. To overcome these problems, many attempts have been made to develop a method of continuous fetal pH assessment. However, it appears unlikely that such instrumentation will be available for clinical use in the near future.

How can fetal scalp stimulation be used as a test of fetal well-being during labor?

Several investigative groups have demonstrated that the so-called fetal scalp stimulation test can often serve as a clinically helpful and simple alternative to fetal scalp pH monitoring. When digital pressure is applied to the baby's head during a vaginal examination or the scalp is lightly pinched with a surgical clamp, a healthy fetus will almost always demonstrate an acceleration of its heart rate by at least 15 beats per minute for at least 15 seconds. When this occurs, a physician can be almost certain that the fetal pH is at least 7.20 and the fetus is healthy. Without such a response, however, there is roughly a 40 to 50 percent chance that the pH is below 7.2 and the fetus is acidotic. To confirm this, a fetal scalp pH determination should be performed immediately.

MRI

How is magnetic resonance imaging (MRI) used obstetrically?

Magnetic resonance imaging (MRI) is an exciting new radiological technique which is in its obstetrical infancy. Like ultrasound, MRI carries no known risks to the fetus or mother since it does not involve ionizing radiation. Although MRI is unlikely to replace ultrasound as a diagnostic technique, most experts foresee its value as a supplement to ultrasound in more clearly identifying abnormal fetal development, ectopic pregnancy, IUGR, placental pathology, premature cervical effacement, and pelvic tumors complicating pregnancy. One distinct advantage of MRI over ultrasound is its ability to measure the planes of the maternal bony pelvis with unsurpassed accuracy. There are situations such as a contemplated vaginal delivery of a baby in the breech position in which such pelvimetry measurements may occasionally prove helpful.

One major disadvantage of MRI is its exorbitant cost, varying between $600 and $1,000 per 45 minutes to 1 hour, with some procedures taking as long as 2 hours to complete. The obstetrical image obtained with MRI is precise but requires that the fetus and mother lie perfectly still. For this reason, its use during the first two trimesters, when fetal movement is most pronounced, is limited. To quiet the fetus, some investigators have reported success by administrating maternal tranquilizers.

Others inject a muscle-paralyzing drug named pancuronium directly into the fetal muscle or umbilical cord under ultrasound visualization.

MRI images of anatomical structures within the fetal brain are unequaled, and the presence of a wide variety of defects suspected on ultrasound can be confirmed at an early stage of pregnancy. Other clearly visualized anatomical sites include the heart and its chambers, the liver, stomach, lungs, and vertebral column. The kidneys are less readily seen. MRI provides clear images of fetal fat stores below the skin surrounding the skull, neck, and extremities. Loss of these fat layers is an indication of nutritional deprivation and an earlier sign of IUGR than any ultrasound finding. Ultrasound's usefulness is also limited in the presence of oligohydramnios, or reduced amniotic fluid volume, because fetal parts become crowded and boundaries between the placenta, uterus, and fetal soft tissues become obscure. In contrast, oligohydramnios tends to improve the quality of MRI because it is associated with less fetal movement. Placental location, shape, maturity, and abnormalities such as placenta previa, abruptio placenta, and placental infarcts are all more clearly visualized with MRI.

Indications for MRI use in obstetrics are expanding rapidly. However, its ultimate value to obstetricians and their patients remains to be determined.

PREVENTION OF PREMATURE LABOR

What are some of the medications used for preventing premature labor?

Preterm labor prior to the thirty-sixth week of pregnancy is unquestionably the main problem confronting the modern obstetrician. Although fewer than 10 percent of infants are premature, they account for 80 percent of all reported deaths of newborns and a significant number of neurologically handicapped infants. Most of the deaths attributed to prematurity are the result of respiratory distress syndrome (RDS) caused by immaturity of the fetal lungs. In an attempt to rapidly mature the lungs prior to delivery, doctors have administered cortisone medications, such as betamethasone, dexamethasone, and hydrocortisone, to susceptible pregnant women (see page 358). This controversial treatment, however, does not inhibit contractions or prevent premature labor and delivery.

While a wide variety of medications have been endorsed as labor-inhibiting drugs, or tocolytics, most have failed miserably. Many of the reports have been inconsistent and contradictory in the criteria used for diagnosing premature labor and less than precise in the statistical methods employed for evaluating drug efficacy.

In the past, a 10 percent solution of intravenous alcohol was the most widely used method of preventing premature births in the United States. Alcohol is believed to inhibit labor by blocking the release of oxytocin, the pituitary gland hormone that stimulates the muscles of the uterus. Unfortunately, the dose needed to stop uterine contractions is quite high and may cause complications for the mother such as nausea, vomiting, restlessness, intoxication, stupor, and even death. Danger to the fetus makes the use of alcohol unacceptable.

Magnesium sulfate is an excellent drug for treating preeclampsia and toxemia. In recent years, it has been used with great success in stopping premature contractions by relaxing the muscles of the uterine wall. Unlike other tocolytics, magnesium sulfate is relatively free of annoying maternal side effects, with the exception of an occasional temporary drop in blood pressure and a sensation of facial flushing. Another great advantage of magnesium sulfate over other tocolytics is that it increases uterine and placental blood flow, making it extremely valuable in cases of suspected uteroplacental insufficiency and intrauterine growth retardation (IUGR).

Since the magnesium sulfate dose is excreted almost entirely by the kidneys, it should not be administered to women with kidney failure. Accumulation of magnesium in the body can depress respirations, and women with a rare muscle disorder named myasthenia gravis should not be given the drug. Its use is also contraindicated when maternal blood calcium levels are low, since magnesium can depress the levels even further. Magnesium sulfate rapidly crosses the placenta, and levels in the fetal circulation parallel maternal levels. Recent continuous Doppler ultrasound studies of the umbilical and uterine arteries have not revealed abnormal changes following maternal magnesium infusions. Of recent concern is a 1991 study by doctors at Washington University School of Medicine in St. Louis, Missouri, in which they found x-ray evidence of abnormal bone mineralization in 6 of 11 newborns whose mothers received intravenous magnesium for more than 7 days during pregnancy. These findings supported two previous reports showing similar bone changes associated with in utero magnesium exposure. The clinical significance of these bone abnormalities is uncertain at the present time, but in one report they had resolved by 45 days of life.

Prostaglandins, found in many body tissues, including the lining of the uterus and fetal membranes, cause severe uterine contractions and are often used for inducing second-trimester abortions and for ripening the cervix for induction of labor. A sudden increase in prostaglandin levels is believed by scientists to be most responsible for initiating and maintaining contractions during labor. Drugs which inhibit prostaglandin release, known as prostaglandin synthetase inhibitors, are capable of preventing premature labor. Aspirin, for example, inhibits prostaglandin release as does ibuprofen (trade names Motrin, Nuprin, and Advil) and naproxen (trade names Anaprox and Naprosyn). All can prolong the onset of labor if taken in relatively high doses during the last weeks of pregnancy, but other factors preclude their use in this fashion. Indomethacin (trade name Indocin) has been used most often and most successfully to inhibit labor. Indomethacin's main drawback, however, is its potential to prematurely close a fetal blood vessel called the ductus arteriosus. This vessel, which normally closes soon after birth, runs between the fetal pulmonary artery and the aorta, and its closure in utero may lead to a very serious and permanent condition known as pulmonary hypertension. Recent Doppler ultrasound flow studies have demonstrated that a degree of ductus arteriosus constriction occurs in a significant number of women treated with indomethacin during the last trimester. However, closure of the vessel is unlikely to occur if indomethacin is used for less than 48 hours and tocolysis is discontinued prior to the thirty-sixth week of pregnancy.

Animal experimentation and human experience suggest that indomethacin may interfere with the normal uterine and placental circulations, causing a decrease in the volume of the amniotic fluid, or oligohydramnios, meconium staining of the amniotic fluid suggestive of fetal distress, and impaired fetal kidney function. If indomethacin is to be used for treating preterm labor, frequent and periodic ultrasounds should be performed to detect the earliest indication of diminished amniotic fluid volume.

The most commonly used group of drugs for inhibiting premature labor are the beta-sympathomimetics. These agents stop contractions and relax the uterus by stimulating special receptors, known as beta receptors, located in the muscle wall. Members of this group include isox-

suprine (trade name Vasodilan), terbutaline (trade names Brethine, Bricanyl, and Brethaire) fenoterol, salbutimol, ritodrine (trade name Yutopar), orciprenaline, and hexoprenaline. Of these preparations, it is ironic that only ritodrine is approved by the FDA as therapy for the inhibition of premature labor, despite the clinical evidence that other tocolytic agents are probably more effective and are associated with a lower incidence of fetal and maternal side effects. In fact, a 1992 multicenter study from Canada of over 700 women in premature labor found no differences in pregnancy prolongation, birth weight, or perinatal complications among women treated with ritodrine and those given a placebo. This lack of FDA approval for excellent tocolytics such as terbutaline and magnesium sulfate has not dissuaded American obstetricians from prescribing these drugs. Contrary to the public's perception, a medication need not be approved by the FDA as a tocolytic for a doctor to use it for that purpose. If it is FDA-approved for other indications, such as terbutaline in the treatment of asthma and magnesium sulfate for the control of toxemia, doctors are not liable or breaking the law if they use the drug for another well-recognized, though nonsanctioned, indication.

A relatively new group of antihypertensive medications, known as calcium channel blockers, have recently been introduced as a means of treating premature labor. Calcium channel blockers prevent calcium from passing into the smooth muscle cells of the uterus, thereby relaxing them. Of the drugs in this group, nifedipine (trade names Procardia and Adalat) has the best tocolytic effect. The major concern surrounding the use of calcium channel blockers is that experimental data suggest that they may decrease uteroplacental blood flow and cause fetal hypoxia and acidosis. Experience with nifedipine remains limited at the present time.

Diazoxide (trade name Hyperstat) is another antihypertensive which is also a potent uterine muscle relaxant. While experience with diazoxide in treating preterm labor is limited, it would appear that a major drawback is the profound drop in maternal blood pressure associated with its use. Aminophylline, classified as a methylxanthine, is one of the most commonly used medications for treating asthma. As a recently introduced tocolytic, aminophylline was found to delay labor for more than 54 hours in 80 percent of a group of women in preterm labor. Tachycardia, or a rapid heart rate, appears to be the only major maternal side effect, occurring in 10 percent of all cases. Fetal tachycardia has also been reported.

What are the side effects and risks of using beta-sympathomimetics to treat premature labor?

As the use of these drugs has become more popular in the treatment of premature labor, the number of side effects and complications associated with their use has also increased. Problems are especially more likely to occur when beta-sympathomimetics are given intravenously in high doses to stop labor contractions, rather than when they are used prophylactically in lower oral doses to prevent contractions from recurring.

A woman's cardiac output during intravenous beta-sympathomimetic therapy can increase by 40 to 60 percent. Of all drugs in this category, ritodrine appears to exert the greatest effects on a woman's cardiovascular system. Shortly after it is administered intravenously, practically all women experience an increase in their heart rate of approximately 20 to 40 beats per minute. The fetal heart rate also increases by less than 10 beats per minute. These changes are easily tolerated by most women and are of no cause for concern.

A person's blood pressure is composed of two numbers: a systolic or higher reading and a diastolic or lower number. Ritodrine will usually raise the systolic blood pressure and lower the diastolic pressure. For example, if a woman's normal blood pressure is 110/70, ritodrine may convert it to 120/60. This too is of no consequence for the vast majority of women. Of far greater concern is sud-

den pulmonary edema, the accumulation of fluid in the lungs. This complication has been observed in as many as 4 to 5 percent of women treated with intravenous ritodrine and a smaller number of those given terbutaline. Whenever cortisone and beta-sympathomimetics are used together, women and their doctors should be alert to the early symptoms of pulmonary edema, such as cough and shortness of breath, so that treatment can be started immediately.

Approximately 10 to 15 percent of women receiving intravenous ritodrine experience either tremors, vomiting, headache, or flushing of the face or body. Palpitations are experienced by 33 percent, while 5 to 10 percent note either nervousness or restlessness. Abnormal heart rhythms have been observed in 1 to 3 percent of ritodrine-treated women, while some studies have found that as many as 20 percent experience some degree of chest pain. Chest pain occurs because beta-sympathomimetics raise the oxygen demands of the heart muscles. For these reasons, beta-sympathomimetics should never be administered to women with a history of heart disease or those with abnormalities of their heart rate or rhythm. Although oral ritodrine and terbutaline cause only a slight increase in the maternal heart rate, their use is still contraindicated if heart disease is present.

Beta-sympathomimetics in general, and terbutaline in particular, may cause significant impairment of glucose tolerance. Other metabolic derangements associated with beta-sympathomimetic therapy include low calcium and potassium levels in the blood (hypocalcemia and hypokalemia) and acidosis. These complications are most likely to occur when the drugs are administered intravenously rather than orally.

Beta-sympathomimetics rapidly cross the placenta, and fetal blood levels equal maternal levels within minutes. In addition to a commonly observed increase in the fetal heart rate, these drugs can, on rare occasions, cause serious cardiovascular complications. The elevated maternal blood glucose and insulin levels caused by beta-sympathomimetics are present in the fetal circulation as well. As a result, the fetal pancreas works overtime to produce even greater amounts of insulin in its attempts to normalize glucose concentrations. Following delivery, the flood of fetal insulin creates abnormally low blood glucose levels, or hypoglycemia, in the newborn. Infants with hypoglycemia must be carefully monitored until their metabolic condition becomes stabilized. Newborn hypocalcemia has also been described following in utero ritodrine and terbutaline exposure. Fortunately, studies to date have shown that infants born to mothers who received beta-sympathomimetics experience no permanent medical, developmental, or neurological defects when examined one and nine years later.

When should tocolytics be used to inhibit labor, and when not?

Tocolytics are not harmless, and their use requires a careful clinical decision by a woman and her doctor as to whether the gain for the mother and child is worth the risk. Inhibition of labor is clearly indicated when the fetus is estimated to weight less than 5½ pounds, the pregnancy is between 20 and 35 weeks in length, the contractions are coming at intervals of 5 to 7 minutes or less, the cervix is 4 centimeters or less dilated, the cervix is thinning out or effacing, and the amniotic membranes are not ruptured. It is important to initiate therapy as soon as possible, since the success rates for all tocolytics are poor if the cervix is more than 4 centimeters dilated or greater than 50 percent effaced.

Under ideal conditions, labor can be successfully delayed for at least ten days in 80 percent of all women treated in the hospital either with intravenous ritodrine, magnesium sulfate, or terbu-taline. Additional valuable days can be gained by switching to oral ritodrine, terbutaline, magnesium preparations, or to a subcutaneous terbutaline infusion prior to hospital discharge. If this is not done, at least 50 percent of women initially treated will have a recurrence of preterm labor within a period of three weeks.

Although use of tocolytics may be attempted when labor is significantly advanced beyond 4 centimeters of cervical dilatation, the possibility of successfully prolonging the pregnancy at that point is less than 10 percent. It is debatable whether or not these drugs should be given if the amniotic membranes are ruptured. If a woman and her doctor elect to pursue this course, they should be aware of the increased risk of fetal and uterine infection when labor is inhibited for periods of time greater than 24 hours. Tocolytics should absolutely not be used when there is intrauterine or fetal infection, since these conditions can only be successfully treated by accomplishing an immediate delivery. Nor should they be used when there is active vaginal bleeding or evidence of a major malformation of the fetus, making it unlikely that the fetus will survive. Beta-sympathomimetics and all other tocolytics should not be used before the twentieth week of pregnancy because their effects on early fetal development are not known. Tocolytic use in the prevention of early spontaneous abortion may also have the undesirable effect of prolonging chromosomally abnormal pregnancies.

Tocolytics have been used most recently during labor as a means of treating fetal distress. By temporarily abolishing contractions, uteroplacental blood flow and oxygen exchange is enhanced, as evidenced by higher umbilical cord blood and fetal scalp pH values. This technique allows valuable time for a fetus to recover and labor to proceed, or for cesarean section to be performed with less urgency.

HOME UTERINE MONITORS

How effective are the new home uterine monitors for detecting preterm labor?

A woman at high risk for preterm labor can now be monitored for uterine contractions outside the hospital setting with a portable electronic tocodynamometer. Readings can be obtained for periods of 1 to 2 hours, twice daily, with the information relayed by telephone to a center staffed by experienced nurses and technicians. If more than four to five contractions are noted per hour, the woman's obstetrician is notified so that tocolytic treatment, usually in the form of a subcutaneous terbutaline pump, can either be initiated or adjusted to quiet the uterine activity. Programs utilizing home monitoring devices also provide daily phone contact with a healthcare professional in which the symptoms and signs of premature labor are constantly reviewed.

The use of home monitoring is based on the findings of several studies showing that women at risk of preterm labor tend to experience more uterine contractions than other women throughout pregnancy, with a sudden surge of activity 24 to 48 hours prior to the effacement and dilatation of the cervix which characterizes true labor. Unfortunately, a woman's perception of these contractions is extremely unreliable. In one report, women detected only 15 percent of the total number of contractions observed on the tocodynamometer. Other researchers have found that women can be trained to the point of detecting as many as 85 percent of their prelabor contractions. In a 1990 study published in the *Journal of Reproductive Medicine*, investigators noted that the prelabor increase in uterine contractions was detected on the electronic monitor an average of 10 hours earlier than the maternal perception of this critical event in almost one-half of the women studied.

Initial trials of home monitoring suggested that the early detection of contractions could reduce the incidence of preterm birth by one-third and also significantly lower the likelihood of premature rupture of the membranes. Monitored women were found to be far more likely than nonmonitored women to initiate tocolytic therapy with the cervix less than 2 centimeters dilated and less than 50 percent effaced, thereby improving the prognosis for stopping labor.

Despite the excitement and aura of using this new gadgetry, the value of home uterine monitoring remains unproven. The cost of the technology ranges between $80 and $150 per day and averages a total of approximately $6,500 per woman using it. Proponents of home monitoring claim that these costs are far less than those incurred in caring for a severely premature infant in a hospital pediatric intensive care unit. Others refute this claim, noting as well that more than 50 percent of women who experience preterm labor have no predisposing risk factors such as a previous history of premature labor, in utero DES exposure, uterine anomalies, or multiple births. Therefore, to diagnose premature contractions in this large group, obstetricians would have to routinely monitor all of their patients. Such a policy would be an economic disaster.

 # FETAL THERAPY

What are some of the newer methods of fetal therapy that have been devised?

In recent years, a host of ingenious surgical and medical methods of fetal therapy have been devised. While some of the more dramatic procedures, such as the in utero repair of a diaphragmatic hernia, have gained worldwide attention, they have had little practical application for the vast majority of practicing obstetricians and their patients. Other less highly touted techniques have proven to be of significant benefit to a far greater number of individuals.

Direct access to the fetal circulation is now possible with percutaneous umbilical cord blood sampling (PUBS; see page 364). This procedure has enabled doctors to transfuse blood into the fetal circulation in cases of erythroblastosis caused by Rh incompatibility and other anemic conditions of the fetus. The PUBS technique has also enabled doctors to diagnose and treat a variety of medical disorders affecting the fetus. For example, abnormally fast fetal heart rates have been successfully controlled by administering digitalis to the mother or by injecting it directly into the fetal umbilical vein. The accurate determination of fetal thyroid status is also possible with PUBS, while ultrasound can detect the presence of a goiter in the fetus.

Intraamniotic injections of thyroxin have also been used to stimulate surfactant production in the lungs of premature infants. However, the more commonly employed method of achieving this goal is to administer intramuscular maternal steroids such as betamethasone and dexamethasone (see page 358). Thyrotropin-releasing hormone (TRH) is produced by the pituitary gland and is responsible for stimulating the thyroid gland to release its hormones. Recent investigative efforts by doctors at Auckland University in New Zealand suggest that maternal use of TRH in addition to betamethasone will enhance fetal lung maturity and reduce the number of days that premature newborns require oxygen or ventilation therapy.

Regulating the diet of the mother can save the baby from a metabolic defect. This was proven in one case in which doctors prevented the death of a baby with a rare genetic disorder in its inability to metabolize vitamin B_{12}. The child's older sister had died of this disease, called methylmalonic ac-

idemia, shortly after birth. When the mother became pregnant again her condition was diagnosed early in her prenatal course, and she was treated with injections of vitamin B_{12} that were almost 5,000 times the normal adult dose during the last trimester. As a result, a healthy female was born; she has maintained her good health on a controlled, B_{12}-supplemented diet. Biotin is another B vitamin that doctors at the University of California have given in high doses to a woman with a rare inherited enzyme disorder known as carboxylase deficiency. As a result, she gave birth to a healthy newborn. Similar success has been reported following maternal albumin ingestion as a means of preventing the complications associated with genetic hypoalbuminemia.

Congenital adrenal hyperplasia is an inherited autosomal recessive enzymatic defect which results in the excessive secretion of male hormones by the adrenal gland beginning as early as the first trimester. Female fetuses affected with this disorder are often born with masculinization of their external genitals. Modern genetic technology has allowed doctors to diagnose congenital adrenal hyperplasia during pregnancy. There are currently 15 case reports in the medical literature which show that if a mother is given steroids such as dexamethasone and hydrocortisone starting in the first trimester, female newborns will demonstrate few if any of these abnormal genital changes.

Several studies have indicated that maternal use of folic acid and other vitamin supplements immediately before and throughout the first trimester may significantly reduce the number of babies born with neural tube defects. Another method of fetal therapy is the use of tocolytic drugs to prevent preterm birth and to stop contractions when full-term labor is complicated by fetal distress. More exciting discoveries are evolving each day.

RH BABIES

How does Rh hemolytic disease develop, and how is it treated?

One of the first fetal problems to be treated successfully in utero was Rh hemolytic disease. An Rh-negative mother may form antibodies, or D immunoglobulins, against the red blood cells of her Rh-positive, or D-positive, fetus. These antibodies cross the placenta and enter the fetal circulation where they destroy the red blood cells, causing severe fetal anemia, heart failure, and even death. For maternal D immunoglobulins to form, D-positive red blood cells must first enter the maternal bloodstream. This is most likely to occur during the last trimester and at delivery of a first pregnancy, but it may also happen to a lesser degree following a spontaneous or induced first- or second-trimester abortion and at the time of an ectopic pregnancy. Statistically, the overall likelihood of a woman developing D immunoglobulins following an induced abortion is approximately 4 to 5 percent, with the risks directly related to the length of gestation. Diagnostic medical procedures such as CVS, amniocentesis, and PUBS, as well as extensive fetal manipulation as occurs with external cephalic version (see page 424), can all increase the incidence of feto-maternal bleeding and the risk of maternal D immunoglobulin formation. Obstetrical hemorrhage occurring in association with abruptio placenta and placenta previa also contributes significantly to this problem. Once a woman becomes sensitized, meaning that she has formed her own maternal antibodies or D immunoglobulins, the condition persists throughout life and presents an extreme hazard to Rh-positive offspring of all subsequent pregnancies.

When blood tests confirm that a pregnant woman is sensitized, antibody blood tests should be obtained at two- to four-week intervals beginning at the sixteenth to eighteenth week of pregnancy. When antibody titres or concentrations remain low, the chances are that the fetus is at minimal risk. High or rising titres, however, are cause for concern and require that bilirubin levels in the amniotic fluid be measured to determine how seriously the fetus is affected. High concentrations of the pigment bilirubin mean that many red blood cells are being destroyed. The interval between periodic amniocenteses and the timing of delivery is based on a graph plotting the bilirubin concentrations and gestational weeks. If the fetus is found to be severely anemic, certain to die, but too immature for immediate delivery, it is possible to transfuse small amounts of fresh adult Rh-negative red blood cells directly into its abdominal cavity under ultrasound guidance. From there, the blood cells are absorbed into the fetal bloodstream, replacing those that were destroyed by maternal antibodies. This procedure must be repeated at ten-day to two-week intervals until the fetus is sufficiently mature to survive outside the uterus. Intraabdominal transfusions can be technically difficult and require considerable skill and expertise. As a result, many physicians have abandoned this procedure in favor of PUBS (see page 364). With this technique, direct access to the fetal circulation is possible as early as the eighteenth gestational week, allowing rapid determination of the fetal blood type and the presence or absence of anemia. If the fetus is anemic, direct blood transfusion into the umbilical vein can be accomplished at that time. Several recently published studies of PUBS-transfused fetuses have demonstrated survival rates of 80 to 95 percent, a remarkable achievement in view of the severity of the fetal condition.

What is RhoGAM, and when should it be given?

Fortunately, Rh incompatibility is infrequently seen today because of the introduction of D immunoglobulin, or Rh-immune globulin, in 1969. More commonly known by its trade name

RhoGAM, this medication consists of Rh antibodies. Other equally effective D immunoglobulin products are Gamulin Rh, HypRho-D, and Rho-D Immune Globulin. When given intramuscularly to an Rh-negative woman within 72 hours after birth or after an abortion, it destroys the Rh-positive fetal cells that may have passed into her bloodstream. RhoGAM prevents the Rh-negative woman from producing her own D immunoglobulins to the Rh-positive cells. If a woman becomes sensitized, meaning that she has already formed her own D immunoglobulins, the injection of RhoGAM becomes valueless and remains so throughout her lifetime. For this reason, RhoGAM injections must be given to all nonsensitized Rh-negative women following birth of each Rh-positive infant. Since the blood type of an early abortus is not determined, RhoGAM must be given to all Rh-negative women at the time of a spontaneous or induced abortion or an ectopic pregnancy. The one exception to this rule is when the father is known to be Rh-negative, since two

Rh-negative parents cannot conceive an Rh-positive infant. Approximately 15 percent of the population is Rh-negative.

Since feto-maternal bleeding is a very real threat following amniocentesis, D immunoglobulin should be given at the time that the procedure is performed during the second or third trimester, as well as when PUBS, CVS, and an external cephalic version of a breech to a head-first position are performed.

Researchers have clearly demonstrated that all nonsensitized Rh-negative women should receive a 300-microgram prophylactic injection of RhoGAM between the twenty-eighth and twenty-ninth weeks of pregnancy and again during the immediate postpartum period if the baby is found to be Rh positive at birth. This has helped to reduce the 2 percent risk of maternal sensitization to 0.3 percent. No ill effects have been noted among infants delivered of mothers who receive RhoGAM in this manner.

 GENETIC DISORDERS

What vital information does CVS and amniocentesis provide about the X and Y sex chromosomes?

The sex of the fetus can easily be determined either with CVS or amniocentesis. Unlike several other prenatal studies which require culturing of the cells obtained over a period of one or more weeks, rapid staining techniques often allow instant identification of the X and Y chromosomes.

The sex of the fertilized egg is determined by the type of sex chromosome present in the head of the sperm. The adult male has two sets of X chromosomes in his body cells; they are called X and Y. The adult woman contains two X sex chromosomes in each of her body cells, but no Y's. Therefore, her egg always contributes an X to the future offspring. If a sperm cell carrying a Y chromosome

fertilizes the X egg, the result is an XX female.

Knowing the sex of the fetus is invaluable in offering genetic counseling to couples at risk of conceiving a child with a so-called X-linked or sex-linked disease. Such diseases are carried on one of a woman's two X chromosomes and appear in the offspring only when the affected chromosome is fertilized by a man's Y chromosome. With few exceptions, only male fetuses inheriting the disease-carrying X will be afflicted with the disease. Those males inheriting the nonaffected X chromosome will be normal. The odds, therefore, of a carrier mother transmitting the disease to her male offspring are 50 percent, but for female offspring they are zero. Each daughter has a 50 percent chance of being a carrier and transmitting the disease to one-half of her sons. No male-to-male

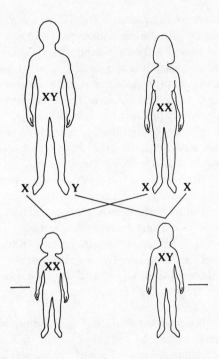

Figure 49 *How X-linked determination works.*

*In the most common form of X-linked
inheritance, the female sex chromosome of an
unaffected gene mother carries one faulty gene
(X) and one normal one (x). The father has one
normal male x and y chromosome complement.
The odds for each male child are: 50 percent risk
of inheriting the faulty X and the disorder
50 percent chance of inheriting normal x and y
chromosomes.*

*The odds for each female child are: 50 percent
risk of inheriting one faulty X to be a carrier like
mother 50 percent chance of inheriting no faulty
gene.*

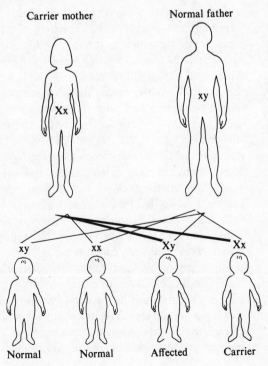

Carrier mother   Normal father

Normal   Normal   Affected   Carrier

transmission of X-linked disorders can occur. That is, a father cannot pass the disorder on to his son. (See Figure 49.)

Color blindness is an example of a benign condition passed on through the X chromosome, but this category also includes deadly diseases, such as a common form of muscular dystrophy known as Duchenne; classic hemophilia, or hemophilia A; hemophilia B; and rare diseases with names such as Hunter syndrome, Lesch-Nyhan syndrome, Fabry's disease, and Menke's disease. Until recently, geneticists were often quite limited in their ability to determine with certainty if a male fetus was affected. As a result, couples were faced with the dilemma of a midtrimester abortion on all male fetuses, while allowing females to survive. Unfortunately, this necessitated aborting healthy males 50 percent of the time, although it prevented the despair of caring for an infant afflicted with one of these terrible diseases. While this grim alternative still remains for many of the families suffering from the more than 200 X-linked diseases, others are now readily diagnosed in utero.

Over the past five years, researchers in the field of molecular biology have made extraordinary advances in the prenatal diagnosis of several X-linked diseases. These advances have been achieved through the discovery of several new techniques, including gene mapping, a process of locating the position of a gene at a specific chromosome site. To date, approximately 3,000 of the more than 100,000 human genes have been mapped. Methods of studying the composition and sequence of fragments of DNA (deoxyribonucleic acid, the active substance of all genes) within the nucleus of fetal cells with CVS and aminocentesis have enabled doctors to diagnose fetal diseases such as Duchenne muscular dystrophy and hemophilia A and B without resorting to more invasive and dangerous techniques such as fetoscopy and PUBS. Scientists have discovered ingenious methods of splitting or cleaving segments of long DNA chains with either bacterial enzymes or pulses of electricity and then analyzing these smaller isolated fragments to determine if the DNA sequences are normal or abnormal. Abnormal DNA markers are often associated with specific genetic disorders, and in some cases it is also possible to identify healthy carriers of the disease trait who are capable of passing it on to their children. DNA sequence studies are directly processed and do not require cell culture, as do many other prenatal CVS and aminocentesis tests. Because of this, test results are usually available in 24 hours or less.

With increasing frequency, couples are requesting amniocentesis merely to know the sex of the their child. Some have requested an abortion based solely on the fact that the fetus, although healthy, is not of the desired sex. Important ethical questions have been raised as to whether or not modern technology should be used to abort potentially healthy offspring because of a couple's sex preference for their child.

Abnormalities of the sex chromosomes make up approximately 20 percent of all chromosomal defects. Approximately 1 out of 950 females are born with the so-called triple X, or super-female chromosomal abnormality. These individuals have three X chromosomes, or a trisomy (threesome), rather than the normal female complement of two. Their total chromosomal count is 47 rather than the usual 46. While many triple-X females have no symptoms and lead perfectly normal lives, 5 to 10 percent may experience infertility, premature menopause, congenital abnormalities, poor coordination, problems with speech and language, delayed neuromuscular development, and mental retardation. At the opposite end of the spectrum are the 1 in 10,000 female infants who are born with only one X chromosome, or monosomy, rather than two, giving them a total of 45 chromosomes. This condition, called ovarian dysgenesis, is characterized by short stature, small streaks of tissue instead of ovaries, infertility, infantile genitals, sparse pubic hair, undeveloped breasts, and a failure to menstruate. About one-third of these young girls will also have multiple congenital deformities, such as webbing of the neck, abnormalities of the heart and its blood vessels, abnormal loss of bone minerals or osteoporosis, bony abnormalities, and visual defects. This constellation of abnormalities is known as Turner's syndrome.

Klinefelter's syndrome is characterized by the presence of an XXY sex chromosome pattern. It occurs as frequently as 1 in 1,000 male births. In addition to having 47 chromosomes, these men are often tall and demonstrate decreased facial and pubic hair, subnormal testosterone levels, abnormally small genitals, minimal if any sperm cell formation, and prominent breasts.

Men with an XYY chromosomal pattern, known as "super-males," also have 47 chromosomes. The incidence of this abnormality is equal to that of Klinefelter's syndrome. Most XYY men are asymptomatic, fertile, and lead normal lives. Others have been described as tall, thin, acneed, and excessively aggressive and violent individuals. There is some evidence that a significant percentage of XYY men are in penal institutions; lawyers for Richard Specks, the mass murderer from Chicago, unsuccessfully claimed that his XYY genetic makeup was responsible for his violent deeds. Recent statistics demonstrate that the likelihood of a 47-chromosome XYY male being incarcerated is approximately ten times that of a 46-chromosome XY male. However, the 96 percent of 47-chromosome XYY males who behave normally refute the argument that these individuals are genetically predestined to a life of crime.

The most recently described sex chromosome abnormality is referred to as the "fragile-X" chromosome. The presence of a small, delicate, constricted spot or apparent break at the end of the long arm of the X chromosome has been found in as many as 1 in 1,500 males, and 10 percent of all mentally retarded males. After Down syndrome, or trisomy 21 (see page 402), the fragile-X syndrome constitutes the most common cause of chromosomally related mental retardation in male children. In addition to a 90 percent incidence of mental retardation, these individuals have large gonads, a long face, and abnormally large ears, and are hyperactive. Girls carrying the fragile-X chromosome tend to be protected by their second unaffected X chromosome. Approximately one-third are unaffected asymptomatic carriers, another one-third have normal IQs but experience learning disabilities, especially in math, and the final one-third demonstrate borderline IQs or appear mildly retarded. In families with a strong history of mental retardation, it is extremely helpful to perform chromosome studies in order to detect this condition. In 1991, geneticists from France and Australia simultaneously discovered the use of DNA analysis to rapidly and accurately determine if the fetus is afflicted with the fragile-X syndrome. Doctors can also tell whether a fetus has healthy genes, is likely to be retarded, or will be a normal carrier of the bad gene. The same test performed on parental blood can determine which parent carries the defective gene and the risk of passing it to their children. When a male fetus is found to have the fragile-X syndrome, the strong likelihood of a retarded infant influences most couples to opt for abortion. Genetic counseling and a decision to continue or terminate the pregnancy are often far more difficult when the fetus with the fragile-X chromosome is female.

It has recently been discovered that as many as 25 percent of sufferers of manic-depressive psychiatric illness carry a defective gene for the disorder at the tip of their X chromosome. Unlike most other X-linked disorders in which females are either asymptomatic or mildly affected, manic-depression is far more common among women than men. This suggests that in this particular situation the presence of the defect on one X chromosome abolishes the protective effect of the normal X. Investigators have also discovered families that carry the gene for manic-depressive illness on chromosome 11 of the 23 pairs.

DOWN SYNDROME AND OTHER AUTOSOMAL TRISOMIES

How do chromosomal defects, such as Down syndrome, develop?

It is estimated that 15,000 infants with chromosomal abnormalities are born each year in the United States. Practically all of these genetic disorders can be diagnosed prenatally by studying the fetal cells obtained at the time of chorionic villus sampling (CVS) or amniocentesis. By far, the most common reason for these procedures is to detect Down syndrome.

Normally, a person has 22 pairs of body, or autosome, chromosomes and one pair of sex chromosomes in each body cell, for a total of 46 chromosomes. Down syndrome is also known as trisomy 21 because affected infants have three chromosomes, rather than the normal two, on the chromosome named number 21. Consequently, these infants have a total count of 47 chromosomes in each of their body cells. Trisomy 21 occurs when the paired number 21 chromosomes fail to divide and separate at the time that either the sperm or egg cell is being formed. This inability of chromosomes to divide normally is called nondisjunction. When one of these cells with an extra chromosome is fertilized by a normal sperm or egg cell, a chromosome trisomy is inevitable. The chances of producing an infant with a trisomy increases with advancing maternal age and less frequently with paternal age over 55. Parents of these infants show a normal chromosomal pattern when their blood cells are analyzed. In 1991, Dr. Stylianos E. Antonarakis of Johns Hopkins Hospital in Baltimore used DNA markers to prove that the extra chromosome 21 is of maternal origin 95 percent of the time. Researchers have used DNA analysis to link the more than 1,000 genes on chromosome 21 to a variety of other conditions such as cancer, leukemia, Alzheimer's disease, visual disturbances, and congenital heart defects.

Three percent of all infants with Down syndrome inherit their extra number 21 chromosome from one parent through a process called translocation. Although carrier parents of children with this condition appear normal, they are genetically abnormal because they are born with a fragment of their twenty-first chromosome attached to another chromosome such as the eighteenth, thirteenth, fifteenth, or twenty-second. Carrier parents produce Down syndrome infants at a frequency ranging from 2 to 100 percent, depending on where the 21 fragment is attached. Unlike Down syndrome caused by nondisjunction, this form of the disease is not related to parental age and can be diagnosed by studying the chromosomes of the affected parent's blood cells. In the case of Down syndrome, the extra amount of chromosome material is responsible for significant fetal damage. It has been estimated that two-thirds of the fetuses with this abnormal chromosome configuration undergo spontaneous abortion, stillbirth, or neonatal death. The remaining one-third who survive present a striking clinical picture, which is easily recognized at birth. Characteristics are mental retardation, short stature, a thick and fissured tongue, low-set ears, slanting and closely set eyes, and abnormal hands and fingers. Many of these infants suffer from congenital heart disease and respiratory infections.

What are my chances of having a baby with Down syndrome or other trisomies?

Although the incidence of Down syndrome and other trisomies increases with each year during the 20s as well as the 30s, after 30 the risk increases perceptibly with each advancing year. As noted in Table 28, a woman's risk of giving birth to a Down syndrome infant is roughly one-half the risk for all chromosomal anomalies at each maternal age.

It should be emphasized that the chromosomal abnormality risks quoted in Table 28 are for

TABLE 28

RISK OF CHROMOSOMAL ABNORMALITIES IN LIVEBORN INFANTS FOR EACH MATERNAL AGE OVER THE AGE OF 30

Maternal Age	Risk for Down Syndrome	Total Risk for Chromosomal Abnormalities
20	1/1,667	1/526
21	1/1,667	1/526
22	1/1,429	1/500
23	1/1,429	1/500
24	1/1,250	1/476
25	1/1,250	1/476
26	1/1,176	1/476
27	1/1,111	1/455
28	1/1,053	1/435
29	1/1,000	1/417
30	1/952	1/385
31	1/909	1/385
32	1/769	1/322
33	1/602	1/286
34	1/485	1/238
35	1/378	1/192
36	1/289	1/156
37	1/224	1/127
38	1/173	1/102
39	1/136	1/83
40	1/106	1/66
41	1/82	1/53
42	1/63	1/42
43	1/49	1/33
44	1/38	1/26
45	1/30	1/21
46	1/23	1/16
47	1/18	1/13
48	1/14	1/10
49	1/11	1/8

live-born infants. However, the prevalence of abnormalities in amniocentesis specimens is approximately 30 percent higher, and even higher in CVS specimens. The reason for this is that many of these chromosomally abnormal fetuses are spontaneously aborted or succumb later in pregnancy.

While the cutoff for performing CVS or amniocentesis for the purpose of diagnosing age-related chromosomal defects has been set at 35, this policy seems somewhat arbitrary and inflexible. It is derived from epidemiological studies showing that the maternal age of 35 is the point at which the risk of a chromosomal abnormality approximately equals or exceeds the small but definite risk of inadvertent fetal loss caused by the procedure. I have never understood the logic behind this reasoning, and I am pleased to see that women under 35 are increasingly availing themselves of CVS and amniocentesis. A minority of geneticists have suggested that the new maternal age cutoff be set at 30, since the risk of a trisomy rises continually from the early 20s.

❧ *AUTOSOMAL DOMINANT AND RECESSIVE INHERITANCE* ❧

How are autosomal recessive and autosomal dominant genetic diseases transmitted from parents to their offspring?

Autosomal recessive diseases are carried by individuals who themselves show no symptoms of the disease. The disease appears in the offspring when those who are carriers of the same harmful gene mate. Under these circumstances, the theoretical risk of giving birth to an affected infant will be one out of four. Two out of four, or 50 percent, will be healthy carriers capable of transmitting the disease, while one out of four will be normal and unaffected. Actual experience, however, does not always follow this theoretical scheme, and many parents have had the misfortune of giving birth to two or more diseased infants in succession. The genetics of autosomal recessive inheritance is demonstrated in Figure 50.

Sickle cell anemia, thalassemia, cystic fibrosis, Tay-Sachs, and phenylketonuria are among the better known autosomal recessive diseases. However, there are several hundred others—serious and rare disorders with names such as Gaucher's, Nieman-Pick, hemochromatosis, maple syrup urine disease, cystinosis, and Pompe's disease.

Unlike autosomal recessive diseases, there are usually no healthy carriers of autosomal dominant conditions, and inheritance in autosomal dominant diseases follows a different pattern. An afflicted person with the disease trait on one of a pair of genes shows symptoms of the disease either at birth or later in life and has a 50 percent chance of transmitting the condition to his or her offspring;

Figure 50

How autosomal recessive inheritance works. Both parents, usually unaffected, carry a normal gene (N) that takes precedence over its faulty recessive counterpart (r). The odds for each child are:

A 25 percent risk of inheriting a "double dose" of r genes, which may cause a serious birth defect.

A 25 percent chance of inheriting two N's, thus being unaffected.

A 50 percent chance of being a carrier, as both parents are.

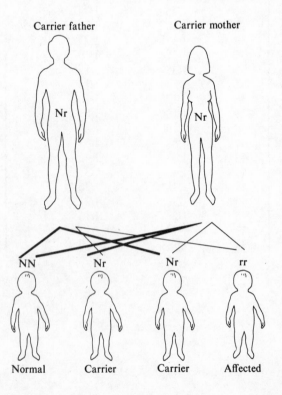

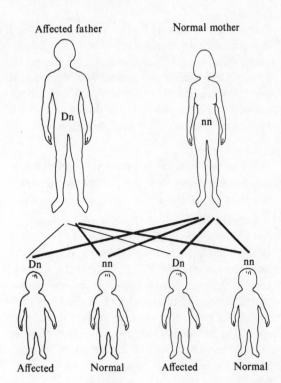

Figure 51

How autosomal dominant inheritance works.

One affected parent has a single faulty gene (D) that dominates its normal counterpart (n). Each child's chances of inheriting either the D or the n from the affected parent are 50 percent.

the other 50 percent are normal, with no chance of passing on the disease. Children who inherit the abnormal gene have symptoms of the disease, regardless of the normal genetic makeup of the unaffected parent, because the dominant gene overwhelms the effect of the normal gene. This is demonstrated in Figure 51.

Examples of some of the many autosomal dominant diseases are acute intermittent porphyria, Huntington's disease, achondroplastic dwarfism, the adult type of polycystic kidney disease, Ehlers-Danlos syndrome, von Willebrand's disease, Marfan's syndrome, and neurofibromatosis.

There is convincing evidence that some autosomal genetic diseases may suddenly appear as a result of a gene change, or mutation, in the sperm or egg of an otherwise healthy parent. Statistically, two-thirds of these mutations occur in the sperm and one-third affect the egg. Even when there is no previous family history of the disorder, once a mu-

tation occurs, the disease is passed to subsequent generations by the afflicted person in the usual pattern of autosomal dominance.

Individuals afflicted with autosomal recessive and autosomal dominant diseases show no obvious gross abnormalities in the appearance of their chromosomes obtained at the time of CVS or amniocentesis. Their disease is caused by specific defects in the composition and sequence of their DNA, the active substance of all genes. Revolutionary molecular biology techniques introduced during the last five years have enabled scientists to separate and analyze DNA fragments and diagnose an even greater number of autosomal recessive and autosomal dominant diseases. Accurate testing of asymptomatic carriers of several autosomal recessive diseases through DNA analysis is now possible, and autosomal dominant conditions such as Huntington's disease can be diagnosed prenatally and early in life prior to the onset of symptoms.

Biochemical laboratory studies have also been used to detect several autosomal recessive metabolic diseases, most notably Tay-Sachs disease. However, despite the availability of genetic and biochemical laboratory studies, there are still hundreds of autosomal dominant and recessive diseases for which there is no method of prenatal detection.

What are some of the newer methods of diagnosing the more common autosomal recessive diseases during pregnancy?

Tay-Sachs disease is 99 times more common in Jewish families than among non-Jews and is always fatal. Approximately 1 in 900 Jewish couples is at risk of having children with Tay-Sachs. Ninety percent of American Jews are of Ashkenazi origin, that is, Jews of Central and Eastern European ancestry, the group that runs the highest risk of carrying Tay-Sachs. Of this group, one out of every 30 men or women will be carriers of the disease. Among the non-Jewish population, one in 150 individuals is a carrier of Tay-Sachs.

Tay-Sachs is caused by the absence of a vital enzyme named hexosaminidase A, which helps to break down fatty chemicals, named glycolipids, in body cells. When hexosaminidase A is absent, a glycolipid named GM_2-ganglioside accumulates, leading to the degeneration and eventual destruction of nerve cells in the brain and other body tissues. Tragically, affected children appear normal at birth; the physical weakness and lack of coordination that are symptoms of the disease don't appear until the child reaches six months of age. From this point, deterioration is rapid and is characterized by blindness, seizures, severe mental retardation, and death by the age of four. There is no cure or treatment for this disease.

Fortunately, scientists have discovered that healthy Tay-Sachs carriers can be identified by means of a simple blood test that measures hexosaminidase A levels. Carriers show a 50 percent reduction in the level of this enzyme. If both parents are known to be carriers before conception, a test for hexosaminidase A levels in cultured CVS or amniotic fluid cells can be performed and an accurate determination made during pregnancy. A woman found to be carrying a Tay-Sachs fetus can be offered the alternative of terminating the pregnancy. With repeated attempts, the odds are that a carrier couple will eventually conceive either an unaffected baby or a healthy carrier.

Routine blood screening to determine whether a woman is a Tay-Sachs carrier is not as accurate when performed during pregnancy as it is before conception. If testing was not done before conception, the father should be tested immediately. If he is a carrier, the mother must then undergo a time-consuming and more specific blood test to determine her hexosaminidase A levels. If this test proves positive, CVS or amniocentesis is mandatory.

As of 1991, the American College of Obstetricians and Gynecologists has recommended that when one partner is Jewish and the other is not, the Jewish partner should be screened first. If he or she is found to be a carrier, the other partner should also be screened. However, during pregnancy it is easier to screen the male partner first.

Cystic fibrosis is the most common lethal inherited disease in America, afflicting approximately 1 in every 2,000 babies born in the United States. Like Tay-Sachs disease, it has an autosomal recessive inheritance pattern and is rare among nonwhite racial groups. Approximately 1 of every 25 Americans is an asymptomatic carrier of the cystic fibrosis gene.

Children with this condition lack the normal body enzymes needed to clear thick mucous secretions from their respiratory tract. As a result, they become prone to respiratory complications and repeated infections and often die in their late teens or early 20s. Despite intensive efforts by scientists to detect healthy carriers of cystic fibrosis and diagnose the disease prenatally, it is only in the last five years that this goal has become a reality. The cystic fibrosis gene is actually a defective gene on the long arm of chromosome 7 that has been inactivated by a mutation or deletion of part of the gene. Geneticists are now able to identify approximately 75 percent of all adult carriers of the disease. The diagnosis of cystic fibrosis in the fetus can sometimes be made between the seventeenth and eighteenth week of gestation, when ultrasound visualization of the fetal abdomen will often reveal meconium-filled, dilated loops of small intestine, a sign confirming the presence of the disease.

Sickle cell disease is a debilitating and often fatal disorder which afflicts approximately one out of every 400 blacks. In this disease, the hemoglobin in the red blood cells is abnormal, causing the cells to be more fragile than unaffected normal cells. Some of the red blood cells actually have a sickle shape; the number of cells with this shape increases as the condition worsens. As many as 9 percent of healthy blacks are carriers of the sickle cell trait, meaning their blood contains 50 percent sickle hemoglobin and 50 percent normal adult hemoglobin. A simple blood test known as hemoglobin electrophoresis can easily detect carriers, while DNA analysis of CVS and amniotic fluid cells can diagnose sickle cell disease in the fetus with an accuracy of virtually 100 percent.

Thalassemia, like sickle cell disease, is an autosomal recessive inherited condition caused by abnormal hemoglobin in the blood. This disease affects many individuals of Mediterranean ancestry, particularly those from Italy or Greece. The two major types of thalassemia are beta-thalassemia and alpha-thalassemia. Beta-thalassemia major, also known as Cooley's anemia and Mediterranean anemia, is a debilitating disease and one of the world's most common inherited disorders. It is estimated that there are close to 250,000 healthy beta-thalassemia carriers in the United States in addition to thousands of severely affected children.

Unlike beta-thalassemia, alpha-thalassemia occurs mainly in Southeast Asian, Chinese, and Filipino populations, but a slightly different variety of this disease is also present in a small number of blacks. Though healthy thalassemia carriers usually suffer from nothing more than a very mild anemia, two carriers have a one in four chance of producing an affected infant suffering from severe anemia, frequent infections, abnormal enlargement of the liver and spleen, and thin, brittle bones.

While the simple hemoglobin electrophoresis test is used to readily diagnose thalassemia in infants, DNA analysis has now made it possible to diagnose the disease in the fetus through CVS and amniocentesis. As with sickle cell anemia, DNA studies have totally replaced more dangerous methods such as fetoscopy, PUBS, and placental aspiration of blood cells.

12

CHILDBIRTH
and the
POSTPARTUM PERIOD

*T*his final chapter presents the most current information concerning the proper management of labor, delivery, and the postpartum period. It is meant to serve as a reference for women eager to carry on a more intelligent dialogue with their doctors. Only with this knowledge can greater participation in obstetrical decisions be achieved.

 ## BODY POSITIONS BEFORE AND DURING LABOR AND DELIVERY

How can a woman's posture during her pregnancy affect the fetus?

When a woman lies flat on her back during the second half of pregnancy, her enlarged uterus flops backward and compresses the aorta and vena cava, the largest artery and vein in the body. This phenomenon has the effect of reducing the volume of blood returned to the heart and the amount which is pumped to the uterus and placenta. Consequently, the fetus receives less oxygen. For this reason, I encourage my patients to lie on their left side when they rest or sleep during the second half of pregnancy. The left side is preferred over the right because the vena cava passes slightly to the right of the midline and is less apt to be compressed if the uterus is tilted to the left.

Fetal growth lags slightly during the last ten weeks prior to delivery. This finding has led to speculation that markedly reduced activity and greater periods of time spent off one's feet may improve fetal growth, particularly during the last few weeks of pregnancy. Support for this position comes from a 1982 report from the Pennsylvania State University College of Medicine. They found that women who worked at "stand-up" jobs throughout pregnancy were at significantly greater risk of giving birth to smaller babies (see page 350).

How can a woman's posture affect the position of her baby at birth, and can exercises influence the fetal position?

There has been much theorizing, but little scientific proof to show, that a woman's posture during pregnancy and labor helps to determine the in utero position of her baby. The size and shape of the pelvis, the location of the placenta, the presence of maternal uterine and pelvic anomalies, the amount of amniotic fluid which is present, the laxity of a woman's pelvic supports, and the presence of fetal anomalies are all factors which have been thought to contribute to the position the fetus assumes in its mother's uterus. More often than not, the reason why a woman's baby assumes an abnormal position, such as breech (buttocks first) or occiput posterior, remains a mystery.

The usual fetal position at the time of delivery is known as the occiput anterior position: the back of the baby's head, or the occiput, is anterior, or forward, and the baby is facing the maternal spine. In this position, the baby's back is closest to the maternal abdominal wall. In the occiput posterior position, the baby is facing in the same direction as the mother and its spine is closest to the maternal spine. This position is also known as a "sunny-side-up" position because the baby's head is facing upward at the moment of birth. Responsible for back labor (low back pain with labor), this position is more difficult and painful than the anterior position because a greater diameter of the fetal head must pass through the pelvis. Most often, the fetal head rotates to an anterior position just before delivery.

Many midwives and childbirth instructors have devised "posturing exercises" for women so that occiput posterior positions can be avoided and rotation of the head to the anterior position can occur without medical intervention. Included among these exercises have been variations of the hands-and-knees posture and pelvic tilting maneuvers. In my experience, the use of these maneuvers has been of no help in rotating the fetal head. Enthu-siastic supporters of these techniques may claim excellent results, but the large majority of occiput posterior positions revert spontaneously to the more favorable anterior position. These exercises are safe and simple, but I believe that they are ineffectual.

Extensive experience with ultrasound has confirmed earlier observations showing that fetal position prior to 26 weeks is as likely to be cephalic, or head-down, as it is to be breech or transverse (sideways) and is totally unrelated to the baby's eventual position at delivery. In contrast, the fetal position at 36 weeks has a predictive accuracy of 97 percent.

What is the ideal maternal position during labor and delivery?

While the standing position may not be the ideal prescription for fetal growth during the last trimester, there is no doubt that it offers great benefits for the woman in labor. As a matter of fact, just about any position is preferred to lying on one's back. In at least 30 percent of women, the supine position has been found to cause uterine occlusion of the common iliac artery, a branch of the aorta, which supplies blood and oxygen to the placenta, resulting in fetal heart rate decelerations, oxygen deprivation, and fetal distress.

Condemnation of the supine position may seem a radical departure from established obstetrical ideas. However, it is well documented that until late in the eighteenth century, most women in the world used an upright position during labor—standing, sitting, kneeling, or squatting, but always with the trunk more vertical than horizontal. The recumbent bed position became widely accepted during the nineteenth and twentieth centuries because it was more convenient for obstetricians to carry out vaginal examinations, forceps applications, and various other maneuvers. The return to the more natural vertical position has been attributed to the research of many doctors, but none has been as influential as Dr. Roberto Caldeyro-Barcia of Montevideo, Uruguay, who concluded that a woman's contractions are stronger and more efficient, but less frequent, when she labors on her side rather than her back and even more efficient when she stands. When mothers were asked to describe if it was more painful to lie down, sit, or stand during labor, they indicated that they were more comfortable when upright. The majority of subsequent studies have supported the benefits of the vertical, or upright, position during labor, including stronger contractions, significantly shorter first and second stages of labor, less discomfort, and less frequent need for narcotic pain relief. In a 1987 study published in the British journal *Lancet*, Dr. Jason Gardosi and his associates at Milton Keynes General Hospital in England followed the progress of labor among 400 women, half of whom were instructed to assume a squatting position, while the other half reclined. Those who squatted had a shorter second stage of labor and were half as likely to require a forceps delivery. Women who squatted also had a higher rate of intact perineums and no episiotomies, although they did experience a slight increase in superficial labial lacerations or tearing which, in most cases, healed quickly without the need for suturing. The most impressive statistic was that 95 percent of the squatting group said that they would assume the same position for subsequent deliveries. Dr. Gardosi and others before him have found that squatting actually helps to enlarge the dimensions of the maternal bony pelvis and allows more room for the passage of the baby's head.

The benefits to a mother and her fetus of walking during labor have been supported by several studies. In one British report of 68 women in spontaneous labor, 34 were randomly assigned to an ambulatory group while the remainder labored in supine positions. Electronic monitoring of the fetal heartbeat and uterine contractions was performed on all patients. Although the number of women studied was small, there were significant differences between the two groups. The ambulatory women experienced much shorter labors, were less likely to require intravenous oxytocin to improve the strength of their contractions, requested less medication for pain relief, delivered babies with significantly higher 1- and 5-minute Apgar scores, and were less likely to experience fetal heart rate abnormalities. The frequency of contractions among ambulatory women was lower, but the strength of their contractions was significantly greater.

When dilatation of the cervix fails to progress during labor, use of intravenous oxytocin often increases the strength and frequency of uterine contractions. Since there are some hazards associated with oxytocin use, it would be nice to employ a natural method of augmenting weak labor contractions. In a report from the University of Southern California School of Medicine published in the *American Journal of Obstetrics and Gynecology* in 1981, doctors studied 14 women who failed to progress during labor because of inadequate contractions. Six were given intravenous oxytocin to improve contraction strength while eight others were asked to walk. Labor progress was slightly better in the ambulatory group, with almost immediate improvement in the uterine contraction strength and frequency. It took 2 hours for the intravenous oxytocin to achieve an effect equal to that achieved simply by walking. Despite the small number of patients studied, the authors concluded that walking was as effective as oxytocin for the enhancement of labor. Certainly, if labor augmentation is needed, walking would appear to be a simpler and safer initial technique to try instead of the use of intravenous oxytocin.

Why is the upright position more efficient than lying on one's back during labor, and are there any hazards associated with its use?

When a woman assumes a vertical position, the effect of gravity on the fetus works harmoniously with the uterine contractions. It has been accurately calculated that gravity adds an additional 35 millimeters of mercury to the pressure exerted by the fetal head on the cervix during the first stage of labor. In addition, the same amount of pressure is exerted on the vaginal tissues during the second stage of labor, when the cervix is fully dilated.

The angle formed by the baby's body and the mother's spine also has an effect on the progress of labor. This angle, referred to as the "drive angle," is greater when a woman is standing than when she is lying on her back, and labor is significantly more efficient when the angle is greater.

In 1987, doctors from Oita Medical College in Japan reported that, for women giving birth for the first time, "sitters" dilated from 5 to 10 centimeters in an average of 59 less minutes than those in the flat or supine position. The second stage, defined as the time from full dilatation to delivery of the baby, was an average of 28 minutes shorter. In addition, the frequency of forceps use was significantly higher for women giving birth for the first time who labored in the supine position. Equally impressive results were noted for multiparous women.

In a 1977 study comparing 189 women laboring in the horizontal position with 126 in the vertical position, doctors studied the incidence of swelling of the tissues of the fetal scalp caused by pressure during labor. When the amniotic membranes were intact, the incidence of swelling was surprisingly higher among those in the former group. In addition, disalignment of the cranial bones, or molding, in the newborn was found not to be related to a woman's position during labor.

Although labor in a vertical position appears to be safe when the amniotic membranes are intact, there are no large studies demonstrating that the added pressure on the fetal scalp does not cause harm if the membranes are ruptured.

What is a birthing chair?

A birthing chair is exactly what its name says it is: a chair in which a woman gives birth. Such devices have been in existence since at least the second century A.D. All sorts of chairs, tables, and boards have been developed over the years to elevate a woman's upper body so that it is in a near-vertical position during labor. Clinical experience suggests that women are most comfortable when their backs are between 30 and 45 degrees from the horizontal position, but in one study labor was shortened by more than 1 hour when the chair was tilted to a 70-degree angle.

Resurgent interest in the birthing chair peaked in the early 1980s with the introduction of highly touted manufactured models having the appearance of modern molded chairs and containing motors capable of elevating, lowering, and tilting the seat. Some chairs cost as much as $5,000. Hundreds of hospitals throughout the United States purchased birthing chairs based on unsubstantiated claims that they would shorten labor and prove more comfortable for delivery, but many of these chairs are now gathering dust in storerooms. One reason for this decline in popularity has been the increasingly widespread use of more comfortable and easily adjustable labor-delivery beds. While most women fit comfortably into the chair, those who are overweight or have large thighs have complained of uncomfortable pressure against the inner part of the leg and thigh. In addition, earlier claims of a more rapid labor and reduced incidence of perineal lacerations with the chair have not been substantiated by clinical experience. In fact, it has been the impression of many obstetricians that there is actually an increase in the severity of both perineal and vaginal lacerations due to the increased pressure on the pelvic tissues. Published reports of severe perineal swelling and greater postpartum blood loss have also helped to dampen enthusiasm for using the birthing chair. Although the chair supposedly can be used with general anesthesia, in fact it is inadequate for this purpose. Until more extensive scientific data are available on the outcome of labor and the pressure effects of the added gravitational force on the fetal head and maternal pelvis created by the sitting position, I will remain skeptical about the merits of the birthing chair.

Is there a preferred maternal position for a cesarean section?

A woman undergoing a cesarean section in the supine position is at the same risk of experiencing compression of the aorta and vena cava as one who labors in this position. This compression can markedly lower the maternal blood pressure as well as impair placental circulation and fetal oxygenation.

These effects may be intensified when epidural or spinal anesthesia is administered. To remedy this problem, most hospitals use operating room tables that tilt at least 15 degrees to the left while a cesarean section is performed. The tilt to the left allows the uterus and its contents to fall away from the vena cava, thereby improving the return circulation from a woman's lower extremities to her heart. Hypotension is prevented, and normal placental blood flow returns.

Many hospitals use specially designed foam rubber wedges, positioned to the left of a mother's pelvis to hold her safely in position at the time of surgery. Some obstetricians have even devised methods of tilting the table to a full lateral or side position so that the cesarean section is performed with the doctor assuming a sitting position. This method, however, has not been endorsed by the majority of physicians.

What are the hazards to the fetus when the mother bears down during the second stage of labor?

It is not unusual to detect early fetal heart rate decelerations, or Type I dips, during the second stage of labor when a woman is bearing down. These decelerations are the result of fetal head compression and are practically always harmless. Characteristically, early fetal heart rate decelerations begin with the onset of the contraction and return to normal with or before the end of the contraction. Prolonged bearing down efforts, however, may be dangerous to the fetus. Research by Dr. Roberto Caldeyro-Barcia of Uruguay suggests that best results are obtained when the bearing down or pushing effort lasts 4 to 5 seconds. Prolonging the attempt for longer than 6 to 7 seconds at a time is ill advised and potentially very dangerous. When bearing down was encouraged for longer than 15 seconds, Dr. Caldeyro-Barcia noted that the fetus was much more likely to experience hypoxia, or lack of oxygen, and a marked deceleration in heart rate. If bearing down efforts are spontaneously and voluntarily performed by a woman, the early fetal heart rate decelerations recover and return to normal after the last pushing effort of each contraction. However, if the pushing is extended and unnatural and each push is prolonged beyond 6 seconds, the fetal heart rate does not have time to recover between contractions.

The mechanism behind the development of fetal distress with prolonged pushing is easily explained. When a woman bears down she holds her breath. This closes the glottis at the opening of the trachea, or windpipe, increasing pressure within the thorax, or chest cavity, which in turn results in a drop in maternal blood pressure. The longer the bearing down effort, or Valsalva maneuver, the more marked the fall of a woman's blood pressure. As a result, there is a decline in the amount of blood reaching the placenta, and the oxygen supplied to the fetus is reduced. This may lead to late decelerations and fetal distress as well as maternal exhaustion, erratic blood pressure changes, and ruptured blood vessels in the conjunctiva of a woman's eyes. These changes occur in all maternal positions, although they are intensified in the supine position.

Rather than showing patience in waiting for women to naturally experience the bearing down reflex following full dilation, too many obstetricians rush the process and encourage pushing efforts far too soon. This attitude is based on the long-held misconception that a second stage of labor lasting longer than 2 hours in a primigravida or 1 hour in a multiparous woman is associated with a higher incidence of fetal acidosis and permanent disability. In fact, just the opposite is true: Setting predetermined time limits has resulted in far too many dangerous forceps deliveries and unnecessary cesarean sections. Recent studies have clearly shown that a second stage of 3 or more hours is not necessarily worrisome, provided that the fetus is monitored electronically and scalp pH determinations are performed when indicated (see Chapter 11). If progress in descent of the fetal head in the pelvis is being made and there is no evidence of fetal distress, labor should be allowed to continue without interference.

Too often, obstetricians and nurses demand that their patients push as hard and as long as they can, and some women are criticized for not being "good pushers." Do not follow this advice. In labor bear down as you feel the need, without trying to produce very strong or prolonged efforts. Furthermore, push less if you are lying on your back. Although the second stage of labor may proceed more slowly when this advice is followed, the risks of cutting the supply of oxygen to the fetus will be reduced significantly.

 # LABOR

How does labor begin?

Some theories have attributed the origin of labor to the mother, while others have implicated the fetus, amniotic membranes, amniotic fluid, and a communication system that exists between a fetus and its mother. Practically all theories, however, agree that prostaglandins, especially prostaglandin F2α (PGF2α) and prostaglandin E (PGE) to a lesser degree, play a significant role in the process. Prostaglandins have the ability to initiate uterine contractions at any stage of gestation, and elevated levels in maternal and fetal plasma, urine, and amniotic fluid coincide with the onset of labor. Researchers have found that fetal membranes and the decidua, or lining layer of the uterine cavity that forms during pregnancy, are the two major sites of increased prostaglandin production at the time of labor. The triggering mechanism for prostaglandin release is believed by many to originate in the fetus. At the end of pregnancy, fetal urine comprises a major portion of the total amniotic fluid volume. Studies have suggested that a substance is excreted by the fetus into the amniotic fluid which interacts with the fetal membranes and provides a signal for starting labor. This substance may eventually prove to be platelet activating fac-

tor (PAF), which is present in the amniotic fluid only during labor. PAF may play a role in prostaglandin synthesis by diffusing into the decidua and fetal membranes or by directly stimulating uterine muscle contractions.

Should a woman be routinely monitored electronically during labor even if she has no obstetrical or medical complications?

Since its introduction more than 20 years ago, electronic monitoring of the fetal heart rate and maternal uterine contractions has been a source of great controversy among women and their obstetricians. Since its inception, those opposed to fetal monitoring have claimed that the technique is at variance with the concept of family-centered childbirth and the return to a more natural, homelike labor environment. Words such as "dehumanizing" and "humiliating" have been used frequently by feminists to describe electronic fetal monitoring. Attachment to the machine's wires and electrodes confines a woman to a bed or chair, is unnatural, detracts from the spontaneity of her birth experience, and has been too frequently associated with a false diagnosis of fetal distress. This false diagnosis has helped contribute to an incredibly high number of unnecessary cesarean sections. While internal fetal monitoring has proven to be more accurate than the external technique (see page 384), it has also been accused of causing a greater incidence of maternal and fetal infection and hemorrhage, as well as a variety of other complications. Finally, those in opposition to monitoring point out the exorbitant costs of using it routinely on all women in labor. Despite these arguments, the use of electronic fetal monitoring has continued unabated, as evidenced by the fact that 75 percent of women giving birth in the United States are monitored to some degree during labor.

When fetal monitoring was first introduced in the early 1970s, it was hailed as the long-awaited panacea for preventing stillbirths, low Apgar scores, neonatal deaths, and cerebral palsy by diagnosing hypoxia and fetal distress at an early stage. Unfortunately, at least nine well-conducted investigative reports published over the past decade have proven beyond a doubt that electronic fetal monitoring has not fulfilled any of its early optimistic expectations. Periodic auscultation, or listening to the fetal heart rate during labor with either a hand-held Doppler ultrasound device or an old-fashioned stethoscope, or fetoscope, is associated with an incidence of stillbirths, low Apgar scores, cerebral palsy, and low IQs equal to that obtained with continuous electronic fetal monitoring. In fact, one 1990 study from the University of Washington School of Medicine, comparing 93 premature infants monitored electronically with 96 monitored with a fetoscope, found that the incidence of cerebral palsy was three times higher in the group monitored electronically. All recent studies have concluded that falsely abnormal electronic fetal monitoring tracings have resulted in a higher incidence of potentially dangerous and difficult emergency forceps deliveries and unnecessary cesarean sections for fetal distress.

In response to the overwhelming evidence refuting the superiority of electronic fetal monitoring over auscultation, the American College of Obste-

tricians and Gynecologists has formulated newer, more liberal guidelines for monitoring fetal well-being during labor. The College now states that intermittent auscultation of the fetal heart at intervals of 15 minutes, preferably following a uterine contraction, during the first stage of labor and 5 minutes during the second stage is equivalent to continuous electronic monitoring in assessing the fetal condition in a high-risk pregnancy. For low-risk women in labor, the College recommends either continuous electronic monitoring or auscultation at intervals of at least every 30 minutes following a contraction in the active phase of the first stage of labor and at least every 15 minutes during the second stage.

Many women are opposed to fetal monitoring because it hampers their movement during labor and confines them to a bed or chair. One way to avoid this restriction is to use the monitor intermittently. On admission to the labor room, an external fetal monitor can be applied for 15 to 30 minutes to be sure that no heart rate abnormalities are present. The machine can then be unhooked and the woman allowed to walk about. Periodic tracings, taken at 30-minute intervals during the first stage of labor, may be the ideal compromise for women who are opposed to continuous monitoring. When potential fetal problems are present, the first-stage monitoring interval should be reduced to 15 minutes. This method of monitoring may be continued throughout labor as long as the fetal heart rate and cervical dilatation remain normal. Following full dilatation and throughout the second stage of labor, the American College of Obstetricians and Gynecologists recommends that the electronic monitor tracing be evaluated at 15-minute intervals for uncomplicated and 5-minute intervals when risk factors are present during labor. Even with the application of the internal scalp electrode, monitoring may still be used intermittently simply by detaching the electrode from the wires leading to the machine. The electrode can then be taped to a woman's inner thigh while she leaves her bed to walk about. Some women are under the false impression that they have to lie perfectly still in bed in order to be monitored adequately. In fact, a change of position involves only a slight adjustment of the external transducer and no changes in the internal instruments. It is also possible to keep the monitor running while the mother is sitting in a chair or even standing near the machine.

What constitutes normal progress during labor?

The historic work of Dr. Emmanuel A. Friedman enables us to understand and evaluate the normal course of labor. Dr. Friedman studied thousands of births and then derived a graph showing the approximate length of time that each phase of labor should last. While these statistics represent averages, from which considerable deviation may occur, they allow for instant evaluation and detection of labor progress, as well as deviations from this normal pattern.

Normal labor is characterized by progressive cervical dilatation and descent of the fetal head in the pelvis. Descent is measured in terms of the relationship between the level of the lowest part of the fetal head and the maternal ischial spines. These two bony projections lie on either side of the pelvis, and a doctor can easily touch them during a vaginal or rectal examination. If the head is at the same level as the spines, the station, or point of descent in the pelvis, is said to be 0, and levels above and below the spines are referred to as minus (−) and plus (+) stations, respectively. A station of −3 means that the leading part of the head is 3 centimeters above the maternal spines, while a +1 station signifies that it is 1 centimeter below. The station of the fetal head at any time during labor can be easily determined during a vaginal examination. Dr. Friedman was able to show that progress in labor could be followed by charting the results of periodic examinations on a labor graph. The results of each examination are plotted on the graph and then joined together to form a continuous line. On such a graph one can readily observe that during normal labor cervical dilatation will follow a characteristic S-shaped curve. In contrast, the line measuring descent of the baby's head will follow a more angulated route. The classic configuration of the normal labor graph is shown in Figure 52. This method has become so successful that many hospitals throughout the world have adopted the Friedman graph for following the progress of all women in labor.

The latent phase of labor (A—B on the curve) begins with the onset of regular uterine contractions and continues until the dilatation line begins to curve upward. In this phase the cervix softens for subsequent active dilatation. Most of the total time that a woman spends in labor is spent in this phase. The cervix during this phase may be as little as 1 centimeter and as much as 4 centimeters dilated. Under normal circumstances, the latent phase should not exceed 20 hours for a woman having her first baby (nullipara or primigravida), or 14 hours for someone who has previously given birth (multipara). Usually, however, the latent phase averages 6.5 hours in primigravidas and slightly less than 5 hours in multiparas.

The active phase of labor (line B—D) is divided into three parts: the acceleration phase (B), in which cervical dilatation begins to increase; the phase of maximum slope (C), which is characterized by rapid cervical dilatation; and the deceleration phase (D), in which the rate of cervical dilatation slows just prior to full dilatation. During the phase of maximum slope, dilatation of the cervix should progress at a rate of no less than 1.2 centimeters per hour for primigravidas and 1.5 centimeters per hour for multiparas. All the phases of labor leading up to full dilatation of the cervix (A through E) make up the first stage of labor.

The second stage of labor (E) begins with full dilatation of the cervix and ends with delivery of the baby. Although there is a great deal of variability, the average length of the second stage of labor will be approximately 50 minutes for a primigravida and 20 minutes for a multiparous woman.

The dotted line, which depicts fetal descent,

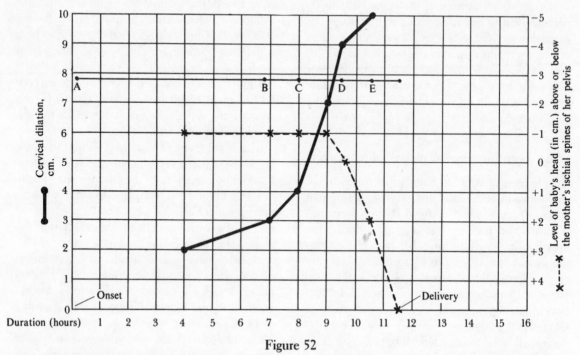

Figure 52

Phases of labor. Characteristic patterns of cervival dilatation and descent charted against elapsed time in labor, showing their component phases: A: latent phase; B-D: active phase; B: acceleration phase; C: phase of maximum slope; D: deceleration phase; E: second stage.

shows that the station of the baby's head rapidly moves downward during the active phase of cervical dilatation.

Couples taking childbirth education courses need not be confused trying to correlate this medical terminology with what they have learned. Most couples are taught that "active labor" is that period of time in which the cervix dilates from 3 to 7 centimeters. During this phase, the contractions are usually very strong, may occur as frequently as every 2 to 3 minutes, and last 1 minute. This period of time corresponds to the acceleration and maximum slope components (B and C) of the active phase. The most difficult part of labor, from 8 to 10 centimeters of cervical dilatation, is commonly referred to by childbirth instructors as the "transition" stage. At this point, contractions are

most intense, lasting as long as 90 seconds and coming as frequently as 1 minute apart. Fortunately, this stage usually lasts only 20 to 45 minutes. The transition stage can be considered as being synonymous with Dr. Friedman's deceleration phase (D).

How do these objective measurements relate to what a woman actually experiences during labor?

Women have described latent phase contractions, which are rhythmic and get stronger as time progresses, in a number of different ways, including pelvic pressure, backache, menstrual-like cramps, and a sensation of tightening in the area over the pubic bone. During this time, contractions are usually tolerated easily, and most women feel quite sociable and able to carry on a conversation between contractions. It is not necessary to time each contraction until the interval from the start of one to the start of another is approximately 5 minutes or less. Since the latent phase of labor may last for several hours, it is usually more comfortable to rest between contractions rather than rush prematurely to the hospital.

During the "active labor" phase, with its more intense and more frequent contractions, most women do not feel like talking and usually become thoughtful, serious, and quiet, and totally preoccupied with their labor. Joking, loud noises, and conversations carried on during contractions are extremely distracting and annoying to a woman at this time, although companionship and sincere encouragement are invaluable and greatly appreciated. As dilatation approaches 7 centimeters, many women have some doubts about their ability to cope with the contractions that lie ahead. This is a normal reaction.

The most difficult part of labor, from 8 to 10 centimeters of cervical dilatation, is commonly referred to by childbirth instructors as the transition stage—Dr. Friedman's deceleration (D) phase. At this point, contractions are most intense, lasting as long as 90 seconds and coming as frequently as 1 minute apart. Fortunately, this stage usually lasts only 20 to 45 minutes. For many women, the contractions during this stage feel almost continuous, making it nearly impossible to relax. Restlessness, extreme irritability, expressions of discomfort, and requests for help and medication are frequent during transition. Hiccups or belching, a feeling of nausea, and a desire to vomit are also frequently expressed as the cervix approaches full dilatation.

Contractions during the second stage of labor (E) are often further apart than those of the transition stage, and they are accompanied by an irresistible urge to bear down and expel the baby. The feelings of insecurity and fear which characterize the transition stage are quickly replaced by a great sense of relief and confidence. A woman feels an almost unbelievable physical strength during this stage, knowing that each of her expulsive efforts is bringing her closer to the successful completion of labor. It is impossible for this male obstetrician to describe the incredible feeling of relief and joy which a woman experiences following the final Herculean effort which results in the birth of her baby.

How can the doctor and patient diagnose and correct an abnormal pattern of cervical dilatation?

Dr. Friedman described four major types of abnormal cervical dilatation patterns: prolonged latent phase, protracted active-phase dilatation, secondary arrest of dilatation, and prolonged deceleration phase.

The latent phase is considered to be prolonged if it exceeds 20 hours in the primigravida or 14 hours in the woman who has previously given birth. Excessive sedation at a point too early in labor is the most common factor associated with this problem. Similarly, administering a conduction anesthetic such as an epidural during the latent phase will also serve to prolong it. In addition, women who begin labor with a rigid, thick, and undilated cervix will be more likely to experience a long and difficult latent phase. Others, for unknown reasons, will have poorly synchronized uterine contractions as the cause of their lack of cervical dilatation.

It is often very difficult for even the most experienced obstetricians to distinguish between false labor and a prolonged latent phase. The correct diagnosis can only be made after several hours of observation. Regardless of the cause of the prolonged latent phase, rest and sedation is the treatment. After 14 or more hours of contractions, most women are exhausted and disheartened by their lack of progress. An intramuscular narcotic should be administered in a dosage which is sufficient to rest both the patient and her uterus for a period of 6 to 8 hours. If, following this rest period, the contractions have stopped, the diagnosis of false labor can be made and the woman can be sent home.

Dr. Friedman found, however, that 85 percent of all women with a prolonged latent phase enter the active phase of labor following this period of therapeutic rest. Of this group, more than 90 percent go on to normal active-phase dilatation of the cervix. Among the small number of women who continue to experience latent-phase labor following sedation, Dr. Friedman recommends initiation of intravenous oxytocin stimulation, provided there are no medical problems in the mother preventing its use. All too often, cesarean sections are performed for "failure to progress," when in reality one is dealing with a benign, though prolonged, latent phase. Nine times out of ten, surgery is unnecessary, since these women spontaneously enter the phase of active cervical dilatation.

Protracted dilatation during the active phase is a rare type of abnormal labor in which cervical dilatation creeps along at a pace which is slower than the minimal normal amount of 1.2 centimeters per hour for primigravidas and 1.5 centimeters per hour for multiparas. It can be caused by excessive sedation, inappropriately early epidural anesthesia, or an abnormal position of the baby. However, in most cases, the cause remains unknown. Measures to speed up labor, such as artificial rupture of the amniotic membranes and intravenous oxytocin stimulation, only serve to complicate matters. Provided that some progress is being made, the best treatment is a hands-off policy. Two-thirds of all women with a protracted active phase eventually experience an uneventful vaginal delivery. However, one-third stop dilating at some point during labor and require a cesarean section because the baby's head size is too large to pass through the maternal pelvis. This condition is known as cephalopelvic, or feto-pelvic, disproportion.

The most ominous of cervical dilatation abnormalities is known as secondary arrest, or cessation of dilatation, during the active phase of labor. Approximately 40 percent of all women experiencing this problem ultimately require a cesarean section because of cephalopelvic disproportion. Other causes of secondary arrest of dilatation during the active phase of labor include sedation and improperly administered conduction anesthesia, such as an epidural. Among women who are believed to have adequate pelvic measurements, the use of intravenous oxytocin at this stage produces progressive dilatation of the cervix and subsequent vaginal delivery at least 80 percent of the time. X-ray pelvimetry can be avoided and oxytocin carefully administered if the pelvic measurements appear to be adequate, there are no significant heart rate abnormalities on the fetal monitor, and there is no evidence of fetal distress. Failure of labor to progress following 3 to 4 hours of good oxytocin-induced contractions would warrant a cesarean section.

When arrest of dilatation is caused by analgesics or conduction anesthesia, rather than cephalopelvic disproportion, the effects of the drugs should be allowed to wear off. Progressive dilatation of the cervix and a successful vaginal delivery usually follow.

The final disorder of cervical dilatation, known as the prolonged deceleration phase, occurs just before full dilatation and is often associated with cephalopelvic disproportion. It can be recognized whenever dilatation of the cervix from approximately 8 or 9 centimeters to 10 centimeters (full dilatation) takes longer than 3 hours in the primigravida or more than 1 hour in the multipara. Management of this problem in a manner similar to that for arrest of labor in the active phase should bring a successful outcome, provided that your obstetrician does not attempt a difficult midforceps delivery after the cervix is fully dilated.

What happens when the baby's head does not descend in the normal way during labor?

The curve for descent of the fetal head during labor follows a flat line until the cervical dilatation curve reaches its maximum upward slope. It normally reaches its own maximum at the onset of the deceleration phase of cervical dilatation. During the second stage of labor, descent is usually progressive and at a rate of no less than 1 centimeter per hour in primigravidas and 2 centimeters in multiparas.

Dr. Friedman has described three abnormalities of fetal descent: failure of descent, protracted descent, and arrest of descent. In a failure of descent situation the baby's head does not drop to a lower position in the pelvis at the time that the cervical deceleration phase begins. This failure is an ominous sign that cephalopelvic disproportion may be present. A protracted descent pattern is often related to a protracted active-phase cervical-dilatation abnormality. The prognosis for vaginal delivery is generally good. Arrest, or cessation of descent for more than 1 hour after it has begun, is the third type of abnormal descent pattern described by Dr. Friedman.

Until recently, it was accepted obstetrical policy in many hospitals to attempt delivery following a maximum of 2 hours of full dilatation in women having their first baby and 1 hour in women who have had a previous baby. Occasionally this rule was followed even if it involved a difficult midforceps operation. It was mistakenly believed that prolongation of the second stage of labor for periods longer than these limits adversely affected the fetus. Recent studies have shown, however, that this is not so. Labor can continue as long as descent is progressing and the fetus is monitored. Given enough time for their descent patterns to evolve, most women with labor abnormalities experience a normal vaginal delivery.

 ## *FORCEPS DELIVERY*

What are obstetric forceps?

Obstetric forceps are paired metallic instruments designed for rotation and/or extraction of the baby's head after full dilatation of the cervix. The blades of the forceps, resembling the end of a shoehorn, are applied against the side of the head, and traction is exerted by pulling on the interlocked handles (see Figure 53).

There are many types of obstetric forceps, most of them named after the doctors who invented them. Some are designed specifically for exerting traction, while others are used primarily for rotating or turning the baby's head into a more favorable position for delivery.

Forceps operations are classified according to the level and position of the head in the birth canal when the blades are applied and bear no relation to

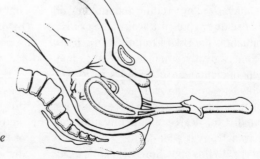

Figure 53

Proper application of forceps to the side of the baby's head.

the type of instrument used. There are three classifications of forceps operations:

1 Low and outlet forceps. With outlet forceps, the scalp is visible at the vaginal opening, without having to separate the labia to see it. With low forceps, the head of the baby rests low on the pelvic floor at station +2 or more, and its face is turned in the direction of the maternal spine. The baby's sagital suture, or the line formed in the middle of the top of the head by the joining of the two parietal bones, must be positioned front to back or at a slight angle in relation to the maternal pelvis if the criteria for a low-forceps delivery are to be met. A low-forceps delivery is usually very easy to perform if carried out by a competent obstetrician.

2 Midforceps. In this more difficult operation, the forceps are applied after the head is engaged, but before the conditions for low forceps have been met. The head is engaged if an imaginary line between the two parietal bones on the top of the baby's skull has descended to a level below the woman's bony pelvic inlet. By definition, the leading part of the fetal skull is above station +2 when midforceps is performed. Any forceps operation requiring significant rotation of the baby's head is also a midforceps operation, regardless of how low in the pelvis the head has descended. Occasionally, a doctor may erroneously believe that the baby's head is engaged when it is not. This is especially likely to occur after a long, difficult labor, characterized by swelling and molding of the fetal head due to pressure against the cervix. In this situation the risk of trauma to the fetus and mother is greatly enhanced. While some midforceps operations are extremely easy to perform, others are quite difficult and hazardous. Unfortunately, an obstetrician is not always able to predict the degree of difficulty until the midforceps delivery is attempted.

3 High forceps. In this operation, the baby's head is not engaged and may even be floating above the pelvic brim. High forceps has no place in modern obstetrics because it carries great risk for a mother and her baby.

Under what circumstances can an obstetrician justify the use of forceps?

Not too long ago, a large part of the "art" of obstetrics centered around the ability of an obstetrician to perform a difficult midforceps delivery soon after a woman's cervix was fully dilated. But it was shown that the number of maternal complications, in the form of cervical and vaginal lacerations and hemorrhage, as well as the number of infant deaths, rose substantially following these difficult maneuvers. Although indications for attempting a forceps operation still remain, many midforceps deliveries have been replaced by more cesarean sections. The tremendous popularity of prepared childbirth education has been a very important factor in reducing the number of women seeking anesthesia, forceps, or other forms of medical interference in the birth process.

Most forceps deliveries are termed "prophylactic" or "elective." Simply translated, this means that they are performed without clear-cut medical reasons. Included among these dubious indications are a desire to reduce a woman's effort and discomfort during the second stage of labor, to save her perineal tissues from overstretching, and to reduce the risk of fetal brain injury from prolonged pushing of the head against an unyielding perineum. In the presence of an uneventful pregnancy and labor, these alleged benefits would appear to be questionable at best. A more likely benefit of "prophylactic" forceps is that it shortens the doctor's stay in the hospital with his or her patient.

Forceps use is indicated if, for a variety of reasons, a woman is unable to push the baby's head out following a prolonged effort. Although there are no absolute and arbitrary rules, a second stage of labor exceeding 3 hours with a regional anesthetic such as an epidural, or 2 hours without an epidural in a woman having her first child, would be considered prolonged. For someone who has previously given birth, a second stage of more than 2 hours with an epidural or more than 1 hour without one would usually be considered to be abnormal. However, it must be emphasized that these are general guidelines and doctors need not rush to perform a forceps delivery simply because the second stage of labor is prolonged. If progress is being made in descent of the fetal head and there is no evidence of distress, it is reasonable to exceed these time limits and await a spontaneous birth. Arrest of progress during the second stage may be caused by fatigue, too much medication, poor uterine contractions, weak abdominal musculature, excessively resistant or inelastic perineal tissues, or a large baby. An abnormal position of the baby's head, such as the occiput posterior or transverse positions, may also be responsible for this problem.

One very important indication for the use of forceps is the diagnosis of fetal distress. Occasionally, an obstetrician must make a decision and weigh the relative risks of an immediate forceps delivery against those of a cesarean section or further delay in hopes that the distress will correct itself. Often, valuable minutes may be lost while preparations are being made for a cesarean section.

Under certain medical conditions, a forceps operation may be preferred to spontaneous vaginal delivery. For example, a woman with heart disease will fare better if she avoids bearing down efforts during the second stage. Similarly, a woman with a history of retinal detachment should not raise her intracranial pressure with excessive pushing. Obstetrical complications, such as severe abruptio placenta, a prolapsed umbilical cord, or intrapartum infection, often demand instant delivery with forceps rather than a prolonged second stage of labor. Forceps are also valuable for delivery of very small babies because they are more prone to develop intracranial hemorrhage as a result of prolonged bearing down efforts.

Isn't a cesarean section safer for a baby than a forceps delivery?

Not always. There is no doubt that a low-forceps delivery is infinitely safer for both mother and child than a cesarean section. Fears of such a procedure are unfounded.

Many doctors believe that if an easy spontaneous or outlet forceps delivery is not possible, a cesarean section should be performed so that the risk of fetal and maternal trauma may be reduced. The research of Dr. Emmanuel Friedman noted 2 deaths per 1,000 spontaneous deliveries, compared with 11 deaths per 1,000 with midforceps and 29 per 1,000 if the midforceps delivery followed a protracted labor. More importantly, Dr. Friedman found that the quality of life also suffers in newborns surviving midforceps deliveries. Speech and hearing disorders at the age of three were 6 per 1,000 following spontaneous vaginal delivery and 33 per 1,000 following arrested labors which were terminated by midforceps. Significantly lower IQ scores have also been noted at the age of four among babies delivered by midforceps. Several more recent studies of midforceps deliveries have not substantiated Dr. Friedman's pessimistic conclusions. For example, in a 1990 article published in the *American Journal of Obstetrics and Gynecology*, Dr. Richard A. Bashore and his associates at the University of California School of Medicine evaluated the maternal and neonatal outcome of 358 midforceps and 486 cesarean deliveries and found no differences in Apgar scores, umbilical cord blood gases, birth trauma, or need for treatment in the neonatal intensive care unit. However, maternal complications in the form of fever, more frequent need for blood transfusions, prolonged hospital stay, deep vein thrombosis, and life-threatening pulmonary embolus were significantly greater among those undergoing cesarean section. While some institutions are replacing the midforceps delivery with greater numbers of cesarean sections, the majority of teaching institutions in the United States and Canada continue to successfully use midforceps and support this policy with convincing data showing lower complications compared to cesarean sections. The judicious and skillful use of forceps can, in properly selected situations, offer a preferable alternative to cesarean sections.

 # *VACUUM EXTRACTION*

What is a vacuum extractor, and how does its safely compare to that of forceps?

As a substitute for midforceps and low-forceps operations, the vacuum extractor has gained wide acceptance in Europe, but not in the United States. To use this instrument, a metal or plastic traction cup is first attached to the back of the baby's scalp. Negative pressure is then built up slowly over several minutes so that the cup adheres firmly to the area of the scalp on which it is attached. After adequate suction is obtained, an obstetrician exerts traction by pulling on a chain which passes through the suction tube.

Theoretically, the vacuum extractor has several advantages over the use of forceps. The overall severity of maternal and fetal injuries is less with this device. The procedure is easy to master. Unlike with forceps, anesthesia is not necessary for its use. In the case of fetal distress, in which a vaginal delivery is imperative, this can be a great advantage.

The vacuum extractor, however, is not harmless. In fact, it may be associated with trauma to the fetal scalp in the form of abrasions and lacerations. Hematomas, or blood clot formations under the skin of the scalp, are known to occur in 10 to 12 percent of infants delivered by vacuum extraction. Deaths following trauma, although extremely rare, have also been reported. Some studies have demonstrated a higher incidence of hemorrhage within the skull and the eyes among babies delivered with this device as well as a greater likelihood of neonatal jaundice. It is advisable not to use the vacuum extractor to deliver premature infants weighing less than 2,500 grams (5½ pounds) because of the greater likelihood of head trauma.

 # *BREECH BIRTHS*

How frequent are breech births, and what are the causes?

The breech, or buttocks-first, position of the baby occurs in 3 to 4 percent of all deliveries, with a much higher incidence noted among premature infants. Many theories have been proposed to explain why the baby assumes a breech position. Factors other than prematurity which appear related to this condition include uterine relaxation in a woman who has several previous children, multi-ple births, excessive amniotic fluid (hydramnios), congenital abnormalities such as hydrocephaly and anencephaly, maternal uterine anomalies, and the location of the placenta. Women with placenta previa, an abnormally low-lying placenta, are more likely to carry a baby in the breech position. Similarly, a placental location in the cornua, or upper lateral part of the uterus, predisposes to a breech position. But the cause of a breech position remains unknown in the vast majority of cases. It also remains a mystery as to why a women who gives birth to one breech will be more likely to do so again.

How is the breech position diagnosed?

The relationship between the legs and buttocks of a fetus in the breech position falls into one of three classifications: frank breech, complete breech, and incomplete breech (see Figure 54).

The frank breech position is the most common and is associated with the lowest number of complications. As the cervix dilates during labor, one or both feet of an incomplete breech may drop down into the vagina through the dilated cervix. This is then known as a single or double footling breech; both conditions are associated with a much higher complication rate than the frank breech and complete breech.

Most experienced obstetricians can diagnose a breech position simply by palpating a woman's abdomen. Often, the patient suspects the diagnosis before her doctor because she detects the hardness of the fetal head in the upper abdomen, accompanied by a greater amount of lower abdominal kicking. If the findings on abdominal palpation are in doubt, a vaginal examination usually confirms the diagnosis. Occasionally, however, the buttocks of a frank breech can confuse an examiner into believing that he or she is palpating the head. Absolute confirmation of a breech can be made by ultrasound or abdominal x-ray examinations. The breech position is probably one of the few remaining valid indications for the use of x-ray pelvimetry. This x-ray examination has the great advantage of being able to demonstrate the relationship between the fetal breech and the bony structures of the maternal pelvis. In addition, it can determine if the head is extended and vaginal delivery would be hazardous. Most recently, the use of computed tomographic pelvimetry has replaced x-ray pelvimetry in some medical centers. This technique is equally accurate but exposes the fetus to only a fraction of the radiation dose used with the conventional x-ray method. Accurate assessment of the diameter and shape of the maternal pelvis is vital if vaginal delivery of a baby in the breech position is contemplated. This important information cannot be obtained with ultrasound. However, fetal anomalies, more common among breech babies, are most readily identified with an ultrasound examination.

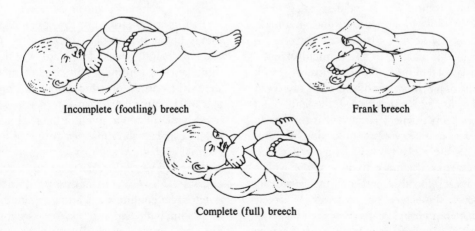

Incomplete (footling) breech

Frank breech

Complete (full) breech

Figure 54 Breech positions.

What problems may be encountered when a baby is in a breech position?

There is no doubt that the prognosis for a fetus in a breech position is considerably worse than that of a head-first position. This is true at every stage of pregnancy. In a report comparing the results of head-first deliveries with more than 1,000 breech births, doctors at the University Hospital in Cleveland noted a ten times greater overall mortality rate in the breech group. In addition, birth defects occurred in 6.3 percent of breech deliveries but only 2.4 percent of nonbreech births. When the same comparison is made between healthy babies weighing more than 5½ pounds, the results, though less striking, are still significant. In one study, conducted at Mount Sinai Hospital in New York City, the death rate was 3 percent among breech babies, compared to less than 1 percent for those in the head-first position.

While trauma to the baby may occur at any time during a vaginal breech delivery, problems are most commonly encountered when the obstetrician attempts to deliver the head. This is especially worrisome in the woman having her first baby. Unfortunately, x-ray pelvimetry demonstrating adequate maternal size is no guarantee that the head will be delivered easily. There is no obstetrical situation which is more frantic and desperately tragic than the inability to successfully and atraumatically deliver the head of a baby in the breech position. Time is crucial in these circumstances, since a delay of 4 or more minutes is likely to result in permanent brain damage due to a lack of oxygen received by the fetus. At this stage, the point of no return has been reached, because it is too late to perform an emergency cesarean section. Entrapment of the breech baby's head by a cervix which is not fully dilated is most likely to occur with a footling breech. In this situation, the legs easily pass through the cervix, but progressively larger, less readily compressible parts must then be delivered. The largest structure, namely the head, may then be unable to pass. Head entrapment is also significantly more common when the baby weighs in excess of 8 pounds. While one would assume that a premature infant, weighing less than 5½ pounds, would be less apt to encounter this problem, the opposite is true. As previously mentioned, there is a disproportion between the large size of the head and the small buttocks of the premature infant. The incidence of head entrapment is greatest among those premature babies who are smallest.

Prolapse, or dropping down of the umbilical cord into the vagina, is an acute emergency requiring immediate delivery. It is far more common among babies in the breech position. Even when prolapse is not present, delivery of the buttocks draws the umbilicus and attached cord into the pelvis and causes compression. Therefore, once the buttocks of the baby has passed the vaginal opening, the rest of its body must be delivered promptly.

Can anything be done to prevent the breech position from developing?

When a breech or transverse (sideways) position is recognized during the last trimester, a growing number of obstetricians have reported great success in turning the baby to the safer and more common head-first position by rotating it through palpation and manipulation over the maternal abdominal wall. This technique, known as external cephalic version, is accomplished by the obstetrician gently lifting the breech out of the pelvis with one hand while pushing the head downward with the other. Simultaneous continuous ultrasound monitoring should be carried out throughout the procedure and for 1 hour following it in order to verify the baby's position and to monitor the fetal heart rate. Fetal heart rate abnormalities during or following external cephalic version, including decelerations or decreased variability, occur in up to 40 percent of cases. This is usually transitory but underscores the need for continuous heart rate monitoring and for prompt intervention by cesarean section if fetal distress is unrelenting.

Successful external cephalic version will reduce

the need for cesarean section by 70 percent among women carrying a baby in the breech position. However, serious complications may arise in a small number of cases. For this reason the procedure must be performed in a hospital with immediate access to an operating room in the event that an emergency cesarean section is necessary. The timing of the procedure is extremely important, and it should not be performed prior to the thirty-seventh week, since a complication necessitating immediate delivery could result in the birth of a premature baby. Spontaneous conversion of the breech to a vertex, or head-first, position occurs 15 to 20 percent of the time prior to the thirty-seventh week, making the version unnecessary.

Some of the complications attributed to attempts at external cephalic version have included compression and knotting of the umbilical cord causing fetal distress, uterine hemorrhage, premature labor, inadvertent rupture of the amniotic membranes, fetal death, and abruptio placenta or premature separation of the placenta. In one study in which 100 external cephalic versions were performed, a significant number of red blood cells were found to pass into the maternal circulation. This so-called feto-maternal hemorrhage is especially significant in women who are Rh negative. To prevent Rh sensitization, a full dose of RhoGAM should be administered when external cephalic version is attempted for these women.

External cephalic version should not be attempted if there is a marked disproportion between the size of the fetus and the maternal pelvis, the breech is too deep in the pelvis to safely lift it out, the abdominal wall or uterus is tense, the amniotic membranes are ruptured, or there is only a minimal amount of amniotic fluid present (oligohydramnios). Other contraindications include uterine anomalies, placenta previa, third-trimester bleeding, a previous cesarean section or other uterine surgery, multiple gestation, a nonreactive nonstress test (see page 384), intrauterine growth retardation, and ultrasound evidence of the umbilical cord around the baby's body or neck. Anesthesia must never be administered when an external cephalic version is attempted because a woman's ability to detect pain is often the best indication that her doctor is exerting too much force.

In the hands of a skilled obstetrician, the success rates for external cephalic version have been reported to be as high as 75 percent for multiparous women and 50 to 60 percent for primigravidas. Spontaneous conversion back to a breech position after successful external cephalic version occurs approximately 5 to 10 percent of the time. When this occurs, the procedure can usually be repeated successfully. The value of cephalic version is evident from several recent studies showing cesarean section rates of 13 to 20 percent among women undergoing successful version compared to 75 to 90 percent for those whose babies remain in the breech position.

Is there any way to predict which breech babies can be safely delivered vaginally and which ones will require cesarean section?

The Zatuchni-Andros Breech Scoring Index was developed by doctors of the same names in an effort to more accurately predict which infants would require cesarean section and which ones could safely deliver vaginally. Points are given for six determining factors: number of previous children, length of pregnancy in weeks, estimated fetal weight, delivery of a previous full-term breech, dilatation of the cervix at the initial vaginal examination in the hospital, and station or level of the breech in relation to the maternal ischial spines. The Breech Scoring Index is a helpful guide which has been used with success by many obstetricians, although it certainly is not infallible.

Whenever vaginal delivery of a breech is contemplated, an obstetrician must consider many different factors, the most important of which is the fetal size. The very large fetus is extremely likely to be traumatized when a vaginal breech delivery is attempted. Although estimates of fetal weight, based on the use of ultrasound, are an aid, these calculations are far from foolproof. If it is determined that the fetus weighs 8 pounds or more, most experts would agree that a cesarean section should be performed. This advice applies even if the mother's pelvis appears to be of normal size or larger than normal.

The adequacy and configuration of the maternal pelvis must be precisely determined before an attempted vaginal delivery of a full-term breech. Even if a minimal amount of pelvic contraction is detected on x-ray or CT pelvimetry, cesarean section is necessary.

Hyperextension or excessive backward tilting of a fetal head may be detected by x-ray in 5 percent of all babies in the breech position. Cesarean section is indicated when the head is hyperextended in order to prevent injury to the baby's neck and spinal cord.

The use of x-ray and ultrasound in the evaluation of a baby in the breech position may help to determine the route of delivery if an abnormality is detected. The diagnosis of a severe defect, incompatible with survival, would be the deciding factor in opting for a vaginal, rather than a cesarean delivery.

While some doctors have advocated the use of oxytocin when needed to induce or improve labor in a woman with a breech, the majority of evidence suggests that this use is associated with lower Apgar scores and higher infant mortality rates. Cesarean section is undoubtedly the much wiser choice.

All infants in the single or double footling position are best delivered by cesarean section because of the possibility of cord prolapse and entrapment of the fetal head when vaginal delivery is attempted.

The extremely premature infant, or one weighing between 1 pound 2 ounces and 3 pounds 5 ounces, is best delivered by cesarean section because it is less traumatic and not associated with entrapment of the head by a cervix which is not fully dilated.

Unfortunately, even if all of these guidelines are followed, the infant may still not fare as well with a vaginal delivery as when a cesarean section is performed. While it is true that a vaginal delivery is safer for the mother than a cesarean section, there is a far greater risk of permanent fetal damage, cerebral palsy, and perinatal mortality following a vaginal breech delivery.

The vast number of babies in the breech position should be managed with a cesarean section. There is little question that fetal trauma, hypoxia, and perinatal deaths can be reduced only by liberalizing the use of cesarean section. In most medical centers, the cesarean section rate for breech births has risen from an average of 10 percent to approximately 75 to 90 percent over the past ten years. The breech position is now the third leading cause for the increase in the number of cesarean sections in the United States. Many obstetricians in teaching positions have expressed concern that young residents in training are not obtaining sufficient opportunities to deliver breeches vaginally. As a result, it is predicted that future specialists will lack this important skill. Perhaps this is a blessing in disguise. I am firmly convinced that the escalating cesarean section rate in the management of breech position is a justifiable development in modern obstetrics.

What are the third and fourth stages of labor, and how should they be managed?

The third stage of labor begins immediately after delivery of the baby and ends with the separation and expulsion of the placenta. In most cases, placental separation occurs within 15 minutes following childbirth, and textbooks define a prolonged third stage of labor as one in which the placenta remains attached to the uterine wall for 30 minutes or more. It is important that your birth attendant be patient and not try to rush this stage by pulling too vigorously on the umbilical cord or pushing too hard on the fundus, or top, or your uterus.

Such premature attempts are not only futile, they can be dangerous.

The classical signs of placental separation are learned by every first-year medical student but too often forgotten by hurried practicing obstetricians. They include a rising up of the fundus in the abdomen as it assumes a globular appearance and a firm consistency, a gush of blood into the vagina from the placental site, and a lengthening of the umbilical cord as the placenta descends. When one or more of these signs is present, the placenta can easily be removed by gentle traction on the cord combined with minimal pressure on the fundus.

Manual removal of the placenta involves inserting a hand into the uterine cavity and gently sweeping it between the placenta and the uterine wall. This procedure is usually indicated if bleeding is excessive or the placenta has not separated in a reasonable amount of time. The definition of "reasonable" varies, but is most often defined as 30 minutes from birth.

A growing number of obstetricians are practicing manual removal sooner and more often than in the past. The rationale for this aggressive approach is that immediate removal reduces blood loss caused by the accumulation of clots behind the partially separated placenta. On the negative side, however, inserting the hand into the uterus can be extremely painful and is most often unnecessary in the vast majority of cases. It is a sound idea for you to discuss your doctor's policy regarding management of the third stage of labor so that you do not have the unwelcome surprise of a rapid manual removal immediately after you deliver.

Several recent studies have demonstrated that manual removal of the placenta can often be avoided if oxytocin is injected directly into the vein of the umbilical cord immediately following delivery. Other protocols to avoid retention of the placenta call for intravenous or intramuscular injections of oxytocin or ergot alkaloids administered simultaneously with the delivery of the baby's shoulders. In a 1991 report published in the *British Journal of Obstetrics and Gynaecology*, doctors from the Netherlands noted equal success in reducing blood loss and the length of the third stage of labor by administering either oxytocin or prostaglandin E2 (see prostaglandin discussion in the following question) intramuscularly immediately after the birth of the baby. Though natural childbirth instructors commonly teach that suckling of the newborn immediately after birth will hasten placental separation and lower the incidence of postpartum hemorrhage, a 1989 study reported in *Lancet* would tend to refute this clinical impression. In this study, when mothers practicing early nursing were compared to a control group, the frequency of postpartum hemorrhage was a statistically insignificant 7.9 percent and 8.4 percent, respectively. Surprisingly, the average blood loss was slightly higher in the suckling group.

The hour immediately following delivery of the placenta is a critical period that has been designated the fourth stage of labor. Even if oxytocin is administered, postpartum hemorrhage as a result of uterine relaxation is most likely to occur at this time. It is vital that the uterine fundus be evaluated frequently during this hour and massaged at the slightest sign of relaxation. It is a wise obstetrician who stays at the hospital during the hour following delivery of the placenta.

 INDUCED LABOR AND PROLONGED PREGNANCY

Should labor be induced, and how?

Labor induction may be classified as being either indicated or elective. Inducing labor is indicated when the medical benefits of delivery to the fetus or mother exceed those of continuing the pregnancy. IUGR, postmaturity syndrome, suspected fetal distress, abruptio placenta, fetal death, premature rupture of the membranes, amniotic membrane infections, preeclampsia, Rh disease, and maternal diseases such as diabetes, hypertension, and kidney disease are among the reasons for indicated induction of labor to benefit the fetus or mother.

Labor can be induced for convenience in a woman who is free of medical or obstetrical complications. Candidates for this elective induction are those with a history of a previous rapid labor or excessive travel time to the hospital. In the not too distant past, it was common practice among obstetricians to electively induce labor for a variety of nonmedical and nonobstetrical reasons, such as a planned vacation or a doctor's desire to avoid working at an inconvenient hour. Several large studies show this inadequate obstetrical care results in higher rates of fetal distress, ruptured uterus, maternal water intoxication due to too much oxytocin, cervical lacerations, birth injuries, postpartum hemorrhage, abruptio placenta, perinatal deaths, respiratory distress syndrome (RDS), and premature births due to miscalculation of the due date by an overanxious physician.

In response to the outcry of some prominent physicians, consumer groups, and the American Foundation for Maternal and Child Health, the FDA in 1978 issued restrictions on the use of oxytocin, the uterine stimulant, for the elective induction of labor. Even with the use of modern monitoring techniques and delicately controlled intravenous infusion pumps, oxytocin use is still more likely than natural labor to be associated with a higher incidence of abnormally powerful, painful, and prolonged uterine contractions. During a natural labor, the interval between uterine contractions allows a reservoir of oxygenated blood to accumulate in sufficient quantities to meet the needs of the fetus before the next contraction takes place. Since oxytocin-induced contractions are often harder and more frequent than normal, there is less time for oxygen to accumulate between contractions, and fetal hypoxia and distress are more likely to result. This in turn leads to a higher incidence of emergency cesarean sections among women undergoing induction of labor. Some women who receive oxytocin experience greater tension of the uterine muscles, which may persist even after the contraction has ended and further reduce the fetal oxygen supply. In one study, 94 percent of the women who were induced required pain relief, compared to only 60 percent of those who labored spontaneously. The excess amount of pain medication required can serve no helpful purpose for a compromised infant. It has been convincingly demonstrated that oxytocin crosses the placenta and enters the fetal circulation, where it produces distinct biochemical and physiological changes. Among these are hyponatremia, or a reduction in the sodium concentration of the newborn infant's blood, and jaundice during the first few days of life. Both these changes are temporary and are of little if any clinical significance.

Labor should not be induced with oxytocin under certain medical and obstetrical conditions. Included among these are a weakened uterus due to a previous cesarean section performed in the classical manner (see page 437) or extensive uterine surgery, placenta previa, infections of the lower genital tract, such as herpes and gonorrhea, some abnormal positions of the baby, and marked disproportion between the large size of the baby and the small size of the maternal pelvis.

A woman who has had five or more previous full-term pregnancies should not undergo oxytocin-induced labor, since her uterus is more likely to rupture under the stimulus of potentially potent contractions. Overdistention of the uterus, as in the case of twins and hydramnios (excessive amounts of amniotic fluid), is a condition in which oxytocin stimulation should be used with extreme caution.

When the cervix is truly ripe for labor, induction can often succeed simply by artificially rupturing the amniotic membranes. This technique, called amniotomy, is easily and painlessly performed by guiding a sterile clamp or stylet through the cervix in order to puncture the amniotic membranes. Amniotomy induces labor successfully, without oxytocin, in at least 90 percent of all women with a Bishop score of 4 or more. (The Bishop Scoring System, named after Dr. Edward Bishop, uses five objective criteria for determining if a woman can successfully undergo induction of labor: cervical dilatation, cervical effacement or thinning out, station of the fetal head, cervical consistency, and cervical position in relation to the vaginal axis.) One distinct advantage of performing amniotomy is that it allows examination of the amniotic fluid for evidence of blood or meconium staining. In addition, it makes possible the placement of an intrauterine pressure catheter and a fetal scalp electrode and the taking of scalp pH blood samples in the high-risk patient. Amniotic membranes should never be ruptured if the baby's head is high in the pelvis, because the sudden release of fluid can cause a prolapse, or dropping down, of the umbilical cord beneath the level of the head. This dire emergency requires immediate delivery, because the cord may then be compressed and fetal oxygenation impaired. The fetal heart tones should always be checked immediately before and after the membranes are ruptured in order to determine what effect the procedure may have on the fetus. Occasionally, a previously undetected low-lying umbilical cord may be compressed as the head descends. This can be detected promptly by the sudden bradycardia, or slowing of the fetal heart rate, and can be relieved by gently elevating the head with the fingers in the vagina, while emergency preparations for cesarean section are made. When amniotomy is performed during labor, it is best accomplished between contractions in order to avoid the potential risk of cord prolapse as the fluid gushes rapidly out of the uterus. Once the amniotic membranes have been artificially ruptured, delivery should be accomplished within 24 hours since the risk of an amniotic membrane infection increases significantly after this time. While most obstetricians view amniotomy as a safe and simple procedure, some authorities, including Dr. Caldeyro-Barcia (see page 412), condemn this common practice as being extremely dangerous. They claim that the fluid-filled membranes provide a liquid cushion that helps to protect the head of the fetus from damage caused by pressure against the pelvis during labor. It has been stated that artificial rupture of the membranes can produce massive tears in brain tissue due to misalignment of the unfused bones of the skull. To date, no studies support this assertion.

Obstetricians often claim that they are able to induce labor by manipulating the amniotic membrane. This technique, known as "stripping of the membranes," consists of inserting the examining finger into the cervix and then separating the amniotic membranes from their lower uterine wall attachment. One advantage of stripping, rather than rupturing the membranes, is that the procedure can easily be performed in a doctor's office, and if it fails, nothing is lost because the membranes have not been ruptured and the risk of infection is practically nonexistent. Unfortunately, there is a paucity of scientific data supporting the efficacy of this method in inducing labor. The most recent report espousing the benefits of membrane stripping was published in 1990 by doctors at the University of Mississippi Medical Center. They performed weekly stripping of the membranes on 90 women beginning at 38 weeks gestation and compared their time of labor onset with a group of 90 women whose membranes were not stripped. Fifty-four percent of those in the "stripped" group delivered within one week compared to only 16 percent of those in the control group. The average number of days from the time of membrane stripping until delivery was equally impressive—8.6 days versus 15, respectively. Of greatest significance was that postdate delivery after 42 weeks occurred in only 3.3 percent of women whose membranes were stripped, compared to 15.6 percent in the control group. While these statistics are impressive, membrane stripping is still too unreliable and unpredictable to use as the sole method of labor induction when medical or obstetrical complications necessitate immediate delivery.

Induction of labor with intravenous oxytocin will only succeed if the cervix is "ripe," meaning that it is slightly dilated and effaced. When medical or obstetrical circumstances necessitate delivery, an "unripe" cervix can be converted to a "ripe" one by inserting one or two applications of introcervical or intravaginal prostoglandin E2 (PGE2) gel.

When is a pregnancy considered prolonged?

A pregnancy is prolonged, or postdated, when it exceeds 42 weeks, two weeks or more beyond the due date. However, based on recent reports, some obstetricians now consider a pregnancy to be prolonged if it exceeds 41 weeks. What makes labor begin remains unknown, and why it is delayed is also a mystery. A small but significant number of infants involved in prolonged pregnancies die or face serious complications. Research has shown that, in the absence of obstetrical intervention, fetal loss doubles after 42 weeks and quadruples at or beyond 44 weeks when compared to pregnancies delivered at 40 weeks. Furthermore, there is evidence that a wide variety of serious fetal and long-term neonatal complications may ensue, including birth trauma, a higher infant mortality up to two years of age, an increase in hospitalization rates in the first three years of life, and disturbances in physical, cognitive, and behavioral development.

To further complicate matters, 40 to 55 percent of all pregnancies are dated incorrectly. This may occur because of a forgotten missed period, a long or unpredictable menstrual cycle, or conception which occurs soon after birth control pills are stopped. The consequences of misdiagnosing a postdate pregnancy can be serious if an obstetrician attempts induction of labor of a 38-week pregnancy erroneously believed to be 42 weeks in length.

What effect can a prolonged pregnancy have on the fetus?

Research has demonstrated that the placenta undergoes degenerative changes with advancing ges-

tational age, and this subjects the fetus to a decrease in the amount of oxygen and nutrients it receives. Metabolic wastes also accumulate. Affected infants are especially sensitive to the stress which labor produces and the degenerative changes described may cause intrauterine growth retardation, fetal distress, asphyxia, passage of meconium (greenish fecal material) in the amniotic fluid, oligohydramnios or a marked decrease in amniotic fluid volume, and even death before or during labor. Without the cushioning effect of the amniotic fluid, the umbilical cord may become compressed and obstruct the oxygen supply to the fetus. This in turn causes vagal nerves to stimulate intestinal movement and passage of meconium into the amniotic fluid. It is estimated that 25 to 30 percent of postdate pregnancies are complicated by meconium staining of the amniotic fluid. The thickness and tenacity of meconium is inversely related to the amount of amniotic fluid present, and in severe cases it has the appearance and consistency of thick pea soup. If this is aspirated or inhaled into the trachea and lungs as a result of fetal or infant gasping, it can obstruct the airway, interfere with gas exchange, and cause severe respiratory distress. A significant finding in postterm newborns is an increase in urine albumin excretion to double the normal value at 40 weeks. This is thought to be a direct response to impaired kidney function caused by a lack of oxygen.

Some postdate babies continue to grow after the fortieth week and reach abnormally large, or macrosomic, weights greater than 4,500 grams (10 pounds). Attempts to deliver these babies vaginally are more apt to be complicated by prolonged labor, difficult forceps procedures, inability to deliver the baby's shoulders, and permanent physical and developmental defects. Although body length and head circumference remain normal in most postterm infants, body length increases in relation to weight and subcutaneous fat is lost. As a result, affected newborns appear long and lean. Only 20 to 30 percent of infants born after the forty-second week of pregnancy display the classic postmaturity or dysmaturity syndrome, consisting of meconium staining of the amniotic fluid, long hair, an overly alert facial expression, extreme loss of subcutaneous fat, long meconium-stained nails, and wrinkled, peeling skin.

The postterm newborn faces the risk of pneumonia caused by meconium aspiration as well as complications resulting from abnormally low blood sugars and calcium levels.

How should a prolonged pregnancy be managed?

To avoid incorrect pregnancy dating, your due date should be firmly established prior to the third trimester. Accurate basal body temperature charts, an early positive pregnancy test, and a first-trimester pelvic examination by a competent physician will help to avoid later discrepancies. Other methods of assessing gestational age include the determination of fetal heart tones at the twelfth gestational week with a Doppler ultrasound device or at the twentieth week with an old-fashioned fetoscope. A woman's perception of her first fetal movements should also be noted. This important event usually occurs at approximately 20 weeks for primigravidas and 18 weeks for multiparas. While all these factors are helpful in confirming a woman's due date, none is as accurate as an ultrasound examination performed during the first or second trimester. Measurements of the fetal crown-rump length, femur length, and biparietal diameter will help to pinpoint the due date within one week. Once the gestational age is established by ultrasound early in pregnancy, it should not be revised later on. Avoiding the hazards of postmaturity is probably one of the most important arguments for advocating routine early ultrasound examinations on all pregnant women.

When it is firmly established that pregnancy is prolonged and the cervix is ripe, induction should be carried out. This can usually be achieved with intravenous oxytocin. When the cervix is unripe, one or two applications of intravaginal or intracervical prostaglandin E2 (PGE2) gel will usually ini-

tiate labor or make the cervix ripe or favorable enough for a successful oxytocin induction (see previous discussion). While most obstetricians hold to the standard of 42 gestational weeks before inducing labor, recent data suggest that 41 weeks may be more appropriate, since the risk to the fetus begins to increase at this point. If your obstetrician is not contemplating induction at 41 weeks, it is still wise for him or her to perform tests for fetal well-being at 41 weeks to detect those infants at risk for postdate complications.

In my opinion, the single most important test for monitoring the condition of a postdate fetus is an ultrasound measurement of the amniotic fluid volume. If adequate amounts of fluid are present, one can reasonably assume that the placenta is functioning adequately and that severe compression of the umbilical cord blood vessels will not occur. At the minimum, this examination should be performed at weekly intervals. However, since the amount of amniotic fluid can diminish quite rapidly, twice-weekly examinations are preferred, although admittedly they are more expensive. Delivery should be initiated whenever decreased amniotic fluid is noted. An ultrasound examination performed for a postdate pregnancy should also include the other components of the biophysical profile such as fetal breathing, muscle tone, and body movements (see page 381) and a view of the placenta for characteristic signs of aging. An ultrasound estimate of the fetal weight is imperative, and the diagnosis of macrosomia (fetal weight greater than 4,500 grams, or 10 pounds) usually warrants a cesarean section rather than an attempt at a vaginal delivery.

In addition to ultrasound, most obstetricians use weekly electronic fetal monitoring when a pregnancy is prolonged (see page 383). Several studies, however, have found that the weekly nonstress test (NST) can be misleading and give false reassurance of fetal well-being in postterm patients. Studies show that perinatal outcome is better with twice-weekly nonstress testing than with weekly testing, especially if combined with ultrasound examinations performed with the same frequency. The contraction stress test (CST), although more cumbersome and time-consuming than the NST, is nevertheless more likely to unmask a problem pregnancy. Many doctors are now performing CSTs rather than NSTs as the initial test for determining the health of the postdate fetus. If the CST is negative, it should be repeated at five- to seven-day intervals, since the chance of fetal death occurring within a week of a normal CST is usually less than 1 percent. If the CST becomes positive, immediate delivery is usually indicated. There is a low incidence of abnormal CSTs in postterm pregnancies; however, if the CST is abnormal, about 60 percent of women will develop fetal distress in labor and 50 percent will require a cesarean section.

A woman whose pregnancy is prolonged beyond 41 weeks should be instructed to count and chart fetal movements each day (see page 380). A reduction in the number of fetal movements is an ominous sign that merits immediate attention.

Whether labor is induced or occurs spontaneously, it is imperative that electronic monitoring be used on any woman whose pregnancy is prolonged. Artificial rupture of the membranes early in labor is helpful in determining the amount of amniotic fluid and whether or not meconium is present.

PREMATURE RUPTURE OF THE AMNIOTIC MEMBRANES

What happens when the bag of waters breaks prematurely, and how can the diagnosis be confirmed?

The spontaneous breaking of the amniotic membranes, or bag of waters, at any time before the onset of labor is an obstetrical problem in approximately 10 percent of all pregnancies. This condition is called premature rupture of membranes (PROM), while the term "preterm rupture of the membranes" has gained popularity in recent years in describing this condition when it occurs earlier than the thirty-sixth gestational week. For most women, labor follows premature rupture of the membranes within a few hours, but the time between the rupture of the membranes and the onset of labor tends to be longer for those who are farthest from their estimated delivery date. Among women with PROM at term, 90 percent will be in spontaneous labor within 24 hours. In contrast, only 50 percent of individuals with preterm rupture of the membranes will be in labor within 24 hours, and 15 to 25 percent will still remain undelivered one week later. The cause of preterm PROM in most cases remains unknown, but there is compelling evidence to suggest that at least one-third of the time it is the result of a local infection and weakening of the amniotic membranes caused by the ascent of bacteria from the cervix or vagina. PROM is also more likely to be associated with hydramnios, multiple births, incompetent cervix, premature separation of the placenta (abruptio placenta), and placenta previa.

While a woman will correctly diagnose premature rupture of her membranes more than 90 percent of the time, an obstetrician must confirm the diagnosis with certainty. Quite often, the pressure of the baby's head on a woman's urinary bladder produces urine which may be mistaken for leakage of amniotic fluid. Similarly, the passage of mucus from the cervix and the increased vaginal secretions which are often noted at the end of pregnancy may confuse the diagnosis. Insertion of a sterile speculum resolves this question and allows visualization of the fluid as it passes from the cervix. Confirmation of the presence of amniotic fluid is easily accomplished by testing its alkalinity through the use of Nitrazine paper or by viewing under a microscope a sample of the dried fluid on a glass slide.

In addition to confirming the diagnosis of PROM, the viewing of the cervix with a sterile speculum can help to determine cervical dilatation and effacement as well as the presence of serious complications such as prolapse, or dropping down, of the umbilical cord or a fetal extremity. Samples of amniotic fluid can also be cultured for possible infection or studied for determinants of fetal lung maturity.

How should a doctor manage PROM?

Although procedures vary from one medical center to the next, most experts recommend induction of labor when the fetus is believed to be at least 36 weeks mature, weighs at least 5½ pounds on ultrasound examination, and amniotic fluid analysis shows that the lungs are mature. Some doctors initiate oxytocin induction immediately following membrane rupture, while others allow time intervals of 6 to 24 hours. This aggressive approach has proven to be successful in reducing the incidence of maternal and fetal infection when the cervix is ripe for induction. However, if the cervix is unripe, attempts at oxytocin induction may actually result in a higher risk of infection, a longer and more difficult labor, failed or unsuccessful induction, and a threefold greater cesarean section rate than when labor occurs spontaneously. To avoid these complications, a growing number of obstetricians are using intravaginal and intracervical prostaglandin to ripen the cervix and induce labor.

A number of obstetricians believe that a conservative, wait-and-see approach to PROM, rather than induction of labor, is both safe and beneficial even if a pregnancy is full term. However, if an obstetrician elects to treat PROM conservatively, he or she must be constantly alerted to any early indications of fetal and maternal infection or fetal distress. A complete blood count should be performed at least every other day, since an elevation in the number of white blood cells often indicates the presence of infection. Fever, abdominal tenderness, or a foul-smelling vaginal discharge are all ominous signs. Although some obstetricians hospitalize women with ruptured membranes, I believe that this regimen is a bit too restrictive and expensive, and it is just as easy to instruct patients to take their temperatures at least twice daily and report any elevation above 37.5°C (99.5°F) immediately. Intercourse and the use of tampons should be strictly prohibited. There is no doubt that the chances of infection are significantly increased if even one digital vaginal examination is performed after the membranes rupture. Such an examination must be strictly avoided until labor has begun or the decision has been made to induce labor. Many women harboring an infection often remain asymptomatic. Amniocentesis for Gram stain and bacterial culture of the amniotic fluid has become a popular method of identifying women with early or occult chorioamnionitis. Despite the fact that the membranes are ruptured, a skilled physician can usually find a residual pocket of fluid on ultrasound and obtain a sample for testing pulmonary maturity and the presence of bacteria. If bacteria are present, delivery is mandatory.

Statistically, 30 percent of all women with preterm PROM give birth to a premature infant. Fetal immaturity as manifested by respiratory distress syndrome (RDS) is by far the most important cause of death of these infants. When a fetus is premature, the obstetrician must balance the risk of delivering it as soon as possible, to avoid the slight risk of infection, against the dangers of not interrupting the pregnancy so that maturation of the fetus can occur in utero.

When the membranes rupture prior to the last six weeks of pregnancy, it is possible that the fetus has a congenital anomaly since this is a condition in approximately 25 percent of such patients. For this reason, an ultrasound examination is very important in deciding whether to wait or to induce labor.

Recent studies by several investigative groups have found that the use of either ampicillin or erythromycin by women with preterm PROM helped to prolong pregnancy for ten days or longer by preventing the development of chorioamnionitis. In a 1990 report published in the *American Journal of Obstetrics and Gynecology*, doctors at the University of Florida Health Science Center administered the antibiotics mezlocillin and ampicillin to 40 women who ruptured membranes at 34 weeks gestation. When compared to an untreated control group, women given antibiotics had a significantly lower incidence of chorioamnionitis, experienced a longer time period from membrane rupture to the onset of labor, and gave birth to babies with higher weights and better Apgar scores. Infection in the newborn, RDS, intraventricular hemorrhage, perinatal deaths, and prolonged hospitalization were also increased in the control group. Further large-scale studies are required before this method of managing preterm PROM can be endorsed.

When a woman's amniotic membranes rupture prior to the twenty-fifth gestational week, the outlook for a successful pregnancy is grim. Only 25 percent of these infants will survive, and many will suffer permanent damage. The lack of amniotic fluid for such a prolonged period of time may result in inadequate development of the lungs, as well as facial and limb deformities.

Whenever the diagnosis of chorioamnionitis is strongly suspected, delivery should be accomplished, regardless of the gestational age. If not, the consequences of delay may be an overwhelming maternal infection and even death. Antibiotics should be administered and delivery accomplished within 24 hours, although an 8-hour time limit is preferable. If induction is unsuccessful or fetal distress occurs, cesarean section should be performed. It is most important that pregnancies complicated by infection be treated at medical centers capable of handling all potential problems.

 # CESAREAN SECTION

What factors account for today's soaring cesarean section rates?

Over the past 20 years, the cesarean section rate in the United States has increased from less than 5 percent to approximately 23 percent, with some medical centers reporting rates as high as 40 percent. In actual numbers, almost 1 million women undergo cesarean section each year, making it the most commonly performed operation in American hospitals. Repeat cesarean section accounts for approximately one-third to 40 percent of this number. The diagnosis of "failure to progress" in labor is responsible for another 25 to 30 percent, fetal distress 5 to 15 percent, and breech and other abnormal fetal positions 10 percent. Miscellaneous conditions such as maternal hypertension and diabetes, multiple births, and placental complications account for the remaining 10 to 20 percent.

The obstetrical management of labor through most of the 1960s differed markedly from today's more sophisticated state of the art. Lacking objective methods of evaluating labor progress, obstetricians frequently made decisions based solely on their personal experience and clinical intuition. Patience was considered the hallmark of good obstetrical care, and labor often lasted for hours and even days, frequently culminating in a difficult midforceps delivery of a severely depressed infant. More often than most obstetricians would care to admit, these maneuvers were responsible for a significant incidence of maternal trauma and permanent fetal damage.

Probably the most important obstetrical contribution of the late 1960s and the 1970s was that of Dr. Emmanuel A. Friedman (see page 415). He was the first to objectively evaluate the labor patterns of thousands of women and establish guidelines for the assessment of normal and abnormal labor, making it possible for obstetricians to rapidly diagnose and remedy labor abnormalities without subjecting a woman to an endless labor. The failure to progress in labor, or dystocia, has become the single most important factor for primary or initial cesarean sections performed in the United States over the past ten years. It has also been one of the main reasons for the decline in fetal and maternal morbidity incurred with prolonged, nonprogressive labor. Through the research of Dr. Friedman and others, the use of difficult forceps delivery has now been replaced by cesarean section when the baby's head fails to descend in the pelvis following full dilatation of the cervix. Unfortunately, too many impatient obstetricians have used the diagnosis of dystocia and failure to progress to justify unnecessary cesarean sections when the situation can be appropriately remedied with the judicious use of oxytocin. In the words of one cynic, failure to progress is too often "failure to wait" on the part of a busy obstetrician.

Changing ideas about maternal nutrition during pregnancy have resulted in the birth of larger babies over the past 20 years. This has contributed to higher cesarean section rates for disproportion between the size of the baby and that of the maternal pelvis. However, true cephalopelvic disproportion, meaning that the baby's head is too big to pass through the maternal pelvis, probably occurs in only 1 to 2 percent of all women in labor. A growing trend among obstetricians has been to perform a primary cesarean section and not allow a trial of labor if a woman is carrying a macrosomic baby, or one estimated to weigh more than 4,500 grams (10 pounds). Statistically, the number of cesarean sections performed for macrosomia has tripled over the last ten years. The reason for performing cesarean sections is to avoid maternal and fetal injury, especially shoulder dystocia, at the time of birth. This potentially catastrophic situation occurs when the baby's head is delivered but its shoulders remain impacted behind the pubic symphysis bone. Some studies quote a 10 percent risk

of shoulder dystocia in babies weighing 4,000 grams (8.8 pounds) and a 30 percent risk for babies over 4,500 grams (10 pounds). Despite this, the logic of this approach is questionable since ultrasound examinations at the end of pregnancy are more likely to overestimate, rather than underestimate, fetal weight. In a 1991 study from the University of Pittsburgh, doctors found that 77 percent of women delivering within three days of an ultrasound examination had babies with birth weights which were below the ultrasound determination and 50 percent of infants diagnosed as macrosomic actually weighed less than 4,000 grams. Even when infants were truly macrosomic, 72 percent were successfully delivered vaginally. Although there were five cases of shoulder dystocia in this group, none of the infants experienced birth trauma or permanent injury as a result.

There is no doubt that the extensive use of electronic fetal monitoring during labor has contributed greatly to the incidence of cesarean sections performed for the incorrect diagnosis of fetal distress. Falsely abnormal nonstress tests (NSTs) and contraction stress tests (CSTs) (see pages 382 and 386) performed in the last trimester also contribute to these alarming statistics. Although confirmation of fetal distress with scalp blood pH determinations during labor and use of ultrasound biophysical profiles in the last trimester could reduce this number significantly (see pages 389 and 381), too few obstetricians take advantage of these important techniques.

The marked increase in cesarean section rates for babies in the breech position is a recent trend based on convincing clinical experience. It is now estimated that 85 percent of all breech births result in cesarean section, compared to 10 percent only 15 years ago. Conversion of a breech to a vertex, or head-first, position through the technique of external cephalic version can be accomplished 70 percent of the time. Unfortunately, too few obstetricians have developed the skills necessary to perform this technique.

Fifteen years ago, 32 weeks of pregnancy (aver-

BIRTH WEIGHT (GRAMS)	PERCENTAGE SURVIVAL
500–750 grams (1 lb. 2 oz.–1 lb.11 oz.)	35–45 percent
750–1,100 grams (1 lb. 11oz.–2 lbs. 4 oz.)	75–80 percent
1,000 grams (2 lbs. 4 oz.)	80–85 percent
1,500 grams (3 lbs. 5 oz.)	90 percent
2,000 grams (4 lbs. 7 oz. or more)	99 percent

age fetal weight of 1700 grams or 3 pounds 12 ounces) was considered the earliest that one could justify the risk of cesarean section, weighed against the benefits for the immature fetus. An obstetrician today is more apt to perform a cesarean section to save a small fetus if ultrasound and clinical history suggest that survival is likely. The following guide summarizes fetal prognosis:

Even in the absence of obvious fetal distress, some doctors have endorsed use of cesarean sections for infants born before the thirty-fifth week and those weighing between 500 and 1,500 grams. One reason for this is that a greater number of premature infants assume a breech position and vaginal delivery is often hazardous because of the larger head diameter when compared to that of the body. As a result, the body of the infant may easily pass through the cervix, but the head may become entrapped at the moment of birth. Some have advocated cesarean sections even when the premature infant is in a head-down position. The reason for this is that smaller babies are more likely to experience intracranial hemorrhage due to pressure on the head caused by uterine muscle contractions and the perineum. Most studies, however, show that there are some potentially serious dangers associated with performing a cesarean section prior to term. Since the cervix is rarely thinned out or effaced at this time, bleeding at the site of the uterine incision can be quite brisk. In addition, either a low vertical or a more extensive classical incision is often needed to deliver the baby (see page 437). Such incisions are weaker and more likely to rupture during a subsequent pregnancy, and they usually preclude an attempt at a subsequent vaginal birth.

With the development of newer and more potent antibiotics, modern blood bank facilities, more sophisticated anesthetic techniques, and improved postpartum care, cesarean section is no longer regarded as a significant risk to a woman. However, we tend to lose sight of the fact that it is still a major abdominal operation accompanied by a significantly higher rate of maternal complications than a vaginal delivery. Occasionally, a couple requests and even demands a cesarean section in preference to the pain and discomfort associated with childbirth. This apparently simple solution is not nearly as innocuous as one would imagine. Even under the most modern and ideal conditions, cesarean section is associated with a four- to fivefold increase in the maternal mortality rate. The most often quoted statistics are that there will be between 4 and 8 maternal deaths per 10,000 cesarean sections, compared to 0.3 per 10,000 following a vaginal birth. The incidence of complications, combined with the longer, more expensive hospital stay, a greater need for blood transfusions, and a prolonged recovery period, makes a cesarean section a far less attractive option than a vaginal birth.

Under what conditions can a woman attempt labor and vaginal delivery following a previous cesarean section?

"Once a cesarean section, always a cesarean section" was first proposed as a clinical dictum by Dr. Edwin B. Craigin in 1916. Until recently, American obstetricians blindly followed this practice, as evidenced by repeat cesarean rates of 86 percent. Thanks to the objections of both consumer advocates and some leading obstetricians, this practice is now being changed in most medical centers. While the majority of women with uterine scars are still being delivered by elective repeat cesarean section, the proportion of vaginal births after cesareans, or VBACs, is increasing dramatically every year.

Evidence to date suggests that between 50 and 85 percent of women who have had cesarean sections should be able to subsequently deliver vaginally if allowed to try. Even when the indication for a primary cesarean section is failure to progress, or dystocia, successful vaginal delivery can be anticipated 70 percent of the time. While proponents of repeat cesarean section may argue that it is easier and safer than a vaginal delivery, statistics do not bear this out. Even under the most ideal conditions, cesarean section has a four- to fivefold higher maternal mortality than vaginal delivery. Cesarean section is a major operation accompanied by a greater blood loss and anesthetic risk than vaginal delivery, and a variety of immediate postoperative problems. Later complications, such as abdominal and pelvic adhesions, may cause intestinal blockage in a small percentage of women years after the surgery has been performed. The newborn mortality rate and the incidence of respiratory distress syndrome (RDS) is higher among babies delivered by cesarean section. Women undergoing cesarean section require significantly more pain medication during the postpartum period and greater amounts of these drugs pass into the breast milk and are ingested by the nursing infant.

Doctors are often too insensitive to the fact that vaginal delivery is far more emotionally satisfying for a woman than cesarean section. Many of my patients have expressed great disappointment and the feeling of having failed because they were unable to experience the physical and psychological "high" of delivering vaginally. The close maternal-infant contact and bonding so vital in the first few days of life is often never realized because the mother suffers from the pain and discomfort of surgery and is sleepy and nauseous from the potent analgesics used. Many women rightfully believe that they have been cheated from experiencing a very special event.

The main argument that proponents of repeat cesarean section have used for years is that rupture or tearing of the previous uterine scar, under the stress of labor contractions, will be accompanied by catastrophic hemorrhage and expulsion of the fetus into the abdominal cavity. This complication, while often a possibility in 1916, is unlikely to happen today. In 1916, all cesarean sections were performed through a **classical incision** into the muscles of the upper uterine segment (see Figure 55). Even after healing, the tissues of the scar from such an incision remain permanently weakened, and uterine expansion during a subsequent pregnancy or labor causes rupture 2 percent of the time. Of this 2 percent, one-half occur during labor and the other half before its onset. The consequences of a classical incision rupture may be truly catastrophic, since the entire uterine wall ruptures. In a complete uterine rupture, the fetus and placenta extrude into the abdominal cavity; the infant mortality rate is between 40 and 75 percent. The maternal mortality from hemorrhage has been estimated at less than 1 percent. Because of the dangers involved, a woman who has had a previous classical cesarean section should never be allowed to attempt labor and vaginal delivery. A repeat cesarean section is the much wiser option. Although still performed today, classical cesarean sections comprise fewer than 5 percent of the total number of cesareans. The operation is occasionally indicated when a baby is premature and the cervix is thick or uneffaced, when the fetal position is unusual, such as a breech or transverse, or when the placenta is covering the preferred incision site over the lower cervix, a condition known as placenta previa.

The so-called **low cervical transverse cesarean section** is performed through the tissues of the

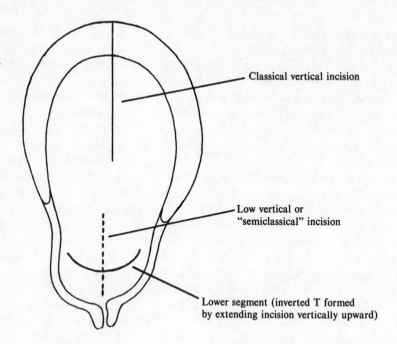

Figure 55 *Types of cesarean section incisions.*

lower uterine segment and cervix. Today, practically all cesareans are of this type. Since connective tissue and only a thin layer of muscle are cut with this incision, it is far less likely to rupture than the classical operation. Another contributing factor is that most of the force of a uterine contraction comes from the upper segment, while the lower segment plays a more passive role. The reported rate of rupture of a low transverse scar is 0.25 to 0.5 percent. Even when it does occur, it hardly ever happens before the onset of labor and is highly unlikely to be catastrophic. It may even go unrecognized because the rupture of a low transverse scar is usually incomplete. At least one tissue layer remains intact, and consequently the baby hardly ever is extruded into the abdominal cavity. Sometimes the uterine tissue layer is so thin that, at the time of a repeat cesarean section, the amniotic fluid and baby can actually be seen through the scar. This phenomenon, appropriately called a

window, is seen in 8 percent of all repeat low transverse cesarean sections. In the rare case when rupture is complete, the perinatal mortality rate can be significant. For this reason, an obstetrician must never be too cavalier in managing the labor of a woman who has had a previous cesarean section. Two articles published in the same 1991 issue of *Obstetrics and Gynecology* graphically illustrate this point. Doctors at the University of Utah Medical Center and Fitzsimmons Army Medical Center in Colorado reported a total of 20 uterine ruptures resulting in death, depression, or permanent neurological damage in three-fourths of the affected infants. Maternal blood loss in the Utah study ranged from 1 to 4 liters, hardly an inconsequential amount.

Despite the rare but potentially serious complication of uterine rupture, clinical studies support the 1988 conclusion of the American College of Obstetricians and Gynecologists that most women with a previous low cervical transverse cesarean section may safely labor and deliver vaginally during a subsequent pregnancy. The College also advised that women with two or more previous cesareans be encouraged to attempt vaginal birth, since there are no data to show that such women are at a greater risk of uterine rupture.

Another type of incision, known as the **inverted T,** usually occurs out of desperation when difficulty is encountered while trying to deliver a baby through a low cervical transverse incision. The base of the T is an ad-lib incision performed to allow more room for the delivery. An inverted T heals into a significantly weaker scar, predisposed to rupture during a future pregnancy.

A small percentage of doctors perform **low vertical,** rather than transverse incisions (see Figure 55). This technique, also known as a **semiclassical incision,** is sometimes helpful for delivering small premature infants, babies in breech or transverse positions, and very large babies. However, this incision is associated with a 1.4 to 4 percent chance of sudden rupture and shock during a subsequent pregnancy or labor. Women with inverted T-type and semiclassical incisions should not be allowed to labor. The four types of incisions discussed are shown in Figure 55.

Knowing the type of incision you had previously is crucial in determining whether or not you should be allowed to labor in a subsequent pregnancy. If you have moved or changed doctors and are contemplating an attempt at a vaginal delivery, it is vital that you secure your previous doctor's operative notes. These are kept on file in the record room of the hospital in which you had your cesarean section. It is only in this way that you will know with certainty the type of incision you received. Many women confuse the scar on their abdominal skin with the type of uterine incision that they received. It is important to understand that a long, vertical scar on the skin is as likely to be associated with a low transverse cervical incision as is a "bikini," or horizontal hairline incision.

Is there any way for a doctor to predict if a transverse low cervical cesarean section scar will hold up when subjected to the stress of labor?

While it has been claimed that certain surgical techniques and the use of specific suture material at the time of cesarean section minimizes scar defects, most obstetricians now believe this is not true. Furthermore, hysterogram and ultrasound are less than ideal predictors of the strength or weakness of the incision. The strength of the previous low cervical transverse incision is only known following a trial of labor during a subsequent pregnancy.

What precautions should be taken when caring for a laboring woman who has had a previous cesarean section?

The same criteria used to assess labor progress for all women should be applied to those undergoing a trial of labor, and you should object to a premature decision to perform a cesarean section. If labor fails to progress, cesarean section should be performed.

Women attempting a vaginal birth following a previous cesarean section for dystocia or failure to progress often ask if their labor will resemble that of a primigravida or a multipara. Based on a preliminary study published in 1990, most women will have labors similar in length or longer than women having their first baby, regardless of when in the course of their previous labor cesarean section was performed for dystocia. This important bit of information should encourage obstetricians to show patience and restraint before resorting to a repeat cesarean.

The use of oxytocin to induce or augment the strength of your contractions during a VBAC attempt is controversial. However, there is no evidence that the incidence of uterine rupture is higher when oxytocin is used judiciously.

You should be admitted to the hospital at the

onset of your earliest contractions and preparations made for immediate cesarean delivery in the event that a uterine rupture is suspected at some point during labor. Adequate emergency preparations include the availability of at least two units of blood for immediate transfusion if needed, an intravenous infusion in a vein of your arm, 24-hour availability of a fully equipped laboratory and blood bank, a readily available anesthesiologist stationed in the hospital, a nearby operating room ready for emergency surgery, and a sufficient number of experienced obstetrical nurses. Most important, your obstetrician should be actively managing your labor at the hospital and not from his or her office. During labor, fetal monitoring is imperative, as is frequent maternal blood pressure and pulse readings, since, occasionally, a rapid pulse is the first sign of a uterine rupture and maternal hemorrhage. Classic signs of uterine rupture include a "tearing" pain in the lower abdomen, tenderness on palpation over the previous scar, a bulge in the abdominal wall over the site of the previous surgery, easily palpable fetal parts through the maternal abdomen, cessation of contractions, ascent rather than descent of the fetal head on vaginal examination, and vaginal bleeding. The advent of fetal monitoring has enabled doctors to identify earlier findings associated with uterine rupture. The use of an intrauterine pressure monitor is a much more sensitive method than clinical symptoms for detecting impending uterine rupture. If this diagnosis is even a remote possibility, it is best to immediately proceed with a cesarean section rather than wait for symptoms to worsen.

Epidural anesthesia, a popular technique used to totally relieve pain during labor, is not recommended by many obstetricians for women undergoing a trial of labor after a previous cesarean section because they fear that, by eliminating all pain, the early symptoms of uterine rupture may not be recognized. However, a growing number of doctors are using epidural anesthesia because they believe that careful monitoring of the fetal heart rate and the strength of uterine contractions will diagnose an impending rupture earlier and more accurately than the symptom of pain over the incision site. An epidural also has the advantage of providing anesthesia if an emergency cesarean section is required.

Although the risk of uterine rupture and obstetrical complications is rare when a woman is allowed a trial of labor, if an emergency does arise, it is best that it happen in a large, well-equipped medical center rather than in a small rural hospital. If you live in an area which lacks a hospital with a modern blood bank, adequate staffing, up-to-date obstetrical facilities, and full-time anesthesia coverage, it is probably best to undergo a repeat cesarean section instead of a trial of labor.

     # EPISIOTOMY

Should I allow my doctor to perform an episiotomy at the time of delivery?

Many women consider an episiotomy to be contrary to their desire for a natural childbirth experience. Despite this, episiotomies are performed in more than 60 percent of all vaginal deliveries and 80 percent of primigravida births. As a result of a number of published articles in recent years that have questioned the wisdom of routine episiotomy, opposition to the procedure is growing.

Briefly stated, an episiotomy is a minor procedure in which an incision is made through the outer vagina and perineum, or the area between the vagina and the rectum. An episiotomy is most often performed as the baby's head is crowning, which means the emerging head is causing the perineum to bulge. If adequate amounts of local anesthesia are used, the performance of the episiotomy and its repair with sutures should both be painless. Childbirth instructors often speak of the natural anesthesia created by the pressure of the baby's head on the perineum during a contraction, stating that if an episiotomy is made during a contraction, it will be painless. Don't believe it! If an episiotomy must be performed, insist that anesthesia be given beforehand. Even if you are lucky enough to experience the natural anesthetic effect, the repair of the episiotomy following delivery is extremely painful in the absence of anesthesia. In addition, injection of a local anesthetic following delivery, when a woman is most sensitive, is often far more painful than if it is given when the baby's head is crowning. The timing of the episiotomy is very important. If done too early, before crowning is evident, bleeding from the incision can be quite brisk. The crowning of the head puts firm pressure against the perineum and its muscles, and the episiotomy site bleeds far less if it is performed at this time. When the episiotomy is made too late, the perineal muscles may be stretching and tearing, thereby defeating the purpose of the procedure.

An incision made exactly in the center is called a median episiotomy, while the mediolateral technique veers off to one side or the other. The median episiotomy has many advantages over the mediolateral, which is extremely painful, is associated with a greater blood loss than the median technique, and leaves a larger and more permanent scar. Proponents of this method claim that it allows more room for difficult deliveries and large babies. However, most experts familiar with both techniques question this. Admittedly, the incidence of extension of the episiotomy into the rectum is greater with the median episiotomy, occurring in 2 to 5 percent of all cases in which this technique is used; it is seen in only 1 percent of all mediolateral episiotomies. However, repair of an extension into the rectum is actually quite simple and is by no means a major catastrophe.

Even the harshest critics of episiotomy concede that it is beneficial under certain circumstances. One of these is shortening the second stage of labor when fetal distress is present and prompt delivery is necessary. Most experts concur that it is also helpful when labor is prolonged and a woman has become exhausted and unable to push the baby out. Breech deliveries often present unique problems and complications; it is best to perform an episiotomy on all women undergoing a vaginal delivery of a baby in the breech position. The use of forceps usually requires an episiotomy. It takes sound judgment on the part of the person delivering the baby to decide if an episiotomy is absolutely indicated.

Obstetricians who are proponents of routine episiotomy claim that it offers other immediate and long-term benefits for both mother and child. However, the medical literature does not support these unsubstantiated premises. In fact, there is some evidence to show that it may cause more harm than good. One of the standard arguments in favor of routine episiotomy is that it prevents excessive stretching and ragged lacerations of the perineal muscles which may result from the pressure of the baby's head and shoulders at the moment of birth. When tears involve the muscles around the rectum they are known as third-degree lacerations, while fourth-degree lacerations extend into the lower portion of the rectum. In recent studies, several investigative groups have found that episiotomies actually increase the incidence of third- and fourth-degree perineal lacerations by initiating a tissue defect and weakness that did not previously exist. While obstetricians generally believe that episiotomy should be performed for most women having their first baby, it is ironic that these are the women who are most likely to suffer severe perineal lacerations resulting from the procedure. In a 1989 study from the Albert Einstein College of Medicine in New York City, doctors reported a twentyfold increase in the frequency of third- and fourth-degree perineal lacerations with the use of episiotomy in women giving birth to their first child. The largest and most recent report evaluating the association between episiotomy and perineal lacerations was conducted by researchers at the National Institutes of Health and the Oklahoma University School of Medicine. After studying 24,000 births, they concluded that women with midline episiotomites were nearly 50 times more likely to suffer severe perineal lacerations than those who did not undergo episiotomy, while women with mediolateral episiotomies had only an eight times greater risk.

The claim that episiotomy prevents cerebral palsy and infant brain damage, by decreasing the amount of time the baby's head pounds against the perineum, is grossly inaccurate, highly unlikely, and certainly not justification for performing an episiotomy.

Myths abound about the effects of episiotomy on a woman's future anatomical appearance and sex life. Some obstetricians claim that prolonged bearing down causes prolapse, or droppage, of the uterus, urinary bladder (cystocele), and rectum (rectocele), and that episiotomy lessens the risk. In fact, the presence of these conditions is more a matter of an inherited predisposition that some women have toward developing weakened pelvic support following childbirth. Some women have given birth to five or more children and still have far healthier vaginal tissues than other women who have had only one child.

The main muscle that is cut at the time of an episiotomy is named the bulbocavernosus. When you consciously contract this muscle, you narrow the vaginal opening and can enhance your sexual enjoyment to some degree. Some obstetricians believe that episiotomy will prevent the tearing, stretching, and weakening of the bulbocavernosus muscle, thereby enhancing a woman's future sexuality. Opponents take the opposite view: that a woman's sexuality may be diminished because these important muscles, and the nerves which supply them, are permanently weakened when episiotomy is performed. There is little in the way of scientific data to show whether the performance or nonperformance of episiotomy ultimately en-

hances or detracts from a woman's sex life. In two recent studies from England, doctors found that women who did not receive episiotomies were significantly less likely to experience pain-free intercourse three months postpartum. In 1991, Dr. Michael Klein and his associates at McGill University in Canada tried to scientifically measure the strength of the bulbocavernosus using a tampon-sized instrument called an electromyographic perineometer. Women whose perineums remained intact during childbirth, meaning no episiotomy and no lacerations, were found to have the strongest muscles, fewer bowel and bladder problems, less pain on intercourse, and earlier resumption of intercourse postpartum. Based on these findings, Dr. Klein concluded that there was no evidence to sustain the claim that episiotomy use prevents stretching of the pelvic floor.

All women, regardless of whether or not they have had an episiotomy, will benefit from muscle setting, or Kegel's exercises, which are very useful in overcoming mild or moderate amounts of bulbocavernosus weakening following childbirth and also strengthen the muscles which surround the vagina, bladder, and rectum following delivery. The simplest Kegel exercise is to tighten the muscles of the buttocks as though trying to prevent the escape of feces from the anus. The same group of muscles is also used to try to stop the flow of urine in midstream. After learning Kegel's exercises, you must practice them at least 100 times per day for a minimum of six months. In addition, each time you pass urine, voluntarily interrupt the flow several times. If you perform these exercises diligently, you will note improvement in your ability to tighten the muscles surrounding the vagina and perineum.

Many women believe that midwives possess a magical ability to avoid unnecessary episiotomies, while obstetricians hunger for a chance to perform the procedure even when it isn't indicated. In addition, it has been said that if women were allowed to squat or sit during delivery, instead of being forced to lie down, episiotomy would be unnecessary because the laboring mother would work with, not against, the forces of gravity. These observations are probably more accurate than obstetricians would care to admit. A 1989 study from Albert Einstein College of Medicine in New York City found that when a woman was positioned on her back with her legs in the stirrups, she was more likely to require an episiotomy than if she was permitted to assume a less conventional position. Several authors have reported lower laceration rates among women who deliver their babies in the lateral, or side, position.

As soon as the baby distends the perineum, a doctor or midwife may place a towel over the woman's rectum and exert upward pressure on the baby's chin through the perineum. Some claim that this technique, known as the Ritgen maneuver, allows a slow and careful delivery of the baby's head and also helps to prevent perineal lacerations. However, excessive pressure placed in this fashion can occasionally force the head upward and cause lacerations around the mother's urethra. Since these lacerations are often more painful and difficult to anesthetize and suture than perineal lacerations, a Ritgen maneuver should be done with

moderation and not in excess. Some midwives and obstetricians prefer not to use the Ritgen maneuver. Instead, they keep the baby's head flexed and push the maternal perineum around the head. This prevents extension of the head until the final moment before birth.

Another technique that has gained great popularity is referred to as "ironing out the perineum"; the perineal muscles are gradually stretched by applying digital pressure against the vaginal wall during the final stages of labor. Some women tolerate this very well, but others find it quite annoying and irritating. It is believed that this procedure decreases the necessity for episiotomy, but there is no proof that it does. Neither has use of various lotions for massaging the perineum been shown to increase its capacity to stretch and accommodate the birth of the baby.

In summary, despite its common application, there is little evidence to support the routine use of episiotomy. The procedure may well increase the incidence of third- and fourth-degree perineal lacerations, and there is no scientific evidence that it prevents relaxation of the pelvic tissues.

ANESTHESIA AND ANALGESIA

How is local anesthesia used in obstetrics?

An anesthetic is any substance that obliterates pain either through induction of unconsciousness (general anesthesia) or by interrupting the pathway of nerves which carry sensations of pain to the brain. The term "balanced anesthesia" refers to a technique in which a combination of drugs, each in a dosage sufficient to produce its own desired effects, is used to achieve a light state of general anesthesia with muscle relaxation and minimal exposure of the fetus to the anesthetic agents. Regional anesthetics, such as pudendal block and epidural,

numb specific regions over the lower half of the body, while local anesthesia obliterates pain over a small and well-defined area such as the skin over the episiotomy site. Analgesics are drugs which relieve or diminish the intense pain without complete loss of sensation or of consciousness. Many of the same drugs that produce anesthesia will provide analgesia at lower doses. Narcotic analgesics, such as morphine, meperidine (trade name Demerol), and fentanyl (trade name Sublimaze), will relieve or diminish the intensity of pain when given intravenously, intramuscularly, subcutaneously (below the skin), and most recently, as an epidural. (The effects of narcotic analgesics have been previously discussed; see Chapter 9.)

I am frequently asked which anesthetic is best, and my standard, but accurate, response is that the perfect anesthetic has not yet been invented. Even the safest of methods may occasionally be associated with undesirable side effects. For this reason, it is encouraging to note the growing number of couples enrolling in childbirth education classes. Regardless of whether one is a Lamaze, Grantly Dick-Read, or Bradley enthusiast, women practicing these methods usually require or request less analgesia and anesthesia during labor and delivery.

The simplest and safest form of anesthesia is the injection of medications, such as procaine (trade name Novocaine), chloroprocaine (trade name Nesacaine), or lidocaine (trade name Xylocaine), just below the skin of the perineum at the site of the episiotomy (see previous discussion). This local anesthetic is administered just as the baby's head is crowning, as the emerging head is causing the perineum to bulge, and relieves pain only for the performance and repair of the episiotomy. Lidocaine is the most commonly used agent for this technique. However, a recent pharmacologic study has shown that when it is used for local perineal anesthesia, considerable amounts rapidly enter the maternal circulation, cross the placenta, and achieve highest levels in the newborn's bloodstream. Although no discernible evidence of adverse effects is likely to be noted in an infant following a maternal perineal injection of lidocaine, chloroprocaine is probably a better choice since little if any enters the baby's circulation.

A pudendal nerve block anesthetizes the outer vagina, vulva, and perineum, or those areas containing branches of the two pudendal nerves. When performed correctly, this popular technique provides adequate perineal anesthesia for spontaneous delivery, as well as the performance and repair of the episiotomy. Although enthusiasts claim that a pudendal block provides adequate anesthesia for a low forceps delivery, most obstetricians would agree that it is less than adequate for

this purpose. To anesthetize the left pudendal nerve, a doctor inserts the left index and middle fingers deep into the left side of the vagina in order to locate the ischial spine. This bony landmark is important because it is in close proximity to the pudendal nerve. A long needle, housed in a protective sleeve or guide, is then inserted between the doctor's fingers and the vaginal wall and advanced to a point just below the spine. The needle is several inches long, but only the last centimeter is inserted below the vaginal surface at this location. The local anesthetic is then injected and the procedure is then repeated on the opposite side.

A paracervical block is the injection of a local anesthetic into the tissues surrounding the cervix. A properly placed paracervical block can completely relieve the pain of cervical dilatation for one to two hours. Repeat injections may be given whenever the pain returns. Specially designed indwelling catheters, which pass out of the vagina and can be strapped to a woman's thigh or abdomen, make it possible to reinject additional amounts every 45 minutes to 1 hour without having to reinsert the needle. Since a paracervical block provides no perineal, vaginal, or vulvar pain relief, another form of anesthesia is needed as the head begins to distend the vagina and perineum following full cervical dilatation.

A spinal, or subarachnoid, block is a frequently used anesthetic technique which provides deep pain relief for either a vaginal delivery or a cesarean section. To perform a spinal block, a long, fine needle is inserted between the bony processes of two adjacent vertebrae in the lower back. The needle is then advanced through the dura, or outer membrane, covering the spinal cord. When the dura has been punctured and the subarachnoid space entered, clear spinal fluid flows through the end of the needle. The anesthetic is then injected through the needle, bringing almost instantaneous relief of pain, numbness over the lower half of the body, loss of voluntary movement of the legs, and an inability to use the abdominal muscles during bearing down efforts.

If a woman is given a spinal block and then maintained in a sitting position for a minute or two after the anesthesia is administered, the medication settles to a lower level and numbs only her vagina, perineum, and inner thighs. This distribution of pain relief, with the exception of the vagina, covers most areas which would come in contact with a saddle if one were riding a horse. A spinal block of this type is appropriately named a saddle block. A saddle block provides excellent anesthesia for a vaginal delivery and forceps operation, and also has the advantage of maintaining some voluntary bearing down efforts of the abdominal wall musculature. Saddle block anesthesia should not be administered for a vaginal delivery until the cervix is completely dilated and the baby's head is deep in the pelvis, because the saddle block interferes with the normal descent of the head, possibly resulting in the need for a difficult mid-forceps delivery.

While an obstetrician is responsible for injecting a paracervical and pudendal nerve block, in most hospitals a spinal anesthetic is usually administered by a trained anesthesiologist. Although the technique of spinal block is extremely easy to learn and master, it may still be associated with serious complications. Patients receiving this form of anesthesia require careful monitoring of their vital signs, and an anesthesiologist should be available throughout the delivery and for at least 30 minutes following its completion.

Severe headache following a spinal block may occur in as many as 10 to 20 percent of all women receiving this form of anesthesia. These headaches are often incapacitating and may last for several days. The cause of spinal headache is believed to be the leakage of spinal fluid from the site of the needle puncture. The risk of this complication can be minimized if a small 25- or 26-gauge needle is used.

With a spinal block, the needle passes through the dura and into the spinal fluid, while the epidural needle is more superficial and does not perforate the dura. Unlike a spinal block, an epidural

or peridural block may be given before the cervix is fully dilated, and it provides excellent anesthesia during the entire active phase of labor, spontaneous vaginal delivery, forceps operations, or cesarean section. An epidural may dull a woman's bearing down reflex during the second stage of labor, but it is less likely to do this than a spinal block. Epidural is rapidly becoming the most widely used form of regional block for relief of pain during labor. In fact, most Lamaze and Dick-Read childbirth instructors now recognize it as a compatible and acceptable addition to the childbirth experience.

Periodic administration of small increments of local anesthesia during the first stage of labor provides epidural analgesia that can later be extended for pain relief during either vaginal delivery or cesarean section. This technique results in a low total dosage and reduces the amount of drug which is transmitted to the fetus throughout labor. The frequency of anesthetic redosing is usually determined by a woman's perception that the painful contractions have returned and are worsening. One drawback to administering an epidural in this fashion is that each time redosing is necessary, one has to locate an anesthesiologist who, in turn, must return to the bedside and reinject the anesthetic. It then may take an additional 10 to 20 minutes for the epidural to reach its previous level of effectiveness. To remedy this situation, a growing number of medical centers are using low-dose infusion pump techniques in which premeasured amounts of a local anesthetic are given at a slow and continuous pace through the epidural catheter, thereby providing more predictable pain relief.

Another modern addition to epidural anesthesia is known as PCEA, or patient-controlled epidural anesthesia. With this technique, the patient pushes a button and a predetermined, computer-regulated amount of local anesthesia is injected into the epidural catheter. A built-in safety mechanism shuts off the flow of medication if a woman pushes the button at too frequent intervals. While some researchers have concluded that women using PCEA will require considerably less local anesthesia than nonusers receiving epidural in the standard fashion, other studies have found just the opposite to be true.

All local anesthetics administered epidurally have the potential to cause a variety of nervous system and cardiovascular complications, most of which are easily remedied (see next question). The likelihood and severity of these problems can be minimized by combining a lower dose of the local anesthetic with a narcotic, such as fentanyl or sufentanil, in the epidural. Some investigators have reported success in relieving pain during the first stage of labor by using only fentanyl in place of a local anesthetic.

One of the greatest advances in the management of postoperative cesarean section pain has been the use of epidural morphine (trade name Duramorph). When Duramorph is injected immediately after the delivery of the baby it can provide pain relief for the first 24 postoperative hours. In contrast, fentanyl's analgesic effect has an average duration of approximately 4 hours. Some anesthesiologists leave the epidural catheter in place for as long as two or three days following a cesarean and periodically inject Duramorph or fentanyl as it is needed.

In addition to an epidural block, peridural anesthesia may also be administered by inserting a needle into the lower end of the sacral bone at the base of the spine. This form of anesthesia is known as a caudal (meaning tail) block. Continuous caudal anesthesia is possible with a plastic catheter. The caudal block technique requires a great deal of skill and uses a far greater quantity of anesthetic than epidurals in order to be effective. In addition, the increased pelvic and abdominal muscle relaxation produced by this technique may impede progress in the second stage of labor. While caudal block was formerly a very popular method of childbirth anesthesia, it has been widely replaced by the simpler and safer epidural technique.

What are some of the drawbacks of using general anesthesia for delivery?

The use of general anesthesia in obstetrics has declined dramatically in recent years. Several large studies show that any general anesthetic given to the mother rapidly crosses the placenta and enters the fetal circulation. Babies exposed to this form of anesthesia are more likely to be depressed at birth than those who are delivered under local, pudendal, spinal, or epidural block.

Childbirth education classes have emphasized the importance of viewing labor and delivery as a shared experience for a couple. A father will be deprived of seeing his baby being born because most hospitals will not allow him in the delivery room or the operating room when general anesthesia is being administered. (Women under general anesthesia are usually unable to bear down or cooperate in the birth of the baby. As a result, forceps are usually required for a vaginal birth.) In addition to preventing a woman from experiencing an unequalled moment of joy when her baby first cries, the drowsiness induced by general anesthesia also hinders early maternal-infant bonding and nursing during the immediate postpartum period.

One of the greatest disadvantages of general anesthesia is the ever-present threat that the contents of the stomach may be vomited and then aspirated into the lungs. The material from the stomach contains undigested food which can cause airway obstruction and death. Even if a woman has fasted, and there is no food in her stomach, aspiration of the strongly acidic stomach secretions may be even more deadly. General anesthesia has become the leading cause of maternal deaths in the United States.

What types of general anesthesia are used in obstetrics?

In addition to eliminating painful sensations, general anesthesia also induces loss of consciousness, muscle movement, and reflex activity. Nitrous oxide, a gas administered through an anesthetic face mask, may be used to provide relief of pain during labor as well as delivery. While nitrous oxide should never be used for minor surgery or dental work during the first trimester because it may be associated with a higher incidence of birth defects, during the first stage of labor a 50 percent concentration mixed with 50 percent oxygen can be inhaled as soon as each uterine contraction begins. It is then withdrawn as the contraction subsides. During the second stage of labor, a woman can take three or four deep breaths of gas, hold the last breath, and then bear down. Nitrous oxide does not affect uterine contractions or prolong labor. Although it is classified as an anesthetic, nitrous oxide cannot provide total pain relief since concentrations required for complete relief provide too little oxygen for a woman and her fetus, and may even be fatal if administered over a period of several minutes. When combined with another anesthetic, it can usually provide adequate pain relief for episiotomy, delivery, and repair of the episiotomy.

Nitrous oxide may also be used effectively for cesarean section or difficult vaginal delivery if combined with an intravenous barbiturate named thiopental and a muscle-paralyzing medication named succinylcholine. This so-called crash induction, or balanced inhalation anesthesia procedure, begins with a small intravenous dose of a drug named D-tubocurarine to block muscle twitching, followed by a rapid intravenous injection of the thiopental to induce instant anesthesia and unconsciousness. Immediately after the thiopental is given, an intravenous injection of succinylcholine is administered in order to prevent movement and allow adequate muscle relaxation so that a plastic breathing tube may be placed in the trachea. The nitrous oxide gas is then given through the tracheal tube in order to maintain an anesthetic that will not depress the infant. A cesarean section incision can usually be made immediately after the tube has been passed into the trachea. This technique provides adequate anesthesia for 15 to 20 minutes, and the baby can almost always be delivered during this period of time. Additional anesthesia can then be added in order to prevent the mother from experiencing any discomfort for the remainder of the procedure. Any competent obstetrician can easily deliver a baby in 3 minutes after the skin incision is made. Rapid delivery in this fashion prevents these drugs from accumulating in the baby's body and causing respiratory depression at birth.

Ethylene is an anesthetic gas which is similar to nitrous oxide in its activity, but it has the distinct disadvantage of an unpleasant odor. It is also more likely to cause nausea and vomiting. As a result, it is rarely used in most obstetrical units.

Cyclopropane is a potent anesthetic gas which until recently was commonly used for both vaginal and cesarean section births. It is highly flammable and explosive, causes abnormal heart rhythms when administered with oxytocin or methergine, may induce an elevation of the blood pressure, and can cause severe maternal and fetal respiratory depression. This last complication may be intensified when cyclopropane is given following the use of narcotics or barbiturates earlier in labor. In addition to these drawbacks, cyclopropane is frequently associated with nausea and vomiting. One might logically ask, "Why on earth would anyone use this terrible anesthetic?" Though it is infrequently used in most hospitals today, in the past it was invaluable in inducing anesthesia rapidly during certain acute obstetrical emergencies.

The group of gases classified as volatile anesthetics include ether, chloroform, halothane (trade name Fluorthane), methoxyflurane (trade name Penthrane), and enflurane (trade name Ethrane). Chloroform and ether will rarely be found or used in a modern obstetrical suite because of unpleasant side effects and complications associated with their use.

Halothane, a potent, rapidly acting anesthetic

gas, has the unique ability to totally relax the uterine muscles. For this reason, it is the anesthetic of choice for those rare situations which require complete uterine relaxation, such as version, or turning, of a second twin or the emergency delivery of a baby in a difficult breech position. Halothane's major advantage, namely the relaxation which it provides, is also its main disadvantage because the uterine muscles may fail to contract following delivery. This may lead to severe postpartum hemorrhage. Attempts to remedy this situation with oxytocin and methergine are often unsuccessful.

Methoxyflurane, better known by the name of Penthrane, is a popular gas for both analgesia and anesthesia at the time of delivery. It is pleasant to breathe and can be self-administered. A woman actually holds the inhaler in her hand and rapidly breathes the Penthrane throughout her contractions. During the second stage of labor, the anesthetic may be inhaled just before the bearing down begins. In proper analgesic concentrations, the gas will cause no harm to a mother or her fetus, but close nursing surveillance is necessary to be sure that too much Penthrane is not inhaled. Although somewhat helpful for relief of pain during a spontaneous vaginal delivery, self-administered Penthrane is totally inadequate if forceps are to be applied. In higher anesthetic concentrations, it may cause maternal and newborn respiratory depression, bradycardia, impairment of kidney and liver function, a drop in blood pressure, an abnormal amount of postpartum uterine relaxation, and a higher incidence of postpartum blood loss. Induction of full anesthesia with Pentrane often takes several minutes; for this reason it is less than adequate when immediate delivery is indicated.

Enflurane is rarely used for complete obstetrical anesthesia because of its many side effects, its possible role in causing impaired kidney function, and its effects on the heart. However, in low concentrations it can provide excellent pain relief when inhaled during contractions in the second stage of labor. In addition to providing rapid analgesia, enflurane is pleasant to breathe and does not cause respiratory depression in the baby.

Thiopental (trade name Pentothal) is a rapidly acting barbiturate which is given intravenously to induce sleep for a cesarean section. It is also given intravenously, although less frequently, for a vaginal delivery combined with a general anesthetic. Ketamine hydrochloride, a relatively new nonbarbiturate anesthetic which can be administered intravenously or intramuscularly, has recently been gaining popularity because, unlike thiopental, it will rarely cause maternal or infant respiratory depression. Barbiturates may impair reflexes in the pharynx and larynx and cause choking, but ketamine in properly administered doses is less likely to do this. Instead, it produces an almost trancelike state in which the patient appears to be awake but experiences amnesia and no pain, an effect termed "dissociative anesthesia" because it selectively interrupts pain pathways to the brain without altering other nervous reflexes. Ketamine has been used as the sole anesthetic for vaginal delivery, for short minor surgical procedures, and for inducing anesthesia prior to administering other agents. It can also be combined with a low-potency anesthetic such as nitrous oxide to enhance its efficacy.

No anesthetic is perfect, and ketamine is certainly not an exception. It can elevate the blood pressure, and women with heart disease and hypertension must be carefully monitored. One of the most serious and common problems associated with ketamine use is bizarre psychological behavior, a reaction reported to occur in as many as 12 percent of women who are anesthetized with this drug. Reactions may range from a pleasant, dreamlike state to hallucinations and delirium. Although no known permanent psychological effects have been reported, the bizarre behavior pattern may last for a few hours and in some cases for as long as 24 hours. Experience with ketamine use for vaginal delivery and cesarean section is limited, but reports suggest that it rapidly crosses the placenta and has the potential to cause some degree of central nervous system depression in the fetus, especially when multiple doses are administered during labor.

How can the complications associated with general anesthesia be decreased?

Given the choice between general anesthesia and one of the local anesthetic techniques, it is the wise woman who selects the second option. If general anesthesia is contemplated, the hazards associated with aspiration of stomach contents into the respiratory tract can be markedly reduced if food is withheld for at least 8 hours before the onset of contractions. Unfortunately, one is never clairvoyant enough to predict when labor will begin, and the fullness of one's stomach is often a matter of chance. However, if your amniotic membranes rupture before the onset of contractions, do not eat any solid foods since it is a good bet that labor will begin within a few hours. Similarly, if you are having contractions suggestive of early labor, don't eat solid foods or drink large quantities of liquid. To neutralize the deadly chemical reaction in the lungs caused by aspiration of acidic gastric juices, women who are to receive a general anesthetic should be given a clear, nonparticulate antacid such as sodium citrate or Bicitra within 30 minutes of the anesthetic induction.

It is essential that all women receiving general anesthesia for vaginal or cesarean delivery have a tube inserted into the trachea immediately after sleep is induced. The most important factor in reducing general anesthetic complications is an attentive, alert, and skilled board-certified anesthesiologist using up-to-date monitoring techniques such as pulse oximetry. The pulse oximeter consists of a sensor attached to both the computer and a patient's fingertip or toe. It is capable of continuously and accurately measuring arterial blood oxygen saturation, respirations, and pulse rate, and can often identify abnormalities in arterial oxygenation before they become serious and potentially irreversible. Experts believe that if pulse oximetry was used extensively it could prevent 50 percent of the annual deaths attributed to general anesthesia. If there is any doubt as to whether a woman has aspirated while under general anesthesia, her arterial blood gases should be measured immediately. Treatment for this potentially catastrophic emergency includes clearing the airway, mechanical ventilation, and providing supportive therapy such as intravenous fluids and drugs to maintain the blood pressure. The use of antibiotics and steroids has both advocates and detractors.

When is general anesthesia more appropriate than spinal, caudal, or epidural anesthesia?

Caudal, epidural, and spinal anesthesia can cause significant lowering of the blood pressure. When administered in the presence of obstetrical hemorrhage, they intensify the problem and create difficulties in supplying blood and oxygen to a woman's vital organs and placenta. For this reason, a general anesthetic is a far better choice in the presence of abruptio placenta, placenta previa, and other conditions which cause heavy bleeding.

Women with severe hypertension and preeclampsia are far more likely to experience a drastic drop in blood pressure following caudal, epidural, and spinal block. This may sound like a good method of treating high blood pressure, but in fact it is extremely dangerous for the maternal and fetal circulation. Proponents of using caudal, epidural, or spinal block in the presence of hypertension maintain that severe complications caused by a drop in blood pressure are unlikely if a woman is carefully monitored and precautions are taken. The choice of anesthesia for the hypertensive woman is not always simple, especially since studies have shown that there may be a tremendous increase in blood pressure accompanying the induction of general anesthesia and insertion of an endotracheal tube. Epidural anesthesia is often the better choice for women with hypertension, preeclampsia, diabetes, or cardiac disease in pregnancy.

Other deterrents to the use of local anesthetic

techniques include the presence of a superficial skin infection at or near the intended puncture site, as well as bony deformities of the spine, previous low back surgery, a blood clotting disorder, a low platelet count, a history of a herniated disc, evidence of neurologic disease, and chronic low back pain of unknown cause.

When fetal distress is extreme and immediate delivery becomes urgent, epidural and caudal anesthesia are extremely poor anesthetic choices. Spinal is better because it takes effect at least twice as fast, but a rapid "crash induction" with general anesthesia is probably the fastest method of delivering the infant.

If anesthesia is needed for a vaginal delivery of a baby in the breech position, general anesthesia is sometimes preferred to spinal or epidural because the head can be more easily manipulated and delivered without trauma. Other abnormal fetal positions requiring uterine relaxation and manipulation may be encountered in the delivery of a second twin. In these situations, no anesthetic compares to halothane. The various local anesthetic techniques are totally inadequate for this type of intrauterine manipulation.

How is patient-controlled analgesia used obstetrically?

Patient-controlled analgesia (PCA) is an innovative technique in which a patient self-administers a preset dose of an intravenous narcotic, through a syringe fixed in a pump linked to a computer. By pressing a button, a woman is able to activate the computer to deliver the analgesic dose instantly. Overmedication or abuse cannot occur with PCA because there is a time period, known as the lock-out interval, when the pump cannot be triggered. The PCA device can also be programmed for a continuous small-dose infusion, with periodic increase as needed. As previously mentioned, patient-controlled analgesia is also gaining popularity as a method of administering patient-controlled epidural anesthesia.

Experience with intravenous PCA for control of pain during labor and in the days following a cesarean section is limited at the present time. Some studies have shown that the total narcotic dose required during labor is less with PCA than when it is given in the standard manner by a nurse following a patient's request. Other studies, however, have not confirmed these findings. In a 1989 study published in *Obstetrics and Gynecology*, doctors from the University of Nebraska reported that they were less than impressed with the supposed benefits of PCA. When compared to a control group of women receiving meperidine for pain in the standard manner, those on PCA meperidine used significantly greater amounts of the drug, and more of their infants required naloxone (Narcan) to reverse the depressive effects on the respiratory system.

On the basis of patient satisfaction scores, most researchers have reported that women who use PCA narcotics during labor appear significantly more satisfied with their level of pain control than women receiving narcotics in the standard nurse-administered fashion.

 NATURAL CHILDBIRTH

What is your opinion of the different methods of natural childbirth?

The term "natural childbirth" had its origins in 1933 with the publication of a book with that same title, written by the English physician Grantly Dick-Read. In this book and in another, *Childbirth Without Fear*, Dick-Read formulated his "fear-tension-pain" theory. Simply stated, he observed that those women who were most fearful experienced the most pain, while those who appeared calm had the easiest labors. The Grantly Dick-Read method, therefore, involved educating women so that they would be more knowledgeable about and less fearful of labor, thereby breaking the vicious cycle of fear, tension, and pain. Grantly Dick-Read further emphasized relaxation and breathing exercises. Today, his method is widely practiced in Britain and Canada, although it is far less popular in the United States.

The Bradley method, named after Robert Bradley, an American physician, has achieved only limited popularity in the United States. Presently, there are approximately 1,200 certified instructors in the United States and an estimated 10,000 to 20,000 births each year among women using this method. Dr. Bradley adopted Grantly Dick-Read's principles and later added an emphasis on "husband-coached" childbirth, in which vital and active participation of the father becomes necessary for success. Bradley classes differ from most other types of childbirth education in many important ways. A special series of eight "early bird meetings" begin as soon as a woman's pregnancy is confirmed. Some of the early pregnancy topics include anatomy, nutrition, and physiology of pregnancy. Regular weekly sessions start at the sixth month of pregnancy to allow parents plenty of time to evaluate their needs and to find cooperative medical care. Unlike the more publicized Lamaze method, Bradley instructors deplore rapid breathing techniques which can, on rare occasions, lead to exhaustion, dizziness, and hyperventilation as well as reduction in the oxygen supplied to the fetus. Instead, the Bradley method emphasizes that mothers continue to breathe normally throughout labor and birth. Bradley instructors teach relaxation training to the woman and her partner so that even under the stress of labor she can relax groups of muscles. Her partner's role is to instruct her and determine if she has indeed achieved a relaxed state. In childbirth classes and practice at home, the couple feel and learn to detect the difference between tense and relaxed muscles; they learn to

achieve immediate relaxation of tense muscles at the first sign of simulated contractions. The father-coach whispers encouragement and praise to the mother in labor. To date, I have seen only a handful of Bradley-coached couples, but I have been most impressed with the success they have achieved.

The most popular method of prepared childbirth in the United States is the Lamaze method, or Psychoprophylaxis. Introduced in France in 1951 by the now-immortalized French obstetrician Fernand Lamaze, the method has made it possible for millions of women to experience controlled childbirth with a minimum of anesthesia. The Lamaze method was first popularized in this country by Marjorie Karmel in 1959 with the publication of her book, *Thank You, Dr. Lamaze.*

With the Lamaze method, a women under the direction of her partner carries out a variety of controlled breathing exercises. The rate of breathing is determined by the strength and frequency of the contractions. By totally focusing on the breathing patterns and a "concentration point," such as a picture on a nearby wall, a woman is able to block out the pain stimuli to that area of the brain which interprets them. Psychoprophylaxis enthusiasts do not deny the existence of pain in labor, but they distract themselves with their controlled breathing techniques so completely that many report painless labor.

Several large studies have documented the medical value of the Lamaze method. One at Northwestern University noted that Lamaze-prepared women had only 25 percent the number of cesarean sections and 20 percent the incidence of fetal distress compared to a group of women who had not undergone childbirth preparation. Infant deaths were 25 percent lower in the Lamaze group, and maternal infection rates and perineal lacerations were also significantly lower. Other studies have concluded that women trained in the Lamaze method were more likely to have a shorter first stage of labor (the time from the onset of regular contractions to full dilatation of the cervix) and required significantly less narcotic medication than those not using this method.

Much has been written about the potentially harmful effects of hyperventilation caused by La-maze breathing, but I believe that this danger has been grossly exaggerated. It is true that excessive rapid breathing can lead to exhaustion, dizziness, muscle spasm, and even a decrease in oxygen supplied to the baby. However, such instances are extremely rare. Furthermore, an attentive nurse or doctor can prevent or correct the problem simply by having a woman breathe into a bag. When the woman rebreathes her exhaled carbon dioxide gas, symptoms associated with rapid breathing quickly disappear.

The term "natural childbirth" should probably be obliterated from the modern obstetrical vocabulary and replaced by more appropriate descriptions such as "prepared," "aware," and "family-centered" childbirth—terms used to describe a number of methods for preparing and educating both mother and father so that pregnancy, labor, and delivery are positive and beautiful experiences, resulting in the birth of a healthy infant. In the past, one of the arguments against Lamaze and other childbirth methods was the lack of flexibility of the instructors who taught them. Couples were instructed to refuse analgesics, and those who requested them often experienced guilt for being such weaklings. Fortunately, a more liberal attitude now prevails, and many childbirth instructors teach that the use of analgesics and epidural block are both integral and acceptable additions to a successful childbirth experience. With refinements in the administration of anesthesia, a growing number of women are delivering babies using breathing and relaxation exercises as well as analgesics to control pain. The definition of natural childbirth has happily evolved and changed so that it now includes any birth in which a woman is awake and delivers vaginally. In other words, you don't have to be consumed with pain to deliver "naturally."

 # GENTLE BIRTH

What is meant by the term "gentle birth"?

Until recently, American obstetricians took great pride in bringing newborns into the world with a vigorous slap on the buttocks while hoisting the baby aloft by its ankles. The latter procedure, reported to cause orthopedic problems for some babies, has been abandoned by most doctors. Thanks to the influence of a French obstetrician named Frederick Leboyer, the slap on the buttocks has been replaced by the more humane and natural "gentle birth" in many delivery rooms throughout the United States.

Leboyer's thesis, outlined in his book, *Birth Without Violence* (1974), is that birth is a violent experience for a baby and is made even more violent by insensitive treatment in the delivery room. Examples of this insensitivity are excessive amounts of noise, bright lights, early clamping of the umbilical cord, and excessive suctioning of the baby's mouth secretions. To correct this trauma, the Leboyer remedy is to darken the delivery room, keep it warm and quiet, and to place the newborn immediately on its mother's abdomen and enhance this skin-to-skin contact by gently massaging the baby at the same time. The umbilical cord is cut approximately 5 minutes later, when it has stopped pulsating. Then the baby is placed in a tepid bath, which Dr. Leboyer claims is a soothing return to the weightlessness of existence in the amniotic fluid.

Many caustic comments came from the medical establishment in response to Dr. Leboyer's unscientific book, but claims that the dim lights and lack of suctioning would endanger the baby have not been substantiated. Furthermore, Dr. Leboyer never advocated abandoning good, sound medical practice when it proves necessary. The pundits may ridicule the simplicity of the Leboyer method, but the contentment noted on the face of a Leboyer baby is the best argument in its defense.

To date, the few published reports evaluating the Leboyer method have all attested to its safety. In 1980, doctors at Pennsylvania State University compared the outcome of pregnancy among 87 mothers delivered by the Leboyer method with a control group using conventional techniques. Mothers and infants in both groups did equally well. Nurses caring for the newborns, when asked to make six subjective assessments of the infants, noted no significant differences between the Leboyer and control group in contentment, "smilability," sleep-wake cycle, sucking ability, reaction to circumcision, and reaction to eye care. Couples participating in Leboyer births are enthusiastic about the method, particularly praising the father's participation and the serene atmosphere of the delivery room.

Dr. David A. Kliot and Dr. Max I. Lilling of the Brookdale Hospital Medical Center in New York, who have attended hundreds of Leboyer births, find this method to be as safe as traditional delivery styles and note medical benefits as well. The maternal abdomen proved to be as effective a heat source as the radiant warmers used in most delivery rooms. In addition, they found that by placing the baby in the prone position on the mother's abdomen and massaging its back, the possibility of aspiration of secretions and mucus into the mouth, nose, throat, and lungs was decreased, and the use of a suction apparatus to remove secretions was rarely needed. The postural drainage achieved in the face-down position effectively cleared the nasopharyngeal cavity. While placing a baby on its mother's abdomen immediately after birth has several positive effects, it should be pointed out that it does have the disadvantage of depriving the newborn of all the blood that it should receive from the placenta. The reason for this is that blood in the umbilical cord does not flow upward, and a transfusion into the newborn's circulation will only occur if it is held below the level of the placenta for 1 to 3 minutes following its birth.

Reports in newspapers and popular women's magazines claiming that Leboyer children are socially and psychologically better adjusted than conventionally delivered infants are based on some very unscientific observations made by a French psychologist. To date, there are no large scientific studies to support these claims.

The natural extension of a "gentle birth" is the immediate nursing of the baby in the delivery room and extensive close contact of the mother with her baby during the early hours and days of life. Both experimental animal studies and observations of human behavior emphasize the importance of early maternal-infant bonding, which is achieved by close physical and emotional contact immediately after birth. Eye-to-eye contact, tactile contact, caressing, and verbal contact all enhance this relationship. Routine eye care with silver nitrate is a hindrance to maternal-infant bonding and should be delayed for at least 1 hour following birth, except when there has been a recent positive gonorrhea culture from the cervix or prolonged rupture of the membranes. Other eye-care options may cause fewer problems in this regard (see page 162).

HOSPITAL BIRTH

How can I make my admission and discharge from the hospital as easy as possible?

Often, the greatest obstacles encountered by a couple electing to have their child in a hospital arise at the time of arrival to the admitting office. Entering an unfamiliar environment for the first time can be unnerving, and under such circumstances it is often difficult to be assertive when dealing with unyielding and narrow-minded hospital employees. Be assertive! Your efforts will be rewarded. Tour and inspect the hospital earlier in your pregnancy so that admission to the delivery room will be less foreboding. You should find out ahead of time which entrance to use, what the admission procedures are, and what financial arrangements are necessary. Many hospitals have preadmission procedures which enable you to complete much of the paperwork during the last two months of pregnancy. It's much easier to attend to these matters before the need is urgent. At the time of admission, if you are faced with a new admissions clerk asking unnecessary and irrelevant questions, the best advice is to insist on seeing the nursing supervisor immediately. Don't let the hospital or obstetrical staff intimidate you.

After being admitted to the hospital, you will be taken to the labor and delivery area. Most hospitals have a variety of labor and birthing rooms, some more attractive and comfortable than others. If you did not make note of this during your previous hospital tour, you should ask to look at the rooms which are available. After you are in the room which you have selected, you will be given a hospital gown to wear and a nurse or resident physician will ask some brief questions about your previous medical and obstetrical history, allergies, medications which you may be taking, the time you last ate, and the exact contents of the meal. This last question is very important since the onset of labor stops the normal digestive processes. If it is

necessary to use general anesthesia for delivery, solid food eaten several hours earlier can be regurgitated and cause a catastrophic emergency. Don't be surprised if an insensitive nurse or doctor pursues the questioning during your contractions. After the brief history is taken, the nurse will ask you for a urine sample and record your pulse, blood pressure, temperature, respiratory rate, and listen to your baby's heart rate. You will probably be given an identification bracelet that lists your name, the date of admission, your doctor's name, and your hospital number. Later, your baby will be given a bracelet in the delivery room with the identical hospital number as yours. You must carefully check this number whenever your baby is brought to you from the nursery.

Vehemently resist any attempt to separate you from your prepared childbirth partner. Equally protest attempts at shaving your entire perineum, the starting of a routine intravenous solution, the total restriction of clear fluids or ice chips, or confinement to bed during the early stages of labor. Shaving of the pubic hair is especially dehumanizing, and it does not decrease your chances of contracting an infection. If anything, it may increase your risk of a hair follicle infection during the uncomfortable period of time when the hair is growing back. Clipping the few hairs between the vagina and rectum will provide your doctor with more than adequate exposure for performance of an episiotomy. All of your special requests should be discussed with your doctor prior to labor and noted on your obstetrical record which he or she forwards to the delivery room during the last month of pregnancy. It is an excellent idea to prepare a typewritten birth plan listing all of your requests. A copy signed by you and your obstetrician should be forwarded to the delivery room with your prenatal records.

An initial pelvic examination by a resident physician, obstetrical nurse, or nurse-midwife may be acceptable and indicated on admission, but if the doctor whose fee you are paying does not arrive within a reasonable amount of time, demand his or her presence in the delivery room. Too many doctors follow the progress of their patients by telephone, and arrive in a blaze of glory only at the very last minute before delivery.

Some physicians believe that an enema should be given in labor because women are often constipated late in pregnancy, and expulsion of the feces during the bearing down stages may contaminate the episiotomy site. It has also been stated that the passage of the baby through the birth canal may be easier if the colon and rectum are empty. I know of no scientific studies to support this claim. However, it is true that an enema given early in labor may occasionally bring on more effective uterine contractions. Some women prefer to take an enema because they fear embarrassment caused by expulsion of feces. For this reason, I allow my patients to decide for themselves if they want an enema. Another option is to take a mild Fleet's enema at home just at the onset of labor, but I do not recommend this for women with a history of very rapid labors. When you are in the hospital, you should avoid an enema if your labor is advanced to a cervical dilatation of 7 centimeters or more, since it will only intensify your discomfort and increase the risk of a delivery which is too rapid and uncontrolled.

While some women thoroughly enjoy the days spent in the hospital following delivery, others are anxious to return as quickly as possible to their more familiar home surroundings. To accommodate the latter group, many hospitals and birthing centers offer an almost immediate release from the hospital following delivery. On rare occasions, I have discharged a healthy mother and her baby as early as three hours following delivery, without apparent ill effects. An early release from the hospital should take place only after the baby has been carefully examined by a qualified pediatrician. Provisions must also be made for careful follow-up of the baby on an almost daily basis during the first few days of life and for proper rest and care for the mother at home.

How long do most women stay in the hospital following delivery?

A small minority of women will opt to leave within 24 hours following childbirth. Most, however, prefer to rest and receive the instructions about nursing and infant care which many hospitals provide. This luxury, however, is rapidly being eliminated by cost-conscious insurance companies and hospitals. Although the American College of Obstetricians and Gynecologists recommends a minimum hospital stay of 48 hours following a vaginal delivery and 96 hours after a cesarean section, many women are being given the "hospital hustle," meaning that they are being asked to leave one day after a vaginal birth and two days after a cesarean. If these arbitrary requirements are not met, insurance companies simply refuse to pay for any additional time spent in the hospital. Some insurance companies have the audacity to start their countdown for hospital coverage at the time of admission to the delivery room, so that a woman who experiences a prolonged labor is allotted less postpartum time in the hospital. Other companies are offering financial incentives to patients, doctors, and hospitals for early discharge; as a result, many women and babies are leaving the hospital before they are ready. These early-discharge policies are destined to get worse, and some experts predict that labor and delivery will be treated virtually as an outpatient procedure within ten years.

Although the long-term medical and psychological consequences of this policy are unknown at this time, a disturbing number of hospital readmissions and serious late-developing problems, such as neonatal jaundice, poor feeding, respiratory distress, and urinary infections, are being uncovered. These cases are likely to increase in number since less time is being spent by nurses in teaching and counseling mothers during the postpartum period.

A couple should carefully review their insurance

policy before conception in order to find out how much time is allowed in the hospital following delivery. It is also important to ask your obstetrician if he or she is willing to recommend an extra day or two if you need it. Medical conditions which most insurance companies will accept as reasonable for extending a stay include excessive bleeding, anemia, adverse reactions to medications, fever, inability to urinate, elevated blood pressure, and pain and discomfort that can't be alleviated with oral analgesics. If you believe that you are being discharged too early, be assertive and express your concerns to your obstetrician and the nurses caring for you. A letter from your obstetrician attesting to your need for staying in the hospital will satisfy the requirements of most insurance companies.

 # HOME BIRTH AND FAMILY-CENTERED FACILITIES

What are the advantages and disadvantages of giving birth at home?

In recent years there has been an alarming increase in the number of women having their babies at home. Estimates are that they make up 2 to 3 percent of all deliveries in the United States and that mortality rates are higher than among babies born in a hospital environment. Dr. Warren H. Pearse, past president of the American College of Obstetricians and Gynecologists, refers to this trend as an example of "maternal trauma" and "child abuse." In a recent review of statistics from all over California, infant deaths were 20 per 1,000 in hospitals and 42.3 per 1,000 at home. The stillbirth rate was 9.9 per 1,000 in hospitals and 25 per 1,000 at home.

The dangers of home delivery to a baby are obvious when one considers that one-third of the infants admitted to newborn intensive care units are born of healthy mothers who developed complications during labor or who experienced problems that were not anticipated. (The rate of complications occurring in apparently normal pregnancies is estimated to be about 7.5 to 10 percent.) Furthermore, trying to transfer a sick infant from the home to the hospital shortly after birth heightens the danger to the baby. One doctor with many years of home-birth experience has recently estimated that, even among carefully screened women, 20 percent attempting birth at home will have to be taken to the hospital during delivery.

Some home-birth advocates acknowledge its hazards but assert that dangerous complications are almost always predictable. Nothing could be further from the truth! Obstetrical emergencies, such as premature separation of the placenta, ruptured uterus, shoulder dystocia, cervical and vaginal lacerations, postpartum hemorrhage due to failure of the uterine muscles to contract, and aspiration of thick meconium by a newborn, often happen suddenly and pose a great threat to both a woman and her infant if they are not expertly managed in a hospital environment. Regardless of the skill and training of the nurse, midwife, or doctor attending a home delivery, the absence of a laboratory, blood bank, monitoring equipment, and special resuscitative procedures places both mother and child in unnecessary jeopardy.

If, despite all logic, you still intend to give birth at home, it is vital that you take certain precautions. Although a rare few uncertified or lay midwives have achieved a limited degree of competence following years of trial and error, most cannot evaluate an abnormal labor pattern. If you do opt for a home birth, please be sure to obtain the services of a certified nurse-midwife. Call the American College of Nurse-Midwives (1522 K

Street NW, Suite 1000, Washington, D.C. 20005; telephone (202) 289-0171) to verify an individual's credentials. In addition, be certain that the mid-wife has adequate back-up coverage of a qualified obstetrician.

Is there a happy medium between home delivery and hospital delivery?

Couples requesting childbirth at home are usually normal individuals who want to avoid the deper-sonalized environment of most hospital delivery rooms and the authoritative attitudes of the doctors and nurses who staff them. These couples reject the contention of some medical authorities that every labor must be monitored routinely with elec-tronic equipment. They would rather chance the greater risks of home delivery than be placed in a typical hospital environment of increasing auto-mation and mechanization. Advocates of home birth deeply believe that this experience confers unmatched psychological advantages on the par-ents, the newborn infant, and its siblings. They especially believe that the bonding between baby and mother can take place more easily at home, in a relaxed environment, supported by close friends.

To discourage this trend of childbirth at home, many hospitals throughout the United States are attempting to find a happy medium by creating a homelike atmosphere within the hospital. This concept, called family-centered maternity/new-born care, tries to include the entire family in the childbearing experience so that all members may benefit. There are childbirth preparation classes and a tour of the hospital's maternity and newborn units before delivery. Labor rooms are converted into bright, attractively decorated rooms which re-semble living rooms or bedrooms, and some hos-pitals have provided family waiting rooms and early-labor lounges near the obstetrical unit where patients in early labor can walk and visit with friends and family members. A vital member of the obstetrical team in many family-centered units

is the nurse-midwife. In addition to participating in delivery of the baby, this individual is skilled at providing prolonged emotional support which, al-though needed, is often not provided by the obste-trician.

A welcome addition to many obstetrical suites has been the "birthing room" equipped with a labor-delivery bed. This unique bed is quite com-fortable during labor, and stirrups can be easily lifted into place when delivery is imminent. This allows a woman the opportunity to give birth in the same bed in which she labors, avoiding transfer to a separate delivery room at a time when she is most uncomfortable. "Birthing rooms" are also equipped with a cribette and warmer for the new-born, as well as emergency resuscitation apparatus if needed.

I have found that a father's clamping and cutting of the umbilical cord and his bathing of the baby following delivery adds immeasurably to his joy and sense of participation in the birth process. If the delivery is uncomplicated, his guiding of the baby out of the birth canal with coparticipation and supervision of the obstetrician is perfectly safe and will be remembered as probably the greatest moment of a young father's life. Assisting in the delivery of a baby under the watchful eye of a doctor is not nearly as dangerous as some obstetri-cians would have you believe. After all, the busiest obstetrician once delivered his or her first baby under the supervision of another doctor.

Family-centered care permits fathers to have ex-tended visiting hours after the birth and gives them the opportunity to assist in the care and feeding of the baby. Many hospitals have provisions for fa-thers to reside in the room throughout a woman's hospital stay. Other children in the family are al-lowed special hours for visiting with their mother and father in a special family room. Flexible "rooming-in" allows mothers and newborns to re-main together in the same room rather than have the newborn separated in a nursery. It also encour-ages breast-feeding immediately after delivery in a quiet environment free of distractions.

Family-centered alternative birth centers (ABCs) have gained great popularity over the past ten years. An ABC may be either hospital-based or located in a converted residence within minutes of a fully-equipped obstetrical unit. Patients are carefully screened for medical or obstetrical complications before they are allowed to deliver in an ABC. These facilities are usually furnished with comfortable sofas and rocking chairs, carpeting, cheerful wallpaper, quilt-covered beds, stereos, televisions, coffee machines, and other items which make the room as cozy and homelike as possible. Equipment, including portable anesthesia machines, is often discreetly concealed behind curtains. In this one room, a woman labors, delivers, and recovers, hence the name LDR, or labor-delivery-recovery room. The initials LDRP means that a woman also receives all of her postpartum care in the same room until she leaves the hospital. Husbands and even siblings are often permitted to stay in the room throughout the hospital course. Many of these women and their babies are discharged within 24 hours, and sometimes as early as 6 hours, following birth. As a result, obstetrical costs often average half that of a traditional hospital delivery. The logistics of using only one room, rather than transferring a woman from a labor room to a delivery suite and then back to a postpartum ward, are far simpler and require less nursing and housekeeping personnel. When the idea of LDRPs was first conceived, planners believed that the ultimate in obstetrical care would be to assign the same nurse to a patient from the time of admission until discharge from the hospital. However, this concept has been less than successful because most skilled obstetrical nurses have expressed little interest in the prospect of administering routine postpartum and early pediatric care.

The obvious advantage of a hospital-based facility is that it can offer both a homelike environment and the security of standby medical expertise and equipment that are necessary to deal with rare, unexpected complications of pregnancy. This would appear to be the most satisfactory compromise for women who are rejecting hospitals for home births.

A free-standing birth center is a separate non-hospital facility organized to provide family-centered maternity care for women judged to be at low risk for obstetrical complications. While this broad definition includes centers that are within seconds of a well-equipped hospital, others located in rural areas are often isolated and dangerously removed from adequate back-up facilities and personnel capable of dealing with unexpected complications. Data suggest that there may be great differences in quality among birth centers. The National Association of Childbearing Centers is an organization which maintains a master list of the approximately 140 centers in the United States. If you choose a free-standing birth center, be sure it is in compliance with the standards of the National Association of Childbearing Centers. Fortunately, most states now regulate free-standing birth centers by licensure, and the services of an accredited facility are covered by health care insurance plans. While estimates vary, it would appear that certified nurse-midwives or students of nurse-midwifery deliver more than 80 percent of the babies at these facilities.

Some studies have shown that women who deliver at free-standing birth centers experience fewer complications, infant deaths, episiotomies, and cesarean sections than women giving birth in hospital obstetrical units, but these statistics may be misleading since women who receive care in birth centers constitute a particularly low-risk group that is constantly being screened throughout pregnancy. Unfortunately, there are no large studies comparing the outcome of women in birth centers with a control group of low-risk women cared for in hospitals. One of the most comprehensive studies of the treatment received in free-standing birth centers was published in the *New England Journal of Medicine* in 1989. It involved almost 12,000 women who were cared for in 84 birth centers; in my opinion, the results were less than comforting. For example, one disturbing statistic was that 21 percent of the women experienced complications classified as serious, and in 8 percent the problem was severe enough to require immediate hospital care for proper treatment. However, the emergencies were so acute and so severe that it was possible to transfer less than half of the women who required it. I believe that this statistic unequivocally proves that instances will occur in which a woman in a free-standing birth center will have a serious complication resulting in an outcome that may be less favorable than if the complication had occurred in a hospital. Unanticipated emergencies, such as acute preeclampsia, fetal distress, shoulder dystocia, postpartum hemorrhage, retained placenta, and meconium aspiration are inevitable, regardless of how carefully women are screened during pregnancy and labor. Another dismal finding in this study was that 29 percent of women giving birth for the first time were transferred to hospitals because of complications during pregnancy, labor, or the postpartum period, compared to only 7 percent for multiparous women. This has prompted some critics to suggest that nulliparous women should be managed only in hospital-based facilities rather than free-standing birth centers. Although the overall intrapartum and neonatal death rate in this study was only 1.3 per 1,000 births, this number is really not that impressive given the fact that these individuals were supposedly at an extremely low risk for an adverse pregnancy outcome. Finally, more than one-third of the 140 free-standing birth centers invited to participate actually did so, suggesting that the statistics of these places may have been more favorable than those who decided not to participate. In fact, the infant mortality rate of five centers not meeting the criteria for the study was a significantly less favorable 7.2 per 1,000 births.

In summary, if you decide to experience childbirth in a free-standing birth center, be sure that it meets the standards of the National Association of Childbearing Centers and that it is within shouting distance of a well-equipped hospital obstetrical unit.

How do you feel about the presence of siblings in the delivery room?

Those who enthusiastically endorse the presence of siblings in the delivery room claim that it provides a unique educational experience for children, fosters family bonding, prevents separation anxiety, and decreases the likelihood of sibling rivalry. However, few if any of these alleged benefits have been proven. Older children are especially disturbed by the pain which their mother is experiencing, and younger children are often totally unable to comprehend the intensity of the birth experience. Even when children are given extensive indoctrination and undergo careful evaluation by trained personnel before labor, results may still be disappointing and unpredictable.

 MIDWIFERY

Can you evaluate the competency of the nurse-midwife?

Modern midwifery is a far cry from the stereotype of the early 1900s in which babies were delivered at home by "grannies" and an assortment of untrained persons. The incompetence of these individuals was reflected in an incredibly high number of maternal and infant deaths. Today's nurse-midwives are well-educated, highly qualified, dedicated professionals who have contributed immeasurably to the practice of modern obstetrics in the United States.

To become a nurse-midwife, one must first graduate from a three- or four-year nursing school and become a registered nurse. Following this, one must get a year's experience in obstetrical nursing and then take a course in nurse-midwifery in one of approximately 20 medical centers offering training programs which are recognized by the American College of Nurse-Midwives. The course of instruction usually lasts for 24 months and includes subjects such as anatomy, physiology, embryology, neonatology, and genetics. Students are required to assist in as many as 40 or 50 deliveries and to manage at least 20 by themselves, under supervision. After graduation, one must take a national certification examination given by the American College of Nurse-Midwives. Passing this test permits the use of the initials C.N.M., for Certified Nurse-Midwife, after the nurse-midwife's name. Unfortunately, many unqualified individuals calling themselves nurse-midwives have capitalized on the public's enthusiasm for home births. If you have elected to deliver your baby at home, carefully check the midwife's credentials.

Nurse-midwives attend only normal, uncomplicated deliveries, and they always work under the supervision of an obstetrician who must be available for immediate consultation. This applies to deliveries which take place in a hospital, at an alternative birth center, or at home. Midwives can give local anesthesia for vaginal delivery, perform episiotomies, and suture vaginal and perineal lacerations. They do not perform complicated deliveries or prescribe medications. Following delivery, midwives are trained to provide full postpartum care.

Since the midwife's expertise is limited to uncomplicated births, one might ask, "Why not use an obstetrician who can treat all complications?" The answer is that a midwife offers invaluable minute-by-minute emotional support, enthusiasm, and family-centered care, which most obstetricians seem incapable of giving. Doctors have been trained to treat diseases with objectivity and detachment, and this can be a great barrier to providing meaningful emotional support to a woman in labor. The overwhelming majority of midwives are women, and patients in labor often remark that they are most comfortable and secure in a first-name relationship with a woman whom they consider to be a friend, rather than an authoritative figure. There are also taboos against the physician, especially if he is a male, giving the intense physical support that the woman in labor often needs. The touching, stroking, and applications of pressure performed by the nurse-midwife can often relieve the stress of labor without use of excessive amounts of analgesics.

Despite official endorsement of certified nurse-midwives by the American College of Obstetricians and Gynecologists, some of the greatest antagonism and scorn of nurse-midwifery has come from board-certified obstetricians who remain highly suspicious of the nurse-midwife's ability and simply cannot understand how some women could prefer an individual less qualified than themselves to deliver their baby. Hopefully, as doctors learn more about the midwife's skills and sense of commitment, some of these negative attitudes will change. As a member of the obstetric team, the special skills of the nurse-midwife can complement those of the physician in meeting the needs of the patient.

 # CIRCUMCISION

What are the advantages and disadvantages of newborn circumcision?

Circumcision is the most commonly performed operation in the United States, with more than 1 million procedures recorded annually. In the 1960s it was estimated that 95 percent of newborn males underwent circumcision, but this percentage has dropped to less than 60 percent as adverse publicity about the procedure surfaced in the 1970s and 1980s and people began to question whether or not it was medically necessary. It is ironic that in the past few years, as the anticircumcision movement has grown and the number of circumcisions has decreased, studies have uncovered several benefits of the procedure. These new reports may once again reverse this trend and increase the number of parents requesting that their newborn be circumcised.

In most hospitals, circumcision is performed on the second day after birth. In some hospitals, the pediatricians do the procedure, while in others it is the job of the obstetricians. The Jewish ritual circumcision, or Brith, is performed on the eighth day of life by a trained religious leader, or mohel. Since few women will remain in the hospital for eight postpartum days, this joyous occasion, for everyone but the baby, is usually celebrated at home.

The operation itself is simple. The prepuce, or skin covering the mushroom-shaped tip of the penis, or glans, is removed by applying a specially designed clamp. The clamp crushes any blood vessels as the skin is being removed. The result of the operation is that the glans of the circumcised male is permanently exposed. In contrast, the uncircumcised male must retract his foreskin in order to expose his glans. In most uncircumcised babies, the foreskin is not fully retractable for at least a year and sometimes as long as five years following birth. Forced retraction and overzealous cleaning should be avoided since it may cause tearing of tissues and exposure of raw skin surfaces. Once the foreskin is easily retractable, a parent can wash beneath it periodically and a boy can be instructed to do this as part of his regular hygiene at puberty.

Advocates of circumcision claim that it prevents phimosis, a condition in which the prepuce adheres to the glans. Occasionally, the prepuce will retract but then can't be repositioned. This condition, known as paraphimosis, causes a painful constriction at the base of the glans. The smegma, or penile secretions, and the inner lining of the prepuce provide a perfect culture medium for a variety of bacteria to adhere and colonize. This, in turn, predisposes uncircumcised men to infections of the urinary tract, balanitis (inflammation of the glans), and posthitis (inflammation of the foreskin). Daily bathing and retraction and cleaning of the glans with soap and water can prevent most of these problems; however, it is estimated that 5 to 10 percent of all males medically require circumcision at a later date. Uncircumcised male diabetics are especially prone to balanitis, as evidenced by a 1990 study showing an incidence of 35 percent. Several types of bacteria colonize and adhere to the inner lining of the prepuce. One organism, named beta-hemolytic streptococcus, is often associated with balanitis and prosthitis and may be sexually transmitted.

It is not surprising that the decrease in the number of newborn circumcisions has coincided with a sharp rise in the incidence of urinary tract infections in infancy. In what has proven to be a monumental study, Dr. Thomas E. Wiswell, a neonatologist at Walter Reed Army Medical Center, followed the first-year medical histories of 220,000 male infants born in army hospitals between 1975 and 1985, and found that uncircumcised male infants had a ten- to twentyfold higher risk than circumcised males of a urinary tract infection within their first years of life. Subsequent studies from Children's Hospital in Boston and researchers in Sweden have confirmed Dr. Wiswell's observations. Dr. James Robert, another expert in this field, has estimated that if no newborn males were circumcised in this country, 20,000 infants would suffer kidney infections annually.

Although cancer of the penis is a rare condition, occurring with a frequency of less than one case per 100,000 adult males, there is no doubt that circumcision plays a significant role in almost completely eliminating a man's susceptibility to this disease. According to one recent national study, there have been approximately 50,000 cases of penile cancer in the United States since 1940, and only nine have occurred in circumcised men. Previous claims of a higher incidence of cervical cancer among wives of uncircumcised men have not been proven, although the human papillomavirus, believed responsible for this disease, can survive for longer periods of time under a foreskin. Similarly, anecdotal reports asserting that uncircumcised men are more prone to gonorrhea, syphilis, and AIDS because of a greater likelihood of their foreskins becoming abraded during coitus have never been proven in any large-scale scientific studies.

From 1971 until 1989, the American Academy of Pediatrics steadfastly held to the view that circumcision was a medically unnecessary operation and that there was "no absolute indication for routine circumcision of newborns." As a result, a growing number of state Medicaid agencies and insurance companies were quick to accept this policy and have refused to pay for newborn circumcision. Recent scientific evidence, however, prompted the Academy in 1989 to alter its statement to read that "properly performed newborn circumcision prevents phimosis, paraphimosis, balanophosphitis, and has been shown to decrease the incidence of cancer of the penis." This revised statement also cites other circumcision-related benefits, such as a lower incidence of urinary tract infections and a reduction in cervical cancer among women. Despite this positive statement, it remains the opinion of many physicians that the only currently valid indications for circumcision are religious preference and the psychological concerns of parents who want their infant to have a penile appearance resembling that of a father or older sibling. More adamant opponents of circumcision, such as the National Organization of Circumcision Resource Centers (NO/CIRC), claim that it is a human rights issue, a harsh and barbaric example of child abuse; they oppose all circumcisions, without exception. These individuals correctly assert that circumcision is the only surgical procedure performed without informed consent of the defenseless victim, most often without benefit of anesthesia.

Some doctors would have you believe that newborns do not feel intense pain, but nothing could be further from the truth. Circumcision is certainly not painless, and individuals observing the procedure for the first time are often appalled at the amount of pain that some infants appear to experience. Although short-lived, the experience certainly is not in keeping with attempts to provide a peaceful and serene environment for all newborns. If anything, this practice recalls a more primitive era of medicine. Studies conducted on newborns suggest that a circumcision without anesthesia affects both psychological and physiological behavior. In one report, changes in sleep patterns, characterized by crying, were noted following the procedure. The endocrine response of newborns supports the behavioral evidence that the operation is stressful. Although the pain and adverse reactions can be almost entirely eliminated with use of a local anesthetic technique known as dorsal penile nerve block (DPNB), it is sad to note that fewer than 25 percent of surveyed physicians employ this humane method.

Physical complications from circumcision occur no more often than 1 in 500 cases, and most of these are rather mild. A family history of bleeding or a blood-clotting defect should postpone circumcision until adequate testing is performed on the newborn. Circumcision should also be delayed if the baby is immature or shows the slightest indication of compromise.

LACTATION SUPPRESSION

If a woman prefers not to nurse her baby, what can she do to relieve breast engorgement and lactation?

Breast engorgement can be relieved with simple measures such as use of a breast binder or good maternity brassiere, ice packs, and mild analgesics. Contrary to popular belief, restricting fluid intake does not decrease breast engorgement and lactation. Discomfort is most pronounced between the second and fourth postpartum day. All signs and symptoms usually subside by the end of the first postpartum week, provided that the breasts are not stimulated by pumping.

Bromocriptine mesylate (trade name Parlodel) is a nonhormonal ergot derivative that has been used effectively to inhibit postpartum lactation and lactation associated with a variety of endocrine disorders. Since an abnormal drop in blood pressure has been reported in as many as 28 percent of postpartum women receiving Parlodel, the first tablet should be taken no earlier than 4 hours following delivery, and only after it is certain that a woman's postdelivery vital signs are stable. While estrogen preparations (see question below) must be taken immediately after delivery if they are to be effective, an advantage of bromocriptine is that it remains effective even when taken days, weeks, or months following childbirth. In addition to these benefits, bromocriptine, unlike estrogens, is not associated with an increase in blood-clotting factors or an abnormal increase in uterine bleeding patterns.

To date, millions of postpartum women have been treated with Parlodel with excellent results. However, it is not free of adverse reactions. In addition to the previously mentioned 28 percent incidence of a drop in blood pressure, it may cause headache, dizziness (8 percent), nausea (7 percent), vomiting (3 percent), fatigue (1 percent), fainting (0.7 percent), diarrhea (0.4 percent), and abdominal cramps (0.4 percent).

Less frequent, but far more dangerous, complications associated with Parlodel use include postpartum seizures, stroke, and myocardial infarction (heart attack). Recent studies have also uncovered a postpartum hypertensive reaction associated with the use of Parlodel in women with a history of pregnancy-induced hypertension or preeclampsia. Scientists have attributed these serious side effects to Parlodel's ergot-like chemical structure, which causes constriction and spasm of arterial smooth muscles. This, in turn, reduces oxygen flow to the brain and heart. For this reason, Parlodel should not be prescribed when a woman has a vasoconstrictive condition such as hypertension, migraine headaches, or Raynaud's disease. To date, fewer than 100 cases of these serious complications have been reported among the millions of women who have used Parlodel for suppression of lactation and breast engorgement.

When a woman takes bromocriptine to inhibit lactation, her ovulatory function and ability to conceive returns earlier than usual. It is, therefore, imperative that she use adequate contraception even if intercourse is resumed as early as the second or third postpartum week.

How safe are estrogens and other hormonal preparations in inhibiting lactation?

Although hormonal preparations have been widely prescribed in the past to inhibit breast engorgement and lactation, they are used infrequently today because they are less than adequate for this purpose and may even be associated with serious side effects. Estrogens remain the most popular medication prescribed, even though they prevent breast engorgement in only 25 percent of all nonnursing women and do not prevent lactation. Natural and synthetic estrogens, including the popular chlortrianisene (trade name Tace), quinestrol, and the infamous DES, have all been used to suppress lactation. All of these preparations, however, may increase a woman's risk of abnormal blood coagulation and the formation of blood clots or thrombi in the veins of the legs and pelvis. On very rare occasions, dislodged clots called emboli may travel to vital organs, such as the lungs, and cause death. It has been estimated that postpartum estrogens may increase the maternal death rate by 1 to 2 deaths per 100,000 women. This may not sound like very much, but even one preventable death should be enough to discourage doctors from prescribing these hormones for lactation suppres-. sion.

Another lactation suppressant infrequently used today contains a long-acting estrogen named estradiol valerate combined with the male hormone testosterone enanthate (trade name Deladumone). For maximum results, it is best administered intramuscularly immediately after delivery. Androgens, or male hormones such as testosterone and fluoxymesterone (trade name Halotestin), reduce breast pain and engorgement but do not affect milk production. The potential for masculinization precludes widespread use of androgens during the postpartum period.

 ## *LACTATION STIMULATION*

Are there any medications that can be used to increase the quantity of a woman's breast milk?

Approximately 20 to 40 percent of mothers willing to breast-feed fail to do so because lactation does not become established or stops too early. If prolactin was available as a pill or injection, it would probably be helpful in stimulating milk production among women who want to nurse but lack an adequate supply of milk. Although this medication does not exist, there are lactation-inducing agents including antidepressants and tranquilizers, such as chlorpromazine (trade name Thorazine) and thioridazine (trade name Mellaril). It is not unusual for even nonpregnant women to experience

lactation following long-term use of these drugs. Maternal side effects of tranquilizers, such as fatigue and drowsiness, may serve as a deterrent to their use.

In addition to its effects on uterine muscle contractions, oxytocin also stimulates cells in the breast, known as myoepithelial cells, to contract. This causes milk "letdown," or ejection from the nipple, and helps to initiate the nursing process. Oxytocin in the form of a nasal spray or tablet placed below the tongue has been used extensively to aid milk ejection. Contrary to popular belief, it will not increase the total yield of milk and should not be used for this purpose.

 ## *POSTPARTUM*

What emotional feelings may be experienced during the postpartum period?

For the majority of women, the euphoria which they experience at the moment of birth continues

throughout the postpartum period. However, for as many as 40 percent, the emotional "high" of childbirth is often followed by varying degrees of postpartum depression, or "blues," usually manifested by one or two crying episodes without apparent cause during the first three to seven postpartum days, and classically on the fifth postpartum day, followed by a rapid recovery with no further difficulties. For other less fortunate individuals, the depression may become deeper, last longer than two weeks, and cause serious psychological impairment requiring professional help. The risk of recurrence of postpartum depression in subsequent pregnancies is believed to be between 25 and 33 percent.

Despite extensive study, the cause of postpartum depression remains a mystery. Some psychiatrists attribute this condition to the many sudden physical, social, and psychological changes which occur immediately following the birth of a child. Other doctors believe it is caused by the dramatic decline in concentration of circulating female hormones, combined with a reduction in a woman's blood volume following childbirth. These factors, in addition to a variety of physical discomforts, such as episiotomy and hemorrhoid pain, "afterbirth" pains caused by contractions of the postpartum uterus, breast engorgement, and lack of sleep, all contribute to the problem. Women who, for a variety of medical reasons, are separated from their infants during the first two days of life are believed to be more susceptible to postpartum depression because they have lost the opportunity to bond with them during this critical time.

Interviews with women suffering from postpartum depression reveal a wide range of concerns. The most commonly reported problem is arguing with their husbands or partners and the strong conviction that a spouse is not as supportive as he could be. For some the reality of caring for a demanding and irritable baby 24 hours a day is far more difficult than they had anticipated, while for others the concern is the change that their bodies have undergone. Some women express feelings of isolation because the baby has suddenly become the focus of everyone's attention.

Women who have had a cesarean section are also more likely to experience depression. Such women often express a feeling of inadequacy and a sense of having deprived their spouse of the birth experience. A great aid for such women has been the emergence of cesarean section support groups. Too often, hospitals isolate babies born by cesarean section in a special nursery. If a baby is healthy and a woman is awake during the cesarean section, she should be allowed to hold her baby as soon as possible after the operation is completed.

While postpartum "blues" usually start when a woman is in the hospital, they may intensify when she arrives home and is confronted with the added burden of household chores, unannounced visitors, a demanding mate, and too little sleep. Of all these factors, a lack of sleep is probably the greatest underlying reason for postpartum depression. For this reason it is vital that you sleep whenever your baby sleeps and nap during the day when your baby does not demand attention. One interesting observation is that postpartum "blues" rarely occur among women who are discharged from the hospital within two days after delivery.

Interestingly, a significant number of fathers also suffer from postpartum "blues." In one study as many as 62 percent of new fathers experienced some form of this feeling. Many interviewed men seemed frustrated by their inability to help cope with the new baby. Others experienced helplessness in caring for the babies themselves, while some who experienced prolonged depression described themselves as "overwhelmed" by the problems that their spouses were having in caring for the infants. A small number of fathers expressed frustration because the amount of time allotted to them with their baby was limited.

Postpartum "blues" can't be prevented, but their intensity and duration can be dramatically reduced. The most important thing you can do is to get help with the housework, shopping, and cooking so that you are free to concentrate on the care of your baby during the first two weeks at home. Don't be afraid to ask for help—there is nothing to be gained by suffering silently. A professional baby nurse is a luxury which is well worth the expense. By caring for your baby, a nurse allows you the opportunity to catch up on your sleep and enjoy leisure time away from the house. A quiet evening out to a favorite restaurant is great therapy for postpartum depression, although you should not expect it to be an instant cure. Discuss your feelings openly with your mate and let him do the same with you. It is through this process of communication that the problems and depression of the early postpartum days can be corrected.

When friends, relatives, nurses, and other helpers have all departed after the first few weeks, you can continue to enjoy your leisure time if you join or form a babysitting co-op with other new mothers. One of the great cures for postpartum depression is a mothers' support group. Such groups are usually made up of a handful of women from the same neighborhood whose children are roughly the same age. Frequently local YMCAs or community centers sponsor such groups. During weekly meetings, a wide range of topics dealing with the physical and emotional concerns of motherhood can be discussed. This will often help you to realize that your problems are not unlike those of other young mothers. While you may have prided yourself on being the perfect cook, homemaker, and lover prior to the birth of your baby, you must accept the fact that the limited number of hours in the day will prevent you from achieving unrealistic and unnecessary goals. Furthermore, make it clear to your partner that he should not demand more than you are capable of giving and that he must actively participate in the management of the household. Assertiveness is the key to preventing and curing postpartum depression.

How do most women feel about sex during the postpartum period?

While a minority of women experience an early return to erotic interest within 4 weeks, do not be surprised if it takes as long as 6 to 12 weeks before your libido returns to its prepregnancy levels (see Chapter 4). One hindrance to complete sexual en-

joyment during the early postpartum weeks is a woman's fear that her episiotomy is not completely healed. In addition, pain with intercourse during the first three months is more likely to occur among women who nurse their babies because their vaginal tissues are thin and fragile due to a lack of estrogen. While some doctors prescribe estrogen cream vaginally twice a week to correct this problem, it is a form of therapy which I don't endorse because significant amounts of the hormone may be absorbed through the vaginal walls and enter the bloodstream and breast milk. Instead, lubricants such as K-Y Jelly, Replens Vaginal Moisturizer, and Lubrin tablets may be used. While these products are not as effective as estrogen cream, they are in my opinion much safer.

In addition to the physical and hormonal changes which occur during the postpartum period, a woman's libido may be dampened by a variety of other factors, such as fatigue, anxiety, lack of sleep, a crying baby, and financial concerns. Patience, love, understanding, communication, and elixir of time will cure an overwhelming number of postpartum sexual problems.

When can intercourse be resumed after childbirth?

Contrary to what most doctors recommend, there is no scientific evidence to show that a couple must wait six weeks before resuming intercourse. Following an uncomplicated vaginal delivery, in which there are no lacerations and no episiotomy is performed, intercourse should be perfectly safe at two weeks postpartum. The stitches of an episiotomy or a sutured laceration usually completely dissolve three weeks following delivery. At that time, intercourse can be attempted gingerly, and if there is no discomfort, there is no need to abstain. Following a cesarean section, the abdominal incision usually takes two weeks to heal, and barring unusual medical complications, intercourse should be safe at this time.

Noncoital lovemaking techniques should be undertaken with caution. The mouth contains a wide variety of potentially harmful bacteria which, when introduced into a vaginal, urethral, or vulvar laceration may be capable of causing an infection. If you are contemplating oral-genital sex prior to three weeks postpartum, I advise that you carefully inspect your vulva and vagina with a hand mirror for evidence of a laceration that has not healed. If you are unable to do this, consult your obstetrician. While some doctors believe that bacteria from a man's mouth may be introduced to the nipple of a nursing mother during lovemaking, there is no scientific evidence to show that this would cause mastitis, or breast inflammation.

Is contraception necessary prior to the six week postpartum examination?

I have never seen a woman who has conceived prior to her six-week postpartum visit, and many studies have confirmed that ovulation rarely occurs before the fifth postpartum week. However, there is scientific evidence which clearly documents ovulation in a nonnursing woman as early as 25 days following a full-term delivery. Although you may have a period prior to your six-week visit, it will most likely be anovulatory, meaning that it will not be preceded by ovulation and the risk of pregnancy. It has been estimated, on the basis of available statistics, that 5 percent of nursing women and 15 percent of nonnursing women ovulate by the sixth postpartum week. By the twelfth postpartum week, the percentages increase to 25 and 40 percent, respectively. At the twenty-fourth postpartum week, the theoretical risk of conception jumps to 65 percent if you nurse and 75 percent if you don't. In actual practice, however, the number of women who conceive is much lower than the above figures, since most couples use some type of contraceptive technique during this time. When this is taken into account, only 1 percent of nursing mothers and 3 percent of nonnurs-

ing mothers conceive within three months of delivery. At six months, conception rates increase to 5 percent and 15 percent, respectively.

Carefully documented research conducted since 1981 has clearly shown that breast-feeding may work far more effectively as a contraceptive when six or more feedings are given every 24 hours, each lasting 10 to 15 minutes, including at least one at night. Nursing practiced in this so-called "push-button" manner may yield pregnancy rates as low as 1 to 2 per 100 women during the first six postpartum months. The reason for this protection is that the frequent suckling of the nipple sends impulses to the hypothalamus in the brain, continually blocking the releasing factors responsible for stimulating the LH (luteinizing hormone) secretion necessary for ovulation. Instead, the pituitary gland is constantly stimulated to produce prolactin, and this prevents follicle growth in the ovary as well as ovulation and menstruation. Studies have shown that prolactin levels drop precipitously when a baby is given supplemental formula feedings.

It is becoming increasingly clear that the pattern of breast-feeding at night may be the major determinant in predicting the return of fertility in lactating women. In one report, doctors found that whenever a woman skipped nursing for a period of 10 to 12 hours at night, ovulation was sure to follow within a short period of time. They found that this 10- to 12-hour hiatus was a more reliable predictor of the return of fertility than were the initiation of supplemental feedings or the return of menses. Another report found that the first period in a nursing woman who gave no supplemental feedings was never preceded by ovulation.

After the sixth postpartum month or the resumption of menses, the effectiveness of breast-feeding as a contraceptive drops significantly. In a 1990 study published in *Lancet*, researchers from Johns Hopkins University noted that a woman would have to breast-feed at least 15 times every 24 hours, for a minimum of 10 minutes each, to achieve a less-than-adequate contraception success rate of 94 percent.

What form of contraception can I use before the six-week postpartum check-up?

Since the risk of pregnancy is minimal during the first six postpartum weeks, the use of condoms and vaginal spermicides in the form of nonprescription aerosol foams, jellies, tablets, creams, and suppositories provides adequate and easy-to-use contraception. When choosing a condom, be sure that it is lubricated so that the sensitive vaginal tissues are not irritated.

All spermicidal agents must be inserted high into the vagina, as close to the cervix as possible, if they are to be effective. It is best to do this within 30 minutes before intercourse, and repeated acts of coitus should be preceded by insertion of additional spermicide. Contraceptive aerosol foam is probably the best of the vaginal spermicides because it is more rapidly distributed throughout the vagina and quickly forms a barrier over the cervix so that intercourse and ejaculation can immediately follow its insertion. Allow creams or jellies slightly more time to adjust to your body temperature and melt, and allow suppositories and tablets at least 10 minutes to completely liquefy. Since intravaginal distribution of jelly, tablets, and suppositories is partially dependent on penile thrusting, a greater chance of pregnancy exists if a man ejaculates quickly after penetration. Foam is also not nearly as messy as the other vaginal spermicides. It is less likely to leak out of the vagina during intercourse and afterward.

The Today Sponge is an excellent postpartum contraceptive option which can be purchased without prescription at any pharmacy. Manufactured by Whitehall Laboratories, Inc., it is a small, round, disposable, soft, comfortable, squeezable vaginal insert. One size fits all. To activate the nonoxynol-9 spermicide in the sponge you must moisten it with tap water immediately before plac-ing it deep in the vagina. Once it is in place, the sponge releases spermicide at a steady rate for up to 30 hours, providing immediate and continuous contraception. Although it must never be left in the vagina for longer than 24 hours, it has the unique advantage over other spermicide-containing contraceptives of not requiring any additional applications of spermicide for as long as it is left in place. To ensure the greatest sperm-killing effect, it is best not to remove the Today Sponge until at least 8 hours after the last coital act. After removal, the sponge should be discarded.

While many women express concern that the sponge's small size will prevent it from adequately covering the cervix and blocking the ascent of sperm, the fact is that this is its least important mechanism of contraceptive action. Far more effective is the dispersion of nonoxynol-9 over the cervix and upper vagina. In addition, laboratory research has shown that the Today Sponge has the capacity to absorb sperm for up to 24 hours.

Can a diaphragm be used during this early postpartum period?

No. Don't try to use your old diaphragm prior to your six-week postpartum visit because, as a result of your changing anatomy and greater sensitivity of your vaginal tissues, it will be difficult to insert and may not adequately cover your cervix. Ask your doctor to recheck your diaphragm size at your six-week visit, since it is quite possible that you will require a larger size than you previously needed. If you intend to lose additional weight, be sure to have your diaphragm size rechecked after each 15 pounds of weight loss.

If you have never used a diaphragm, your doctor can measure or fit you for the correct size at the time of your postpartum visit. The prescription for the specific type and size and the spermicidal cream or jelly to be used with it is then filled by a pharmacist. The actual measuring for the diaphragm takes only a few minutes, but once the size is determined, it is the obligation of your doctor to explain the simple anatomy involved, as well as the proper insertion technique. You should practice inserting the diaphragm without assistance, and your doctor should then do a vaginal examination to check the position. Regardless of how many failures are encountered, don't leave the office until you are satisfied and fully understand the insertion technique. Occasionally, when a woman has become discouraged at several unsuccessful insertion attempts, I tell her to practice in the privacy of her home and then return to the office on another day wearing the diaphragm so that we can be sure that it is inserted correctly. But remember that other contraception should be used during this learning period. Once the insertion technique is learned, it becomes extremely simple and is never forgotten.

What is a cervical cap, and how effective is it as a postpartum contraceptive?

A cervical cap looks like a small diaphragm but fits securely over the cervix rather than against the vaginal walls. While cervical caps have been created from many different materials and fashioned into a variety of inventive shapes over the years, the latex rubber Prentif Cavity-Rim Cervical Cap is the only one approved by the FDA. The cap is held in place and exerts its contraceptive effect by adhering to the cervix and preventing the entry of sperm from the vagina. For greater efficacy, spermicidal cream or jelly should be placed inside the cap before it is inserted. Once inserted, it can remain in place for up to 48 hours without the reapplication of spermicide. Since the size of the cervix continues to decrease during the first two postpartum months, it would be foolish to be fitted for a cervical cap during this time. Studies of the cervix show that it is far more changeable in size and shape well beyond the immediate postpartum period than previously believed. It is now known that a woman's cervical cap size fluctuates not only

during the monthly cycle, but during sexual excitation and orgasm as well. While some reports have noted cervical cap pregnancy rates equal to those experienced with the diaphragm, others have found higher rates caused by slippage during intercourse and activities requiring intense straining and bearing down. In various studies, dislodgement has been reported in anywhere from 20 to 31 percent of cap-users, tripling the risk of these women for an accidental pregnancy. Current researchers now know that as many as 10 percent of women wearing cervical caps need at least two different sizes to accommodate the changes in their cervix each month.

What problems may be encountered if I use birth control pills during the postpartum period?

Aside from permanent sterilization, no other method of birth control approaches the efficacy of oral contraceptives. If you are not nursing and your doctor can't find a medical reason for not prescribing the Pill, it can be started on or before your six-week postpartum visit. Practically all birth control pills contain estrogen combined with a synthetic progesterone-like chemical known as a progestin (see Chapter 1). Minipills such as Micronor and Nor-Q.D. contain only a progestin. Measurable amounts of both estrogens and progestins have been detected in the breast milk of women using combination birth control pills. In addition, research has demonstrated that the estrogen is capable of reducing the quantity of a woman's breast milk by inhibiting the action of prolactin in breast-tissue receptors. Despite this, the overwhelming majority of women are able to successfully nurse their babies while using one of the low-dose estrogen formulations currently on the market. The progestin-only minipill, on the other hand, does not appear to adversely affect the quantity of milk produced. As a result, many obstetricians prescribe the minipill as their first choice of contraception for nursing women. Other doctors are reluctant to do this because no large-scale studies have been conducted to prove that small amounts of progestins ingested in the milk over a prolonged period of time are harmless to a nursing infant.

The American Academy of Pediatrics endorses the use of combination oral contraceptives for nursing women after effective lactation is well established at least four weeks following delivery. This will minimize the reduction in milk quantity as well as lower the risks associated with intravascular blood clotting and thromboembolism during the immediate postpartum period. Women in the immediate postpartum days have a higher risk of thromboembolic disease than do nonpregnant women, regardless of whether or not they use oral contraceptives. The use of combination oral contraceptives can cause changes in coagulation factors that can further predispose to this potentially serious condition during the first four postpartum weeks.

How effective and safe are Norplant and Depo-Provera as postpartum contraceptives?

Norplant is a long-acting reversible, hormonal contraceptive for women that was approved by the FDA in 1990. It consists of six matchstick-sized Silastic capsules, each containing 35 milligrams of the progestin levonorgestrel, which are surgically inserted under the skin of a woman's upper arm under local anesthesia. The slow release of 30 micrograms daily provides excellent contraception for up to five years, with pregnancy rates reported at less than 1 percent annually.

The 30 micrograms of levonorgestrel released daily from Norplant is only 20 percent of the 150-microgram dose found in a single low-dose combination birth control pill such as Nordette and Levlen. As a result, little of the drug enters the breast milk. Similarly, exposure of a fetus to this dose of levonorgestrel in the event of an accidental pregnancy is unlikely to affect fetal genital development associated with progestin use or cause birth defects. Nevertheless, the capsule should be immediately removed if pregnancy occurs.

The insertion of Norplant immediately after delivery would appear to be the ideal contraceptive for a woman who is either medically unable or emotionally unwilling to use alternative methods of birth control. Women considering sterilization, but not yet ready for permanent contraception, will also benefit from using Norplant. In addition, the absence of estrogen from Norplant markedly reduces the risk of postpartum thromboembolic disease associated with combination birth control pills. However, since there are no studies describing the effects of Norplant insertion prior to the sixth postpartum week, its manufacturer cautions against its use earlier than this time in nursing women.

Norplant is less than ideal for the vast majority of women. Its drawbacks include a 60 percent incidence of menstrual irregularities and less frequent side effects such as depression, headache, acne, weight gain, ovarian cysts, and infection and tissue trauma at the insertion site. In addition, the capsules can occasionally be seen and are often palpable below the skin of the upper arm, especially in thin women. The cost of Norplant, including $350 for the device, the $200 insertion fee, and follow-up and removal fees, can raise its total cost to $600 to $1,000.

Depo-Provera is the trade name for an intramuscular progestin named medroxyprogesterone acetate which was approved as a contraceptive by the FDA in 1992. When 150 milligrams of Depo-Provera is given every three months, it will successfully prevent pregnancy in 99 to 100 percent of all women who use it. Though small amounts of the drug have been detected in breast milk, no adverse effects have been reported in nursing infants. The manufacturer suggests that Depo-Provera not be started until nursing is well-established at six weeks postpartum. Unpredictable uterine bleeding and weight gain are the chief disadvantages of Depo-Provera.

What is your opinion of the intrauterine device as a method of postpartum contraception?

An intrauterine device (IUD) is inserted into the endometrial cavity and left there for varying periods of time for the purpose of contraception (see page 7). The progesterone-releasing Progestasert and the copper-releasing ParaGard are both T-shaped and the only two IUDs approved for use by the FDA. Of the two, the ParaGard is superior since it is effective for eight years, while the Progestasert must be changed annually.

In the past, a variety of IUDs were designed specifically for the purpose of insertion at the time of a full-term birth. Despite these efforts, expulsion rates for all IUDs remain significantly higher at this time. Opinions differ as to whether uterine perforation is more likely to occur when IUDs are inserted during the immediate postpartum period. In one study of almost 1,700 postpartum women who had IUDs inserted prior to discharge from the hospital, the author reported no uterine perforations. Other reports have not been as favorable. However, all studies agree that expulsion and perforation rates can be minimized if the person inserting the device is skilled, gentle, and able to place it in as high a position as possible within the endometrial cavity. In a 1984 report studying data on 2,595 IUD insertions, doctors found a significantly higher probability of expelling the device when it was inserted between 10 minutes and 36 hours following delivery of the placenta. In contrast, expulsion rates were lowest for IUDs inserted within the first 10 minutes. Other studies have found that the best time for postpartum IUD insertion is between the fourth and the eighth week.

The obvious advantages of an IUD are its extremely low pregnancy rate of less than one pregnancy per 100 women who use the device annually and the convenience of not having to take precautions in preparation for each coital act. However, before you receive an IUD, be sure to carefully read and understand its accompanying booklet, which describes the unlikely but serious complications which you may encounter. For example, the risk of infection is less than 2 percent, but if it occurs it may be quite serious.

What advice do you have for couples seeking permanent sterilization?

Emotionally, a woman may believe that she wants a tubal ligation, or tying of her tubes, immediately following a difficult nine months of pregnancy and a painful labor. However, studies show that she may later regret this decision. In one report, a significant number of women who requested postpartum sterilization but had surgery delayed for various reasons, declined to undergo the operation when given the opportunity at a later date. For this reason, it is best not to have the surgery if there is even the slightest doubt. Nothing is lost by waiting.

An abdominal tubal ligation during the immediate postpartum period is extremely easy to perform. Under either general or local anesthesia, an incision of an inch or less is made just under the navel and a small segment of each tube is then tied and cut. When a tubal ligation is performed immediately after delivery or on the following day, a woman can return home two to four days later. This lengthens her total postpartum hospitalization time an average of only one to two days.

Instead of the traditional abdominal tubal ligation, many doctors now perform postpartum tubal sterilization through a viewing instrument called a laparoscope (see page 367) which is inserted through the umbilicus. Using this instrument, a doctor can block the tubes by burning them or by applying special bands or clips. In my experience with this technique, I have found that patients have experienced significantly less discomfort and a shorter hospitalization than those undergoing the traditional abdominal procedure. There is also the added benefit of no visible scar. One great advantage of laparoscopy over abdominal postpartum tubal ligation is that it may be performed on the first or second day following delivery rather than immediately after. This gives a woman more time to decide if she really wants the operation.

Vasectomy means cutting of the vas deferens, the two tubes which carry sperm from each testicle in the male. While vasectomy is a minor surgical procedure, it is the simplest, surest, and safest surgical or medical method known to prevent unwanted pregnancy. Unlike tubal sterilization, vasectomy may be performed easily in a doctor's office under local anesthesia. There is no doubt that the incidence and severity of complications associated with tubal sterilization far exceed those related to vasectomy.

All too often, vasectomy is still looked upon with skepticism and fear, and misinformation about the operation is widespread. Many individuals mistakenly believe that vasectomy causes such ill effects as the inability to ejaculate, loss of fertility, inability to achieve orgasm, hair loss, premature aging, and a change in voice pitch. Vasectomy has even been accused of causing skin disease, kidney, lung, and liver diseases, narcolepsy (inability to stay awake), and multiple sclerosis. Sadly, such misinformation has been responsible for many men's avoidance of this simple and relatively harmless procedure.

       POSTPARTUM WEIGHT LOSS

How much weight does a woman normally lose following childbirth?

Despite emptying their uterus of a baby, placenta, and amniotic fluid, many women are shocked and dismayed to find that they weigh the same or more immediately after delivery. However, by the fifth postpartum day weight loss will begin and steadily continue for most women over the next ten postpartum weeks. In fact, the average woman will lose weight throughout the first four months. By the time of the standard six-week postpartum visit, the average weight loss ranges between 20 and 25 pounds, with the amount often higher among women who elect to breast-feed. Weight loss appears to be less successful for individuals who have other children and those who have undergone a cesarean section.

In a 1988 multicenter study published in *Obstetrics and Gynecology*, researchers found that the amount of weight permanently retained postpartum is directly related to the number of pounds above 20 that a woman gains throughout her pregnancy as well as short time intervals from one pregnancy to the next. This study also confirmed the

findings of previous reports demonstrating that most women remain permanently heavier after pregnancy than before, and at least one in ten retains excessive weight of 15 pounds or more. Half of the more than 7,000 women studied in this report retained an average of 2 pounds in the two years between the beginning of one pregnancy and the beginning of the next. One interesting and important observation was that if a woman did not work diligently to achieve her prepregnancy weight within a year after delivery, she was unlikely to lose the weight after this time.

What exercises do you recommend for improving physical fitness during the postpartum period?

There is no scientific indication that exercise during pregnancy and the postpartum period is responsible for sagging breasts or prolapse of the urinary bladder or uterus. Factors such as obesity and lack of good muscle tone probably contribute more to these conditions than any form of exercise. However, since activity levels of most women decline dramatically during the last trimester of pregnancy, the prudent course is to resume all forms of previous exercise gradually and carefully until you reach your prepregnancy levels of stamina and conditioning.

If you continue your prenatal exercises after you give birth (see Chapter 3), you will increase your muscle tone and strength. Exercise can begin on the first day after you give birth and can build in frequency and intensity with each subsequent day. You should let your body be your guide. If you feel pain or have unusual symptoms, you shouldn't be doing that particular exercise, that many repetitions, or that long a routine. If your pregnancy and delivery was complicated or you required a cesarean section, you may need to delay your return to exercise; you should consult with your obstetrician before resuming physical conditioning.

New mothers often complain that they still look several months pregnant just after delivery. This is because it takes several weeks for the uterus to shrink to its prepregnancy size. Another reason is the loss of muscle tone in the abdomen after it was stretched so much during pregnancy. Accept the fact that it takes time and effort for your abdominal muscles to regain their normal elasticity.

... *Bibliography* ...

Chapter 1
CONTRACEPTION AND CONCEPTION

1. Harlap, S.; Shiono, P. H.; and Ramcharan, S. "Congenital abnormalities in the offspring of women who used oral contraceptives around the time of conception." *International Journal of Fertility* 30,2(1985): 39–47.

2. Janerich, D. T.; Piper, J. M.; and Glebatis, D. M. "Oral contraceptives and congenital limb-reduction defects." *New England Journal of Medicine* 291(1974): 697–700.

3. Katz, Z., et al. "Teratogenicity of progestogens given during the first trimester of pregnancy." *Obstetrics and Gynecology* 65(1985): 775.

4. Shapiro, H. I. *The Birth Control Book.* New York: Prentice Hall Press, 1988, pp. 63–64.

5. Bracken, M. B. "Oral contraception and congenital malformations in offspring: A review and meta-analysis of the prospective studies." *Obstetrics and Gynecology* 76(1990): 552–556.

6. Simpson, J. L. "Contraception and fetal risk." *Dialogues in Contraception* 3(1991): 1–2.

7. Rothman, K. J. "Fetal loss, twinning, and birth weight after oral contraceptive use." *New England Journal of Medicine* 297(1977): 468–471.

8. World Health Organization Task Force on Oral Contraceptives. "A randomized, double-blind study of two combined and two progesterone-only oral contraceptives." *Contraception* 25(1982): 243.

9. Skolnick, J. L., et al. "Rifampin, oral contraceptives, and pregnancy." *Journal of the American Medical Association* 236(1976): 1382.

10. Murphy, A. A., et al. "The effect of tetracycline on levels of oral contraceptives." *American Journal of Obstetrics and Gynecology* 164(1991): 28–33.

11. Franks, A. L., et al. "Contraception and ectopic pregnancy risk." *American Journal of Obstetrics and Gynecology* 163(1990): 1120–1123.

12. Andrews, W. C. "Pregnancy, the Pill, and postpartum contraception." *Dialogues in Contraception* 2(1988): 1–3.

13. Powell-Beard, L.; Lei, K. Y.; and Shenker, L. "Effect of long-term oral contraceptive therapy before pregnancy on maternal and fetal zinc and copper status." *Obstetrics and Gynecology* 69(1987): 26–31.

14. Lammer, E. J., and Cordero, J. F. "Exogenous sex hormone exposure and the risk for major malformations." *Journal of the American Medical Association* 225(1986): 3128.

15. "Contraceptives and congenital anomalies." ACOG committee opinion, number 62, September, 1988.

16. Kricker, A., et al. "Congenital limb reduction deformities and use of oral contraceptives." *American Journal of Obstetrics and Gynecology* 155(1986): 1072–1078.

17. Wolner-Hanssen, P. "Oral contraceptive use modifies the manifestations of pelvic inflammatory dis-

ease." *British Journal of Obstetrics and Gynaecology* 93(1986): 619.

18. Lewin, T. "Implanted birth control device renews debate over forced contraception." *The New York Times*, Thursday, 1991, p. A20.

19. Pollack, A. "Norplant—What you should know about the new contraceptive." *Medical Aspects of Human Sexuality*, January 1991.

20. Wilson, J. C. "A prospective New Zealand study of fertility after removal of copper intrauterine contraceptive devices for conception and because of complications: A four-year study." *American Journal of Obstetrics and Gynecology* 160(1989): 391–396.

21. Burkman, R. T. "Association between intrauterine device and pelvic inflammatory disease." *Obstetrics and Gynecology* 57(1981): 269–275.

22. Barber, H.R.K. "Contraceptives versus abortifacients." *The Female Patient* 15(1990): 13–14.

23. Sivin, I. "Dose- and age-dependent ectopic pregnancy risks with intrauterine contraception." *Obstetrics and Gynecology* 78(1991): 291–296.

24. Lee, N. C.; Rubin, G. L.; and Borucki, R. "The intrauterine device and pelvic inflammatory disease revisited: New results from the women's health study." *Obstetrics and Gynecology* 72(1988): 1–6.

25. Jovanovic, R., et al. "Preventing infection related to insertion of an intrauterine device." *Journal of Reproductive Medicine* 33(1988): 347–352.

26. "The intrauterine device." ACOG Technical Bulletin, number 104, May 1987.

27. Kirshon, B.; Poindexter, A. N.; and Spitz, M. R. "Pelvic adhesions in intrauterine device users." *Obstetrics and Gynecology* 71(1988): 251–253.

28. Batzer, F. R., and Corson, S. L. "Diagnostic techniques used for ectopic pregnancy." *Journal of Reproductive Medicine* 31(1986): 86–92.

29. Cramer, D. W., et al. "Tubal infertility and the intrauterine device." *New England Journal of Medicine* 312(1985): 941–947.

30. Daling, J. R., et al. "Primary tubal infertility in relation to the use of an intrauterine device." *New England Journal of Medicine* 312(1985): 937–940.

31. Friberg, J., et al. "Chlamydia trachomatis attached to spermatozoa recovered from the peritoneal cavity of patients with salpingitis." *Journal of Reproductive Medicine* 32(1987): 120–122.

32. Haukkamaa, M., et al. "Bacterial flora of the cervix in women using different methods of contraception." *American Journal of Obstetrics and Gynecology* 154(1986): 520–524.

33. Layde, P. M., et al. "Failed intrauterine device contraception and limb reduction deformities." *Fertility and Sterility* 31(1979): 18–20.

34. Lee, N. C., et al. "Type of intrauterine device and the risk of pelvic inflammatory disease." *Obstetrics and Gynecology* 62(1983): 1–6.

35. Randic, L., et al. "Return to fertility after IUD removal for planned pregnancy." *Contraception* 32(1985): 711–717.

36. Vessey, M., et al. "Outcome of pregnancy in women using different methods of contraception." *British Journal of Obstetrics and Gynaecology* 86(1979): 548.

37. Schwarz, R. H., and Mead, P. B. "A new look at IUD-associated infections." *Contemporary OB/GYN*, October 1991, pp. 65–69.

38. Grimes, D. A. "IUDs and pelvic infection." *American Journal of Gynecologic Health* 3, May/June 1989, pp. 23–26.

39. Cordero, J. F., and Layde, P. M. "Vaginal spermicides, chromosomal abnormalities, and limb reduction defects." *Family Planning Perspectives* 15(1983): 16–18.

40. Jick, H.; Walker, A. M.; and Rothman, K. J. "Vaginal spermicides and congenital disorders." *Journal of the American Medical Association* 245(1981): 1329–1332.

41. McBride, G. "Putting a better cap on the cervix." *Journal of the American Medical Association* 243(1980): 1617–1618.

42. Mills, J. L., et al. "Are there adverse effects of periconceptional spermicide use?" *Fertility and Sterility* 43(1985): 442.

43. Bracken, M. B. "Spermicidal contraceptives and poor pregnancy outcomes: The epidemiologic evidence against an association." *American Journal of Obstetrics and Gynecology* 151(1985): 552–556.

44. Warburton, D., et al. "Lack of association between spermicide use and trisomy." *New England Journal of Medicine* 317(1987): 478–482.

45. Louik, C., et al. "Maternal exposure to spermicides in relation to certain birth defects." *New England Journal of Medicine* 317(1987): 474–478.

46. Klonoff-Cohen, H. S., et al. "An epidemiologic

study of contraception and preeclampsia." *Journal of the American Medical Association* 262(1989): 3143–3147.

47. Mills, J. L., et al. "Barrier contraceptive methods and preeclampsia." *Journal of the American Medical Association* 265(1991): 70–73.

48. Cousins, L., et al. "Reproductive outcome of women exposed to diethylstilbestrol in-utero." *Obstetrics and Gynecology* 56(1980): 70–76.

49. Barnes, A. B., et al. "Fertility and outcome of pregnancy in women exposed in-utero to diethylstilbestrol." *New England Journal of Medicine* 302(1980): 609–613.

50. Berger, M. J., and Alder, H. M. "Intractable primary infertility in women exposed to diethylstilbestrol in utero." *Journal of Reproductive Medicine* 31(1986): 231–234.

51. Berger, M. J., and Goldstein, D. P. "Impaired reproductive performance in DES-exposed women." *Obstetrics and Gynecology* 55(1980): 25–27.

52. Bibbo, M., et al. "A twenty-five year follow-up study of women exposed to diethylstilbestrol during pregnancy." *New England Journal of Medicine* 298(1978): 763.

53. Eisenberg, E. "Fertility problems of DES daughters." *Contemporary OB/GYN* 21(1983): 197–199.

54. Gill, W. B.; Schumacher, G. F. B.; and Bibbo, M. "Structural and functional abnormalities in the sex organs of male offspring of mothers treated with diethylstilbestrol (DES)." *Journal of Reproductive Medicine* 16(1976): 147–153.

55. Goldstein, D. P. "Incompetent cervix in offspring exposed to diethylstilbestrol in utero." *Obstetrics and Gynecology* 52(1978): 73s–75s.

56. Kaufman, R. H., et al. "Upper genital tract changes and pregnancy outcome in offspring exposed in utero to diethylstilbestrol." *American Journal of Obstetrics and Gynecology* 137(1980): 299–308.

57. Kaufman, R. H., et al. "Upper genital tract abnormalities and pregnancy outcome in diethylstilbestrol-exposed progeny." *American Journal of Obstetrics and Gynecology* 148(1984): 973–984.

58. "DES daughters: The risks in their childbearing years." Symposium, *Contemporary OB/GYN* 26, (July 1985), pp. 204–232.

59. Thorp, J. M., Jr., et al. "Antepartum and intra-partum events in women exposed in utero to diethylstilbestrol." *Obstetrics and Gynecology* 76 (1990): 828–832.

60. Levy, M. J., and Stillman, R. J. "Reproductive surgery and the DES uterus." Update on surgery, *Contemporary OB/GYN*, 1990, pp. 97–102.

61. Ludmir, J., et al. "Management of the diethylstilbestrol-exposed pregnant patient. A prospective study." *American Journal of Obstetrics and Gynecology* 157(1987): 665–669.

62. Linn, S., et al. "Adverse outcomes of pregnancy in women exposed to diethylstilbestrol in utero." *Journal of Reproductive Medicine* 33(1988): 3–7.

63. Michaels, W. H., et al. "Ultrasound surveillance of the cervix during pregnancy in diethylstilbestrol-exposed offspring." *Obstetrics and Gynecology* 73(1989): 230–238.

64. Iffy, L., and Wingate, M. B. "Risks of rhythm method of birth control." *Journal of Reproductive Medicine* 5(1970): 11–15.

65. James, W. H. "Down's syndrome and parental coital rate." *Lancet* 2(1978): 895.

66. Moscati, I. M., and Becak, W. "Down's syndrome and frequency of intercourse." *Lancet* 2(1978): 629–630.

67. Juberg, R. C. "Origin of chromosomal abnormalities: Evidence for delayed fertilization in meiotic nondisjunction." *Human Genetics* 64(1983): 122.

68. Cates, W., Jr. "Late effects of induced abortion." *Journal of Reproductive Medicine* 22(1979): 207–212.

69. Slater, P. E.; Vavies, A. M.; and Harlap, S. "The effect of abortion method on the outcome of subsequent pregnancy." *Journal of Reproductive Medicine* 26(1981): 123–128.

70. Harlap, S., et al. "A prospective study of spontaneous fetal losses after induced abortions." *New England Journal of Medicine* 301(1979): 677–681.

71. Levin, A. A., et al. "Association of induced abortion with subsequent pregnancy loss." *Journal of the American Medical Association* 243(1980): 2495–2499.

72. Freijka, T. "Induced abortion and fertility." *Family Planning Perspectives* 17(1985): 230–234.

73. "Methods of midtrimester abortion." ACOG Technical Bulletin, number 109, October 1987.

74. Kaunitz, A. M., et al. "Abortions that fail." *Obstetrics and Gynecology* 66(1985): 533–537.

75. DeStefano, F., et al. "Risk of ectopic pregnancy following tubal sterilization." *Obstetrics and Gynecology* 60(1982): 326–329.

76. Henderson, S. R. "The reversibility of female sterilization with the use of microsurgery: A report on 102 patients with more than one year of follow-up." *American Journal of Obstetrics and Gynecology* 149(1984): 57–65.

77. Soderstrom, R. N. "Sterilization failures and their causes." *American Journal of Obstetrics and Gynecology* 152(1985): 395–403.

78. Spivak, M. M.; Librach, C. L.; and Rosenthal, D. M. "Microsurgical reversal of sterilization: A six-year study." *American Journal of Obstetrics and Gynecology* 154(1986): 355–361.

79. Khandwala, S. D. "Laparoscopic sterilization—A comparison of current techniques." *Journal of Reproductive Medicine* 33(1988): 463–466.

80. Holt, V. L., et al. "Tubal sterilization and subsequent ectopic pregnancy—A case-control study." *Journal of the American Medical Association* 266(1991): 242–246.

81. Silber, S. J., and Cohen, R. "Microsurgical reversible of tubal sterilization: Factors affecting pregnancy rate, with long-term follow-up." *Obstetrics and Gynecology* 64(1984): 679–682.

82. Davis, M. R. "Recurrent ectopic pregnancy after tubal sterilization." *Obstetrics and Gynecology* 68(1986): 44S–45S.

83. Hulka, J. F., and Halme, J. "Sterilization reversal: Results of 101 attempts." *American Journal of Obstetrics and Gynecology* 159(1988): 767–774.

84. "Sterilization." ACOG Technical Bulletin, number 113, February 1988.

Chapter 2
PREPREGNANCY AND EARLY PREGNANCY

1. Reade, J. M., and Ratzan, R. M. "Access to information—Physicians' credentials and where you can't find them." *New England Journal of Medicine* 321(1989): 466–468.

2. Merkatz, I. R. "Preconception care." *OBG Management*, November 1991, pp. 20–27.

3. Moos, M. K., and Cefalo, R. C. "Preconception counseling." *Medical Aspects of Human Sexuality*, March 1990, pp. 45–48.

4. Jack, B. W., and Culpepper, L. "Preconception care." *Journal of the American Medical Association* 264(1990): 1147–1149.

5. Mitzmiller, J. L., et al. "Preconception care of diabetes." *Journal of the American Medical Association* 265(1991): 731–736.

6. Doshi, M. L. "Accuracy of consumer performed in-home tests for early pregnancy detection." *American Journal of Public Health* 76(1986): 512.

7. Guerrero, R. "Type and time of insemination within the menstrual cycle and the human sex ratio at birth." *Studies of Family Planning* 6(1975): 367–371.

8. Harlap, S. "Gender of infants conceived on different days of the menstrual cycle." *New England Journal of Medicine* 300(1979): 1445–1448.

9. Kellokumpu-Lehtinen, P., and Pelliniemi, L. J. "Sex ratio of human conceptuses." *Obstetrics and Gynecology* 64(1984): 220–222.

10. Yasin, S. Y., and Beydoun, S. N. "Pregnancy outcome at greater than twenty weeks' gestation in women in their forties." *Journal of Reproductive Medicine* 33(1988): 209–212.

11. Fonteyn, V. J., and Isada, N. B. "Nongenetic implications of childbearing after age thirty-five." *Obstetrical and Gynecological Survey* 43(1988): 709–719.

12. Berkowitz, G. S., et al. "Delayed childbearing and the outcome of pregnancy." *New England Journal of Medicine* 322(1990): 659–664.

13. Martel, M., et al. "Maternal age and primary cesarean section rates: A multivariate analysis." *American Journal of Obstetrics and Gynecology* 156(1987): 305–308.

14. Lehmann, D. K., and Chism, J. "Pregnancy outcome in medically complicated and uncomplicated patients aged 40 years or older." *American Journal of Obstetrics and Gynecology* 157(1987): 738–742.

15. Redwine, F. O. "Pregnancy in women over 35." *The Female Patient* 13(1988): 30–36.

16. Tuck, S. M.; Yudkin, P. L.; and Turnbull, A. C. "Pregnancy outcome in elderly primigravidae with and without a history of infertility." *British Journal of Obstetrics and Gynaecology* 95(1988): 230.

17. Fride, A., et al. "Older maternal age and infant mortality in the United States." *Obstetrics and Gynecology* 72(1988): 152–157.

18. Chervenak, J. L., and Kardon, N. B. "Advancing

maternal age: The actual risks." *The Female Patient* 16(1991): 17–24.

19. Davidson, J. R., and Fukushima, T. "The age extremes for reproduction: Current implications for policy change." *American Journal of Obstetrics and Gynecology* 152(1985): 467–473.

20. Naeye, R. L. "Maternal age, obstetric complications, and the outcome of pregnancy." *Obstetrics and Gynecology* 61(1983): 210–215.

21. Lieberman, E., et al. "The association of interpregnancy interval with small for gestational age births." *Obstetrics and Gynecology* 74(1989): 1–5.

22. Kovacs, B. W., et al. "Prenatal determinations of paternity by molecular genetic 'fingerprinting.' " *Obstetrics and Gynecology* 75(1990): 474–478.

23. Kolins, N. D., and Walker, R. H. "Laboratory determination of parentage." *Obstetrical and Gynecological Survey* 43(1988): 590–595.

24. Roberts, D. F.; Papiha, S. S.; and Bhattacharya, S. S. "A case of disputed maternity." *Lancet* 2(1987): 478.

25. Massop, K. M., and Anderson, T. L. "Trends in teenage pregnancy." *Journal of Reproductive Medicine* 32(1987): 830–832.

26. Park, G. L. "The duration of pregnancy." *Lancet* 2(1968): 1388.

27. Mittendorf, R., et al. "The length of uncomplicated human gestation." *Obstetrics and Gynecology* 75(1990): 929–932.

28. Bagger, P. V., et al. "The precision and accuracy of symphysis—Fundus distance measurements during pregnancy." *Acta Obstetrics and Gynecology of Scandinavia* 64(1985): 371.

29. Klebanoff, M. A., et al. "Epidemiology of vomiting in early pregnancy." *Obstetrics and Gynecology* 66(1985): 612–616.

30. Sahakian, V., et al. "Vitamin B6 is effective therapy for nausea and vomiting of pregnancy. A randomized, double-blind placebo-controlled study." *Obstetrics and Gynecology* 78(1991): 33–37.

31. Tierson, F. D.; Olsen, C. L.; and Hook, E. B. "Nausea and vomiting of pregnancy and association with pregnancy outcome." *Obstetrics and Gynecology* 155(1986): 1017–1022.

32. Samsioe, G., et al. "Does position and size of corpus luteum have any effect on nausea of pregnancy?" *Acta Obstetrics and Gynecology of Scandinavia* 65(1986): 427.

33. Wilcox, A. J., et al. "Incidence of early loss of pregnancy." *New England Journal of Medicine* 319(1988): 189–194.

34. Campana, M.; Serra, A.; and Neri, G. "Role of chromosome aberrations in recurrent abortion: A study of 269 balanced translocations." *American Journal of Medical Genetics* 24(1986): 341.

35. Strobino, B. A., and Pantel-Silverman, J. "First-trimester vaginal bleeding and the loss of chromosomally normal and abnormal conceptions." *American Journal of Obstetrics and Gynecology* 157(1987): 1150–1154.

36. Clark, S. L. "Bleeding during early pregnancy." *The Female Patient* 14(1989): 74–82.

37. Strobino, B., and Pantel-Silverman, J. "Gestational vaginal bleeding and pregnancy outcome." *American Journal of Epidemiology* 129(1989): 806.

38. Williams, M. A., et al. "Adverse infant outcomes associated with first-trimester vaginal bleeding." *Obstetrics and Gynecology* 78(1991): 14–18.

39. Batzofin, J. H.; Fielding, W. L.; and Friedman, E. A. "Effect of vaginal bleeding in early pregnancy on outcome." *Obstetrics and Gynecology* 63(1984): 515–518.

40. Simpson, J. L. "Genetic causes of spontaneous abortion." *Contemporary OB/GYN*, September 1990, pp. 25–40.

41. Fayez, J. A. "Evaluation and management of recurrent early pregnancy losses." *The Female Patient* 13(1988): 100–112.

42. Sachs, E. S., et al. "Chromosome studies of 500 couples with two or more abortions." *Obstetrics and Gynecology* 65(1985): 375–378.

43. McDonough, P. G. "Repeated first trimester pregnancy loss: Evaluation and planned management." *American Journal of Obstetrics and Gynecology* 153(1985): 1–6.

44. Daya, S.; Ward, S.; and Burrows, E. "Progesterone profiles in luteal phase defect cycles and outcome of progesterone treatment in patients with recurrent spontaneous abortion." *American Journal of Obstetrics and Gynecology* 158(1988): 225–232.

45. Vlaanderen, R. W., and Treffers, P. E. "Prognosis of subsequent pregnancies after recurrent spontaneous abortion in first trimester." *British Medical Journal* 295(1987): 92.

46. Carp, H. J. A., et al. "Recurrent miscarriage: A

review of current concepts. Immune mechanisms and results of treatment." *Obstetrical and Gynecological Survey* 45(1990): 657–666.

47. Michaels, W. H., et al. "Ultrasound differentiation of the competent from the incompetent cervix: Prevention of preterm delivery." *American Journal of Obstetrics and Gynecology* 154(1986): 537–546.

48. Schott, J. R.; Rote, N. S.; and Branch, D. W. "Immunologic aspects of recurrent abortion and fetal death." *Obstetrics and Gynecology* 70(1987): 645–653.

49. McIntyre, J. A., et al. "Immunologic testing and immunotherapy in recurrent spontaneous abortion." *Obstetrics and Gynecology* 67(1986): 169–173.

50. Thomas, M. L., et al. "H.L.A. sharing and spontaneous abortion in humans." *American Journal of Obstetrics and Gynecology* 151(1985): 1053–1058.

51. Harger, J. H.; Rabin, B. S.; and Marchese, S. G. "The prognostic value of antinuclear antibodies in women with recurrent pregnancy losses: A prospective controlled study." *Obstetrics and Gynecology* 73(1989): 419–423.

52. Ober, C., et al. "Prenatal effects of maternal-fetal HLA compatibility." *American Journal of Reproductive Immunology and Microbiology* 15(1987): 141.

53. Moore, T. R., and Resnik, R. "Preventing fetal wastage caused by lupus anticoagulant antibodies." *Contemporary OB/GYN*, November 1987, pp. 127–141.

54. Beckerman, K. P. "What is the lupus anticoagulant?" *Contemporary OB/GYN*, June 1988, pp. 67–86.

55. Cashner, K. A.; Christopher, C. R.; and Dysert, G. A. "Spontaneous fetal loss after demonstration of a live fetus in the first trimester." *Obstetrics and Gynecology* 70(1987): 827–830.

56. Goldstein, S. R., et al. "Very early pregnancy detection with endovaginal ultrasound." *Obstetrics and Gynecology* 72(1988): 200–204.

57. Bromley, B., et al. "Small sac size in the first trimester: A predictor of poor fetal outcome." *Radiology* 178(1991): 375.

58. Steinkampf, M. P. "Transvaginal sonography." *Journal of Reproductive Medicine* 33(1988): 931–937.

59. MacKenzie, W. E.; Holmes, D. S.; and Newton, J. R. "Spontaneous abortion rates in ultrasonographically viable pregnancies." *Obstetrics and Gynecology* 71(1988): 81–83.

60. Cullen, M. T., et al. "Transvaginal ultrasonographic detection of congenital anomalies in the first trimester." *American Journal of Obstetrics and Gynecology* 163(1990): 466–475.

61. Reece, E. A., et al. "Dating through pregnancy: A measure of growing up." *Obstetrical and Gynecological Survey* 44(1988): 544–547.

62. Ward, H. "Review of the development and current status of techniques for monitoring embryonic and fetal development in the first trimester of pregnancy." *American Journal of Medical Genetics* 35(1990): 157.

63. Daya, S., et al. "Early pregnancy assessment with transvaginal ultrasound scanning." *Canadian Medical Association Journal* 144(1991): 441.

64. Nyberg, D. A., et al. "Early pregnancy complications: Endovaginal sonographic findings correlated with human chorionic gonadotropin levels." *Radiology* 167(1988): 619.

65. Nyberg, D. A., et al. "Abnormal pregnancy: Early diagnosis by ultrasound and serum chorionic gonadotropin levels." *Radiology* 158(1986): 393.

66. "Ectopic pregnancy." ACOG Technical Bulletin, number 126, March 1989.

67. Stabile, I., and Grudainaskas, J. G. "Ectopic pregnancy: A review of incidence, etiology, and diagnostic aspects." *Obstetrical and Gynecological Survey* 45(1990): 335–346.

68. Taylor, R. N. "Ectopic pregnancy and reproductive technology." *Journal of the American Medical Association* 259(1988): 1862.

69. Batzer, F. R. "The use of sonography in the diagnosis and management of ectopic pregnancy." *American Journal of Gynecological Health* 5(1991): 29–32.

70. Neiger, R., et al. "Diagnosis of ectopic pregnancy using transvaginal ultrasound scanning." *Journal of Reproductive Medicine* 34(1989): 52–54.

71. Romero, R., et al. "The value of serial human chorionic gonadotropin testing as a diagnostic tool in ectopic pregnancy." *American Journal of Obstetrics and Gynecology* 155(1986): 392–394.

72. Hallatt, J. G. "Tubal conservation in ectopic pregnancy: A study of 200 cases." *American Journal of*

Obstetrics and Gynecology 154(1986): 216–221.

73. "New reproductive technologies." ACOG Technical Bulletin, number 140, March 1990.

74. Martin, M. C. "Gonadotropin releasing hormone agonists and the induction or augmentation of ovulation." *Journal of Reproductive Medicine* 34(1989): 1034–1038.

75. Levran, D., et al. "Pregnancy potential of human oocytes—The effect of cryopreservation." *New England Journal of Medicine* 323(1990): 1153–1156.

76. Hill, G. A., et al. "Complications of pregnancy in infertile couples: Routine treatment versus assisted reproduction." *Obstetrics and Gynecology* 75(1990): 790.

77. Wilson, A. L.; Fenton, L. J.; and Munson, D. P. "State reporting of live births of newborns weighing less than 500 grams—Impact on neonatal mortality rates." *Pediatrics* 78(1986): 850–854.

Chapter 3
SPORTS AND PHYSICAL FITNESS

1. "Women and exercise." ACOG Technical Bulletin, number 87, September 1985.

2. Varrassi, G., et al. "Effects of physical activity on maternal plasma B-endorphin levels and perception of labor pain." *American Journal of Obstetrics and Gynecology* 160(1989): 707–712.

3. Clapp, J. F. "Maternal heart rate in pregnancy." *American Journal of Obstetrics and Gynecology* 152(1985): 659–660.

4. Schaefer, C. F. "Possible teratogenic hyperthermia and marathon running." *Journal of the American Medical Association* 241(1979): 1892.

5. Jones, R. L. "Thermoregulation during aerobic exercise in pregnancy." *Obstetrics and Gynecology* 65(1985): 340–345.

6. Driscoll, C. E., et al. "Women in sports: Guidelines for patient fitness." *The Female Patient* 13(1988): 41–51.

7. Wight, S. E. "Exercise during pregnancy: Yes or no?" *The Female Patient* 11(1986): 73–84.

8. Wong, S. C., and McKenzie, D. C. "Cardiorespiratory fitness during pregnancy and its effect on outcome." *International Journal of Sports Medicine* 8(1987): 79–83.

9. Artel, R., et al. "Exercise prescription in pregnancy: Weight-bearing versus non-weight-bearing

exercise." *American Journal of Obstetrics and Gynecology* 161(1989): 464–469.

10. Jovanovic-Peterson, L.; Durak, E. P.; and Peterson, C. M. "Randomized trial of diet versus diet plus cardiovascular conditioning on glucose levels in gestational diabetes." *American Journal of Obstetrics and Gynecology* 161(1989): 415–419.

11. Artel, R., et al. "Pulmonary responses to exercise in pregnancy." *American Journal of Obstetrics and Gynecology* 154(1986): 378–383.

12. Clapp, J. F. "The effects of maternal exercise on early pregnancy outcome." *American Journal of Obstetrics and Gynecology* 161(1989): 453–457.

13. Beckmann, C. R. B., and Beckmann, C. A. "Effect of a structured antepartum exercise program on pregnancy and labor outcome in primiparas." *Journal of Reproductive Medicine* 35(1990): 704–718.

14. Clapp, J. F. "The course of labor after endurance exercise during pregnancy." *American Journal of Obstetrics and Gynecology* 163(1990): 1799–1805.

15. Kulpa, P. J.; White, B. M.; and Visscher, R. "Aerobic exercise in pregnancy." *American Journal of Obstetrics and Gynecology* 156(1987): 1395–1403.

16. Kollings, C., and Curet, L. B. "Fetal heart rate response to maternal exercise." *American Journal of Obstetrics and Gynecology* 151(1985): 498–501.

17. Clapp, J. F. "Fetal heart rate response to running in mid pregnancy and late pregnancy." *American Journal of Obstetrics and Gynecology* 153(1985): 251–252.

18. South-Paul, J. E.; Rajapopa, K. R.; and Tenholder, M. F. "The effect of participation in a regular exercise program upon aerobic capacity during pregnancy." *Obstetrics and Gynecology* 71(1988): 175–178.

19. Artil, R., et al. "Fetal heart rate responses to maternal exercise." *American Journal of Obstetrics and Gynecology* 155(1986): 729–733.

20. Carpenter, M. W., et al. "Fetal heart rate response to maternal exertion." *Journal of the American Medical Association* 259(1988): 3006–3009.

21. Morrow, R. J.; Ritchie, J. W. K.; and Bull, S. B. "Fetal and maternal hemodynamic responses to exercise in pregnancy assessed by Doppler ultrasonography." *American Journal of Obstetrics and Gynecology* 160(1989): 138–140.

22. Durak, E. P.; Govanovic-Peterson, L.; and Peter-

son, C. M. "Comparative evaluation of uterine response to exercise on five aerobic machines." *American Journal of Obstetrics and Gynecology* 162(1990): 755–756.

23. Watson, W. J., et al. "Fetal response to maximal swimming and cycling exercise during pregnancy." *Obstetrics and Gynecology* 77(1991): 382–386.

24. Veille, J. C., et al. "Umbilical artery waveform during bicycle exercise in normal pregnancy." *Obstetrics and Gynecology* 73(1989): 957–960.

25. Eichner, E. R. "Anemia in female athletes." *Your Patient and Fitness* 3(1989): 3–11.

26. Siegel, A. J. "Exercise-related hematuria." *Journal of the American Medical Association* 242(1979): 1610.

27. Voitk, A. J., et al. "Carpal tunnel syndrome in pregnancy." *Canadian Medical Association Journal* 128(1983): 277.

28. Moran, J. J. M. "Stress fractures in pregnancy." *American Journal of Obstetrics and Gynecology* 158(1988): 1274–1277.

29. Berg, G., et al. "Low back pain during pregnancy." *Obstetrics and Gynecology* 71(1988): 71–75.

30. "Safety guidelines for women who exercise." ACOG Home Exercise Program, May 1986.

31. Hall, D. D., and Kaufmann, D. A. "Effects of aerobic and strength conditioning on pregnancy outcomes." *American Journal of Obstetrics and Gynecology* (1987): 1199–1203.

32. Clark, C. S., et al. "Gastroesophageal reflux induced by exercise in healthy volunteers." *Journal of the American Medical Association* 261(1989): 3599–3601.

33. Brody, J. E. "Cross-country skiing: A booming, high-intensity aerobic sport suitable for nearly all ages." *The New York Times*, Thursday, January 4, 1990, p. B8.

34. Shangold, M. M. "Advising women about exercise: What to tell your patients." *The Female Patient* 12(1987): 57–65.

35. Newhall, J. F., Jr. "Scuba diving during pregnancy: A brief review." *American Journal of Obstetrics and Gynecology* 140(1981): 893–894.

36. Bolton, M. E. "Scuba diving and fetal well-being: A survey of 208 women." *Undersea Biomedical Research* 7(1980).

37. Rippe, J. M., et al. "Walking for health and fitness." *Journal of the American Medical Association* 259(1988): 2720–2724.

38. Brody, J. E. "Beset by pain, a jogger turns to fitness walking and finds new fulfillment." *The New York Times*, Thursday, March 9, 1989, p. B7.

39. Katz, J. "Liquid refreshment for the outer you." *The New York Times*, Monday, June 12, 1989, p. C11.

40. Katz, V. L., et al. "Fetal and uterine responses to immersion and exercise." *Obstetrics and Gynecology* 72(1988): 225–230.

41. McMurray, R. G., et al. "The effect of pregnancy on metabolic responses during rest, immersion, and aerobic exercise in the water." *American Journal of Obstetrics and Gynecology* 158(1988): 481–486.

Chapter 4
SEXUALITY DURING PREGNANCY

1. Masters, W. H., and Johnson, Z. E. *Human Sexuality Response*, Boston: Little, Brown, 1966.

2. Debrovner, C. H. "Vaginal lubrication." *Medical Aspects of Human Sexuality*, November 1975, pp. 35–42.

3. Schnarch, D. M. "Inhibited sexual desire." *The Female Patient* 14(1989): 83–86.

4. "Common sexual complaints—How to elicit and evaluate them." Forum, *The Female Patient* 13(1988): 41–48.

5. Gelman, D. "Not tonight—A common plea." *Newsweek*, Winter 1988, pp. 10–12.

6. Sanderson, M. O., and Maddock, J. W. "Guidelines for assessment and treatment of sexual dysfunction." *Obstetrics and Gynecology* 73(1989): 130–134.

7. Reamy, K., and White, S. E. "Sexuality in pregnancy and the puerperium: A review." *Obstetrical and Gynecological Survey* 40(1985): 1–11.

8. Gameron, G. W. "Helping couples cope with sexual changes pregnancy brings." *Contemporary OB/GYN*, February 1983, pp. 23–34.

9. Wagner, N. N., and Solberg, D. A. "Pregnancy and sexuality." *Medical Aspects of Human Sexuality*, March 1974, pp. 44–66.

10. Naeye, R. L. "Coitus late in pregnancy linked to

antepartum bleeds." *British Journal of Obstetrics and Gynaecology* 88(1981): 765–770.

11. Falicove, C. J. "Sexual adjustment during first pregnancy and postpartum." *American Journal of Obstetrics and Gynecology* 117(1973): 991–1000.

12. Perkins, R. P. "Sexuality in pregnancy: What determines behavior?" *Obstetrics and Gynecology* 59(1982): 189–198.

13. Wales, D. "The impact of childbirth on sexual functioning." *The Female Patient*, September 1979, pp. 44–51.

14. Javert, C. T. "Repeated abortion—Results of treatment with 100 patients." *Obstetrics and Gynecology* 3(1954): 420.

15. Goodlin, R. C.; Keller, D. W.; and Raffin, M. "Orgasm during late pregnancy." *Obstetrics and Gynecology* 38(1971): 916–920.

16. Wagner, N. N.; Butler, J. C.; and Sanders, J. B. "Prematurity and orgasmic coitus during pregnancy: Data on a small sample." *Fertility and Sterility* 27(1976): 911–915.

17. Rayburn, W. F., and Wilson, E. A. "Coital activity and premature delivery." *American Journal of Obstetrics and Gynecology* 137:972–974.

18. Goodlin, R. C. "Orgasm and premature labor." *Lancet* 2(1969): 646.

19. Perkins, R. P. "Sexual behavior and response in relation to complications of pregnancy." *American Journal of Obstetrics and Gynecology* 134(1979): 498–505.

20. Goodlin, R. C.; Schmidt, W.; and Creedy, D. C. "Uterine tension and fetal heart rate during maternal orgasm." *Obstetrics and Gynecology* 39(1972): 125–127.

21. Grudzinskas, J. G.; Watson, C.; and Chard, T. "Does sexual intercourse cause fetal distress?" *Lancet* 2(1979): 692–693.

22. Naeye, R. L. "Coitus and associated amniotic fluid infections." *New England Journal of Medicine* 301(1979): 1198–1200.

23. Neilson, J. P., and Mutambira, M. "Coitus, twin pregnancy, and preterm labor." *American Journal of Obstetrics and Gynecology* 160(1989): 416–418.

24. Romem, Y.; Sires, C.; and Artal, R. "Effects of seminal ejaculate on the biomechanical properties of choreoamniotic membranes." *Journal of Reproductive Medicine* 34(1989): 221–224.

25. Brustman, L. E. "Changes in the pattern of uterine contractility in relationship to coitus during pregnancies at low and high risk for preterm labor." *Obstetrics and Gynecology* 73(1989): 166–167.

26. Klebanoff, M. A.; Nugent, R. P.; and Rhodes, G. G. "Coitus during pregnancy: Is it safe?" *Lancet* 2(1984): 914.

27. Jenson, J. D. "Anal coitus by married couples." *Medical Aspects of Human Sexuality*, July 1975, p. 115.

28. Swerglow, H. "Significance of relaxed anal sphincter during rectal examination." *Medical Aspects of Human Sexuality*, January 1980, p. 121.

29. Aronson, M. E. "Fatal air embolism caused by bizarre sexual behavior during pregnancy." *Medical Aspects of Human Sexuality*, December 1969, pp. 33–39.

30. DeCherney, W. A., and DeCherney, A. H. "Hazardous and safe douching." *Medical Aspects of Human Sexuality*, September 1977, pp. 77–78.

31. Bray, P.; Myers, A. M.; and Cowley, R. A. "Orogenital sex as a cause of nonfatal air embolism in pregnancy." *Obstetrics and Gynecology* 61(1983): 653–657.

32. Renshaw, D. C. "Breastfeeding and postpartum sexuality." *The Female Patient* 12(1987): 37–42.

33. Masters, W. H. "Diminished sexual response after childbirth." *Clinical Practice in Sexuality* 4(1988): 24.

Chapter 5
BAD HABITS

1. MacGregor, S. N., and Keith, L. G. "Substance abuse in pregnancy—A practical management plan." *The Female Patient* 14(1989): 49–63.

2. Hatch, E. E., and Bracken, M. B. "Effect of marijuana use in pregnancy on fetal growth." *American Journal of Epidemiology* 124(1986): 986.

3. Nahas, G. G. "Marijuana, pregnancy and breast feeding." *Journal of the American Medical Association* 242(1979): 1299.

4. Hingson, R., et al. "Effects of maternal drinking and marijuana use on fetal growth and development." *Pediatrics* 70(1982): 539.

5. Zuckerman, B., et al. "Effects of maternal marijuana and cocaine use on fetal growth." *New England Journal of Medicine* 320(1989): 762–768.

6. Wu, T., et al. Pulmonary hazards of smoking marijuana as compared with tobacco." *New England Journal of Medicine* 318(1988): 347–351.

7. Hoff, C., et al. "Trend associations of smoking with maternal, fetal, and neonatal mobility." *Obstetrics and Gynecology* 68(1986): 317–321.

8. Chow, W., et al. "Maternal cigarette smoking and tubal pregnancy." *Obstetrics and Gynecology* 71(1988): 167–170.

9. Rigotti, N. A. "Cigarette smoking and body weight." *New England Journal of Medicine* 320(1989): 931–932.

10. Nelson, N. M., and Stillman, R. J. "Smoking and reproductive health." 1(1987): 6–10.

11. Chatterjee, M. S., et al. "Amniotic fluid cadmium and thiocyanate in pregnant women who smoke." *Journal of Reproductive Medicine* 33(1988): 417–420.

12. Pinette, M. C., et al. "Maternal smoking and accelerated placental maturation." *Obstetrics and Gynecology* 73(1989): 379–382.

13. Brown, H. L., et al. "Premature placental calcification in maternal cigarette smokers." *Obstetrics and Gynecology* 71(1988): 914–916.

14. Hauth, J. C., et al. "Passive smoking and thiocyanate concentrations in pregnant women and newborns." *Obstetrics and Gynecology* 63(1984): 519–522.

15. McLaren, N. M., and Nieburg, P. "Fetal tobacco syndrome and other problems caused by smoking during pregnancy." *Medical Aspects of Human Sexuality*, March 1989, pp. 58–62.

16. Lindblad, A.; Marsal, K.; and Andersson, K. "Effect of nicotine on human fetal blood flow." *Obstetrics and Gynecology* 72(1988): 371–381.

17. Morrow, R. J.; Ritchi, J. W. K.; and Bull, S. B. "Maternal cigarette smoking: The effects on umbilical and uterine blood flow velocity." *American Journal of Obstetrics and Gynecology* 159(1988): 1069–1071.

18. Eriksen, P. S., et al. "Acute effects of maternal smoking on fetal breathing and movements." *Obstetrics and Gynecology* 61(1983): 367–371.

19. White, E., et al. "Maternal smoking and infant respiratory distress syndrome." *Obstetrics and Gynecology* 67(1986): 365–369.

20. Kuhnert, P. M., et al. "The effect of smoking on placental and fetal zinc status." *American Journal of Obstetrics and Gynecology* 157(1987): 1241–1246.

21. Metcoff, J., et al. "Smoking in pregnancy: Relation of birth weight to maternal plasma carotene and cholesterol levels." *Obstetrics and Gynecology* 74(1989): 302–308.

22. Fielding, J. E., and Phenow, K. J. "Health effects of involuntary smoking." *New England Journal of Medicine* 319(1988): 1452–1460.

23. Tager, I. B., et al. "Longitudinal study of the effect of maternal smoking on pulmonary function in children." *New England Journal of Medicine* 309(1983): 699.

24. Haddow, J. E., et al. "Second-trimester serum nicotine levels in nonsmokers in relation to birth weight." *American Journal of Obstetrics and Gynecology* 159(1988): 481–484.

25. Naeye, R. L., and Peters, E. C. "Mental development of children whose mothers smoked during pregnancy." 64(1984): 601–607.

26. Benowitz, N. L., et al. "Influence of smoking fewer cigarettes on exposure to tar, nicotine, and carbon monoxide." *New England Journal of Medicine* 315(1986): 1310.

27. Kozlowski, L. T., et al. "Comparing tobacco cigarette dependence with other drug dependencies." *Journal of the American Medical Association* 216(1989): 898–901.

28. Benowitz, N. L. "Nicotine replacement therapy during pregnancy." *Journal of the American Medical Association* 266(1991): 3174–3177.

29. Tonnesen, P., et al. "A double-blind trial of a 16-hour transdermal nicotine patch in smoking cessation." *New England Journal of Medicine* 325(1991): 311–315.

30. Hughes, J. R., et al. "Nicotine vs. placebo gum in general medical practice." *Journal of the American Medical Association* 261(1989): 1300–1305.

31. Hogue, C. J. R.; Zahniser, S. C.; and Dalmat, M. E. "You can help your ob patients stop smoking." *Contemporary OB/GYN*, August 1987, pp. 130–143.

32. Frank, E., et al. "Predictors of physicians' smoking cessation advice." *Journal of the American Medical Association* 266(1991): 3139–3144.

33. Mullen, T. D.; Quinn, V. P.; and Ershoff, D. H. "Maintenance of nonsmoking postpartum by women who stopped smoking during pregnancy."

American Journal of Public Health 80(1990): 992.

34. Hadi, H. A.; Hill, J. A.; and Castillo, R. A. "Alcohol and reproductive function: A review." *Obstetrical and Gynecological Survey* 42(1987): 69–73.

35. Ewing, J. A. "Detecting alcoholism—The CAGE questionnaire." *Journal of the American Medical Association* 252(1984): 1905–1907.

36. Erskine, R. L. A., and Ritchie, J. W. K. "The effect of maternal consumption of alcohol on human umbilical artery blood flow." *American Journal of Obstetrics and Gynecology* 154(1986): 318–321.

37. Kaufman, M. H. "Ethanol-induced chromosomal abnormalities at conception." *Nature* 302(1983): 258.

38. Ernhart, C. B., et al. "Alcohol teratogenicity in the human: A detailed assessment of specificity, critical period, and threshold." *American Journal of Obstetrics and Gynecology* 156(1987): 33–39.

39. Urfer, F. N., et al. "Low levels of blood alcohol and fetal myocardial function." *Obstetrics and Gynecology* 64(1984): 401–404.

40. Serdula, M., et al. "Trends in alcohol consumption by pregnant women." *Journal of the American Medical Association* 265(1991): 876–879.

41. Stokes, E. J. "Alcohol abuse screening—What to ask your female patient." *The Female Patient* 14(1989): 17–23.

42. Mills, J. L., and Graubard, B. I. "Is moderate drinking during pregnancy associated with an increased risk for malformations?" *Pediatrics* 80(1987): 309.

43. Danis, R. P., and Keith, L. "Fetal alcohol syndrome: Incurable but preventable." *Contemporary OB/GYN*, March 1983, pp. 57–68.

44. Ioffe, S., and Chernick, V. "Maternal alcohol ingestion and the incidence of respiratory distress syndrome." *American Journal of Obstetrics and Gynecology* 156(1987): 1231–1235.

45. Minella, J. A., and Beauchamp, G. K. "The transfer of alcohol to human milk." *New England Journal of Medicine* 325(1991): 981–985.

46. Little, R. E., et al. "Maternal alcohol use during breastfeeding and infant mental and motor development at one year." *New England Journal of Medicine* 321(1989): 425–430.

47. Gawin, F. H., and Ellinwood, E. H., Jr. "Cocaine and other stimulants." *New England Journal of Medicine* 318(1988): 1173–1182.

48. Lang, E. R., et al. "Cocaine-induced coronary-artery vasoconstriction." *New England Journal of Medicine* 321(1989): 1557–1562.

49. Levine, S. R., et al. "Cerebrovascular complications of the use of 'crack' form of alkaloidal cocaine." *New England Journal of Medicine* 323(1990): 699–704.

50. Rosenak, D., et al. "Cocaine—Maternal use during pregnancy and its effects on the mother, the fetus, and the infant." *Obstetrical and Gynecological Survey* 45(1990): 348–358.

51. Phibbs, C. S.; Bateman, D. A.; and Schwartz, R. M. "The neonatal costs of maternal cocaine use." *Journal of the American Medical Association* 266(1991): 1521–1526.

52. Woods, J. R.; Plessinger, M. A.; and Clark, K. E. "Effect of cocaine on uterine blood flow and fetal oxygenation." *Journal of the American Medical Association* 257(1987): 957–961.

53. MacGregor, S. N., et al. "Cocaine use during pregnancy—Adverse perinatal outcome." *American Journal of Obstetrics and Gynecology* 157(1987): 686–690.

54. Hoskins, I. A., et al. "Relationship between antepartum cocaine abuse, abnormal umbilical artery Doppler velocimetry, and placental abruption." *Obstetrics and Gynecology* 78(1991): 279–282.

55. Perlow, J. H.; Schlossberg, D. L.; and Strassner, H. T. "Intrapartum cocaine use." 35(1990): 978–980.

56. Little, B. B., and Snell, L. M. "Brain growth among fetuses exposed to cocaine in utero: Asymmetrical growth retardation." *Obstetrics and Gynecology* 77(1991): 361–364.

57. Chasnoff, I. J., et al. "Temporal patterns of cocaine use in pregnancy." *Journal of the American Medical Association* 261(1989): 1741–1744.

58. Greenland, V. C.; Delke, I.; and Minkoff, H. L. "Vaginally administered cocaine overdose in a pregnant woman." *Obstetrics and Gynecology* 74(1989): 476–478.

59. Little, B. B., et al. "Cocaine abuse during pregnancy: Maternal and fetal implications." *Obstetrics and Gynecology* 73(1989): 157–160.

60. Thatcher, S. S., et al. "Cocaine use and acute

rupture of ectopic pregnancies." *Obstetrics and Gynecology* 74(1989): 478–480.

61. Neerhof, M. G., et al. "Cocaine abuse during pregnancy: Peripartum prevalence and perinatal outcome." *American Journal of Obstetrics and Gynecology* 161(1989): 633–638.

62. Chazotte, C.; Forman, L.; and Gandhi, J. "Heart rate patterns in fetuses exposed to cocaine." *Obstetrics and Gynecology* 78(1991): 323–325.

63. Cherukuri, R., et al. "A cohort study of alkaloidal cocaine ('crack') in pregnancy." *Obstetrics and Gynecology* 72(1988): 147–151.

64. Mastrogiannis, D. S., et al. "Perinatal outcome after recent cocaine usage." *Obstetrics and Gynecology* 76(1990): 8–11.

65. Burkett, G.; Yasin, S.; and Palow, D. "Perinatal implication of cocaine exposure." *Journal of Reproductive Medicine* 35(1990): 35–42.

66. Graham, K., et al. "Determination of gestational cocaine exposure by hair analysis." *Journal of the American Medical Association* 262(1989): 3328–3330.

67. Yaziji, R. A.; Odem, R. R.; and Polakoski, K. L. "Demonstration of specific binding of cocaine to human spermatozoa." *Journal of the American Medical Association* 266(1991): 1956–1959.

68. Oro, A. S., and Dixon, S. D. "Perinatal cocaine and methamphetamine exposure: Maternal and neonatal correlates." *Journal of Pediatrics* 111(1987): 571.

69. Von Almen, W. F., and Miller, J. M., Jr. "Ts and blues in pregnancy." *Journal of Reproductive Medicine* 31(1986): 236–239.

70. Little, B. B.; Snell, L. M.; and Gilstrap, L. C. "Methamphetamine abuse during pregnancy: Outcome and fetal effects." *Obstetrics and Gynecology* 72(1988): 541–544.

71. Trager, J. "A plea not to make a pariah of 'ecstasy.'" *Medical Tribune*, December 29, 1988, pp. 12–14.

72. Dowling, G. P.; McDonough, E. T.; and Bost, R. O. "Eve and ecstasy." *Journal of the American Medical Association* 257(1987): 1615–1617.

73. Dorrance, D. L.; Janiger, O.; and Teplitz, R. L. "Effect of peyote on human chromosomes." *Journal of the American Medical Association* 234(1975): 299–302.

74. Golden, N. L.; Sokol, R. J.; and Rubin, I. L.

"Angel dust: Possible effects on the fetus." *Pediatrics* 55(1980): 18.

75. Kaufman, A. R., et al. "Phencyclidine in umbilical cord blood: Preliminary data." *American Journal of Psychiatry* 140(1983): 450.

76. Little, B. B., et al. "Maternal and fetal effects of heroin addiction during pregnancy." *Journal of Reproductive Medicine* 35(1990): 159–162.

77. Ronkin, S., et al. "Protecting mother and fetus from narcotic abuse." *Contemporary OB/GYN*, March 1988, pp. 178–187.

78. Edelin, K. C., et al. "Methadone maintenance in pregnancy: Consequences to care and outcome." *Obstetrics and Gynecology* 71(1988): 399–403.

79. Archie, C. L., et al. "The effects of methadone treatment on the reactivity of nonstress test." *Obstetrics and Gynecology* 74(1989): 254–255.

80. Dole, V. P. "Implications of methadone maintenance for theories of narcotic addiction." *Journal of the American Medical Association* 260(1988): 3025–3029.

Chapter 6
SEXUALLY TRANSMITTED DISEASES

1. Isacman, S. H., and Closen, M. L. "Diagnosis of STDs: Physician responsibilities." *Medical Aspects of Human Sexuality*, November 1989, pp. 18–22.

2. Bracero, L. A., and Wormser, G. P. "Serologic tests for syphilis." *Medical Aspects of Human Sexuality*, May 1989, pp. 74–80.

3. Mascola, L., et al. "Congenital syphilis: Why is it still occurring?" *Journal of the American Medical Association* 252(1984): 1719.

4. Schwebke, J. R. "Syphilis in the 90s." *Medical Aspects of Human Sexuality*, April 1991, pp. 44–49.

5. Rolfs, R. T., and Nakashima, A. K. "Epidemiology of primary and secondary syphilis in the United States, 1981 through 1989." *Journal of the American Medical Association* 264(1990): 1432–1437.

6. Wendel, G. D. "We can and must prevent congenital syphilis." *Contemporary OB/GYN*, September 1985, pp. 151–165.

7. Handsfield, H. H. "Old enemies—Combatting syphilis and gonorrhea in the 1990s." *Journal of*

the American Medical Association 264(1990): 1451–1452.

8. Sweet, R. L. "Acute salpingitis treatment—An update." *Contemporary OB/GYN*, December 1991, pp. 43–52.

9. Schwarcz, S. K., et al. "National surveillance of anti-microbial resistance in Neisseria gonorrhoeae." *Journal of the American Medical Association* 264(1990): 1413–1417.

10. Laga, M., et al. "Prophylaxis of gonococcal and chlamydial ophthalmia neonatorum—A comparison of silver nitrate and tetracycline." *New England Journal of Medicine* 318(1988): 653–657.

11. Pastorek, J. G. "Antimicrobial therapy for PID." *Contemporary OB/GYN*, April 1989, pp. 31–42.

12. Minkoff, H. L. "Preventing damage from nonviral STDs." *Contemporary OB/GYN*, February 1988, pp. 137–152.

13. Sandstrom, K. I., et al. "Microbial causes of neonatal conjunctivitis." *Journal of Pediatrics* 105(1984): 706.

14. Hammerschlag, M. R., et al. "Efficacy of neonatal ocular prophylaxis for the prevention of chlamydial and gonococcal conjunctivitis." *New England Journal of Medicine* 320(1989): 769–772.

15. Paavonen, J. "Chlamydial disease during pregnancy." *Contemporary OB/GYN*, March 1991, pp. 91–96.

16. Amortejui, A. J., and Meyer, M. P. "Enzyme immunoassay for detection of Chlamydia trachomatis from the cervix." *Obstetrics and Gynecology* 65(1985): 523–526.

17. FitzSimmons, J., et al. "Chlamydial infections in pregnancy." *Journal of Reproductive Medicine* 31(1986): 19–22.

18. Ryan, G. M., Jr., et al. "Chlamydia trachomatis infection in pregnancy and effect of treatment on outcome." *American Journal of Obstetrics and Gynecology* 162(1990): 34–39.

19. Cohen, I.; Veille, J-C.; and Calkins, B. M. "Improved pregnancy outcome following successful treatment of chlamydial infection." *Journal of the American Medical Association* 263(1990): 3160–3163.

20. Campbell, W. T., and Dodson, M. G. "Clindamycin therapy for Chlamydia trachomatis in women." *Fertility and Sterility* 53(1990): 620.

21. Sweet, R. L., et al. "Chlamydia trachomatis infection and pregnancy outcome." *American Journal of Obstetrics and Gynecology* 156(1987): 824–833.

22. Crombleholme, W. "Neonatal chlamydial infections." *Contemporary OB/GYN*, August 1991, pp. 57–60.

23. Bell, T. A., et al. "Chronic Chlamydia trachomatis infections in infants." *Journal of the American Medical Association* 267(1992): 400–402.

24. Schachter, J., et al. "Experience with the routine use of erythromycin for Chlamydial infections in pregnancy." *New England Journal of Medicine* 314(1986): 276.

25. "Perinatal herpes simplex virus infections." ACOG Technical Bulletin, Number 122, November 1988.

26. Harger, J. H. "Genital herpes infections." *Contemporary OB/GYN*, May 1990, pp. 83–91.

27. Peng, T. C. C., and Johnson, T. R. B. "Herpes simplex virus in the pregnant patient." *The Female Patient* 14(1989): 27–39.

28. Maslow, A. S., and Bobitt, J. R. "Herpes in pregnancy: Exploring clinical options." *Contemporary OB/GYN*, October 1988, pp. 44–61.

29. Brock, B. V., et al. "Frequency of asymptomatic shedding of herpes simplex virus in women with genital herpes." *Journal of the American Medical Association* 263(1990): 418–420.

30. Prober, C. G. "Use of routine viral cultures at delivery to identify neonates exposed to herpes simplex virus." *New England Journal of Medicine* 318(1988): 887–891.

31. Simkovich, J. W., and Soper, D. E. "Operative delivery for intra-partum genital herpes virus infection." *American Journal of Gynecologic Health* 1(1987): 13–16.

32. Harger, J. H. "Indications for antepartum HSV screening cultures." *Infections in Surgery*, January 1989, pp. 24–31.

33. Gibbs, R. S. "Herpes simplex virus infections in pregnancy." *Contemporary OB/GYN*, May 1991, pp. 85–86.

34. Gibbs, R. S., et al. "Management of genital herpes infections in pregnancy." *Obstetrics and Gynecology* 71(1988): 779.

35. Minkoff, H. L. "Herpesvirus infection during and after pregnancy." *Medical Aspects of Human Sexuality*, April 1988, pp. 38–46.

36. Brown, Z. A., et al. "Effects on infants of a first episode of genital herpes during pregnancy." *New England Journal of Medicine* 317(1987): 1246–1251.

37. Brown, Z. A., et al. "Neonatal herpes simplex virus infection in relation to asymptomatic maternal infection at the time of labor." *New England Journal of Medicine* 324(1991): 1247–1252.

38. Whitley, R., et al. "Predictors of morbidity and mortality in neonates with herpes simplex virus infections." *New England Journal of Medicine* 324(1991): 450.

39. Brock, B. V., et al. "Frequency of asymptomatic shedding of herpes simplex virus in women with genital herpes." *Journal of the American Medical Association* 263(1990): 418.

40. Straus, S. E., et al. "Acyclovir suppression of frequently recurring genital herpes." *Journal of the American Medical Association* 260(1988): 2227–2230.

41. Kaplowitz, L. G., et al. "Prolonged continuous acyclovir treatment of normal adults with frequently recurring genital Herpes simplex virus infection." *Journal of the American Medical Association* 265(1991): 747.

42. Frenkel, L. M., et al. "Pharmacokinetics of acyclovir in the term human pregnancy and neonate." *American Journal of Obstetrics and Gynecology* 164(1991): 569–576.

43. Baker, D. A., et al. "One-year suppression of frequent recurrences of genital herpes with oral acyclovir." *Obstetrics and Gynecology* 73(1989): 84–86.

44. Brown, Z. A., and Baker, D. A. "Acyclovir therapy during pregnancy." *Obstetrics and Gynecology* 73(1989): 526–530.

45. Meisels, A.; Morin, C.; and Fortier, M. "Rethinking common terminology for HPV." *Contemporary OB/GYN*, August 1988, pp. 84–98.

46. Gall, S. A. "Update on HPV infection and how to manage it." *Contemporary OB/GYN*, October 1991, pp. 37–48.

47. Gordon, A. N. "New STD menace: HPV infection." *Medical Aspects of Human Sexuality*, February 1990, pp. 18–23.

48. Nuovo, G. J., and Pedemonte, B. M. "Human papillomavirus types and recurrent cervical warts." *Journal of the American Medical Association* 263(1990): 1223–1226.

49. "Human papillomavirus—What role does it play in cervical cancer?" *The Female Patient* 15(1990): 17–28.

50. Ferenczy, A. "To contain spread of condyloma—treat your patient's partner." *Contemporary OB/GYN*, June 1986, pp. 51–69.

51. Schneider, A., et al. "Human papillomaviruses in women with a history of abnormal Papanicolaou smears and in their male partners." *Obstetrics and Gynecology* 69(1987): 554–561.

52. Mitchell, H.; Drake, M.; and Medley, G. "Prospective evaluation of risk of cervical cancer after cytological evidence of human papillomavirus." *Lancet* 1(1986): 573.

53. Garden, J. M. "Papillomavirus in the vapor of carbon dioxide laser-treated verrucae." *Journal of the American Medical Association* 259(1988): 1199–1202.

54. Friedman-Kien, A. E., et al. "Natural interferon alfa for treatment of condylomata acuminata." *Journal of the American Medical Association* 259(1988): 533–538.

55. Matsunaga, J.; Bergman, A.; and Bhatia, N. N. "Genital condylomata acuminata in pregnancy: Effectiveness, safety, and pregnancy outcome following cryotherapy." *British Journal of Obstetrics and Gynaecology* 94(1987): 168.

56. Patsner, B. "A patient-applied topical solution for genital warts." *Contemporary OB/GYN*, December 1991, pp. 27–29.

57. Baker, D. A., et al. "Topical podofilox for the treatment of condylomata acuminata in women." *Obstetrics and Gynecology* 76(1990): 656–659.

58. Schwartz, D. B., et al. "Genital condylomas in pregnancy: Use of trichloroacetic acid and laser therapy." *American Journal of Obstetrics and Gynecology* 158(1988): 1407–1416.

59. Sedlacek, T. V., et al. "Mechanisms for human papillomavirus transmission at birth." *American Journal of Obstetrics and Gynecology* 161(1989): 55–59.

60. Fife, K. H.; Rogers, R. E.; and Zwickl, B. W. "Symptomatic and asymptomatic cervical infections with human papillomavirus during pregnancy." *Journal of Infectious Diseases* 156(1987): 904.

61. Shah, K. V.; Kashima, H. K.; and Buscema, J. "Reducing mortality from respiratory papillomas." *Contemporary OB/GYN*, April 1987, pp. 65–74.

62. Ferenczy, A.; Bergeron, C.; and Richart, R. M. "Human papillomavirus DNA in CO_2 laser-generated plume of smoke and its consequences to the surgeon." *Obstetrics and Gynecology* 75(1990): 114–118.

63. Gall, S. A.; Hughes, C. E.; and Trofatter, K. "Interferon for the therapy of condyloma acuminatum." *American Journal of Obstetrics and Gynecology* 153(1985): 157–163.

64. Towers, C. V., and Keegan, K. A., Jr. "The many forms of viral hepatitis." *Contemporary OB/GYN*, August 1987, pp. 39–49.

65. Alter, M. J., et al. "Hepatitis B virus transmission between heterosexuals." *Journal of the American Medical Association* 256(1986): 1307–1310.

66. Kane, M. A., et al. "Routine prenatal screening for hepatitis B surface antigen." *Journal of the American Medical Association* 259(1988): 408–409.

67. Pastorek, J. G. "Hepatitis B screening during pregnancy." *Contemporary OB/GYN*, November 1989, pp. 36–48.

68. Scheig, R. "The hepatitis viruses: Who's at risk?" *Medical Aspects of Human Sexuality*, March 1991, pp. 20–26.

69. Alter, M. J., et al. "Risk factors for acute non-A, non-B hepatitis in the United States and association with hepatitis C virus infection." *Journal of the American Medical Association* 264(1990): 2231–2235.

70. Cohen, M., and Cohen, H. "Current recommendations for viral hepatitis." *Contemporary OB/GYN*, November 1990, pp. 56–79.

71. Butterfield, C. R., et al. "Routine screening for hepatitis B in an obstetrics population." *Obstetrics and Gynecology* 76(1990): 25–27.

72. "Guidelines for hepatitis B virus screening and vaccination during pregnancy." ACOG Committee Opinion, number 78, January 1990.

73. Hoffnagle, J. H. "Toward universal vaccination against hepatitis B virus." *New England Journal of Medicine* 321(1989): 1333–1334.

74. Clarke, J. A., et al. "Intradermal inoculation with Heptavax-B." *Journal of the American Medical Association* 262(1989): 2567–2571.

75. Alter, M. J., et al. "Importance of heterosexual activity in the transmission of hepatitis B and non-A, non-B hepatitis." *Journal of the American Medical Association* 262(1989): 1201–1205.

76. Stevens, C. E., et al. "Epidemiology of hepatitis C virus." *Journal of the American Medical Association* 263(1990): 49–53.

77. Bensadath, J., et al. "Hepatitis virus infection and labrea hepatitis." *Journal of the American Medical Association* 258(1987): 479–483.

78. Fowler, K. B., and Pass, R. F. "Sexually transmitted diseases in mothers of neonates with congenital cytomegalovirus infection." *Journal of Infectious Diseases* 164(1991): 259.

79. Noble, R. C. "Sexually transmitted cytomegalovirus infection." *Medical Aspects of Human Sexuality*, October 1987, pp. 18–27.

80. Larsen, J. W., Jr. "Cytomegalovirus infection during pregnancy." *Contemporary OB/GYN*, May 1991, pp. 89–96.

81. Bhumbra, M. A. "Cytomegalovirus infections and the pregnant woman." *Infections in Surgery*, November 1989, pp. 390–409.

82. Stagno, S., et al. "Primary cytomegalovirus infection in pregnancy." *Journal of the American Medical Association* 256(1986): 1904–1908.

83. Yow, M. D., et al. "Epidemiological characteristics of cytomegalovirus infection in mothers and their infants." *American Journal of Obstetrics and Gynecology* 158(1988): 1189–1195.

84. Hohlfield, P., et al. "Cytomegalovirus fetal infection: Prenatal diagnosis." *Obstetrics and Gynecology* 78(1991): 615–618.

85. Gellin, B., and Broome, C. V. "Listeriosis." *Journal of the American Medical Association* 261(1989): 1313–1320.

86. Cruikshank, D. P., and Warenski, J. C. "First-trimester maternal Listeria monocytogenes sepsis and chorioamnionitis with normal neonatal outcome." *Obstetrics and Gynecology* 73(1989): 469–471.

87. Boucher, M., and Yonekura, M. L. "Perinatal listeriosis—Early onset: Correlation of antenatal manifestations and neonatal outcome." *Obstetrics and Gynecology* 68(1986): 593–597.

88. Greenspoon, J. S.; Wilcox, J. G.; and Kirschbaum, T. H. "Group B. streptococcus: The effectiveness of screening and chemoprophylaxis."

Obstetrical and Gynecological Survey 46(1991): 499–508.

89. Minkoff, H., and Mead, P. "An obstetric approach to the prevention of early-onset group B B-hemolytic streptococcal sepsis." *American Journal of Obstetrics and Gynecology* 154(1986): 973–977.

90. Newton, E., and Clark, M. "Group B streptococcus and preterm rupture of membranes." *Obstetrics and Gynecology* 71(1988): 198–202.

91. Romero, R., et al. "Is there an association between colonization with group B streptococcus and prematurity?" *Journal of Reproductive Medicine* 34(1989): 797–801.

92. Minkoff, H. L. "How we can prevent group B B-beta hemolytic streptococcal sepsis." *Contemporary OB/GYN*, October 1986, pp. 100–109.

93. Gotoff, S. P. "Prophylaxis for early-onset group B strep." *Contemporary OB/GYN*, November 1988, pp. 25–40.

94. Dinsmoor, M. J. "Group B. streptococcus still poses a challenge." *Contemporary OB/GYN*, May 1990, pp. 93–104.

95. "Vulvovaginitis." ACOG Technical Bulletin, number 135, November 1989.

96. Thomason, J. L., and Gelbart, S. M. "Trichomonas vaginalis." *Obstetrics and Gynecology* 74(1989): 536–540.

97. Krieger, J. N., et al. "Diagnosis of trichomoniasis." *Journal of the American Medical Association* 259(1988): 1223–1227.

98. Keith, L. G., et al. "The possible role of Trichomonas vaginalis as a 'vector' for the spread of other pathogens." *International Journal of Fertility* 31(1986): 272–277.

99. Hammill, H., and Kaufman, R. H. "Vaginal candiasis: Tailoring the treatment." *The Female Patient* 14(1989): 49–51.

100. Witkin, S. S. "Chronic recurrent vaginal candidiasis." *Contemporary OB/GYN*, July 1990, pp. 56–67.

101. Horowitz, B. J.; Edelstein, S. W.; and Lippman, L. "Sexual transmission of candida." *Obstetrics and Gynecology* 69(1987): 883–886.

102. Duff, P., et al. "Amoxicillin treatment of bacterial vaginosis during pregnancy." *Obstetrics and Gynecology* 77(1991): 431–434.

103. Sobel, J. D. "Bacterial vaginosis: Assessment and treatment." *Medical Aspects of Human Sexuality*, June 1990, pp. 42–46.

104. Gibbs, R. S., et al. "Microbiologic and serologic studies of Gardnerella vaginalis in intra-amniotic infection." *Obstetrics and Gynecology* 70(1987): 187–190.

105. Whalley, P. J. "Value of creating UTI during pregnancy." *Contemporary OB/GYN*, May 1986, pp. 134–146.

106. Gilstrap, L. C., and Cox, S. M. "An aggressive approach to UTI during pregnancy." *Contemporary OB/GYN*, November 1987, pp. 23–28.

107. Jacobi, P., and Paldi, E. "Asymptomatic bacteriuria in pregnancy." *American Journal of Gynecologic Health* 3(1989): 17–20.

108. Campbell-Brown, M., et al. "Is screening for bacteriuria in pregnancy worth while?" *British Medical Journal* 294(1987): 1579.

109. "Human immune deficiency virus infections." ACOG Technical Bulletin, number 123, December 1988.

110. Magallon, D. T. "Counseling patients with HIV infections." *Medical Aspects of Human Sexuality*, June 1987, pp. 37–55.

111. Friedland, G. H., and Klein, R. S. "Transmission of the human immunodeficiency virus." *New England Journal of Medicine* 317(1987): 1125–1134.

112. Francis, D. P., and Chin, J. "The prevention of acquired immunodeficiency syndrome in the United States." *Journal of the American Medical Association* 257(1987): 1357–1366.

113. Quinn, T. C.; Zacarias, F. R. K.; and St. John, R. K. "AIDS in the Americas—An emerging public health crisis." *New England Journal of Medicine* 320(1989): 1005–1007.

114. "Human immunodeficiency virus infection: Physicians' responsibilities." ACOG Committee Opinion, number 85, September 1990.

115. Sloan, E. M., et al. "HIV testing." *Journal of the American Medical Association* 266(1991): 2861–2866.

116. Saag, M. S., and Weaver, B. L. "HIV in primary care: Guidelines for the '90s." *Medical Aspects of Human Sexuality*, November 1991, pp. 42–51.

117. Grohmann, S. M., and MacDonell, K. B. "Predicting the course of HIV infection." *Medical*

Aspects of Human Sexuality, January 1992, pp. 22–30.

118. Bolognesi, D. P. "Prospects for prevention of an early intervention against HIV." *Journal of the American Medical Association* 261(1989): 3007–3012.

119. Chamberland, M. E., et al. "Health care workers with AIDS." *Journal of the American Medical Association* 266(1991): 3459–3462.

120. Friedland, G. H. "Early treatment for HIV—The time has come." *New England Journal of Medicine* 322(1990): 1000–1002.

121. Volberding, P. A., et al. "Zidovidine in asymptomatic human immunodeficiency virus infection." *New England Journal of Medicine* 322(1990): 941–949.

122. Lange, J. M. A., et al. "Failure of zidovidine prophylaxis after accidental exposure to HIV-1." *New England Journal of Medicine* 322(1990): 1375–1377.

123. Lambert, J. S., et al. "2,3-dideoxyinosine (ddI) in patients with the acquired immunodeficiency syndrome or AIDS-related complex." *New England Journal of Medicine* 322(1990): 1333–1340.

124. Menitov, J. E. "The decreasing risk of transfusion-associated AIDS." *New England Journal of Medicine* 321(1989): 966–968.

125. Callaghan, J. J., et al. "Autologous blood transfusion." *Infections in Surgery*, April 1989, pp. 132–135.

126. Lindenbaum, C. R., et al. "Safety of predeposit autologous blood donation in the third trimester of pregnancy." *Journal of Reproductive Medicine* 35(1990): 537–540.

127. Axelrod, F. B.; Pepkowitz, S. H.; and Goldfinger, D. "Establishment of a schedule of optimal preoperative collection of autologous blood." *Transfusion* 29(1989): 677.

128. Addiss, S. S. "Recommendations on HIV education, counseling, and testing for women." *Connecticut Medicine* 55(1991): 583–584.

129. Allen, J. R., and Setlow, V. P. "Heterosexual transmission of HIV—A view of the future." *Journal of the American Medical Association* 266(1991): 1695–1696.

130. Howard, L. C., et al. "Transmission of human immunodeficiency virus by heterosexual contact with reference to antenatal screening." *British Journal of Obstetrics and Gynaecology* 96(1989): 135–139.

131. Hearst, N., and Hulley, S. B. "Preventing the heterosexual spread of AIDS." *Journal of the American Medical Association* 259(1988): 2428–2432.

132. Haverkos, H. W., and Edelman, R. "The epidemiology of acquired immunodeficiency syndrome among heterosexuals." *Journal of the American Medical Association* 260(1988): 1922–1928.

133. Padian, N., et al. "Male-to-female transmission of human immunodeficiency virus." *Journal of the American Medical Association* 258(1987): 788–790.

134. Padian, N. S.; Shiboski, S. C.; and Jewell, N. P. Female-to-male transmission of human immunodeficiency virus." *Journal of the American Medical Association* 266(1991): 1664–1667.

135. Shapiro, C. N., et al. "Review of human immunodeficiency virus infection in women in the United States." *Obstetrics and Gynecology* 74(1989): 800–814.

136. Holmes, V. F., and Fernandez, F. "HIV in women: Current impact and future implications." *The Female Patient* 13(1988): 47–54.

137. Minkoff, H. L., and DeHovitz, J. A. "Care of women infected with the human immunodeficiency virus." *Journal of the American Medical Association* 266(1991): 2253–2258.

138. Quinn, M., et al. "Prevalence of HIV infection in child-bearing in the United States." *Journal of the American Medical Association* 265(1991): 1704–1708.

139. Chu, S. Y.; Buehler, J. W.; and Berkelman, R. L. "Impact of the human immunodeficiency virus epidemic on mortality in women of reproductive age, United States." *Journal of the American Medical Association* 264(1990): 225–229.

140. Minkoff, H. L. "Funding AIDS: What every physician should know." *The Female Patient* 12(1987): 49–64.

141. Ellerbrook, T. V., et al. "Epidemiology of women with AIDS in the United States, 1981 through 1990." *Journal of the American Medical Association* 265(1991): 2971–2975.

142. Minkoff, H. L. "Care of pregnant women in-

fected with immunodeficiency virus." *Journal of the American Medical Association* 258(1987): 2714–2717.

143. Selwyn, P. A., et al. "Prospective study of human immunodeficiency virus infection and pregnancy outcomes in intravenous drug users." *Journal of the American Medical Association* 261(1989): 1289–1294.

144. Sachs, B. P.; Tuomala, R.; and Frigoletto, F. "Acquired immunodeficiency syndrome: Suggested protocol for counseling and screening in pregnancy." *Obstetrics and Gynecology* 70(1987): 408–411.

145. Koonin, L. M., et al. "Pregnancy-associated deaths due to AIDS in the United States." *Journal of the American Medical Association* 261(1989): 1306–1309.

146. Biggar, R. J., et al. "Immunosuppression in pregnant women infected with human immunodeficiency virus." *American Journal of Obstetrics and Gynecology* 161(1989): 1239–1244.

147. Maury, W.; Potts, B. J.; and Rabson, A. B. "HIV-1 infection of first-trimester and term human placental tissue: A possible mode of maternal-fetal transmission." *Journal of Infectious Diseases* 160(1989): 583.

148. Blanche, S., et al. "A prospective study of infants born to women seropositive for human immunodeficiency virus type 1." *New England Journal of Medicine* 320(1989): 1643–1648.

149. Katz, S. L., and Wilfert, C. M. "Human immunodeficiency virus infection of newborns." *New England Journal of Medicine* 320(1989): 1687–1688.

150. Novick, L. F., et al. "HIV seroprevalence in newborns in New York State." *Journal of the American Medical Association* 261(1989): 1745–1750.

151. Pizzo, P. A. "Emerging concepts in the treatment of HIV infection in children." *Journal of the American Medical Association* 262(1989): 1989–1992.

152. Nanda, D., and Minkoff, H. L. "Managing HIV infection during gestation." *Contemporary OB/ GYN,* January 1991, pp. 19–28.

153. Seltzer, V., and Benjamin, F. "Breast-feeding and the potential for human immunodeficiency virus transmission." *Obstetrics and Gynecology* 75(1990): 713–715.

154. Quinn, T. C., et al. "Early diagnosis of perinatal HIV infection by detection of viral-specific IgA antibodies." *Journal of the American Medical Association* 266(1991): 3439–3442.

155. Connor, E. "Advances in early diagnosis of perinatal HIV infection." *Journal of the American Medical Association* 266(1991): 3474–3475.

156. Imagawa, D. T., et al. "Human immunodeficiency virus type I infection in homosexual men who remain seronegative for prolonged periods." *New England Journal of Medicine* 320(1989): 1458–1462.

157. Haseltine, W. A. "Silent HIV infections." *New England Journal of Medicine* 320(1989): 1487–1488.

158. Rogers, M. F., et al. "Use of polymerase chain reaction for early detection of the proviral sequences of the human immunodeficiency virus in infants born to seropositive mothers." *New England Journal of Medicine* 320(1989): 1649–1654.

Chapter 7
TRAVEL

1. Barry, M., and Bia, F. "Pregnancy and travel." *Journal of the American Medical Association* 261(1989): 728.

2. Crosby, W. M. "Trauma during pregnancy: Maternal and fetal injury." *Obstetrical and Gynecological Survey* 29(1974): 683–698.

3. Crosby, W. M. "Trauma in the pregnant patient." *Connecticut Medicine* 50(1986): 251–258.

4. Pearlman, M. D.; Tintinalli, J. E.; and Lorenz, R. P. "Blunt trauma during pregnancy." *New England Journal of Medicine* 323(1990): 1609.

5. Stafford, P. A.; Biddinger, P. W.; and Zumwalt, R. E. "Lethal intrauterine fetal trauma." *American Journal of Obstetrics and Gynecology* 159(1988): 485–489.

6. Williams, J. K., et al. "Evaluation of blunt abdominal trauma in the third trimester of pregnancy: Maternal and fetal considerations." *Obstetrics and Gynecology* 75(1990): 33–37.

7. Sherer, D. M., and Schenker, J. G. "Accidental injury during pregnancy." *Obstetrical and Gynecological Survey* 44(1989): 330–337.

8. "Trauma during pregnancy." ACOG Technical Bulletin, number 161, November 1991.

9. Bickers, R. G., and Wennberg, R. P. "Fetomaternal transfusion following trauma." *Obstetrics and Gynecology* 61(1983): 258–259.

10. Fakhoury, G. W., and Gibson, J. R. M. "Seat belt hazards in pregnancy. Case report." *British Journal of Obstetrics and Gynaecology* 93(1986): 395–396.

11. Schoenfeld, A., et al. "Seat belts in pregnancy and the obstetrician." *Obstetrical and Gynecological Survey* 42(1987): 275–281.

12. "Automobile passenger restraints for children and pregnant women." ACOG Technical Bulletin, number 151, January 1991.

13. Levin, D. P. "G.M. is challenged over seat belts." *The New York Times*, Saturday, December 15, 1990, p. 48.

14. Huch, R., et al. "Physiologic changes in pregnant women and their fetuses during jet air travel." *American Journal of Obstetrics and Gynecology* 154(1986): 996–1000.

15. Warren, M. P. "Effects of space travel on reproduction." *Obstetrical and Gynecological Survey* 44(1989): 35–37.

16. McCullough, R. E.; Reeves, J. T.; and Liljegren, R. L. "Fetal growth retardation and increased infant mortality at high altitudes." *Archives of Environmental Health* 32(1977): 36–39.

17. Cotton, E. K., et al. "Re-evaluation of birth at high altitude." *American Journal of Obstetrics and Gynecology* 138(1980): 220–222.

18. Hershey, D. W., and Vieiera, L. "Problems of pregnancy at high altitude." *Contemporary OB/GYN*, 23(1984): 47–50.

19. Unger, C., et al. "Altitude, low birth weight, and infant mortality in Colorado." *Journal of the American Medical Association* 259(1988): 3427–3432.

20. Fried, F. A. "Sickle cell anemia and plane travel." *Consultant*, November 1979, pp. 16–17.

21. Montgomery, A. B.; Mills, J.; and Luce, J. M. "Incidence of acute mountain sickness at intermediate altitude." *Journal of the American Medical Association* 261(1989): 732–734.

22. Johnson, T. S., and Rock, P. B. "Acute mountain sickness." *New England Journal of Medicine* 319(1988): 841–844.

23. Bartsch, P., et al. "Prevention of high-altitude pul-

monary edema by nifedipine." *New England Journal of Medicine* 325(1991): 1284–1289.

24. "Lyme disease during pregnancy." ACOG Committee Opinion, number 99, November 1991.

25. Steere, A. C. "Lyme disease." *New England Journal of Medicine* 321(1989): 586–596.

26. Williams, C. L., and Strobino, B. A. "Lyme disease transmission during pregnancy." *Contemporary OB/GYN*, June 1990, pp. 48–64.

27. Makeover, M. E. "Tick, tick, tick." *New York Magazine*, May 22, 1989, pp. 77–78.

28. Schoen, R. T. "Treatment of Lyme disease." *Connecticut Medicine* 52(1988): 641–643.

29. Dennis, D. T. "Lyme disease—Tracking an epidemic." *Journal of the American Medical Association* 266(1991): 1269–1270.

30. Carter, M. L., et al. "Occupational risk factors for infection with parvovirus B19 among pregnant women." *Journal of Infectious Diseases* 163(1991): 282.

31. Gillespie, S. M., et al. "Occupational risk of parvovirus B19 infection for school day-care personnel during an outbreak of erythema infectiosum." *Journal of the American Medical Association* 263(1990): 2061–2065.

32. Anderson, L. J., and Torok, T. J. "Human parvovirus B19." *New England Journal of Medicine* 321(1989): 536–538.

33. Rodis, J. F., et al. "Human parvovirus infection in pregnancy." *Obstetrics and Gynecology* 72(1988): 733–737.

34. Anand, A. "Human parvovirus infection in pregnancy and hydrops fetalis." *New England Journal of Medicine* 316(1987): 183.

35. Taylor, R. B. "Health care for the international traveler." *The Female Patient* 12(1987): 39–50.

36. Brody, A. E. "Preparing for health problems before traveling abroad can assure a happy vacation." *The New York Times*, Health Section, Thursday, June 15, 1989, p. B12.

37. Sobel, D. "Pesticides studied in fight against Lyme disease." *The New York Times*, Environment Section, Tuesday, April 18, 1989, p. C4.

38. "Immunization during pregnancy." ACOG Technical Bulletin, number 160, October 1991.

39. Amstey, M. S. "Immunization in pregnancy." *Contemporary OB/GYN*, October 1989, pp. 15–17.

40. Freij, B. J., and Sever, J. L. "When is immunization in pregnancy really needed?" *Contemporary OB/GYN*, May 1986, pp. 48–58.

41. Insel, R. A. "Maternal immunization to prevent neonatal infections." *New England Journal of Medicine* 319(1988): 1219–1220.

42. Amstey, M. S.; Insel, R. A.; and Pichichero, M. E. "Neonatal passive immunization by maternal vaccination." *Obstetrics and Gynecology* 63(1984): 105–109.

43. White, S., and Larsen, B. "Measles in pregnancy." *Contemporary OB/GYN*, September 1990, pp. 57–62.

44. Enders, G., et al. "Outcome of confirmed periconceptional maternal rubella." *Lancet* 1(1988): 1445.

45. Horstmann, D. M. "Surveillance for rubella." *Contemporary OB/GYN*, October 1989, pp. 43–61.

46. Miller, C. L.; Miller, E.; and Waight, P. A. "Rubella susceptibility and the continuing risk of infection in pregnancy." *British Medical Journal* 294(1987): 1277.

47. Baker, D. A. "Dangers of varicella-zoster virus infection." *Contemporary OB/GYN*, April 1990, pp. 51–57.

48. Esmonde, T. F.; Herdman, G.; and Anderson, G. "Chicken-pox pneumonia: An association with pregnancy." *Thorax* 44(1989): 812.

49. Sterner, G., et al. "Varicella-zoster infections in late pregnancy." *Scandinavian Journal of Infectious Diseases* 71(1990): 30.

50. Gershon, A. "Chickenpox: How dangerous is it?" *Contemporary OB/GYN*, March 1988, pp. 41–56.

51. Alkalay, A.; Pomerance, J. J.; and Rimoin, D. L. "Fetal varicella syndrome." *Journal of Pediatrics* 111(1987): 320.

52. Amstey, M. S. "Confronting influenza in pregnancy." *Contemporary OB/GYN*, November 1985, pp. 33–38.

53. Apuzzio, J. J. "Preventing and treating viral influenza during pregnancy." *Contemporary OB/GYN*, November 1990, pp. 51–54.

54. Douglas, R. G., Jr. "Prophylaxis and treatment of influenza." *New England Journal of Medicine* 322(1990): 443–448.

55. Hoffman, S. L. "Prevention of malaria." *Journal of the American Medical Association* 265(1991): 398–399.

56. Lackritz, E. M., et al. "Imported plasmodium falciparum malaria in American travelers to Africa." *Journal of the American Medical Association* 265(1991): 383–385.

57. Rosenthal, E. "Outwitted by malaria, desperate doctors seek new remedies." *The New York Times*, Science Section, Tuesday, February 12, 1991, p. C1.

58. Moran, J. S., and Bernard, T. W. "The spread of chloroquine-resistant malaria in Africa." *Journal of the American Medical Association* 262(1989): 245–248.

59. Lobel, H. O., et al. "Effectiveness and tolerance of long-term malaria prophylaxis with mefloquine." *Journal of the American Medical Association* 265(1991): 361–364.

60. Ericsson, C. D. "Traveler's diarrhea: How to keep it in check." *The Female Patient* 13(1988): 66–73.

61. Ericsson, C. D., et al. "Treatment of traveler's diarrhea with sulfamethoxazole and trimethoprim and loperamide." *Journal of the American Medical Association* 263(1990): 257–261.

62. DuPont, H. L., et al. "Prevention of travelers' diarrhea by the tablet formulation of bismuth subsalicylate." *Journal of the American Medical Association* 257(1987): 1347–1350.

63. Avery, M. E., and Snyder, J. D. "Oral therapy for acute diarrhea—The underused simple solution." *New England Journal of Medicine* 323(1990): 891–894.

64. D'Alauro, F., et al. "Intestinal parasites and pregnancy." *Obstetrics and Gynecology* 66(1985): 639–643.

65. Watson, P. T. "Treating parasitic infections during pregnancy." *Contemporary OB/GYN*, April 1987, pp. 20–21.

66. Lee, R. V. "GI parasites: How hazardous in pregnancy?" *Contemporary OB/GYN*, March 1987, pp. 137–149.

Chapter 8
NUTRITION

1. Naeye, R. L. "Weight gain and the outcome of pregnancy." *American Journal of Obstetrics and Gynecology* 135(1979): 3–9.

2. Brown, J. E., et al. "Influence of pregnancy weight gain on the size of infants born to underweight women." *Obstetrics and Gynecology* 57(1981): 13–17.

3. Gormican, A.; Valentine, J.; and Satter, E. "Relationships of maternal weight gain, prepregnancy weight, and infant birthweight." *Journal of the American Diet Association* 77(1980): 662–667.

4. Institute of Medicine. *Nutrition During Pregnancy.* Washington, D.C.: National Academy Press, 1990.

5. Cobe, P. "Eating and gaining weight during pregnancy." *Expecting*, Spring 1991, pp. 22–28.

6. Ravussin, E., et al. "Reduced rate of energy expenditure as a risk factor for body-weight gain." *New England Journal of Medicine* 318(1988): 467–472.

7. Abrams, B. F., and Laros, R. K., Jr. "Prepregnancy weight, weight gain, and birth weight." *American Journal of Obstetrics and Gynecology* 154(1986): 503–509.

8. Van Der Spuy, Z. M., et al. "Outcome of pregnancy in underweight women after spontaneous and induced ovulation." *British Medical Journal* 296(1988): 962.

9. Roberts, S. B., et al. "Energy expenditure and intake of infants born to lean and overweight mothers." *New England Journal of Medicine* 318(1988): 461–466.

10. Turner, M. T., et al. "The influence of birth weight on labor in nulliparas." *Obstetrics and Gynecology* 76(1990): 159–162.

11. Ruge, S., and Andersen, T. "Obstetric risks in obesity. An analysis of the literature." *Obstetrical and Gynecological Survey* 40(1985): 57–60.

12. Garbaciak, J. A., Jr., et al. "Maternal weight and pregnancy complications." *American Journal of Obstetrics and Gynecology* 152(1985): 238–245.

13. Kliegman, R. M., and Gross, T. "Perinatal problems of the obese mother and her infant." *Obstetrics and Gynecology* 66(1985): 299–305.

14. Kitay, D. Z., and Lincoln, G. H. "When is a patient 'obese'—and why?" *Contemporary OB/GYN*, September 1987, pp. 96–99.

15. Murray, J. L., and Bernfield, M. "The differential effect of prenatal care on the incidence of low birth weight among blacks and whites in a prepaid healthcare plan." *New England Journal of Medicine* 319(1988): 1385–1391.

16. Shiono, P. H., et al. "Birth weight among women of different ethnic groups." *Journal of the American Medical Association* 255(1986): 48.

17. Swales, J. D. "Dietary salt and hypertension." *Lancet* 1(1980): 1177–1179.

18. Lindheimer, M. D. "Current concepts of sodium metabolism and use of diuretics in pregnancy." *Contemporary OB/GYN*, 15(1980): 207–216.

19. Belongia, E. A., et al. "An investigation of the cause of the eosinophilia-myalgia syndrome associated with tryptophan use." *New England Journal of Medicine* 323(1990): 357–365.

20. Narod, S.A.; Sanjose, S. D.; and Victora, C. "Coffee during pregnancy: A reproductive hazard?" *American Journal of Obstetrics and Gynecology* 164(1991): 1109–1114.

21. Fenster, L., et al. "Caffeine consumption during pregnancy and fetal growth." *American Journal of Public Health* 81(1991): 458–461.

22. Tyrala, E. E., and Dodson, W. E. "Caffeine secretion into breast milk." *Archives of Disease in Childhood* 54(1979): 787–800.

23. Moghissi, K. S. "Risks and benefits of nutritional supplements during pregnancy." *Obstetrics and Gynecology* 58(1981): 68S–78S.

24. Chez, R. A., and Pitkin, R. M. "Nutritional supplements during pregnancy." *Contemporary OB/GYN*, 19(1982): 199–201.

25. "Use of folic acid for prevention of spina bifida and other neural tube defects—1983–1991, CDC Report." *Journal of the American Medical Association* 266(1991): 1190–1191.

26. Kitay, D. Z. "Folic acid deficiency in pregnancy." *Modern Medicine*, June 15, 1970, pp. 77–84.

27. Smithells, R. W., et al. "Possible prevention of neural tube defects by periconceptional vitamin supplementation." *Lancet* 1(1980): 339–340.

28. Kruikshank, D. P. "Don't overdo nutritional supplements during pregnancy." *Contemporary OB/GYN*, February 1986, pp. 101–119.

29. Belizan, J. M., et al. "Calcium supplementation to prevent hypertensive disorders of pregnancy." *New England Journal of Medicine* 325(1991): 1399–1405.

30. Villar, J., and Repke, J. T. "Calcium supplementation during pregnancy may reduce preterm de-

livery in high-risk populations." *American Journal of Obstetrics and Gynecology* 163(1990): 1124–1131.

31. Sikorski, R.; Juszkiewicz, T.; and Paszkowski. "Zinc status in women with premature rupture of membranes at term." *Obstetrics and Gynecology* 76(1990): 675–677.

32. Broun, E. R., et al. "Excessive zinc ingestion." *Journal of the American Medical Association* 264(1990): 1441–1443.

33. "Public health service report on fluoride benefits and risks. Report from the Centers for Disease Control." *Journal of the American Medical Association* 266(1991): 1061–1066.

34. Boffey, P. M. "New artificial sweetener approved." *The New York Times*, Health Section, July 28, 1988, p. B5.

35. London, R. S. "Saccharin and aspartame—Are they safe to consume during pregnancy?" *Journal of Reproductive Medicine* 33(1988): 17–21.

36. Counsel on Scientific Affairs. "Saccharin—Review of safety issues." *Journal of the American Medical Association* 254(1985): 2622–2624.

37. Politzer, B. "Sweet—Sugar and artificial sweeteners." *American Health*, September 1991, pp. 40–42.

38. Long, P. "What America eats." *Hippocrates*, May/June 1989, pp. 39–45.

39. Crosby, W. H. "Can a vegetarian be well nourished?" *Journal of the American Medical Association* 233(1975): 898.

Chapter 9
MEDICATIONS

1. *Physician's Desk Reference*, 46th ed. Montvale, N.J.: Medical Economics Company, Inc., 1991.

2. Briggs, G. G.; Freeman, R. K.; and Yaffe, S. J. *Drugs in Pregnancy and Lactation*, 3rd ed. Baltimore, MD: Williams and Wilkins, 1990.

3. Mattison, D. R., et al. "Effects of drugs and chemicals on the fetus." *Contemporary OB/GYN*, March 1989, pp. 163–176.

4. Karboski, J. A. "Medication selection for pregnant women." *The Female Patient* 16(1991): 69–76.

5. Mattison, D. R., et al. "Effects of drugs and chemicals on the fetus, Part II." April 1989, pp. 97–110.

6. Aselton, P., et al. "First-trimester drug use and congenital disorders." *Obstetrics and Gynecology* 65(1985): 451–455.

7. Rayburn, W. F., and Lavin, J. P., Jr. "Drug prescribing for chronic medical disorders during pregnancy: An overview." *American Journal of Obstetrics and Gynecology* 155(1986): 565–569.

8. Koren, G., et al. "Perception of teratogenic risk by pregnant women exposed to drugs and chemicals during the first trimester." *American Journal of Obstetrics and Gynecology* 160(1989): 1190–1194.

9. Niebyl, J. R. "Drugs with potential fetal toxicity." *Contemporary OB/GYN*, April 1991, pp. 68–77.

10. Neibyl, J. R. "Drugs with little or no potential fetal toxicity." *Contemporary OB/GYN*, May 1991, pp. 71–79.

11. Scalli, A. R. "Safe medications during pregnancy." *Contemporary OB/GYN*, November 1983, pp. 40–50.

12. Friedman, J. M., et al. "Potential human teratogenicity of frequently prescribed drugs." *Obstetrics and Gynecology* 75(1990): 594–599.

13. Scialli, A. R., and Fabro, S. "What drugs are safe during nursing?" *Contemporary OB/GYN*, June 1984, pp. 211–220.

14. Beall, M. H. "Breastfeeding: Some drug admonitions." *Contemporary OB/GYN*, February 1987, pp. 49–54.

15. Darr, M. S., and Taylor, R. B. "A practical guide to drugs in breast milk." *The Female Patient* 13(1988): 42–52.

16. Knothe, H., and Dette, G. A. "Antibiotics in pregnancy: Toxicity and teratogenicity." *Infection* 13(1985): 49.

17. Miller, R. D. "Prescribing antibiotics for pregnant patients." *Contemporary OB/GYN*, February 1983, pp. 55–58.

18. Weinstein, L. "Proper use of antibiotics during pregnancy." *Contemporary OB/GYN*, September 1985, pp. 137–146.

19. Mercer, L. J. "Use of expanded spectrum cephalosporins for the treatment of obstetrical and gynecological infections." *Obstetrical and Gynecological Survey* 43(1988): 569–574.

20. McNeeley, S. G. "Aminoglycosides in Ob/Gyn infections." *Infections in Surgery*, August 1989, pp. 272–276.

21. Hill, L. M. "Fetal distress secondary to

vancomycin-induced maternal hypotension." *American Journal of Obstetrics and Gynecology* 153(1985): 74–75.

22. Cunha, B. A. "Nitrofurantoin: An update." *Obstetrical and Gynecological Survey* 44(1989): 399–404.

23. Donowitz, G. R., and Mandell, G. L. "Beta-lactam antibiotics." *New England Journal of Medicine* 318(1988): 490–498.

24. Hooper, D. C., and Wolfson, J. S. "Fluoroquinolone antimicrobial agents." *New England Journal of Medicine* 324(1991): 384–392.

25. Andersen, R. C., and Goldstein, E. J. C. "Newer quinolone antimicrobials." *Infections in Surgery*, October 1988, pp. 613–621.

26. Jager-Roman, E., et al. "Pharmokinetics and tissue distribution of metronidazole in the newborn infant." *Journal of Pediatrics* 100(1982): 651.

27. Medchill, M. T., and Gillum, M. "Diagnosis and management of tuberculosis during pregnancy." *Obstetrical and Gynecological Survey* 44(1989): 81–84.

28. Meyer, L. J., et al. "Acyclovir in human breast milk." *American Journal of Obstetrics and Gynecology* 158(1988): 586–588.

29. Lau, R. J.; Amery, M. G.; and Galinsky, R. E. "Unexpected accumulation of acyclovir in breast milk with estimation of infant exposure." *Obstetrics and Gynecology* 69(1987): 468–471.

30. Rayburn, W., et al. "Acetaminophen pharmokinetics: Comparison between pregnant and nonpregnant women." *American Journal of Obstetrics and Gynecology* 155(1986): 1353–1356.

31. "FDA: Labeling for oral and rectal over-the-counter aspirin and aspirin-containing drug products. Final rule." *Federal Register* 55(1990): 27776–27784.

32. Sibai, B. M., and Amon, E. A. "How safe is aspirin use during pregnancy?" *Contemporary OB/GYN*, July 1988, pp. 73–82.

33. Werler, M. M.; Mitchell, A. A.; and Shapiro, S. "The relation of aspirin use during the first trimester of pregnancy to congenital cardiac defects." *New England Journal of Medicine* 321(1989): 1639–1642.

34. Rudolph, A. M. "Effects of aspirin and acetaminophen in pregnancy and the newborn." *Archives of Internal Medicine* 141(1981): 358.

35. Schiff, E., et al. "The use of aspirin to prevent pregnancy-induced hypertension and lower the ratio of thromboxane A2 to prostacyclin in relatively high risk pregnancies." *New England Journal of Medicine* 321(1989): 351–356.

36. Mamopoulos, M., et al. "Maternal indomethacin therapy in the treatment of polyhydramnios." *American Journal of Obstetrics and Gynecology* 162(1990): 1225–1229.

37. Goldenberg, R. L.; Davis, R. O.; and Baker, R. C. "Indomethacin-induced oligohydramnios." *American Journal of Obstetrics and Gynecology* 160(1989): 1196–1197.

38. Goldstein, J., and Kappy, K. A. "Treating non-rheumatoid arthritis during pregnancy." *Contemporary OB/GYN*, July 1989, pp. 89–105.

39. Moise, K. J., Jr., et al. "Indomethacin in the treatment of premature labor." *New England Journal of Medicine* 319(1988): 327–331.

40. Dudley, D.K.L., and Hardie, M. J. "Fetal and neonatal effects of indomethacin used as a tocolytic agent." *American Journal of Obstetrics and Gynecology* 151(1985): 181–184.

41. Roberts, W. E.; Norman, P. F.; and Morrison, J. "Pros and cons of meperidine for intrapartum analgesia." *Contemporary OB/GYN*, April 1984, pp. 69–76.

42. Morrison, J. C., et al. "Meperidine metabolism in the parturient." *Obstetrics and Gynecology* 59(1982): 359–364.

43. Pittman, K. A., et al. "Human perinatal distribution of butorphanol." *American Journal of Obstetrics and Gynecology* 138(1980): 797–800.

44. "Naloxone use in newborns." *ACOG* Committee Opinion, number 65, February 1989.

45. Arduini, D., et al. "Effect of naloxone on fetal behavior near term." *American Journal of Obstetrics and Gynecology* 156(1987): 474–478.

46. Walters, W.A.W. "The management of nausea and vomiting during pregnancy." *Medical Journal of Australia* 147(1987): 290.

47. Rayburn, W. F., and Hoffman, K. L. E. "Gestational nausea: A role for antiemetics?" *Contemporary OB/GYN*, September 1986, pp. 163–174.

48. Ross, P. E. "Case against anti-nausea drug overturned." *The New York Times*, Wednesday, September 28, 1988, p. A20.

49. Smith, C. V., et al. "Effect of a single dose of oral

pseudoephedrine on uterine and fetal Doppler blood flow." *Obstetrics and Gynecology* 76(1990): 803–806.

50. Baxi, L. V., et al. "Fetal heart rate changes following maternal administration of a nasal decongestant." *American Journal of Obstetrics and Gynecology* 153(1985): 799–800.

51. Blackburn, G. L., et al. "Determinants of the pressor effect of phenylpropanolamine in health subjects." *Journal of the American Medical Association* 261(1989): 3267–3272.

52. Greenberger, P. A., and Patterson, R. "Beclomethasone dipropionate for severe asthma during pregnancy." *Annals of Internal Medicine* 98(1983): 478.

53. Bonds, P. J. "A new approach to the treatment of asthma." 321(1989): 1517–1526.

54. Fitzsimons, R.; Greenberger, P. A.; and Patterson, R. "Outcome of pregnancy in women requiring corticosteroids for severe asthma." *Journal of Allergy and Clinical Immunology* 78(1986): 349.

55. Brar, H. S. "Medications for asthma during pregnancy." *Contemporary OB/GYN*, September 1986, pp. 145–160.

56. Carter, B. L.; Driscoll, C. E.; and Smith, G. D. "Theophylline clearance during pregnancy." *Obstetrics and Gynecology* 68(1986): 555–559.

57. Cooper, D. S. "Antithyroid drugs: To breast feed or not to breast feed." *American Journal of Obstetrics and Gynecology* 157(1987): 234–235.

58. Danziger, Y.; Pertzelan, A.; and Mimouni, M. "Transient congenital hypothyroidism after topical iodine in pregnancy and lactation." *Archives of Diseases in Childhood* 62(1987): 295.

59. Ang, M. S.; Thorp, J. A.; and Parisi, V. M. "Maternal lithium therapy and polyhydramnios." *Obstetrics and Gynecology* 76(1990): 517–518.

60. Krause, S.; Ebbesen, F.; and Lange, A. P. "Polyhydramnios with maternal lithium treatment." *Obstetrics and Gynecology* 75(1990): 504–506.

61. Kerns, L. L. "Treatment of mental disorders in pregnancy: A review of psychotropic drug risks and benefits." *Journal of Nervous and Mental Diseases* 174(1986): 652.

62. Powers, P. S. "Psychiatric disorders in pregnant women." *Medical Aspects of Human Sexuality*, May 1989, pp. 47–54.

63. Laegreid, L., et al. "Teratogenic effects of benzodiazepine use during pregnancy." *Journal of Pediatrics* 114(1989): 126.

64. Buttino, L., Jr., and Freeman, R. K. "Seizure disorders of pregnancy." *Contemporary OB/GYN*, June 1985, pp. 62–86.

65. Tropper, P. "Guide to correct ob use of antiseizure drugs." *Contemporary OB/GYN*, June 1986, pp. 133–144.

66. Hiilesmaa, V. K.; Bardy, A.; and Teramo, K. "Obstetric outcome in women with epilepsy." *American Journal of Obstetrics and Gynecology* 152(1985): 499–504.

67. Meadown, S. R. "Epilepsy in pregnancy: What are the hazards?" *Contemporary OB/GYN*, November 1989, pp. 51–58.

68. Buehler, B. A., et al. "Prenatal prediction of risk of the fetal hydantoin syndrome." *New England Journal of Medicine* 322(1990): 1567.

69. Jones, K. L., et al. "Pattern of malformations in the children of women treated with carbamazepine during pregnancy." *New England Journal of Medicine* 320(1989): 1661–1666.

70. Weinbaum, P. J., et al. "Prenatal detection of a neural tube defect after fetal exposure to valproic acid." *Obstetrics and Gynecology* 67(1986): 31S–33S.

71. Rosa, F. W. "Spina bifida in infants of women treated with carbamazetine during pregnancy." *New England Journal of Medicine* 324(1991): 674–677.

72. Hanssens, M., et al. "Fetal and neonatal effects of treatment with angiotensin-converting enzyme inhibitors in pregnancy." *Obstetrics and Gynecology* 78(1991): 128–134.

73. Reece, E. A., and Hobbins, J. C. "Diabetic embryopathy: Pathogenesis, prenatal diagnosis and prevention." *Obstetrical and Gynecological Survey* 41(1986): 325–334.

74. Dicker, D., et al. "Spontaneous abortion in patients with insulin-dependent diabetes mellitus: The effect of preconceptional diabetic control." *American Journal of Obstetrics and Gynecology* 158(1988): 1161–1164.

75. "Management of diabetes mellitus in pregnancy." *ACOG Technical Bulletin*, number 92, May 1986.

76. Thompson, D. J., et al. "Prophylactic insulin in

the management of gestational diabetes." *Obstetrics and Gynecology* 75(1990): 960–964.

77. Mills, J. L., et al. "Lack of relation of increased malformation rates in infants of diabetic mothers to glycemic control during organogenesis." *New England Journal of Medicine* 318(1988): 671.

78. Leikin, E.; Jenkins, J. H.; and Graves, W. L. "Prophylactic insulin in gestational diabetes." *Obstetrics and Gynecology* 70(1987): 587–591.

79. Coustan, D. R. "Is insulin necessary for gestational diabetes?" *Contemporary OB/GYN*, June 1987, pp. 35–51.

80. Hoegsberg, V., and Coustan, D. R. "Gestational diabetes—Diagnosis and current management." *The Female Patient* 12(1987): 67–71.

81. Lott, I. T., et al. "Fetal hydrocephalus and ear anomalies associated with maternal use of isotretinoin." *Journal of Pediatrics* 105(1984): 597.

82. Benke, P. J. "The isotretinoin teratogen syndrome." *Journal of the American Medical Association* 251(1984): 3267.

83. Rothman, K. F., and Pochi, P. E. "Use of oral and topical agents for acne in pregnancy." *Journal of the American Academy of Dermatology* 16(1988): 431.

84. Blakeslee, S. "Skin cream as anticancer agent: Experts are cautious about its use." *The New York Times*, March 2, 1989, p. B15.

85. Pierce, C. "Controversy over fetal accutane exposure continues. *Ob. Gyn. News*, June 15–30, 1989, pp. 2–18.

Chapter 10
ENVIRONMENTAL AND OCCUPATIONAL HAZARDS OF PREGNANCY

1. Chamberlain, G., and Garcia, J. "Pregnant women at work." *Lancet* 1(1983): 228.

2. Bond, M. B. "Reproductive hazards in the workplace." *Contemporary OB/GYN*, September 1986, pp. 57–66.

3. Freund, E., et al. "Mandatory reporting of occupational diseases by clinicians." *Journal of the American Medical Association* 262(1989): 3041–3044.

4. Saurel-Cubizolles, M. J., and Kaminski, M. "Pregnant women's working conditions and their changes during pregnancy: A national study in France." *British Journal of Industrial Medicine* 236(1987): 236.

5. Chamberlain, G. "Effect of work during pregnancy." *Obstetrics and Gynecology* 65(1985): 747–750.

6. McDonald, A. D., et al. "Prematurity and work in pregnancy." *British Journal of Industrial Medicine* 45(1988): 56.

7. Chavkin, W. "Work and pregnancy. Review of the literature and policy discussion." *Obstetrical and Gynecological Survey* 41(1986): 467–471.

8. Zuckerman, B. S., et al. "Impact of maternal work outside the home during pregnancy on neonatal outcome." *Pediatrics* 77(1986): 459.

9. Oakley, A. "Does maternal work harm children?" *Contemporary OB/GYN*, April 1984, pp. 122–127.

10. Katz, V. L., et al. "Catecholamine levels in pregnant physicians and nurses: A pilot study of stress and pregnancy." *Obstetrics and Gynecology* 77(1991): 338–342.

11. Miller, N. H.; Katz, V. L.; and Cefalo, C. "Pregnancies among physicians." *Journal of Reproductive Medicine* 34(1989): 790–796.

12. Klebanoff, M. A.; Shiono, P. H.; and Rhodes, G. G. "Outcomes of pregnancy in a national sample of resident physicians." *New England Journal of Medicine* 323(1990): 1040–1045.

13. Schwartz, R. W. "Pregnancy in physicians: Characteristics and complications." *Obstetrics and Gynecology* 66(1985): 672–675.

14. Sayres, M., et al. "Pregnancy during residency." *New England Journal of Medicine* 314(1986): 418.

15. Schnall, P. L., et al. "The relationship between 'job strain,' workplace diastolic blood pressure, and left ventricular mass index." *Journal of the American Medical Association* 263(1990): 1929–1935.

16. Mamelle, N.; Laumon, B.; and Lazar, P. "Prematurity and occupational activity during pregnancy." *American Journal of Epidemiology* 119(1984): 309.

17. Klebanoff, M. A.; Shiono, P. H.; and Carey, C. "The effect of physical activity during pregnancy on preterm delivery and birth weight." *American Journal of Obstetrics and Gynecology* 163(1990): 1450–1456.

18. Easterling, T. R.; Schmucker, B. C.; and Ben-

detti, T. J. "The hemodynamic effects of orthostatic stress during pregnancy." *Obstetrics and Gynecology* 72(1988): 550–552.

19. Veille, J. C., et al. "The effect of exercise on uterine activity in the last eight weeks of pregnancy." *American Journal of Obstetrics and Gynecology* 151(1985): 727–730.

20. Lalande, N. N., et al. "Is occupational noise exposure during pregnancy a risk factor of damage to the auditory system of the fetus?" *American Journal of Industrial Medicine* 10(1986): 427–435.

21. Hartikainen-Sorri, A. L., et al. "No effect of experimental noise exposure on human pregnancy." *Obstetrics and Gynecology* 77(1991): 611–615.

22. Perera, F. P. "Molecular epidemiology: A new tool in assessing risks of environmental carcinogens." *Cancer Journal for Clinicians* 40(1990): 277–286.

23. Ballard, R. "Chemical dangers to reproduction." *Contemporary OB/GYN*, December 1989, pp. 63–75.

24. Ballad, R. "Chemical dangers to reproduction—What the clinician can do." *Contemporary OB/GYN*, January 1990, pp. 129–134.

25. Longo, L. D. "Environmental pollution and pregnancy: Risks and uncertainties for the fetus and infant." *American Journal of Obstetrics and Gynecology* 137(1980): 162–173.

26. Thaler, I.; Goodman, J. D. S.; and Dawes, G. S. "Effects of maternal cigarette smoking on fetal breathing and fetal movement." *American Journal of Obstetrics and Gynecology* 138(1980): 282–287.

27. Manning, F. A., and Platt, L. D. "Maternal hypoxemia and fetal breathing movements." *Obstetrics and Gynecology* 53(1979): 758–760.

28. "Are Hair Dyes Safe?" *Consumer Reports*, August 1979, pp. 456–460.

29. Koren, G., and Bologa, M. "Teratogenic risk of hair care products." *Journal of the American Medical Association* 262(1989): 2925.

30. LoCicero, J.; Quebbeman, E. J.; and Nichols, R. L. "Health hazards in the operating room." *Medical Tribune*, October 27, 1988, p. 34.

31. Mazze, R. L., et al. "Reproduction and fetal development in mice chronically exposed to nitrous oxide." *Teratology* 26(1982): 11–16.

32. Scialli, A. R., and Lione, A. "Environmental toxicants and adverse pregnancy outcome." *Contemporary OB/GYN*, August 1989, pp. 120–129.

33. McMichael, A. J., et al. "Port Pirie cohort study: Environmental exposure to lead and children's abilities at the age of four years." *New England Journal of Medicine* 319(1988): 468–475.

34. Blakeslee, S. "Research on birth defects shifts to flaws in sperm." *The New York Times*, Tuesday, January 1, 1991, pp. 1, 36.

35. Rempel, D. "The lead-exposed worker." *Journal of the American Medical Association* 262(1989): 532–534.

36. Melkonian, R., and Baker, D. "Risks of industrial mercury exposure in pregnancy." *Obstetrical and Gynecological Survey* 43(1988): 637–640.

37. "Are mercury fillings worse for dentists than for their patients?" *Medical Tribune*, Wednesday, January 21, 1987, p. 23.

38. Agocs, M. M., et al. "Mercury exposure from interior latex paint." *New England Journal of Medicine* 323(1990): 1096–1101.

39. Baffos, F., et al. "Prenatal management of 746 pregnancies at risk for congenital toxoplasmosis." *New England Journal of Medicine* 318(1988): 271–275.

40. Alford, C. A. "Chronic congenital infections of man." *Yale Journal of Biological Medicine* 55(1982): 187.

41. Brown, H. L., and Pastorek, J. G. "Toxoplasmosis in pregnancy." *Infections in Surgery*, July 1989, pp. 234–255.

42. Sever, J. L. "Toxoplasmosis." *Contemporary OB/GYN*, March 1990, pp. 13–17.

43. Sever, J. L. "TORCH infections: The list keeps growing." *Contemporary OB/GYN*, March 1989, pp. 65–72.

44. Bogue, C. W., et al. "Antibiotic therapy for cat-scratch disease?" *Journal of the American Medical Association* 262(1989): 813–816.

45. Gillespie, S. M., et al. "Occupational risk of human parvovirus B19 infection for school and day-care personnel during an outbreak of erythema infectiosum." *Journal of the American Medical Association* 263(1990): 2061.

46. Pickering, L. K., and Reves, R. R. "Occupational risks for child-care providers and teachers." *Journal of the American Medical Association* 263(1990): 2096–2097.

47. Mossman, K. L. "Ultrasound and x-rays in pregnancy: How safe are they?" *Contemporary OB/GYN*, May 1984, pp. 175–196.

48. Brent, R. L. "Microwave and ultrasound." *Contemporary OB/GYN*, September 1987, p. 1925.

49. Nordstrom, S.; Burke, E.; and Gustavsson, L. "Reproductive hazards among workers at high voltage substations." *Bioelectromagnetics* 4(1983): 91–101.

50. Wertheimer, N., and Leaper, E. "Possible effects of electric blankets and heated waterbeds on fetal development." *Bioelectromagnetics* 7(1986): 13–22.

51. Wertheimer, N., and Leeper, E. "Fetal loss associated with two seasonal sources of electromagnetic field exposure." *American Journal of Epidemiology* 129(1989): 220–224.

52. Schnorr, T. M., et al. "Video display terminals and the risk of spontaneous abortion." *New England Journal of Medicine* 324(1991): 727–733.

53. Blackwell, R., and Chang, A. "Video display terminals and pregnancy. A review." *British Journal of Obstetrics and Gynaecology* 95(1988): 446.

54. Lewin, T. "Pregnant women increasingly fearful of VDTs." *The New York Times*, Sunday, July 10, 1988, p. 19.

55. "Injuries associated with ultraviolet tanning devices—Wisconsin." *Journal of the American Medical Association* 261(1989): 3519–3520.

56. Ridley, W. J., et al. "Role of antenatal radiography in the management of breech deliveries." *British Journal of Obstetrics and Gynaecology* 89(1982): 342.

57. Parsons, M. T., and Spellacy, W. N. "Prospective randomized study of x-ray pelvimetry in the primigravida." *Obstetrics and Gynecology* 66(1985): 76–78.

58. Brent, R. L. "Ionizing radiation." *Contemporary OB/GYN*, August 1987, pp. 20–29.

59. Neel, J. V. "Update on the genetic effects of ionizing radiation." *Journal of the American Medical Association* 266(1991): 698–701.

60. Benter, Y.; Horlatsch, N.; and Koren, G. "Exposure to ionizing radiation during pregnancy: Perception of teratogenic risk and outcome." *Teratology* 43(1991): 109.

61. Festag, E. "The biologic effects of low-level radiation." *Journal of the American Medical Association* 259(1988): 1327.

62. Drugan, A., and Evans, M. I. "Exposure of the pregnant patient to ionizing radiation." *Contemporary OB/GYN*, October 1988, pp. 16, 21.

63. "Radionuclides in pregnancy." *Reproductive Toxicology* 5(1986): 17–22.

64. Walker, J. S. "The controversy over radiation safety—A historical overview." *Journal of the American Medical Association* 262(1989): 664–668.

65. Hendee, W. R., and Doege, T. C. "Radiation emergencies and the practicing physician." *Journal of the American Medical Association* 258(1987): 677.

66. Moore, M. M., and Shearer, W. R. "Fetal dose estimates for CT pelvimetry." *Radiology* 171(1989): 265.

67. Adelstein, S. J. "Uncertainty and relative risks of radiation exposure." *Journal of the American Medical Association* 258(1987): 655–657.

68. Yoshimoto, Y. "Cancer risk among children of atomic bomb survivors." *Journal of the American Medical Association* 264(1990): 596–600.

69. Gori, G., et al. "Radioactivity in breast milk and placentas during the year after Chernobyl." *American Journal of Obstetrics and Gynecology* 159(1988): 1232–1234.

70. Goldsmith, M. F. "Multiple efforts directed at defining, eliminating excess radiation." *Journal of the American Medical Association* 258(1987): 577–579.

71. Wald, M. L. "New estimates increase radiation risk in flight." *The New York Times*, Monday, February 19, 1990, p. A11.

72. Wald, M. L. "Radiation exposure is termed a big risk for airplane crews." *The New York Times*, Wednesday, February 14, 1990, pp. A1, A18.

73. Harley, N. H., and Harley, J. H. "Potential lung cancer risk from indoor radon exposure." *Cancer Journal for Clinicians* 40(1990): 265–275.

74. Council on Scientific Affairs. "Radon in homes." *Journal of the American Medical Association* 258(1987): 668–672.

75. Paul, M., and Himmelstein, J. "Reproductive hazards in the workplace: What the practitioner needs to know about chemical exposures." *Obstetrics and Gynecology* 71(1988): 921–935.

76. Taylor, P. R.; Stelma, J. M.; and Lawrence, C. E. "The relation of polychlorinated biphenyls to birth weight and gestational age in the offspring of occupationally exposed mothers." *American Journal of Epidemiology* 129(1989): 395–406.

77. Luoma, J. R. "Scientists are unlocking secrets of dioxins' devastating power." *The New York Times*, Tuesday, May 15, 1990, p. C4.

78. McGuire, R. "Dioxin in mother's milk far above safe levels." *Medical Tribune*, Wednesday, December 3, 1986, pp. 1, 8, 39.

79. Simons, M. "Concern rising over harm from pesticides in third world." *The New York Times*, Tuesday, May 30, 1989, p. C4.

80. Svensson, B. G., et al. "Exposure to dioxins and dibenzofurans through the consumption of fish." *New England Journal of Medicine* 324(1991): 8–12.

81. Bailar, J. C. "How dangerous is dioxin?" *New England Journal of Medicine* 324(1991): 260–262.

82. Fingerhut, M. A., et al. "Cancer mortality in workers exposed to 2, 3, 7, 8, - tetrachlorodibenzo-p-dioxin." *New England Journal of Medicine* 324(1991): 212–218.

83. Mastroiacovo, P., et al. "Birth defects in the Seveso area after TCDD contamination." *Journal of the American Medical Association* 259(1988): 1668–1672.

84. Wolfe, W. H., et al. "Health status of air force veterans occupationally exposed to herbicides in Vietnam." *Journal of the American Medical Association* 264(1990): 1824–1831.

85. Mossman, B. D., and Gee, J. B. "Asbestos-related diseases." *Journal of Reproductive Medicine* 320(1989): 1721–1730.

86. "Formaldehyde—Report from Council on Scientific Affairs." *Journal of the American Medical Association* 261(1989): 1183–1187.

87. Enders, L. J. "Analyzing formaldehyde's effect on reproduction." *Contemporary OB/GYN*, February 1987, pp. 79–86.

88. Mallov, J. S. "MBK neuropathy among spray painters." *Journal of the American Medical Association* 235(1976): 1455–1457.

89. Stewart, R. D., and Hake, C. L. "Paint-remover hazard." *Journal of the American Medical Association* 235(1976): 398–401.

90. McCann, M. "The impacts of hazards in art on female workers." *Preventive Medicine* 7(1978): 338–348.

91. Prust, S. L. "MDs stress health dangers in artistic work." *American Medical News*, February 6, 1987, p. 30.

92. Frey, D. L. "Pregnancy and work." *Expecting*, Spring 1989, pp. 24–28.

93. O'Connell, M. "Maternity leave arrangements: 1961–85." *Current Population Reports*, Series P-23, No. 165, 1990.

94. Holmes, S. A. "House passes measure on family lead." *The New York Times*, Friday, May 11, 1990, p. B6.

95. Becker, M. E. "Can employers exclude women to protect children?" *Journal of the American Medical Association* 264(1990): 2113–2117.

96. Taylor, S., Jr. "Job rights backed in pregnancy case." *The New York Times*, Wednesday, January 14, 1987, pp. 1, B10.

Chapter 11
THE NEW OBSTETRICAL TECHNOLOGY

1. Crandall, B. F.; Lebherz, T. B.; and Tabsh, K. "Maternal age and amniocentesis: Should this be lowered to 30 years?" *Obstetrics and Gynecology* 42(1987): 150–152.

2. Savona-Ventura, C. "Amniocentesis for fetal maturity." *Obstetrical and Gynecological Survey* 42(1987): 717–723.

3. Simpson, J. L. "Risks of chromosomal abnormalities." *Contemporary OB/GYN*, January 1988, pp. 21–22.

4. Penso, C. A., et al. "Early amniocentesis: Report of 407 cases with neonatal follow-up." *Obstetrics and Gynecology* 76(1990): 1032–1036.

5. Hanson, F. W., et al. "Amniocentesis before 15 weeks' gestation: Outcome, risks, and technical problems." *American Journal of Obstetrics and Gynecology* 156(1987): 1524–1531.

6. Weiner, S. A., and Weinstein, L. "Fetal pulmonary maturity and antenatal diagnosis of respiratory distress syndrome." *Obstetrical and Gynecological Survey* 42(1987): 75–80.

7. Socol, N. L. "The tap test: Confirmation of a simple, rapid, inexpensive, and reliable indicator of fetal pulmonary maturity." *American Journal of Obstetrics and Gynecology* 162(1990): 218–222.

8. Zachman, R. D., et al. "Lecithin: Sphingomyelin ratio in the amniotic fluid of male and female fetuses." *Journal of Reproductive Medicine* 34(1989): 203–206.

9. Gabbe, S. G. "Latest methods of determining fetal lung maturity." *Contemporary OB/GYN*, February 1990, pp. 89–91.

10. Knight, J. A.; Miya, T.; and Wu, J. T. "Standard lecithin/sphingomyelin and phosphatidylglycerol techniques compared with immunologic slide test." *Obstetrics and Gynecology* 65(1985): 840–842.

11. Doyle, L. W., et al. "Antenatal steroid therapy and 5-year outcome of extremely low birth weight infants." *Obstetrics and Gynecology* 73(1989): 743–746.

12. Cummings, J. J., D'Eugenio, D. B.; and Gross, S. J. "A controlled trial of dexamethasone in preterm infants at high risk of bronchopulmonary dysplasia." *New England Journal of Medicine* 320(1989): 1505–1510.

13. Morales, W. J., et al. "The effect of antenatal dexamethasone administration in the prevention of respiratory distress syndrome in preterm gestations with premature rupture of membranes." *American Journal of Obstetrics and Gynecology* 154(1986): 591–595.

14. Davis, J. M., et al. "Changes in pulmonary mechanics after the administration of surfactant to infants with respiratory distress syndrome." *New England Journal of Medicine* 319(1988): 476–479.

15. Kendig, J. W., et al. "A comparison of surfactant as immediate prophylaxis and as rescue therapy in newborns of less than 30 weeks' gestation." *New England Journal of Medicine* 324(1991): 865–871.

16. Vidyasagar, D. "Treating RDS with bovine surfactant." *Contemporary OB/GYN*, August 1988, pp. 135–141.

17. Owen, J.; Henson, B. V.; and Hauth, J. C. "A prospective randomized study of saline solution amnioinfusion." *American Journal of Obstetrics and Gynecology* 162(1990): 1146–1149.

18. Wenstrom, K. D., and Parsons, M. T. "The prevention of meconium aspiration in labor using amnioinfusion." *Obstetrics and Gynecology* 73(1989): 647–650.

19. Fisk, N. M., et al. "Diagnostic and therapeutic transabdominal amnioinfusion in oligohydram-nios." *Obstetrics and Gynecology* 78(1991): 270–277.

20. Ogita, S., et al. "Transcervical amnioinfusion of antibiotics: A basic study for managing premature rupture of membranes." *American Journal of Obstetrics and Gynecology* 158(1988): 23–27.

21. "Chorionic villus sampling." ACOG Committee Opinion, number 69, November 1989.

22. Rhoads, G. G., et al. "The safety and efficacy of chorionic villus sampling for early prenatal diagnosis of cytogenetic abnormalities." *New England Journal of Medicine* 320(1989): 609–617.

23. Rodeck, C. H., and Morsman, J. M. "First-trimester chorion biopsy." *British Medical Bulletin* 39(1983): 338.

24. Brambati, B., et al. "Genetic diagnosis before the eighth gestational week." *Obstetrics and Gynecology* 77(1991): 318–321.

25. Burton, B. K.; Schulz, C. J.; and Burd, L. I. "Limb anomalies associated with chorionic villus sampling." *Obstetrics and Gynecology* 79(1992): 726–730.

26. Hogdall, C. K., et al. "Transabdominal chorionic sampling in the second trimester." *American Journal of Obstetrics and Gynecology* 158(1988): 345–349.

27. Chieri, P. R., and Aldini, A. J. R. "Feasibility of placental biopsy in the second trimester for fetal diagnosis." *American Journal of Obstetrics and Gynecology* 160(1989): 581–583.

28. Cullen, M. T., et al. "Embryoscopy: Description and utility of a new technique." *American Journal of Obstetrics and Gynecology* 162(1990): 82.

29. Rodeck, C. H., and Nicolades, K. H. "Fetoscopy." *British Medical Bulletin* 42(1986): 296.

30. Benacerraf, B. R., et al. "Fetal abnormalities: Diagnosis or treatment with percutaneous umbilical blood sampling under continuous ultrasound guidance." *Radiology* 166(1988): 105.

31. Amon, E., et al. "Ultrasonically guided direct umbilical cord blood sampling." *Journal of Reproductive Medicine* 32(1987): 951–955.

32. Hobbins, J. C., et al. "Percutaneous umbilical blood sampling." *American Journal of Obstetrics and Gynecology* 152(1985): 1–6.

33. Appleman, Z., and Golbus, M. S. "Screening for hemoglobinopathies before delivery." *Contemporary OB/GYN*, April 1986, pp. 129–146.

34. Shah, D. M., and Boehm, F. H. "Fetal blood gas analysis from cordocentesis for abnormal fetal heart rate patterns." *American Journal of Obstetrics and Gynecology* 161(1989): 374–376.

35. Weiner, C. P. "Cordocentesis for diagnostic indication: Two years' experience." *Obstetrics and Gynecology* 70(1987): 664–667.

36. Pearce, J. M., and Chamberlain, G. V. P. "Ultrasonically guided percutaneous umbilical blood sampling in the management of intrauterine growth retardation." *British Journal of Obstetrics and Gynaecology* 94(1987): 318.

37. Seeds, J. W. "PUBS: Important new aids for prenatal diagnosis." *Contemporary OB/GYN*, February 1988, pp. 117–133.

38. Josten, B. E., et al. "Umbilical cord blood pH and Apgar scores as an index of neonatal health." *American Journal of Obstetrics and Gynecology* 157(1987): 843–848.

39. Thorp, J. A., et al. "Routine umbilical cord blood gas determinations?" *American Journal of Obstetrics and Gynecology* 161(1989): 600–605.

40. Boesel, R. R.; Olson, A. E.; and Johnson, J. W. C. "Umbilical cord blood studies help assess fetal respiratory status." *Contemporary OB/GYN*, November 1986, pp. 63–74.

41. "Maternal serum alpha-fetoprotein." ACOG Committee Opinion, number 76, December 1989.

42. Crandell, B. F., and Matsumoto, M. "Routine amniotic fluid alpha-fetoprotein assay: Experience with 40,000 pregnancies." *American Journal of Medical Genetics* 24(1986): 143.

43. Stiller, R. J., et al. "Elevated maternal serum alpha-fetoprotein concentration and fetal chromosomal abnormalities." *Obstetrics and Gynecology* 75(1990): 994–997.

44. Lindgley, L. H.; Albright, S. G.; and Seeds, J. W. "Prenatal screening with alpha-fetoprotein: Informed choices, increased challenges." *The Female Patient* 12(1987): 85–103.

45. Drugan, A., et al. "A normal ultrasound does not obviate the need for amniocentesis in patients with elevated serum alpha-fetoprotein." *Obstetrics and Gynecology* 72(1988): 627–630.

46. Lemire, R. J. "Neural tube defects." *Journal of the American Medical Association* 259(1988): 558–562.

47. Katz, V. L.; Chescheir, N. C.; and Cefalo, R. C. "Unexplained elevations of maternal serum alpha-fetoprotein." *Obstetrical and Gynecological Survey* 45(1990): 719–726.

48. Nadel, A. S., et al. "Absence of need for amniocentesis in patients with elevated levels of maternal serum alpha-fetoprotein and normal ultrasonographic examinations." *New England Journal of Medicine* 323(1990): 557–561.

49. Garver, K. L., and Buerkle, A. M. "Controversies in maternal serum alpha-fetoprotein screening." *The Female Patient* 14(1989): 87–97.

50. Watson, W. J., et al. "The role of ultrasound in evaluation of patients with elevated maternal serum alpha-fetoprotein. A review." *Obstetrics and Gynecology* 78(1991): 123–127.

51. Kelly, J. C.; Petrocik, E.; and Wassman, E. R. "Amniotic fluid acetylcholinesterase ratios in prenatal diagnosis of fetal abnormalities." *American Journal of Obstetrics and Gynecology* 161(1989): 703–705.

52. Simpson, J. L., et al. "Maternal serum alpha-fetoprotein screening. Low and high values for detection of genetic abnormalities." *American Journal of Obstetrics and Gynecology* 155(1986): 593–597.

53. Davis, R. O., et al. "Decreased levels of amniotic fluid alpha-fetoprotein associated with Down syndrome." *American Journal of Obstetrics and Gynecology* 153(1985): 541–544.

54. Wald, N. J., et al. "Maternal serum screening for Down syndrome in early pregnancy." *British Medical Journal* 297(1988): 883.

55. MacDonald, M. L.; Wagner, R. M.; and Slotnick, R. N. "Sensitivity and specificity of screening for Down syndrome with alpha-fetoprotein, hCG, unconjugated estriol, and maternal age." *Obstetrics and Gynecology* 77(1991): 63–68.

56. "Ultrasound in pregnancy." ACOG Technical Bulletin, number 116, May 1988.

57. Quinlan, R. W. "Ultrasonography: A decade of advances." *The Female Patient* 11(1986): 113–116.

58. Ewigman, B.; LeFevre, M.; and Hesser, J. "A randomized trial of routine prenatal ultrasound." *Obstetrics and Gynecology* 76(1990): 189–194.

59. Benacerraf, B. R.; Gelman, R.; and Frigoletto, F. D., Jr. "Sonographic identification of second-

trimester fetuses with Down's syndrome." *New England Journal of Medicine* 317(1987): 371–376.

60. Toi, A.; Simpson, G. F., and Filly, R. A. "Ultrasonically evident fetal nuchal skin thickening: Is it specific for Down syndrome?" *American Journal of Obstetrics and Gynecology* 156(1987): 150–153.

61. Brumfield, C. J., et al. "Sonographic measurements and ratios in fetuses with Down syndrome." *Obstetrics and Gynecology* 73(1989): 644–646.

62. Crane, J. P., and Gray, D. L. "Sonographically measured nuchal skin fold thickness as a screening tool for Down syndrome: Results of a perspective clinical trial." *Obstetrics and Gynecology* 77(1991): 533–536.

63. Evans, M. I., et al. "Selective first-trimester termination in octuplet and quadruplet pregnancies: Clinical and ethical issues." *Obstetrics and Gynecology* 71(1988): 289–296.

64. Hobbins, J. C. "Selective reduction—A perinatal necessity?" *New England Journal of Medicine* 318(1988): 1062–1063.

65. Berkowitz, R. L., et al. "Selective reduction of multifetal pregnancies in the first trimester." *New England Journal of Medicine* 318(1988): 1043–1047.

66. Reece, E. A., et al. "Can ultrasonography replace amniocentesis in fetal gender determination during the early second trimester?" *American Journal of Obstetrics and Gynecology* 156(1987): 579–581.

67. Plattner, G., et al. "Fetal sex determination by ultrasound scan in the second and third trimesters." *Obstetrics and Gynecology* 61(1983): 454–458.

68. Reece, E. A., et al. "Dating through pregnancy: A measure of growing up." *Obstetrical and Gynecological Survey* 44(1989): 544–554.

69. Vintzileos, A. M., et al. "Value of fetal ponderal index in predicting growth retardation." *Obstetrics and Gynecology* 67(1986): 584–588.

70. Villar, J., and Belizan, J. M. "The evaluation of the methods used in the diagnosis of intrauterine growth retardation." *Obstetrical and Gynecological Survey* 41(1986): 187–198.

71. Chervenak, J. L., et al. "Macrosomia in the postdate pregnancy: Is routine ultrasonographic screening indicated?" *American Journal of Obstetrics and Gynecology* 161(1989): 753–756.

72. Moya, F., et al. "Ultrasound assessment of the postmature pregnancy." *Obstetrics and Gynecology* 65(1985): 319–321.

73. Hirata, G. I., et al. "Ultrasonographic estimation of fetal weight in the clinically macrosomic fetus." *American Journal of Obstetrics and Gynecology* 162(1990): 238–242.

74. Weiner, C. P., et al. "Ultrasonic fetal weight prediction: Role of head circumference and femur length." *Obstetrics and Gynecology* 65(1985): 812–816.

75. Vintzileos, A. M., et al. "The ultrasound femur length as a predictor of fetal length." *Obstetrics and Gynecology* 64(1984): 779–782.

76. Chervenak, F. A. "Diagnosis and management of intrauterine growth retardation." *The Female Patient* 13(1988): 78–79.

77. Thacker, S. B., and Berkelman, R. L. "Assessing the diagnostic accuracy and efficacy of selective antepartum fetal surveillance techniques." *Obstetrical and Gynecological Survey* 41(1986): 121–136.

78. Ott, W. J. "Defining altered fetal growth by second-trimester sonography." *Obstetrics and Gynecology* 75(1990): 1053–1058.

79. Hegge, F. N., et al. "Fetal malformations commonly detectable on ultrasound." *Journal of Reproductive Medicine* 35(1990): 391–398.

80. Bracero, L. A.; Bracero, P. S.; and Fakhry, J. "Fetal ultrasound: Interpreting anomalous signs." *The Female Patient* 12(1987): 80–88.

81. Rosendahl, H., and Kivinen, S. "Antenatal detection of congenital malformations by routine ultrasonography." *Obstetrics and Gynecology* 73(1989): 947–950.

82. Filly, R. A., et al. "Detection of fetal central nervous system anomalies: A practical level of effort for a routine sonogram." *Radiology* 172(1989): 403.

83. O'Brien, G. D. "Limits of ultrasound screening for anomalies." *Contemporary OB/GYN,* July 1989, pp. 51–57.

84. Donnenfeld, A. E., and Mennuti, M. T. "Second trimester diagnosis of fetal skeletal dysplasias." *Obstetrical and Gynecological Survey* 42(1987): 199–216.

85. Perone, N. "A practical guide to fetal echocardiography." *Contemporary OB/GYN,* January 1988, pp. 55–81.

86. Copell, J. A.; Pilu, J.; and Kleinman, C. S. "Con-

genital heart disease and extracardiac anomalies: Associations and indications for fetal echocardiography." *American Journal of Obstetrics and Gynecology* 154(1986): 1121–1132.

87. Kleinman, C. S., et al. "Fetal echocardiography—A tool for evaluation of in utero cardiac arrhythmias and monitoring of in utero therapy: Analysis of 71 patients." *American Journal of Cardiology* 51(1983): 237.

88. Smith, C. S. C.; Weiner, S.; and Bolognese, R. J. "Amniotic fluid volume: Importance and assessment." *The Female Patient* 15(1990): 85–94.

89. Shenker, L., et al. "Fetal cardiac Doppler flow studies in prenatal diagnosis of heart disease." *American Journal of Obstetrics and Gynecology* 158(1988): 1267–1273.

90. Newnham, J. P., et al. "An evaluation of the efficacy of Doppler flow velocity waveform analysis as a screening test in pregnancy." *American Journal of Obstetrics and Gynecology* 162(1990): 403–410.

91. Maulik, D., et al. "The diagnostic efficacy of the umbilical artery systolic/diastolic ratio as a screening tool: A prospective blinded study." *American Journal of Obstetrics and Gynecology* 162(1990): 1518–1525.

92. Rochelson, B. L., et al. "The clinical significance of Doppler umbilical artery velocimetry in the small for gestational age fetus." *American Journal of Obstetrics and Gynecology* 156(1987): 1223–1226.

93. Berkowitz, G. S., et al. "Doppler umbilical velocimetry in the prediction of adverse outcome in pregnancies at risk for intrauterine growth retardation." *Obstetrics and Gynecology* 71(1988): 742–746.

94. Jurkovic, D., et al. "Transvaginal color Doppler assessment of the uteroplacental circulation in early pregnancy." *Obstetrics and Gynecology* 77(1991): 365–369.

95. Brary, H. S.; Platt, L. D.; and Paul, R. H. "Fetal umbilical blood flow velocity waveforms using Doppler ultrasonography in patients with late decelerations." *Obstetrics and Gynecology* 73(1989): 363–365.

96. Malcus, P., et al. "Umbilical artery Doppler velocimetry as a labor admission test." *Obstetrics and Gynecology* 77(1991): 10–16.

97. Erskine, R. L. A., and Ritchie, J. W. K. "Umbilical artery blood flow characteristics in normal and growth-retarded fetuses." *British Journal of Obstetrics and Gynaecology* 92(1985): 605.

98. Jaffe, R., and Warsof, S. L. "Color Doppler imaging in obstetrics and gynecology." *The Female Patient* 16(1991): 85–91.

99. Stark, C. R., et al. "Short- and long-term risks after exposure to diagnostic ultrasound in utero." *Obstetrics and Gynecology* 63(1984): 194–200.

100. Reece, E. A., et al. "The safety of obstetric ultrasonography: Concern for the fetus." *Obstetrics and Gynecology* 76(1990): 139–145.

101. Agustsson, P., and Patel, N. B. "The predictive value of fetal breathing movements in the diagnosis of preterm labor." *British Journal of Obstetrics and Gynaecology* 94(1987): 860.

102. Vintzileos, A. M., et al. "Fetal breathing as a predictor of infection in premature rupture of the membranes." *Obstetrics and Gynecology* 67(1986): 813–817.

103. Devoe, L. D.; Ruedrich, D. A.; and Searle, N. S. "Value of observation of fetal breathing activity in antenatal assessment of high-risk pregnancy." *American Journal of Obstetrics and Gynecology* 160(1989): 166–171.

104. Roberts, A. B., et al. "Fetal breathing movements after preterm premature rupture of the membranes." *American Journal of Obstetrics and Gynecology* 164(1991): 821–825.

105. Sadovsky, E. "Monitoring fetal movement: A useful screening test." *Contemporary OB/GYN*, April 1985, pp. 123–135.

106. Rabinowitz, R.; Persitz, E.; and Sadovsky, E. "The relation between fetal heart rate accelerations and fetal movements." *Obstetrics and Gynecology* 61(1983): 16–18.

107. Schifrin, B. S., and Clement, D. "Why fetal monitoring remains a good idea." *Contemporary OB/GYN*, February 1990, pp. 70–86.

108. Vintzileos, A. M., et al. "Fetal biophysical profile and the effect of premature rupture of the membranes." *Obstetrics and Gynecology* 67(1986): 818–823.

109. Manning, F. A., et al. "Fetal biophysical profile score and nonstress test: A comparative trial." *Obstetrics and Gynecology* 64(1984): 326–331.

110. Jones, T. B., and Frigoletto, F. D. "Fetal con-

dition and the biophysical profile." *Postgraduate Radiology* 5(1985): 47.

111. Vintzileos, A. M. "The relationships among the fetal biophysical profile, umbilical cord pH, and Apgar scores." *American Journal of Obstetrics and Gynecology* 157(1987): 627–631.

112. Roussis, P.; Troiano, N. H.; and Shah, D. M. "Fetal assessment—Nonstress and contraction stress testing." *The Female Patient* 15(1990): 33–40.

113. Devoe, L. D., et al. "The nonstress test as a diagnostic test: A critical reappraisal." *American Journal of Obstetrics and Gynecology* 152(1985): 1047–1053.

114. Phelan, J. P., et al. "Continuing role of the nonstress test in the management of postdates pregnancy." *Obstetrics and Gynecology* 64(1984): 624–628.

115. Boehm, F. H., et al. "Improved outcome of twice weekly nonstress testing." *Obstetrics and Gynecology* 67(1986): 566–568.

116. Small, M. L., et al. "An active management approach to the postdate fetus with a reactive nonstress test and fetal heart rate decelerations." *Obstetrics and Gynecology* 70(1987): 636–639.

117. Clark, S. L. "How a modified NST improves fetal surveillance." *Contemporary OB/GYN*, May 1990, pp. 45–48.

118. Clark, S. L.; Sabey, P.; and Jolley, K. "Nonstress testing with acoustic stimulation and amniotic fluid volume assessment: 5793 tests without unexpected fetal death." *American Journal of Obstetrics and Gynecology* 160(1989): 694–697.

119. Romero, R.; Mazor, M.; and Hobbins, J. C. "A critical appraisal of fetal acoustic stimulation as an antenatal test for fetal well-being." *Obstetrics and Gynecology* 71(1988): 781–785.

120. Thomas, R. L., et al. "Preterm and term fetal cardiac and movement responses to vibratory acoustic stimulation." *American Journal of Obstetrics and Gynecology* 161(1989): 141–145.

121. Gagnon, R., et al. "Effects of low-frequency vibration on human term fetuses." *American Journal of Obstetrics and Gynecology* 161(1989): 1479–1485.

122. Smith, C. V. "Continuing experience with the fetal acoustic stimulation tests." *Journal of Reproductive Medicine* 33(1988): 365–368.

123. Sherer, D. M.; Menashe, M.; and Sadovsky, E. "Severe fetal bradycardia caused by external vibratory acoustic stimulation." *American Journal of Obstetrics and Gynecology* 159(1988): 334–335.

124. Ohel, G., et al. "Neonatal auditory acuity following in utero vibratory acoustic stimulation." *American Journal of Obstetrics and Gynecology* 157(1987): 440–441.

125. Stein, J. L., et al. "Nipple stimulation for labor augmentation." *Journal of Reproductive Medicine* 35(1990): 710–714.

126. Rosenzweig, B. A., et al. "Comparison of the nipple stimulation and exogenous oxytocin contraction stress tests." *Journal of Reproductive Medicine* 34(1989): 950–954.

127. Modanlou, H. D. "Guide to sinusoidal FHR patterns." *Contemporary OB/GYN*, August 1983, pp. 94–98.

128. Anyaegbunam, A., et al. "The significance of antepartum variable decelerations." *American Journal of Obstetrics and Gynecology* 155(1986): 707–710.

129. "Assessment of fetal and newborn acid-base status." ACOG Technical Bulletin, number 127, April 1989.

130. Clark, S. L., and Paul, R. H. "Intrapartum fetal surveillance: The role of fetal scalp blood sampling." *American Journal of Obstetrics and Gynecology* 153(1985): 717–720.

131. Clark, S. L. "Do we still need fetal scalp blood sampling?" *Contemporary OB/GYN*, March 1989, pp. 75–86.

132. Kay, H. H., and Spritzer, C. E. "Preliminary experience with magnetic resonance imaging in patients with third-trimester bleeding." *Obstetrics and Gynecology* 78(1991): 424–429.

133. Wenstrom, K. D., et al. "Magnetic resonance imaging of fetuses with intracranial defects." *Obstetrics and Gynecology* 77(1991): 529–532.

134. Kopelman, J. N., et al. "Computed tomographic pelvimetry in the evaluation of breech presentation." *Obstetrics and Gynecology* 66(1986): 455–458.

135. Graber, D. A. "Dilemmas in the pharmacological management of preterm labor." *Obstetrical and Gynecological Survey* 44(1989): 512–517.

136. Andersen, H. F., et al. "Prediction of risk for

preterm delivery by ultrasonographic measurement of cervical length." *American Journal of Obstetrics and Gynecology* 163(1990): 659–667.

137. Niebyl, J. R. "Averting preterm labor with first-line tocolytics." *Contemporary OB/GYN*, December 1988, pp. 65–78.

138. Besinger, R. E., and Niebyl, J. R. "The safety and efficacy of tocolytic agents for the treatment of preterm labor." *Obstetrical and Gynecological Survey* 45(1990): 415–431.

139. Katz, V. L., and Seeds, J. W. "Fetal and neonatal cardiovascular complications from B-sympathomimetic therapy for tocolysis." *American Journal of Obstetrics and Gynecology* 161(1989): 1–4.

140. Kopelman, J. N.; Duff, P.; and Read, J. A. "Randomized comparison of oral terbutaline and ritodrine for preventing recurrent preterm labor." *Journal of Reproductive Medicine* 34(1989): 225–230.

141. Leveno, K. J.; Little, B. B.; and Cunningham, G. "The national impact of ritodrine hydrochloride for inhibition of preterm labor." *Obstetrics and Gynecology* 76(1990): 12–15.

142. Beall, M. H., et al. "A comparison of ritodrine, terbutaline, and magnesium sulfate for the suppression of preterm labor." *American Journal of Obstetrics and Gynecology* 153(1985): 854–859.

143. Holcomb, W. L., Jr.; Shackelford, G. D.; and Petri, R. H. "Magnesium tocolysis and neonatal bone abnormalities: A controlled study." *Obstetrics and Gynecology* 78(1991): 611–614.

144. Neibyl, J. R., and Witter, F. R. "Neonatal outcome after indomethacin treatment for preterm labor." *American Journal of Obstetrics and Gynecology* 155(1986): 747–749.

145. Lam, F., et al. "Use of the subcutaneous terbutaline pump for long-term tocolysis." *Obstetrics and Gynecology* 72(1988): 810–812.

146. Lam, F. "Miniature pump infusion of terbutaline—An option in preterm labor." *Contemporary OB/GYN*, January 1989, pp. 52–70.

147. "Strategies to prevent prematurity: Home uterine activity monitoring." ACOG Committee Opinion, number 74, November 1989.

148. Gonen, R.; Braithwaite, N.; and Milligan, J. E. "Fetal heart rate monitoring at home and trans-

mission by telephone." *Obstetrics and Gynecology* 75(1990); 464–468.

149. Katz, M.; Newman, R. B.; and Gill, P. J. "Assessment of uterine activity in ambulatory patients at high risk of preterm labor and delivery." *American Journal of Obstetrics and Gynecology* 154(1986): 44–47.

150. Newman, R. B.; Campbell, B. A.; and Stramm, S. L. "Objective tocodynanometry identifies labor onset earlier than subjective maternal perception." *Obstetrics and Gynecology* 76(1990): 1089–1092.

151. Main, D. M., et al. "Controlled trial of a preterm labor detection program: Efficacy and costs." *Obstetrics and Gynecology* 74(1989): 873–877.

152. Morrison, J. C., et al. "Prevention of preterm birth by ambulatory assessment of uterine activity: A randomized study." *American Journal of Obstetrics and Gynecology* 156(1987): 536–643.

153. Iams, J. D., et al. "A prospective random trial of home uterine activity monitoring in pregnancies at increased risk of preterm labor." *American Journal of Obstetrics and Gynecology* 157(1987): 638–643.

154. Longaker, M. T., et al. "Maternal outcome after open fetal surgery." *Journal of the American Medical Association* 265(1991): 737–741.

155. Evans, M. I., et al. "Fetal surgery in the 1990s." *American Journal of Diseases in Childhood* 143(1990): 1431.

156. Harrison, M. R., et al. "Successful repair in utero of a fetal diaphragmatic hernia after removal of herniated viscera from the left thorax." *New England Journal of Medicine* 322(1990): 1582–1584.

157. Pang, S., et al. "Prenatal treatment of congenital adrenal hyperplasia due to 21-hydroxylase deficiency." *New England Journal of Medicine* 322(1990): 111–114.

158. Davidson, K. M., et al. "Successful in utero treatment of fetal goiter and hypothyroidism." *New England Journal of Medicine* 324(1991): 543–547.

159. Reuss, A., et al. "Non-invasive management of fetal obstructive uropathy." *Lancet* 2(1988): 949.

160. Arthur, R. J., et al. "Bilateral fetal uropathy:

What is the outlook?" *British Medical Journal* 298(1989): 1419.

161. Sarno, A. P., Jr., and Phelan, J. P. "Intrauterine resuscitation of the fetus." *Contemporary OB/GYN*, July 1988, pp. 43–52.

162. "Prevention of D isoimmunization." ACOG Technical Bulletin, number 147, October 1990.

163. "Management of isoimmunization in pregnancy." ACOG Technical Bulletin, number 148, October 1990.

164. Rousseau, F., et al. "Direct diagnosis by DNA analysis of the fragile X syndrome of mental retardation." *New England Journal of Medicine* 325(1991): 1673–1681.

165. Sutherland, G. R., et al. "Prenatal diagnosis of fragile X syndrome by direct detection of the unstable DNA sequence." *New England Journal of Medicine* 325(1991): 1720–1722.

166. Arahata, K., et al. "Mosaic expression of dystrophin in symptomatic carriers of Duchenne's muscular dystrophy." *New England Journal of Medicine* 320(1989): 138–142.

167. Korf, B. R. "Molecular diagnosis of Duchenne/Becker muscular dystrophy." *Contemporary OB/GYN*, July 1990, pp. 27–54.

168. Linden, M. G., et al. "47, XXX: What is the prognosis?" *Pediatrics* 82(1988): 619.

169. Antonarakis, S. E., et al. "Parental origin of the extra chromosome in trisomy 21 as indicated by analysis of DNA polymorphisms." *New England Journal of Medicine* 324(1991): 872–876.

170. King, C. R. "Prenatal diagnosis of genetic disease with molecular genetic technology." *Obstetrical and Gynecological Survey* 43(1988): 493–506.

171. Caskey, C. T. "New molecular techniques for DNA analysis." *Contemporary OB/GYN*, May 1991, pp. 27–49.

172. Antonarakis, S. E. "Diagnosis of genetic disorders at the DNA level." *New England Journal of Medicine* 320(1989): 153–162.

173. Meyers, C. M., and Elias, S. "Genetic screening for mendelian disorders." *Contemporary OB/GYN*, August 1990, pp. 56–82.

174. King, C. R. "Genetic linkage: The basis of human gene mapping." *Obstetrical and Gynecological Survey* 44(1989): 177–188.

175. Triggs-Raine, B. L., et al. "Screening for carriers of Tay-Sachs disease among Ashkenazi Jews." *New England Journal of Medicine* 323(1990): 6–12.

176. "Screening for Tay-Sachs disease." ACOG Committee Opinion, number 93, March 1991.

177. Nugent, C. E., et al. "Prenatal diagnosis of cystic fibrosis by chorionic villus sampling using 12 polymorphic deoxyribonucleic acid markers." *Obstetrics and Gynecology* 71(1988): 213–215.

178. Gilbert, F., et al. "Prenatal diagnostic options in cystic fibrosis." *American Journal of Obstetrics and Gynecology* 158(1988): 947–952.

179. Levy, H. L., Kaplan, G. N.; and Erickson, A. M. "Comparison of treated and untreated pregnancies in a mother with phenylketonuria." *Journal of Pediatrics* 100(1982): 876.

180. Koshy, M., et al. "Prophylactic red-cell transfusions in pregnant patients with sickle cell disease: A randomized cooperative study." *New England Journal of Medicine* 319(1988): 1447.

181. Grossman, L. K., et al. "Neonatal screening and genetic counseling for sickle cell trait." *American Journal of Diseases in Childhood* 139(1985): 241.

182. Gehlbach, D. L., and Morgenstern, L. L. "Antenatal screening for thalassemia minor." *Obstetrics and Gynecology* 71(1988): 801–803.

183. Parfrey, P. S., et al. "The diagnosis and prognosis of autosomal dominant polycystic kidney disease." *New England Journal of Medicine* 323(1990): 1085–1090.

184. Kogan, S. C.; Doherty, M.; and Gitschier, J. "An improved method for prenatal diagnosis of genetic diseases by analysis of amplified DNA sequences: Application to hemophilia A." *New England Journal of Medicine* 317(1987): 985.

Chapter 12

CHILDBIRTH AND THE POSTPARTUM PERIOD

1. Carlson, J. M., et al. "Maternal position during parturition in normal labor." *Obstetrics and Gynecology* 68(1986): 443–447.

2. Lupe, P. J., and Gross, T. L. "Maternal upright posture and mobility in labor—A review." *Obstetrics and Gynecology* 67(1986): 727–733.

3. Johnson, N.; Johnson, V. A.; and Gupta, J. K. "Maternal positions during labor." *Obstetrical and Gynecological Survey* 46(1991): 428–433.

4. Chen, S-Z, et al. "Effects of sitting position on uterine activity during labor." *Obstetrics and Gynecology* 69(1987): 67–73.

5. Dundes, L. "The evolution of the maternal birthing position." *American Journal of Public Health* 77(1987): 636.

6. Hughey, M. J. "Fetal position during pregnancy." *American Journal of Obstetrics and Gynecology* 153(1985): 885–886.

7. Stewart, P., and Calder, A. A. "Posture in labour: Patients' choice and its effect on performance." *British Journal of Obstetrics and Gynaecology* 91(1984): 1091.

8. Abitbol, M. M. "Supine position in labor and associated fetal heart rate changes." *Obstetrics and Gynecology* 65(1985): 481–486.

9. Cooperstock, M.; England, J. E.; and Wolfe, R. A. "Circadian incidence of labor onset hour in preterm birth and chorioamnionitis." *Obstetrics and Gynecology* 70(1987): 852–855.

10. Kilpatrick, S. J., and Laros, R. K., Jr. "Characteristics of normal labor." *Obstetrics and Gynecology* 74(1989): 85–87.

11. Newman, R. B., et al. "Maternal perception of prelabor uterine activity." *Obstetrics and Gynecology* 68(1986): 765–769.

12. Wuitchik, M.; Bakal, D.; and Lipshitz, J. "The clinical significance of pain and cognitive activity in latent labor." *Obstetrics and Gynecology* 73(1989): 35–41.

13. Chazotte, C., and Cohen, W. R. "Drug use selection for latent-phase labor." *Contemporary OB/GYN*, March 1987, pp. 73–84.

14. Peisner, D. B., and Rosen, M. G. "Transition from latent to active labor." *Obstetrics and Gynecology* 68(1986): 448–451.

15. Hillard, P. A. "How to tell if you're in labor." *Parents*, January 1986, pp. 96–98.

16. Schauberger, C. W. "False labor." *Obstetrics and Gynecology* 68(1986): 770–772.

17. MacDonald, D., et al. "The Dublin randomized controlled trial of intrapartum fetal heart rate monitoring." *American Journal of Obstetrics and Gynecology* 152(1985): 524–539.

18. Shy, K. K., et al. "Effects of electronic fetal-heart-rate monitoring, as compared with periodic auscultation, on the neurologic development of premature infants." *New England Journal of Medicine* 322(1990): 588.

19. Colditz, P. B., and Henderson-Smart, D. J. "Electronic fetal heart rate monitoring during labour: Does it prevent perinatal asphyxia and cerebral palsy?" *Medical Journal of Australia* 153(1990): 88.

20. Freeman, R. "Intrapartum fetal monitoring—A disappointing story." *New England Journal of Medicine* 322(1990): 624–626.

21. "Intrapartum fetal heart rate monitoring." ACOG Technical Bulletin, number 132, September 1989.

22. Schifrin, B. S. "Electronic fetal monitoring and malpractice." *The Female Patient* 15(1990): 79–82.

23. Greenland, S., et al. "Effects of electronic fetal monitoring on rates of early neonatal death, low Apgar score, and cesarean section." *Acta Obstetrics and Gynecology of Scandinavia* 64(1985): 75.

24. Sandmire, H. F. "Whither electronic fetal monitoring?" *Obstetrics and Gynecology* 76(1990): 1130–1133.

25. Herbert, W. N. P., et al. "Clinical aspects of fetal heart ascultation." *Obstetrics and Gynecology* 69(1987): 574–577.

26. Ellison, P. H., et al. "Electronic fetal heart monitoring, auscultation, and neonatal outcome." *American Journal of Obstetrics and Gynecology* 164(1991): 1281–1289.

27. Patterson, R. M. "Estimation of fetal weight during labor." *Obstetrics and Gynecology* 65(1985): 330–332.

28. Porreco, R. P., and Troyer, L. R. "Meeting the challenge of dystocia in primigravidas." *Contemporary OB/GYN*, October 1990, pp. 54–63.

29. Friedman, E. A. "Failure to progress in labor." *Contemporary OB/GYN*, December 1989, pp. 42–52.

30. Bottoms, S. F.; Hirsch, V. J.; and Sokol, R. J. "Medical management of arrest disorders of labor: A current overview." *American Journal of Obstetrics and Gynecology* 156(1987): 935–939.

31. Steer, P. J.; Carter, M. C.; and Beard, R. W. "The effect of oxytocin infusion on uterine activity levels in slow labour." *British Journal of Obstetrics and Gynaecology* 92(1985): 1120.

32. Cardozo, L., and Pearce, J. M. "Oxytocin in active-phase abnormalities of labor: A randomized study." *Obstetrics and Gynecology* 75(1990): 152–157.

33. Carpenter, M. W., et al. "Practice environment is associated with obstetric decision making regarding abnormal labor." *Obstetrics and Gynecology* 70(1987): 657–662.

34. Akoury, H. A., et al. "Active management of labor and operative delivery in nulliparous women." *American Journal of Obstetrics and Gynecology* 158(1988): 255–258.

35. MacDonald, D. W. "Active management of labor: A unified policy." *Contemporary OB/GYN*, January 1985, pp. 161–169.

36. Turner, M. J.; Brassil, M.; and Gordon, H. "Active management of labor associated with a decrease in the cesarean section rate in nulliparas." *Obstetrics and Gynecology* 71(1988): 150–154.

37. White, D. R. "Does mother know best? Maternal assessment of relative fetal size in utero." *British Journal of Obstetrics and Gynaecology* 95(1988): 135.

38. "Dystocia." ACOG Technical Bulletin, number 137, December 1989.

39. Akoury, H. A., et al. "Oxytocin augmentation of labor and perinatal outcome in nulliparas." *Obstetrics and Gynecology* 78(1991): 227–230.

40. Boyd, M. E.; Usher, R. H.; and McLean, F. H. "Fetal macrosomia: Prediction, risks, proposed management." *Obstetrics and Gynecology* 61 (1983): 715–721.

41. Niswander, K. R. "Does substandard obstetric care cause cerebral palsy?" *Contemporary OB/GYN*, October 1987, pp. 42–60.

42. Chez, R. A. "Effect of labor on intelligence of the offspring." *Obstetrics and Gynecology* 77(1991): 777–778.

43. Roemer, F. J.; Rowland, D. Y.; and Nuamah, I. F. "Retrospective study of fetal effects of prolonged labor before cesarean delivery." *Obstetrics and Gynecology* 77(1991): 653–658.

44. Chaney, R. H., et al. "Birth injury as the cause of mental retardation." *Obstetrics and Gynecology* 67(1986): 771–775.

45. "Operative vaginal delivery." ACOG Technical Bulletin, number 152, February 1991.

46. Hagadorn-Freathy, A. S.; Yeomans, E. R.; and Hankins, G. D. V. "Validation of the 1988 ACOG forceps classification system." *Obstetrics and Gynecology* 77(1991): 356–360.

47. "Obstetric forceps." ACOG Committee Opinion, number 71, August 1989.

48. Bashore, R. A.; Phillips, W. H., Jr.; and Brinkman, C. R. "A comparison of the morbidity of midforceps and cesarean delivery." *American Journal of Obstetrics and Gynecology* 162(1990): 1428–1435.

49. Dierker, L. J., et al. "Midforceps deliveries: Long-term outcome of infants." *American Journal of Obstetrics and Gynecology* 154(1986): 764–768.

50. Harris, B. A., Jr. "Forceps and vacuum delivery." *The Female Patient* 16(1991): 39–50.

51. Berkus, M. D., et al. "Cohort study of silastic obstetric vacuum cup deliveries—Safety of the instrument." *Obstetrics and Gynecology* 66(1985): 503–508.

52. Flanagain, T. A., et al. "Management of term breech presentation." *American Journal of Obstetrics and Gynecology* 156(1987): 492.

53. Gimovsky, M. L., and Petrie, R. A. "Breech presentation: Alternatives to routine C/S." *Contemporary OB/GYN*, January 1992, pp. 35–48.

54. Confino, E., et al. "The breech dilemma. A review." *Obstetrical and Gynecological Survey* 40(1985): 330–337.

55. Tatum, R. K., et al. "Vaginal breech delivery of selected infants weighing more than 2000 grams." *American Journal of Obstetrics and Gynecology* 152(1985): 145–155.

56. Mahomed, K.; Seeras, R.; and Coulson, R. "External cephalic version at term. A randomized controlled trial using tocolysis." *British Journal of Obstetrics and Gynaecology* 98(1991): 8.

57. Yeast, J. D., and Garite, T. J. "External version for breech fetuses—A neglected alternative?" *Contemporary OB/GYN*, March 1985, pp. 45–52.

58. Ferguson, J. E.; Armstrong, M. A.; and Dyson, D. C. "Maternal and fetal factors affecting success of antepartum external cephalic version." *Obstetrics and Gynecology* 70(1987): 722.

59. Fortunato, S. J.; Mercer, L. J.; and Guzick, D. S. "External cephalic version with tocolysis: Factors associated with success." *Obstetrics and Gynecology* 72(1988): 58–61.

60. Combs, C. A., and Laros, R. K., Jr. "Prolonged

third stage of labor: Morbidity and risk factors." *Obstetrics and Gynecology* 77(1991): 863–867.

61. Prendiville, W. J., et al. "The Bristol third stage trial: Active versus physiological management of third stage of labor." *British Medical Journal* 297(1988): 1295.

62. Poeschmann, R. P.; Doesburg, W. H.; and Eskes, T. K. "A randomized comparison of oxytocin, sulprostone, and placebo in the management of the third stage of labour." *American Journal of Obstetrics and Gynecology* 98(1991): 528–530.

63. Bullough, C. H.; Msuku, R. S.; and Karande, L. "Early suckling and postpartum haemorrhage: Controlled trial in deliveries by traditional birth attendants." *Lancet* 2(1989): 522–525.

64. Lagrew, D. C., and Freeman, R. K. "Management of postdate pregnancy." *American Journal of Obstetrics and Gynecology* 154(1986): 8.

65. Lang, J., et al. "Prolonged pregnancy: The management debate." *British Medical Journal* 297 (1988): 715.

66. Shapiro, H., and Lyons, E. "Late maternal age and postdate pregnancy." *American Journal of Obstetrics and Gynecology* 160(1989): 909–912.

67. Shime, J., et al. "The influence of prolonged pregnancy on infant development at one and two years of age: A prospective controlled study." *American Journal of Obstetrics and Gynecology* 154(1986): 341–345.

68. Bochner, C. J., et al. "The efficacy of starting postterm antenatal testing at 41 weeks as compared with 42 weeks of gestational age." *American Journal of Obstetrics and Gynecology* 159(1988): 550–554.

69. Smith, C. I. "Postterm pregnancy: Monitoring versus intervention." *The Female Patient* 15 (1990): 19–32.

70. Dyson, D. C.; Miller, P. D.; and Armstrong, M. A. "Management of prolonged pregnancy: Induction of labor versus antepartum fetal testing." *American Journal of Obstetrics and Gynecology* 156(1987): 928–934.

71. Arias, F. "Postdatism and the law—The minimum standards." *The Female Patient* 14(1989): 28–37.

72. Guidetti, D. A.; Divon, M. Y.; and Langer, O. "Postdate fetal surveillance: Is 41 weeks too early?" *American Journal of Obstetrics and Gynecology* 161(1989): 91–93.

73. Usher, R. H., et al. "Assessment of fetal risk in postdate pregnancies." *American Journal of Obstetrics and Gynecology* 158(1988): 259–264.

74. Fisk, N. M. "Modifications to selective conservative management in preterm premature rupture of membranes." *Obstetrical and Gynecological Survey* 43(1988): 328–333.

75. Toth, M., et al. "The role of infection in the etiology of preterm birth." *Obstetrics and Gynecology* 71(1988): 723–726.

76. Romero, R., et al. "Can antimicrobials prevent preterm delivery?" *Contemporary OB/GYN*, November 1989, pp. 81–92.

77. Vintzileos, A. M. "Premature rupture of the membranes: A management rationale." *The Female Patient* 13(1988): 68–83.

78. Dodson, M. G., and Fortunato, S. J. "Microorganisms and premature labor." *Journal of Reproductive Medicine* 33(1988): 87–94.

79. Clark, S. L. "Managing PROM: A continuing controversy." *Contemporary OB/GYN*, June 1989, pp. 49–55.

80. "Premature rupture of membranes." ACOG Technical Bulletin, number 115, April 1988.

81. Cotton, D. B., et al. "Use of amniocentesis in preterm gestation with ruptured membranes." *Obstetrics and Gynecology* 63(1984): 38–43.

82. Johnston, M. M., et al. "Antibiotic therapy in preterm premature rupture of membranes: A randomized, prospective, double-blind trial." *American Journal of Obstetrics and Gynecology* 163(1990): 743–747.

83. Wagner, M. V., et al. "A comparison of early and delayed induction of labor with spontaneous rupture of membranes at term." *Obstetrics and Gynecology* 74(1989): 93–97.

84. Romero, R.; Mazor, M.; and Oyarzun, E. "Role of intraamniotic infection in preterm labor." *Contemporary OB/GYN*, December 1988, pp. 94–106.

85. Morales, W. J. "Why tocolysis and steroids have a place in PROM management." *Contemporary OB/GYN*, August 1991, pp. 73–82.

86. Nelson, L. H., et al. "Premature rupture of membranes: A prospective, randomized evaluation of steroids, latent phase, and expectant management." *Obstetrics and Gynecology* 66(1985): 55–57.

87. "Induction and augmentation of labor." ACOG Technical Bulletin, number 157, July 1991.

88. Cummiskey, K. C., and Dawood, M. Y. "Induction of labor with pulsatile oxytocin." *American Journal of Obstetrics and Gynecology* 163(1990): 1868–1874.

89. Sorensen, S. S.; Brocks, V.; and Lenstrup, C. "Induction of labor and cervical ripening by intracervical prostaglandin E2." *Obstetrics and Gynecology* 65(1985): 110–114.

90. Zanini, A., et al. "Pre-induction cervical ripening with prostaglandin E2 gel: Intracervical versus intravaginal route." *Obstetrics and Gynecology* 76(1990): 681–683.

91. Williams, J. K., et al. "Use of prostaglandin E2 topical cervical gel in high-risk patients: A critical analysis." *Obstetrics and Gynecology* 66(1985): 769–772.

92. Rayburn, W. "Prostaglandin E2 gel for cervical ripening and induction of labor: A critical analysis." *American Journal of Obstetrics and Gynecology* 160(1989): 529–534.

93. McColgin, S. W.; Patrissi, G. A.; and Morrison, J. C. "Stripping the fetal membranes at term." *Journal of Reproductive Medicine* 35(1990): 811–814.

94. Jovanovic, R. "Incisions of the pregnant uterus and delivery of low-birthweight infants." *American Journal of Obstetrics and Gynecology* 152(1985): 971.

95. Schifrin, B. S., and Clement, D. "Cesarean birth: What accounts for the increase?" *The Female Patient* 11(1986): 47–64.

96. Berkowitz, G. S., et al. "Effect of physician characteristics on the cesarean birth rate." *American Journal of Obstetrics and Gynecology* 161(1989): 146–149.

97. Goyert, G. L., et al. "The physician factor in cesarean birth rates." *New England Journal of Medicine* 320(1989): 706–709.

98. Myers, S. A., and Gleicher, N. "A successful program to lower cesarean section rates." *New England Journal of Medicine* 319(1988): 1511–1516.

99. Gould, J. B.; Davey, B.; and Stafford, R. S. "Socioeconomic differences in rates of cesarean section." *New England Journal of Medicine* 321(1989): 233–239.

100. Kirkinen, P. "Multiple cesarean sections: Outcomes and complications." *British Journal of Obstetrics and Gynaecology* 95(1988): 778.

101. Barber, H. R. K. "Is there a cesarean-section epidemic?" *The Female Patient* 14(1989): 10–12.

102. Halperin, M. E.; Moore, D. C.; and Hannah, W. J. "Classical versus low-segment transverse incision for preterm cesarean section: Maternal complications and outcome of subsequent pregnancies." *British Journal of Obstetrics and Gynaecology* 95(1988): 990.

103. "Guidelines for vaginal delivery after a previous cesarean section." ACOG Committee Opinion, number 64, October 1988.

104. Stovall, T. G., et al. "Trial of labor in previous cesarean section patients, excluding classical cesarean sections." *Obstetrics and Gynecology* 70(1987): 713–717.

105. Flamm, B. L., et al. "Oxytocin during labor and previous cesarean section: Results of a multicenter study." *Obstetrics and Gynecology* 70(1987): 709–712.

106. Allen, R. E., et al. "Pelvic floor damage and childbirth: A neurophysiological study." *British Journal of Obstetrics and Gynaecology* 97(1990): 770.

107. Goodlin, R. C. "On protection of the maternal perineum during birth." *Obstetrics and Gynecology* 62(1983): 393–394.

108. Buekens, P., et al. "Episiotomy and third-degree tears." *British Journal of Obstetrics and Gynaecology* 92(1985): 820.

109. Shiono, P.; Klebanoff, M. A.; and Carey, J. C. "Midline episiotomies: More harm than good?" *Obstetrics and Gynecology* 75(1990):765–770.

110. Thorp, J. M., Jr., et al. "Selected use of midline episiotomy: Effect on perineal trauma." *Obstetrics and Gynecology* 70(1987): 260–262.

111. Thorp, J. M., Jr., and Bowes, W. A., Jr. "Episiotomy: Can its routine use be defended?" *American Journal of Obstetrics and Gynecology* 160(1989): 1027–1030.

112. Haadem, K., et al. "Anal sphincter function after delivery rupture." *Obstetrics and Gynecology* 70(1987): 53–56.

113. "Obstetric anesthesia and analgesia." ACOG Technical Bulletin, number 112, January 1988.

114. Santos, A. C. "Obstetric use of local anesthet-

ics." *Contemporary OB/GYN*, December 1983, pp. 46–59.

115. Phillipson, E., and Kuhnert, B. R. "Chloroprocaine use in modern obstetrics." *Contemporary OB/GYN*, May 1986, pp. 115–130.

116. Zagorzycki, M. T. "General anesthesia in cesarean section: Effect on mother and neonate." *Obstetrical and Gynecological Survey* 39(1984): 134–137.

117. Akhter, J. E. "Cesarean section—Regional or general anesthesia?" *Contemporary OB/GYN*, August 1987, pp. 51–62.

118. Malinow, A. M., and Ostheimer, G. W. "Anesthesia for the high-risk parturient." *Obstetrics and Gynecology* 69(1987): 951–962.

119. Corke, B. C., and Spielman, F. J. "Problems associated with epidural anesthesia in obstetrics." *Obstetrics and Gynecology* 65(1985): 837–839.

120. Viscomi, C. M., et al. "Fetal heart rate variability after epidural fentanyl during labor." *Anesthesia and Analgesia* 71(1990): 679.

121. Niv, D., et al. "Augmentation of bupivacaine analgesia in labor by epidural morphine." *Obstetrics and Gynecology* 67(1986): 206–209.

122. Gibson, W. P. "Epidural fentanyl for pain of labor." *Contemporary OB/GYN*, October 1986, pp. 111–123.

123. McIntosh, D. G., and Rayburn, W. F. "Patient-controlled analgesia in obstetrics and gynecology." *Obstetrics and Gynecology* 78(1991): 1129–1135.

124. Viscomi, C., and Eisenach, J. C. "Patient-controlled epidural analgesia during labor." *Obstetrics and Gynecology* 77(1991): 348–352.

125. Wright, W. C. "Continuous epidural block for ob anesthesia." *Contemporary OB/GYN*, November 1991, pp. 89–98.

126. Podlas, J., and Breland, B. D. "Patient-controlled analgesia with nalbuphine during labor." *Obstetrics and Gynecology* 70(1987): 202–204.

127. Gribble, R. K., and Meier, P. R. "Effect of epidural analgesia on the primary cesarean rate." *Obstetrics and Gynecology* 78(1991): 231–234.

128. Kotelko, D. M., et al. "Epidural morphine analgesia after cesarean delivery." *Obstetrics and Gynecology* 63(1984): 409–413.

129. Murphy, J. F., et al. "Obstetric analgesia, anesthesia, and the Apgar score." *Anesthesia* 39(1984): 760.

130. "Naloxone use in newborns." ACOG Committee Opinion, number 70, August 1989.

131. Beecham, C. T. "Natural childbirth—A step backward?" *The Female Patient* 14(1989): 37–40.

132. Rooks, J. P., et al. "Outcomes of care in birth centers." *New England Journal of Medicine* 321(1989): 1804–1811.

133. Lieberman, E., and Ryan, K. J. "Birth-day choices." *New England Journal of Medicine* 321(1989): 1824–1825.

134. Clark, L. "When children watch their mothers deliver." *Contemporary OB/GYN*, August 1986, pp. 69–75.

135. Eakins, E. S. "Free-standing birth centers in California." *Journal of Reproductive Medicine* 34(1989): 960–970.

136. Machol, L. "Single-room maternity care gains converts." *Contemporary OB/GYN*, November 1989, pp. 62–70.

137. McCann, K. "The modern midwife." *American Baby*, January 1989, pp. 50–51.

138. Horner, E. N. "Bonding: Just another buzz word?" *Contemporary OB/GYN*, October 1985, pp. 105–108.

139. England, M. J., et al. "Suppression of lactation." *Journal of Reproductive Medicine* 33(1988): 630–632.

140. Ruch, A., and Duhring, J. L. "Postpartum myocardial infarction in a patient receiving bromocriptine." *Obstetrics and Gynecology* 74(1989): 448–451.

141. Kletzky, O. A.; Borenstein, R.; and Mileikowsky, G. M. "Pergolide and bromocriptine for the treatment of patients with hyperprolactinemia." *American Journal of Obstetrics and Gynecology* 154(1986): 431–435.

142. Charles, D., and Larsen, B. "How colostrum and milk protect the newborn." *Contemporary OB/GYN*, July 1984, pp. 143–165.

143. Riaha, N. C. L. "Why NCR infants thrive on human milk." *Contemporary OB/GYN*, June 1985, pp. 112–123.

144. Abraham, S., et al. "Recovery after childbirth: A preliminary prospective study." *Medical Journal of Australia* 152(1990): 9.

145. Kendell, R. E., et al. "Day-to-day mood changes after childbirth: Further data." *British Journal of Psychiatry* 145(1984): 620.

146. O'Hara, M. W. "Social support, life events, and depression during pregnancy and the puerperium." *Archives of General Psychiatry* 43(1986): 569.

147. Stang, H. J., et al. "Local anesthesia for neonatal circumcision." *Journal of the American Medical Association* 259(1988): 1507–5111.

148. Poland, R. L. "The status of circumcision of newborns." *New England Journal of Medicine* 322(1990): 1308–1315.

149. Arnett, R. M.; Jones, S.; and Horger, E. O. "Effectiveness of 1 percent lidocaine dorsal penile nerve block in infant circumcision." *American Journal of Obstetrics and Gynecology* 163(1990): 1074–1080.

150. Anand, K. J. S., and Hickey, P. R. "Pain and its effects in the human neonate and fetus." *New England Journal of Medicine* 317(1987): 1321–1348.

151. Gray, R. H., et al. "Risk of ovulation during lactation." *Lancet* 335(1990): 25.

152. Rosner, A. E., and Schulman, S. K. "Birth interval among breast-feeding women not using contraceptives." *Pediatrics* 86(1990): 747.

153. Gray, R. H., et al. "Postpartum return of ovarian activity in nonbreastfeeding women monitored by urinary assays." *Journal of Clinical Endocrinology and Metabolism* 64(1987): 645.

154. Debrovner, C. H., and Winikoff, B. "Trends in postpartum contraceptive choice." *Obstetrics and Gynecology* 63(1984): 65–70.

155. McIntyre, S. L., and Higgins, J. E. "Parity and use-effectiveness with the contraceptive sponge." *American Journal of Obstetrics and Gynecology* 155(1986): 796–801.

156. Richwald, G. A., et al. "Effectiveness of the cavity-rim cervical cap: Results of a large clinical study." *Obstetrics and Gynecology* 74(1989): 143–148.

157. Sulak, P. J. "Oral contraceptives in the puerperium." *International Journal of Fertility* 36(1991): 87–89.

158. Greene, G. W., et al. "Postpartum weight change: How much of the weight gained in pregnancy will be lost after delivery?" *Obstetrics and Gynecology* 71(1988): 701–707.

Index